Injury & Trauma Sourcebook
Learning Disabilities Sourcebook, 2nd Edition
Leukemia Sourcebook
Liver Disorders Sourcebook
Lung Disorders Sourcebook
Medical Tests Sourcebook, 3rd Edition
Men's Health Concerns Sourcebook, 2nd Edition
Mental Health Disorders Sourcebook, 3rd Edition
Mental Retardation Sourcebook
Movement Disorders Sourcebook
Multiple Sclerosis Sourcebook
Muscular Dystrophy Sourcebook
Obesity Sourcebook
Osteoporosis Sourcebook
Pain Sourcebook, 3rd Edition
Pediatric Cancer Sourcebook
Physical & Mental Issues in Aging Sourcebook
Podiatry Sourcebook, 2nd Edition
Pregnancy & Birth Sourcebook, 2nd Edition
Prostate Cancer Sourcebook
Prostate & Urological Disorders Sourcebook
Reconstructive & Cosmetic Surgery Sourcebook
Rehabilitation Sourcebook
Respiratory Disorders Sourcebook, 2nd Edition
Sexually Transmitted Diseases Sourcebook, 3rd Edition
Sleep Disorders Sourcebook, 2nd Edition
Smoking Concerns Sourcebook
Sports Injuries Sourcebook, 3rd Edition
Stress-Related Disorders Sourcebook, 2nd Edition
Stroke Sourcebook, 2nd Edition
Surgery Sourcebook, 2nd Edition
Thyroid Disorders Sourcebook
Transplantation Sourcebook

Traveler's Health Sourcebook
Urinary Tract & Kidney Diseases & Disorders Sourcebook, 2nd Edition
Vegetarian Sourcebook
Women's Health Concerns Sourcebook, 2nd Edition
Workplace Health & Safety Sourcebook
Worldwide Health Sourcebook

Teen Health Series

Abuse and Violence Information for Teens
Alcohol Information for Teens
Allergy Information for Teens
Asthma Information for Teens
Body Information for Teens
Cancer Information for Teens
Complementary & Alternative Medicine Information for Teens
Diabetes Information for Teens
Diet Information for Teens, 2nd Edition
Drug Information for Teens, 2nd Edition
Eating Disorders Information for Teens
Fitness Information for Teens, 2nd Edition
Learning Disabilities Information for Teens
Mental Health Information for Teens, 2nd Edition
Pregnancy Information for Teens
Sexual Health Information for Teens, 2nd Edition
Skin Health Information for Teens
Sleep Information for Teens
Sports Injuries Information for Teens, 2nd Edition
Stress Information for Teens
Suicide Information for Teens
Tobacco Information for Teens

Childhood Diseases and Disorders SOURCEBOOK

Second Edition

Health Reference Series

Second Edition

Childhood Diseases and Disorders SOURCEBOOK

Basic Consumer Health Information about the Physical, Mental, and Developmental Health of Pre-Adolescent Children, Including Facts about Infectious Diseases, Asthma, Allergies, Diabetes, and Other Acute and Chronic Conditions Affecting the Gastrointestinal Tract, Ears, Nose, Throat, Liver, Kidneys, Heart, Blood, Brain, Muscles, Bones, and Skin

Along with Reports on Recommended Childhood Vaccinations, Wellness Guidelines, a Glossary of Related Medical Terms, and a List of Resources for Parents

Edited by
Sandra J. Judd

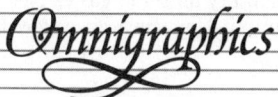

P.O. Box 31-1640, Detroit, MI 48231

Bibliographic Note

Because this page cannot legibly accommodate all the copyright notices, the Bibliographic Note portion of the Preface constitutes an extension of the copyright notice.

Edited by Sandra J. Judd

Health Reference Series

Karen Bellenir, *Managing Editor*
David A. Cooke, M.D., *Medical Consultant*
Elizabeth Collins, *Research and Permissions Coordinator*
Cherry Stockdale, *Permissions Assistant*
EdIndex, Services for Publishers, *Indexers*

* * *

Omnigraphics, Inc.

Matthew P. Barbour, *Senior Vice President*
Kevin M. Hayes, *Operations Manager*

* * *

Peter E. Ruffner, *Publisher*

Copyright © 2009 Omnigraphics, Inc.
ISBN 978-0-7808-1031-0

Library of Congress Cataloging-in-Publication Data

Childhood diseases and disorders sourcebook : basic consumer health information about the physical, mental, and developmental ... / edited by Sandra J. Judd. -- 2nd ed.
   p. cm. -- (Health reference series)
  Includes bibliographical references and index.
  Summary: "Provides basic consumer health information about the physical and mental health of pre-adolescent children including common illnesses and injuries, disease prevention and screening, and wellness promotion. Includes index, glossary of related terms, and other resources"--Provided by publisher.
  ISBN 978-0-7808-1031-0 (hardcover : alk. paper) 1. Pediatrics. 2. Children--Health and hygiene. 3. Children--Diseases. I. Judd, Sandra J.
  RJ61.C5427 2009
  618.92--dc22

                                                                  2008047331

Electronic or mechanical reproduction, including photography, recording, or any other information storage and retrieval system for the purpose of resale is strictly prohibited without permission in writing from the publisher.

The information in this publication was compiled from the sources cited and from other sources considered reliable. While every possible effort has been made to ensure reliability, the publisher will not assume liability for damages caused by inaccuracies in the data, and makes no warranty, express or implied, on the accuracy of the information contained herein.

This book is printed on acid-free paper meeting the ANSI Z39.48 Standard. The infinity symbol that appears above indicates that the paper in this book meets that standard.

Printed in the United States

Table of Contents

Visit www.healthreferenceseries.com to view *A Contents Guide to the Health Reference Series*, a listing of more than 14,000 topics and the volumes in which they are covered.

Preface xiii

Part I: Introduction to Children's Health and Safety

Chapter　1—Child Health Statistics 3
Chapter　2—Preparing Your Child for Visits to the Doctor 9
Chapter　3—How to Give Medicine to Children 15
Chapter　4—Recommended Childhood Vaccinations 19
Chapter　5—Promoting Wellness 27
　　　　　　 Section 5.1—Nutrition for the School-Aged
　　　　　　　　　　　　 Child 28
　　　　　　 Section 5.2—Physical Fitness and Health 33
　　　　　　 Section 5.3—Healthy Sleep Habits 35
　　　　　　 Section 5.4—The Importance of
　　　　　　　　　　　　 Handwashing 37
Chapter　6—Preventing Childhood Injuries 39
　　　　　　 Section 6.1—Preventing Burns 40
　　　　　　 Section 6.2—Preventing Drowning 42
　　　　　　 Section 6.3—Preventing Falls 44
　　　　　　 Section 6.4—Preventing Poisoning 46
　　　　　　 Section 6.5—Preventing Airway Obstruction
　　　　　　　　　　　　 Injuries 48

Section 6.6—Preventing Bicycle Injuries 50
Section 6.7—Preventing Motor Vehicle
Injuries 51
Chapter 7—Fever in Children 53
Chapter 8—Medical Emergencies 57
Section 8.1—Is It a Medical Emergency? 58
Section 8.2—First Aid for Common
Emergencies 61

Part II: Common Childhood Infections and Related Concerns

Chapter 9—Foodborne Illness 65
Chapter 10—Streptococcal Bacterial Infections 75
Section 10.1—Group A Streptococcal
Infections 76
Section 10.2—Pneumococcal Disease 79
Section 10.3—Rheumatic Fever 83
Section 10.4—Scarlet Fever 86
Section 10.5—Strep Throat 88
Section 10.6—Impetigo 90
Chapter 11—Other Bacterial Infections 93
Section 11.1—Cat Scratch Disease 94
Section 11.2—Diphtheria 98
Section 11.3—*Haemophilus Influenzae*
Type B 100
Section 11.4—Lyme Disease 102
Section 11.5—Methicillin Resistant
Staphylococcus Aureus (MRSA)/
Oxacillin Resistant Staph 107
Section 11.6—Mycoplasma Infection 110
Section 11.7—Tetanus 112
Section 11.8—Tuberculosis 115
Section 11.9—Whooping Cough (Pertussis) ... 118
Chapter 12—Viral Infections 121
Section 12.1—Chickenpox 122
Section 12.2—Common Cold 124
Section 12.3—Croup 131

        Section 12.4——Fifth Disease 133
        Section 12.5——Hand, Foot, and Mouth
                            Disease 136
        Section 12.6——Infectious Mononucleosis 140
        Section 12.7——Influenza 142
        Section 12.8——Measles 145
        Section 12.9——Mumps 147
        Section 12.10—Rabies 149
        Section 12.11—Rubella (German Measles) 152
        Section 12.12—Warts 155

Chapter 13—Encephalitis 159
Chapter 14—Meningitis 163
Chapter 15—Pneumonia 167
Chapter 16—Reye Syndrome 173
Chapter 17—Parasitic and Fungal Infections 177
        Section 17.1——Ascariasis 178
        Section 17.2——*Baylisascaris* Infection 180
        Section 17.3——Cryptosporidiosis 182
        Section 17.4——Giardiasis 188
        Section 17.5——*Hymenolepis* (Dwarf
                            Tapeworm) Infection 193
        Section 17.6——Pediculosis (Head Lice) 195
        Section 17.7——Pinworm Infection 202
        Section 17.8——Scabies 204
        Section 17.9——Swimmer's Itch 207
        Section 17.10—Tinea 209
        Section 17.11—Toxocariasis 212

Part III: Common Childhood Medical Conditions

Chapter 18—Allergies 217
        Section 18.1——Allergic Reactions in Kids..... 218
        Section 18.2——Food Allergies 228
Chapter 19—Blood and Circulatory Disorders 233
        Section 19.1——Anemia 234
        Section 19.2——Sickle Cell Anemia 239
        Section 19.3——Thalassemia 242

  Section 19.4—Hemophilia 244
  Section 19.5—Thrombocytopenia 247
  Section 19.6—Thrombophilia 256
  Section 19.7—von Willebrand Disease 259

Chapter 20—Cancer 263
  Section 20.1—Leukemia 264
  Section 20.2—Lymphoma 269
  Section 20.3—Neuroblastoma 276
  Section 20.4—Sarcoma 279

Chapter 21—Cardiovascular Disorders 283
  Section 21.1—Arrhythmia 284
  Section 21.2—Heart Murmurs 290
  Section 21.3—Hyperlipidemia
        (High Cholesterol) 292
  Section 21.4—Hypertension 297
  Section 21.5—Kawasaki Disease 302

Chapter 22—Diabetes 305

Chapter 23—Ear, Nose, and Throat Disorders 315
  Section 23.1—Enlarged Adenoids 316
  Section 23.2—Hearing Loss 319
  Section 23.3—Nosebleeds 322
  Section 23.4—Obstructive Sleep Apnea 324
  Section 23.5—Otitis Media
        (Ear Infection) 327
  Section 23.6—Perforated Eardrum 333
  Section 23.7—Sinusitis 335
  Section 23.8—Swimmer's Ear 344
  Section 23.9—Tonsillitis 347

Chapter 24—Endocrine and Growth Disorders 351
  Section 24.1—Constitutional Growth Delay ... 352
  Section 24.2—Growth Hormone Deficiency 354
  Section 24.3—Hypothyroidism 357
  Section 24.4—Idiopathic Short Stature 359
  Section 24.5—Precocious Puberty 361

Chapter 25—Gastrointestinal Disorders 365
  Section 25.1—Abdominal Pain 366

Section 25.2—Appendicitis 370
Section 25.3—Celiac Disease 374
Section 25.4—Cyclic Vomiting Syndrome ... 377
Section 25.5—Diarrhea 381
Section 25.6—Encopresis
(Constipation and Soiling) 387
Section 25.7—Gastroenteritis 390
Section 25.8—Gastroesophageal Reflux 393
Section 25.9—Irritable Bowel Syndrome 397
Section 25.10—Lactose Intolerance 399

Chapter 26—Kidney and Urologic Disorders 403
Section 26.1—Bedwetting and Urinary
Incontinence 404
Section 26.2—Childhood Nephrotic
Syndrome 409
Section 26.3—Hemolytic Uremic
Syndrome 413
Section 26.4—Urinary Tract Infections 415

Chapter 27—Liver Disorders 423
Section 27.1—Alpha-1 Antitrypsin
Deficiency 424
Section 27.2—Autoimmune Hepatitis 428

Chapter 28—Musculoskeletal Disorders 431
Section 28.1—Bowlegs and Knock-Knee 432
Section 28.2—Flat Feet 435
Section 28.3—Growing Pains 438
Section 28.4—Intoeing 440
Section 28.5—Juvenile Rheumatoid
Arthritis 442
Section 28.6—Juvenile Dermatomyositis 446
Section 28.7—Marfan Syndrome 452
Section 28.8—Muscular Dystrophy 455
Section 28.9—Osgood-Schlatter Disease 460
Section 28.10—Scoliosis 462

Chapter 29—Neurological Disorders 469
Section 29.1—Brain Tumors 470
Section 29.2—Cerebral Palsy 485

   Section 29.3—Epilepsy 492
   Section 29.4—Febrile Seizures 499
   Section 29.5—Headache 503
   Section 29.6—Neurofibromatosis 508
   Section 29.7—Tourette Syndrome 515
Chapter 30—Respiratory and Lung Conditions 523
   Section 30.1—Asthma 524
   Section 30.2—Bronchitis 528
   Section 30.3—Cystic Fibrosis 531
Chapter 31—Skin Conditions 539
   Section 31.1—Eczema/Atopic Dermatitis 540
   Section 31.2—Psoriasis 543
Chapter 32—Vision Problems 547
   Section 32.1—Amblyopia 548
   Section 32.2—Conjunctivitis (Pinkeye) 550
   Section 32.3—Far- and Nearsightedness 553
   Section 32.4—Retinitis Pigmentosa 555
   Section 32.5—Strabismus 557

Part IV: Developmental and Pediatric Mental Health Concerns

Chapter 33—Autism Spectrum Disorders 561
Chapter 34—Attention Deficit Hyperactivity Disorder 577
Chapter 35—Auditory Processing Disorder 583
Chapter 36—Developmental Delay 587
Chapter 37—Dyslexia 591
Chapter 38—Fragile X Syndrome 595
Chapter 39—Learning Disabilities 601
Chapter 40—Stuttering 607
Chapter 41—Anxiety Disorders 611
Chapter 42—Bipolar Disorder 615
Chapter 43—Conduct Disorder 619
Chapter 44—Depression 623
Chapter 45—Obsessive-Compulsive Disorder 629

Chapter 46—Oppositional Defiant Disorder 641

Part V: Additional Help and Information

Chapter 47—Glossary of Terms Related to Childhood
          Diseases and Disorders 647

Chapter 48—Resource List for Parents 653

Index **669**

Preface

About This Book

According to the Federal Interagency Forum on Child and Family Statistics, a study of data from 2006 found that 9 percent of children aged five to seventeen experienced activity limitation resulting from one or more chronic health conditions. Five percent of children aged four to seventeen were reported by a parent to have definite or severe difficulties with emotions, concentration, behavior, or being able to get along with others. Additionally, 17 percent of children aged six to seventeen were overweight, a key predictor of future health problems.

Childhood Diseases and Disorders Sourcebook, Second Edition, provides up-to-date information about the most common disorders affecting the physical, mental, and developmental health of pre-adolescent children, including infectious diseases, asthma and allergies, developmental and growth disorders, anxiety and depressive disorders, and disorders affecting the blood, brain, muscles, bones, skin, and internal organs. Guidelines for maintaining wellness and information about recommended childhood vaccinations are also included, along with a glossary of related terms and a list of resources to which parents can turn for further information.

How to Use This Book

This book is divided into parts and chapters. Parts focus on broad areas of interest. Chapters are devoted to single topics within a part.

Part I: Introduction to Children's Health and Safety provides basic information for parents about preparing children for visits to the doctor, giving medicine to children, and identifying a medical emergency. It describes basic nutritional and physical fitness requirements for maintaining health and provides tips for avoiding common childhood injuries. It also provides a detailed description of recommended childhood vaccinations.

Part II: Common Childhood Infections and Related Concerns describes the most common bacterial and viral infections affecting children, including the common cold, influenza, chickenpox, measles, pneumonia, meningitis, and foodborne illnesses. Common symptoms, disease progression, treatment techniques, and prevention tips are discussed.

Part III: Common Childhood Medical Conditions details common conditions affecting children's skin, muscles, bones, and internal organs. These include asthma and allergies, ear infections and other disorders of the ear, nose, and throat, diabetes, lactose intolerance and other gastrointestinal disorders, bedwetting, cardiovascular disorders, problems with vision, and musculoskeletal disorders. Growth disorders and childhood cancers are also discussed.

Part IV: Developmental and Pediatric Mental Health Concerns provides information about learning disabilities, stuttering, dyslexia, attention deficit hyperactivity disorder, autism, and other disorders that affect learning and childhood development. It also describes common mental health concerns affecting children, including anxiety disorders, obsessive-compulsive disorder, and depression. Tips for recognizing these disorders, along with a discussion of treatment options, are provided.

Part V: Additional Help and Information includes a glossary of terms related to childhood diseases and disorders and a directory of organizations able to provide additional help and support.

Bibliographic Note

This volume contains documents and excerpts from publications issued by the following U.S. government agencies: Centers for Disease Control and Prevention (CDC); Department of Health and Human Services (HHS); Food and Drug Administration (FDA); National Diabetes Education Program (NDEP); National Dissemination Center for Children with Disabilities (NICHCY); National Eye Institute (NEI); National Heart, Lung, and Blood Institute (NHLBI); National Human

Genome Research Institute (NHGRI); National Institute of Allergy and Infectious Diseases (NIAID); National Institute of Arthritis and Musculoskeletal and Skin Diseases (NIAMS); National Institute of Child Health and Human Development (NICHD); National Institute of Diabetes and Digestive and Kidney Diseases (NIDDK); National Institute of Neurological Disorders and Stroke (NINDS); National Institute on Deafness and Other Communication Disorders (NIDCD); and the Substance Abuse and Mental Health Services Administration (SAMHSA).

In addition, this volume contains copyrighted documents from the following organizations: A.D.A.M., Inc.; Allen ENT and Allergy; American Academy of Dermatology; American Academy of Family Physicians; American Academy of Orthopaedic Surgeons; American Headache Society; American Heart Association; American Liver Foundation; Asthma and Allergy Foundation of America; Cedars-Sinai Medical Center; Children's Healthcare of Atlanta; Children's Hospital of Philadelphia; Cincinnati Children's Hospital Medical Center; City of Miami, Department of Fire-Rescue; Cleveland Clinic; Cystic Fibrosis Foundation; Dartmouth-Hitchcock Medical Center; Florida Department of Health—Children's Medical Services; Illinois Department of Public Health; Immunization Action Coalition; Indiana State Department of Health; International Food Information Council Foundation; Leukemia and Lymphoma Society; MAGIC Foundation; March of Dimes; Massachusetts General Hospital-School Psychiatry Program; MCW HealthLink; NAMI: The Nation's Voice on Mental Illness; National Brain Tumor Foundation; National Center for Learning Disabilities; National Hemophilia Foundation; National Psoriasis Foundation; National Sleep Foundation; Nemours Foundation; New Hampshire Department of Health and Human Services; New Zealand Dermatological Society; Safe Kids Worldwide; Seattle Cancer Care Alliance; St. Luke's Cataract and Laser Institute; University of Colorado Health Sciences Center; University of Michigan Health System; University of Nebraska-Lincoln Extension; Virginia Department of Health; and the Wisconsin Department of Health and Family Services;

Full citation information is provided on the first page of each chapter. Every effort has been made to secure all necessary rights to reprint the copyrighted material. If any omissions have been made, please contact Omnigraphics to make corrections for future editions.

Acknowledgements

Thanks go to the many organizations, agencies, and individuals who have contributed materials for this *Sourcebook* and to medical consultant Dr. David Cooke and document engineer Bruce Bellenir. Special thanks go to managing editor Karen Bellenir and permissions coordinator Liz Collins for their help and support.

About the Health Reference Series

The *Health Reference Series* is designed to provide basic medical information for patients, families, caregivers, and the general public. Each volume takes a particular topic and provides comprehensive coverage. This is especially important for people who may be dealing with a newly diagnosed disease or a chronic disorder in themselves or in a family member. People looking for preventive guidance, information about disease warning signs, medical statistics, and risk factors for health problems will also find answers to their questions in the *Health Reference Series*. The *Series*, however, is not intended to serve as a tool for diagnosing illness, in prescribing treatments, or as a substitute for the physician/patient relationship. All people concerned about medical symptoms or the possibility of disease are encouraged to seek professional care from an appropriate healthcare provider.

A Note about Spelling and Style

Health Reference Series editors use *Stedman's Medical Dictionary* as an authority for questions related to the spelling of medical terms and the *Chicago Manual of Style* for questions related to grammatical structures, punctuation, and other editorial concerns. Consistent adherence is not always possible, however, because the individual volumes within the *Series* include many documents from a wide variety of different producers and copyright holders, and the editor's primary goal is to present material from each source as accurately as is possible following the terms specified by each document's producer. This sometimes means that information in different chapters or sections may follow other guidelines and alternate spelling authorities. For example, occasionally a copyright holder may require that eponymous terms be shown in possessive forms (Crohn's disease *vs.* Crohn disease) or that British spelling norms be retained (leukaemia *vs.* leukemia).

Locating Information within the Health Reference Series

The *Health Reference Series* contains a wealth of information about a wide variety of medical topics. Ensuring easy access to all the fact sheets, research reports, in-depth discussions, and other material contained within the individual books of the series remains one of our highest priorities. As the *Series* continues to grow in size and scope, however, locating the precise information needed by a reader may become more challenging.

A Contents Guide to the Health Reference Series was developed to direct readers to the specific volumes that address their concerns. It presents an extensive list of diseases, treatments, and other topics of general interest compiled from the Tables of Contents and major index headings. To access *A Contents Guide to the Health Reference Series*, visit www.healthreferenceseries.com.

Medical Consultant

Medical consultation services are provided to the *Health Reference Series* editors by David A. Cooke, M.D. Dr. Cooke is a graduate of Brandeis University, and he received his M.D. degree from the University of Michigan. He completed residency training at the University of Wisconsin Hospital and Clinics. He is board-certified in Internal Medicine. Dr. Cooke currently works as part of the University of Michigan Health System and practices in Ann Arbor, MI. In his free time, he enjoys writing, science fiction, and spending time with his family.

Our Advisory Board

We would like to thank the following board members for providing guidance to the development of this series:

Dr. Lynda Baker,
Associate Professor of Library and Information Science,
Wayne State University, Detroit, MI

Nancy Bulgarelli,
William Beaumont Hospital Library, Royal Oak, MI

Karen Imarisio,
Bloomfield Township Public Library, Bloomfield Township, MI

Karen Morgan,
Mardigian Library, University of Michigan-Dearborn,
Dearborn, MI

Rosemary Orlando,
St. Clair Shores Public Library, St. Clair Shores, MI

Health Reference Series *Update Policy*

The inaugural book in the *Health Reference Series* was the first edition of *Cancer Sourcebook* published in 1989. Since then, the *Series* has been enthusiastically received by librarians and in the medical community. In order to maintain the standard of providing high-quality health information for the layperson the editorial staff at Omnigraphics felt it was necessary to implement a policy of updating volumes when warranted.

Medical researchers have been making tremendous strides, and it is the purpose of the *Health Reference Series* to stay current with the most recent advances. Each decision to update a volume is made on an individual basis. Some of the considerations include how much new information is available and the feedback we receive from people who use the books. If there is a topic you would like to see added to the update list, or an area of medical concern you feel has not been adequately addressed, please write to:

Editor
Health Reference Series
Omnigraphics, Inc.
P.O. Box 31-1640
Detroit, MI 48231
E-mail: editorial@omnigraphics.com

Part One

Introduction to Children's Health and Safety

Chapter 1

Child Health Statistics

In 2003, 84.1 percent of children were in excellent or very good health, according to parent reports. Males were slightly less likely to be in excellent or very good health than females (83.5 versus 84.7 percent). The percent of children in excellent or very good health decreases with increased age: 86.0 percent of children under age five were in excellent or very good health, compared to 83.8 percent of six- to eleven-year-olds and 82.6 percent of twelve- to seventeen-year-olds.

The rate of children in excellent or very good health varies by several other factors, including family income and race and ethnicity. Non-Hispanic white children were the most likely to be in excellent or very good health (90.7 percent) while Hispanic children were the least likely (64.4 percent). Children with family incomes below 100 percent of the federal poverty level (FPL) were least likely to be reported by parents to be in excellent or very good health (66.8 percent), followed by those with family incomes of 100 to 199 percent of FPL (80.9 percent), and those with family incomes of 200 to 399 percent of FPL (90.2 percent); children with family incomes of 400 percent of FPL or above were the most likely to be in excellent or very good health (93.8 percent).

Excerpted from "Child Health USA 2005," U.S. Department of Health and Human Services, Health Resources and Services Administration, Maternal and Child Health Bureau, 2005.

Asthma

Asthma is a disease in which the airways become blocked or narrowed. It is triggered by allergies or other factors, and symptoms include wheezing, chest tightness, and shortness of breath. In 2003, almost 8 percent of children in the United States were affected by asthma. This includes all children whose parents reported that a doctor ever told them the child had asthma and that the child still has asthma, and children who, in the past year, used asthma medication, had moderate or severe difficulties combined with an attack, or had been hospitalized for asthma.

In 2003, males were more likely to be affected by asthma than females (9.2 versus 6.6 percent). A greater proportion of children ages six to eleven years and twelve to seventeen years were affected by asthma (8.8 and 8.7 percent, respectively) than children from birth to age five (6.2 percent). Non-Hispanic black children were most likely to be affected by asthma, while Hispanic children were least likely to be affected. Children with lower family incomes were more likely to be affected than children with higher family incomes.

The effects of asthma also vary by insurance status. Children with public insurance were more likely to be affected by asthma than children with private insurance (10.6 versus 7.2 percent); of children with no insurance, 5.0 percent were affected in the ways described above. It is important to note that uninsured children may be less likely to have access to doctors and prescription drugs, which may affect whether parents report that their child has been affected by asthma.

Mental Health

In 2003, almost 10 percent of children in the United States had moderate to severe socio-emotional problems. This includes children whose parents reported that they have moderate to severe difficulties with emotions, concentration, behavior, or getting along with others.

Rates of socio-emotional difficulties vary by a number of factors, including sex, age, race/ethnicity, family income, and insurance type. In 2003, a greater proportion of males under age eighteen experienced socio-emotional difficulties than their female counterparts (11.3 versus 6.9 percent). Children of multiple races had the highest rate of socio-emotional problems (12.7 percent) followed by non-Hispanic black children (11.6 percent), and non-Hispanic white children (9.0 percent); Hispanic children had the lowest rate (8.3 percent).

Older children were more likely to experience socio-emotional difficulties than younger children, with twelve- to seventeen-year-olds experiencing the highest rate (10.9 percent) and three- to five-year olds experiencing the lowest rate (4.9 percent). Rates declined consistently with increased family income: children with family incomes below 100 percent of the poverty level experienced the highest rate (14.0 percent), while children with family incomes at or above 400 percent of the poverty level experienced the lowest rate (6.1 percent). Children with public insurance had a higher rate of socio emotional problems than children with private insurance (14.9 versus 7.0 percent); they also had a higher rate than children without insurance (8.0 percent).

Pediatric Acquired Immunodeficiency Syndrome (AIDS)

At the end of 2003, 9,419 cases of Acquired Immunodeficiency Syndrome (AIDS) in children younger than 13 had been reported in the United States since the beginning of the epidemic. Pediatric AIDS cases represented just over 1 percent of all cases ever reported.

In 2003, an estimated 59 new AIDS cases were diagnosed among children, almost 100 percent of which were transmitted before or during birth (perinatal transmission). Since 1993, the number of new cases of pediatric AIDS due to perinatal transmission has declined substantially, and from 1999 to 2003 the number of new cases among children under thirteen years of age, regardless of transmission method, decreased 68 percent. A major factor in this decline is the increasing use of treatment before, during, and after pregnancy to reduce perinatal transmission of the Human Immunodeficiency Virus (HIV), the virus that causes AIDS. In 1994, the U.S. Public Health Service recommended this treatment for all HIV-positive pregnant women, and in 1995 routine HIV counseling and voluntary testing for all pregnant women was recommended. It is expected that the perinatal transmission rate will continue to decline with increased use of aggressive treatments and obstetric procedures, such as elective cesarean section.

Racial and ethnic minorities are disproportionately represented among pediatric AIDS cases. As of 2003, the number of pediatric AIDS cases ever reported among non-Hispanic white children was less than one-third the number among non-Hispanic black children, and 25 percent less than that among Hispanic children.

Vaccine-Preventable Diseases

The number of reported cases of vaccine-preventable diseases has decreased steadily over the past decade. The number of cases of *H. Influenzae* among children under five years of age increased from 2002 to 2003, but the number of cases of measles, mumps, pertussis, and Hepatitis A and B decreased over the same period. It is important to note that since most Hepatitis B infections among infants and young children are asymptomatic, the reported number of cases likely underestimates the incidence of Hepatitis B in these age groups. In 2003, the highest number of cases of pertussis (3,700) was reported since 1964; however, the number of cases among children under five decreased by almost 10 percent. Of all pertussis cases, 17 percent were among infants under six months of age who are too young to have received the full schedule of pertussis vaccine.

Although much progress has been made in reducing the number of reported cases of vaccine-preventable diseases, several of these diseases are still common. The number of cases of pertussis, Hepatitis A, and *H. Influenzae* remain substantial and indicate a continuing need to promote immunization efforts. Since childhood vaccination for Hepatitis A was recommended in 1996 for children living in high-risk areas, the number of cases has decreased; in 2003, it reached the lowest rate ever recorded (2.7 cases per 100,000). Rates of Hepatitis A have shown the greatest decline among children in states where routine vaccination was recommended, suggesting that immunization policies are having a positive impact on the incidence of the disease.

Hospitalization

In 2003, there were 3.7 million hospital discharges among children ages one to twenty-one, or 4.4 discharges per 100 children. This represents little change from 2002. Hospital discharge rates generally decrease until about age seven and increase during later adolescence.

While injuries are the leading cause of death among children older than one year, they accounted for only 9 percent of hospital discharges among children one to fourteen years old in 2003. Diseases of the respiratory system were the major cause of hospitalization for children one to nine years of age, accounting for 34 percent of discharges. Pregnancy and childbirth accounted for 67 percent of discharges of young women ages fifteen to twenty-one. Mental disorders were the second leading cause of hospitalization for adolescents.

Overall, there has been a significant decrease in hospital discharge rates among children over the past twenty years. From 1985 to 2003, there was a 33 percent decrease in discharge rates for children ages one to fourteen years. During this period, hospital discharge rates for diseases of the respiratory system declined 35 percent for children in this age group.

Child Mortality

In 2003, 11,841 children between the ages of one and fourteen years died of various causes; this was 190 fewer than the previous year. The overall death rate among one- to four-year-olds was 31.1 per 100,000, and the rate among five- to fourteen-year-olds was 16.9 per 100,000. The leading cause of death among one- to four-year-olds continues to be unintentional injury, which accounted for 34.2 percent of all deaths in this age group in 2003. The next most common cause of death was congenital malformations (birth defects), followed by malignant neoplasms (cancer), homicide, and diseases of the heart. Unintentional injury was also the leading cause of death among five- to fourteen-year-olds in 2003, accounting for 37.0 percent of deaths among this age group. This was followed by malignant neoplasms, congenital malformations, homicide, suicide, and diseases of the heart.

Childhood Deaths Due to Injury

In 2003, unintentional injuries caused the deaths of 1,679 children aged one to four years and 2,562 children aged five to fourteen years. In 2003, motor vehicle crashes, drowning, and fires and burns were the most common causes of unintentional injury death among children aged one to four years. Motor vehicle crashes were the most common cause of unintentional injury death among children aged five to fourteen years, followed by deaths due to drowning, suffocation, and fires and burns.

In addition, 342 children aged one to four years were the victims of homicide in 2003, and 565 children aged five to fourteen years were the victims of homicide or suicide.

Chapter 2

Preparing Your Child for Visits to the Doctor

When children anticipate "going to the doctor," many become worried and apprehensive about the visit. Whether they're going to see their primary care doctor or a specialist—and whether for a routine exam, illness, or special problem—kids are likely to have fears, and some may even feel guilty.

Some fears and guilty feelings surface easily, so that children can talk about them. Others are harbored secretly and remain unspoken. In preparation for a physician's examination, you can help your child express these fears and overcome them.

Most Common Fears and Concerns about Medical Exams

Things that often top children's lists of concerns about going to the doctor include:

- **Separation:** Children often fear that their parents may leave them in the examining room and wait in another room. The fear of separation from the parent during mysterious examinations

---

"Preparing Your Child for Visits to the Doctor," January 2005, reprinted with permission from www.kidshealth.org. Copyright © 2005 The Nemours Foundation. This information was provided by KidsHealth, one of the largest resources online for medically reviewed health information written for parents, kids, and teens. For more articles like this one, visit www.KidsHealth.org, or www.TeensHealth.org.

is most common in children under seven years old, but it may be frightening to older children through ages twelve or thirteen.

- **Pain:** Children may worry that a part of the examination or a medical procedure will hurt. They especially fear they may need an injection, particularly children ages six through twelve.

- **The doctor:** Unfortunately, one of a child's concerns may be the doctor's manner. A child may misinterpret qualities such as speed, efficiency, or a detached attitude and read into them as sternness, dislike, or rejection.

- **The unknown:** Apprehensive about the unknown, children also worry that their problem may be much worse than their parents are telling them. Some who have simple problems suspect they may need surgery or hospitalization; some who are ill worry that they may die.

In addition, kids often harbor feelings of guilt. They may believe that their illness or condition is punishment for something they've done or neglected to do. Children who feel guilty may also believe that examinations and medical procedures are part of their punishment.

What Can I Do to Help?

As a parent, you can help by encouraging your child to express his or her fears and by addressing them in words that your child understands and isn't likely to misinterpret. Below are some practical ways to do this.

Explain the Purpose of the Visit

If the upcoming appointment is for a regular health checkup, explain that: "It's a 'well-child visit.' The doctor will check on how you're growing and developing. The doctor will also ask questions and examine you to make sure that your body is healthy. And you'll get a chance to ask any questions you want to about your body and your health." Also, stress that all healthy children go to the doctor for such visits.

If the visit is to diagnose and treat an illness or other condition, explain—in very nonthreatening language—that the doctor "needs to examine you to find out how to fix this and help you get better."

Address any Guilty Feelings Your Child May Have

If your child is going to the doctor because of an illness or other condition, he or she may have unspoken feelings of guilt about it.

Preparing Your Child for Visits to the Doctor

Discuss the illness or condition in neutral language and reassure your child that it isn't his or her fault: "This isn't caused by anything you did or forgot to do. Illnesses like this happen to many children. Aren't we lucky to have doctors who can find the causes and who know how to help us get well?"

If you, your spouse, other relatives, or friends had (or have) the same condition, share this information. Knowing that you and many others have been through the same thing may help relieve your child's guilt and fear.

If your child needs a doctor's attention because of a condition that resulted in ridicule or rejection by other children (or even by adults), you'll need to double your efforts to relieve shame and blame.

Head lice, embarrassing scratching caused by pinworm, and involuntary daytime wetting are examples of conditions that are often misunderstood by others. Even if you've been very supportive, you should reassure your child again, before the visit to the doctor, that the condition is not his or her fault and that many children have had it.

Of course, if your child has suffered an injury after disregarding safety rules, it's a good idea to point out (as matter-of-factly as possible) the cause-and-effect relationship between the action and the injury. However, you should still try to relieve guilt. You could say, "You probably didn't understand the danger involved in doing that, but I'm sure you understand now, and I know you won't do it that way again."

If your child repeatedly disobeys rules and becomes injured, speak to your child's doctor. This sort of worrisome behavior pattern needs a closer look.

In any of these cases, though, be sure to explain, especially to young children, that going to the doctor for an examination is not a punishment. Be sure your child understands that adults go to doctors just like children do and that the doctor's job is to help people stay healthy and fix any problems.

Tell Your Child What to Expect during a Routine Exam

You can use a doll or teddy bear to show your young child how the nurse will measure height and weight. It also helps to show your child how the doctor will:

- look in his or her mouth (and will need to hold the tongue down with a special stick for just a few seconds to see the throat);
- look at his or her eyes and into his or her ears;
- listen to his or her chest and back with a stethoscope.

And it helps to explain to your child that the doctor may also:

- tap or press on his or her tummy to listen to or feel what's inside;
- look quickly to see that the "private areas" are healthy;
- tap on his or her knees;
- look at his or her feet.

It's important for parents to let their kids know that what they've taught them about the privacy of their bodies is still true, but that doctors, nurses, and parents must sometimes examine all parts of the body. Emphasize, though, that these people are the only exceptions.

Tell Your Child What to Expect during Other Exams

If your child is going to the doctor because of an illness or medical condition or is going to visit a specialist, you may not even know what to expect during the examination.

When you're calling to make the appointment, you can ask to speak to the doctor or a nurse to find out, in a general way, what will take place during the office visit and exam. Then you can explain some of the procedures and their purpose in gentle language, appropriate to your child's age level. Your child will feel more secure if he or she understands what's going to take place and why it's necessary.

Be honest, but not brutally honest. Let your child know if a procedure is going to be somewhat embarrassing, uncomfortable, or even painful, but don't go into alarming detail.

Reassure your child that you'll be beside him or her and that the procedure is truly necessary to fix—or find out how to fix—the problem. (Adolescents may prefer to be examined without a parent or with only a same-sex parent or same-sex chaperone present. That preference should be honored.)

Children can cope with discomfort or pain more easily if they're forewarned, and they'll learn to trust you if you're honest with them.

Admit to your child if you don't know much about the illness or condition, but assure him or her that you'll both be able to ask the doctor questions about it. Write down your child's questions.

If a blood sample will be taken during or after the examination, be careful how you explain this. Some young children worry that "taking blood" means that all their blood will be taken. Let your child know that the body contains a great deal of blood and that only a very little bit of it (usually no more than one or two teaspoons [about ten milliliters]) will be taken for testing.

Preparing Your Child for Visits to the Doctor

Again, make certain that your child understands that the visit, with its embarrassing or uncomfortable procedures, is not a punishment for any misbehavior or disobedience.

Involve Your Child in the Process

Gathering information for the doctor: If the situation isn't an emergency, allow your child to contribute to a list of symptoms that you create for the doctor. Include all symptoms you've observed, no matter how unrelated they may seem to the problem at hand. Also, before the visit, prepare a history (in the form of a list) of your child's previous illnesses and medical conditions and a history of illnesses and medical conditions among close members of the family (parents, siblings, grandparents, aunts, and uncles).

Writing down questions: Ask your child to think of questions that he or she would like to ask the doctor. Write them down and give them to the doctor. Or, if kids are old enough, they can write down and ask the questions themselves. If the problem has occurred before, list the things that have worked and the things that haven't worked in previous treatment. Your child will be reassured by your active role in his or her medical care and will learn from your example. At the same time, you'll be prepared to give the doctor information vital to making an informed diagnosis. Doctors report that this information is very helpful in determining diagnoses.

Choose a Doctor Who Relates Well to Children

Because your child's doctor is your best ally in helping your child cope with health examinations, it's important to carefully select a doctor. Of course, you want a doctor who's knowledgeable and competent. However, you also want a doctor who understands children's needs and fears and who communicates easily with children, in a friendly manner, and without talking down to them.

In the course of a physical examination, the doctor inspects, taps, and probes various parts of the body—procedures that may be embarrassing (or even physically uncomfortable) for your child. A good rapport between doctor and patient can minimize these feelings.

If your child's doctor seems critical, uncommunicative, disinterested, or unsympathetic, do not be afraid to change doctors. Ask for recommendations from other parents in your area or from other doctors whose opinions you trust. If your child's illness or condition requires a specialist, ask your child's doctor to recommend someone who's knowledgeable, experienced, and friendly.

After all, adults want these characteristics in their own physicians, so as a parent you should serve as your child's advocate in seeking this type of care.

Chapter 3

How to Give Medicine to Children

Do You Know How to Give Medicine to Children?

If you are caring for a child who needs medicine, it's important that you know how to give the medicine the right way.

Over-the-Counter Drugs

Over-the-counter drugs are also called OTC drugs. They are medications you can buy without a doctor's prescription. You usually find them on drugstore shelves, or in supermarkets and other stores. OTC drugs have information on the bottle or box. Always read this information before using the medicine. This information tells you the following things:

- How much to give
- How often to give it
- What is in the medication
- Warnings about using the drug
- If the drug is safe for children.

If no dose is given on the bottle or package for children under twelve years old, ask your doctor or pharmacist:

Reprinted from the U.S. Food and Drug Administration, 2005.

- Is it OK to give the medicine to my child?
- How much should I give my child and when?

If the medicine has alcohol in it, as some cough and cold syrups do, you may want to ask the doctor if it's OK for your child to take it.

Before buying the product, make sure the safety seal is not broken. If it's broken or torn, buy another box or bottle with an unbroken seal. Show the product with the broken seal to the pharmacist or sales person.

If your child has a cold, flu, or chickenpox, do not give your child any product with aspirin or similar drugs called salicylates unless your doctor tells you to. Aspirin and other salicylates given to children with symptoms of cold, flu, or chickenpox can cause a rare but sometimes deadly condition called Reye syndrome. Instead of aspirin or other salicylates, you can give your child acetaminophen (sold as Tylenol®, Datril®, and other brands).

When the Doctor Prescribes the Medicine

If a doctor prescribes a drug for your child, before you leave the doctor's office ask any questions you have about the drug. Some of these questions may be as follows:

- What is the drug and what is it for?
- Will this drug cause a problem with other drugs my child is taking?
- How often does my child need to take this medicine?
- How many days or weeks does my child need to take this medicine?
- What if I miss giving my child a dose?
- How soon will the drug start working?
- What side effects does it have?
- What should I do if my child gets any of these side effects?
- Should I stop giving the medicine when my child gets better?
- Is there a less expensive generic version that I can use?

When you get the medicine, check to see if it's the color and size you expected from the doctor's description. If not, ask the pharmacist about it. When filling a prescription, the pharmacist will often give

How to Give Medicine to Children

you printed information with the medicine. If you don't understand the information, or if you have questions, ask the pharmacist. If you still have questions, call your doctor.

How to Measure

Liquid medicines usually come with a cup, spoon, or syringe to help measure the right dose. Be sure to use it. The devices that come with the medicine are better for measuring than kitchen spoons because the amount of medicine kitchen spoons hold can differ a lot. For example, one kitchen teaspoon could hold nearly twice as much as another.

The numbers on the side of measuring instruments are usually small, so read them carefully. Here are the most common types of dosing instruments and tips for using them:

Dosage cups: For children who can drink from a cup without spilling. Look closely at the numbers on the side to make sure you get the dose right. Measure out the liquid with the cup at eye level on a flat surface.

Cylindrical dosing spoons: For children who can drink from a cup but are likely to spill. The spoon looks like a wide straw with a small spoon at the top. Measure the liquid in the spoon at eye level. Have the child sip the medicine from the spoon.

Droppers: For children who can't drink from a cup. Put the medicine into the dropper and measure at eye level. Give to the child quickly before the medicine drips out.

Syringes: For children who can't drink from a cup. You can squirt the medicine into the back of the child's mouth where it's less likely to spill out. Some syringes come with caps to prevent the medicine from leaking out. Be sure to remove these caps before giving the medicine to the child, or the child could choke on the cap. Throw away the cap or place it out of reach of children. You can fill a syringe with the right dose and leave it capped for a babysitter to give to your child later. Make sure you tell the sitter to remove the cap before giving the medicine to your child. It's best to use syringes specially made to give medicines to children. But if you find you have to use a hypodermic syringe, always remove the needle first.

Chapter 4

Recommended Childhood Vaccinations

Vaccines have contributed to a significant reduction in many childhood diseases, such as diphtheria, polio, measles, and whooping cough. It is now rare for American children to experience the devastating effects of these illnesses. Infant deaths due to childhood diseases have nearly disappeared in the United States and other countries with high vaccination coverage. But the germs that cause vaccine-preventable diseases and death still exist, and can be passed on to people who are not protected by vaccines.

Ensuring the safety and effectiveness of vaccines is one of the Food and Drug Administration's top priorities. Vaccines are developed in accordance with the highest safety standards; they must be safe to give to as many people as possible.

Like any medicine, vaccination has benefits and risks, and no vaccine is 100 percent effective in preventing disease. Most side effects of vaccines are usually minor and short-lived. A child may feel soreness at the injection site or experience a low-grade fever. Serious vaccine reactions are extremely rare, but they can happen. For example, signs of severe allergic reaction can include swelling, itching, weakness, dizziness, and difficulty breathing.

"But parents should also know that the risk of being harmed by a vaccine is much smaller than the risk of serious illness that comes with infectious diseases," says Norman Baylor, Ph.D., director of the

---

Reprinted from "A Parent's Guide to Kids' Vaccines," U.S. Food and Drug Administration, January 28, 2008.

Office of Vaccine Research and Review in the Food and Drug Administration's (FDA) Center for Biologics Evaluation and Research (CBER). "Vaccination is an important step to get children off to a healthy start."

Vaccines may contain live, attenuated (but weakened) or killed (inactivated) forms of disease-causing bacteria or viruses, or components of these microorganisms. They trigger a response by the body's immune system when injected or given by mouth. Vaccines stimulate the body to make antibodies—proteins that specifically recognize and target the disease-causing bacteria and viruses, and help eliminate them from the body.

Steps to Take when You Vaccinate

Review the vaccine information sheets: These sheets explain to vaccine recipients, their parents, or their legal representatives both the benefits and risks of a vaccine. Health practitioners are required by law to provide them.

Talk to your doctor about the benefits and risks of vaccines: Learn the facts about the benefits and risks, along with the potential consequences of not vaccinating against certain diseases. Some parents are surprised to learn that children can die of measles, chicken pox, and other vaccine-preventable diseases.

Tell your doctor about bad reactions: Before your child receives a vaccine, tell your doctor if you, your child, or a sibling has ever had a bad reaction to a vaccine. If your child or a sibling has had an allergic reaction or other severe reaction to a dose of vaccine, talk with your health care provider about whether that vaccine should be taken again.

Ask about conditions under which your child should not be vaccinated: This might include being sick or having a history of certain allergic or other adverse reactions to previous vaccinations or their components. For example, eggs are used to grow influenza (flu) vaccines, so a child who is allergic to eggs should not get a flu vaccine.

Report adverse reactions: Adverse reactions and other problems related to vaccines should be reported to the Vaccine Adverse Event Reporting System, which is maintained by FDA and the Centers for Disease Control and Prevention. For a copy of the vaccine reporting form, call 1-800-822-7967, or report online to www.vaers.hhs.gov

Recommended Childhood Vaccinations

Commonly Used Vaccines

Diphtheria, Tetanus, Pertussis (DTaP) Vaccine

What it's for: Protects against the bacterial infections diphtheria, tetanus (lockjaw), and pertussis (whooping cough). Tripedia®, Infanrix®, and DAPTACEL® are licensed for children six weeks to seven years old. Diphtheria can infect the throat, causing a thick covering that can lead to problems with breathing, paralysis, or heart failure. Tetanus can cause painful tightening of the muscles, seizures, and paralysis. Whooping cough causes severe coughing spells and can lead to pneumonia, seizures, brain damage, and death.

Common side effects: Mild fever, redness, soreness or swelling at the injection site, fussiness or crying more than usual.

Tell your health care provider beforehand if: Your child is moderately or severely ill, or has had a severe reaction to a previous shot or has a known sensitivity to ingredients of the vaccine, including latex.

Tetanus, Diphtheria, Pertussis (Tdap) Vaccine

What it's for: Boostrix® is licensed for use for people ages ten to eighteen years. Adacel® is licensed for people ages eleven years and older, up to age sixty-four. Protects against the bacterial infections diphtheria, tetanus (lockjaw), and pertussis (whooping cough).

Common side effects: Mild fever, pain and redness at injection site, headache, tiredness.

Tell your health care provider beforehand if: Your child has had any allergic reaction to any vaccine that protects against diphtheria, tetanus, or pertussis diseases, any ingredient contained in the vaccine, or to latex.

Haemophilus influenzae *Type b (Hib) Vaccine*

What it's for: Protects against Hib disease, which can cause meningitis (an infection of the covering of the brain and spinal cord), pneumonia (lung infection), severe swelling of the throat, and infections of the blood, joints, bones, and covering of the heart. Approved for children who are at least two months old.

Common side effects: Redness, warmth, or swelling at site of injection, fever.

Tell your health care provider beforehand if: Your child is moderately or severely ill, or has ever had a life-threatening allergic reaction to a previous dose of Hib vaccine.

Hepatitis A Vaccine

What it's for: Protects against liver disease caused by the hepatitis A virus. Hepatitis A can cause mild "flu-like" illness, jaundice (yellow skin or eyes), severe stomach pains, and diarrhea. A person who has hepatitis A can easily pass the disease to others within the same household. Havrix® and VAQTA® are licensed for use in children ages twelve months and up.

Common side effects: Soreness at the injection site, headache, loss of appetite, tiredness.

Tell your health care provider beforehand if: Your child has ever had a severe allergic reaction to a previous dose of the vaccine.

Hepatitis B Vaccine

What it's for: Protects against liver disease caused by the hepatitis B virus. Hepatitis B can lead to liver damage, liver cancer, and death. Recombivax HB® and Engerix-B® are licensed for use in babies at birth.

Common side effects: Soreness at injection site and fever.

Tell your health care provider beforehand if: Your child is moderately or severely ill or has ever had a life-threatening allergic reaction to baker's yeast used for making bread, or to a previous dose of the vaccine.

Human Papillomavirus (HPV) Vaccine

What it's for: Gardasil® is licensed for the prevention of cervical cancer, abnormal and precancerous cervical lesions, abnormal and precancerous vaginal and vulvar lesions, and genital warts in females ages nine to twenty-six.

Common side effects: Pain, redness or swelling, itching at the site of injection, dizziness, fainting.

Recommended Childhood Vaccinations

Tell your health care provider beforehand if: Your child has had an allergic reaction to yeast or another component of HPV vaccine, or to a previous dose of the vaccine.

Influenza (Flu) Vaccine—Inactivated Shot

What it's for: Protects children six months and older against the influenza virus strains contained in the vaccine. Influenza is a contagious respiratory illness caused by the influenza virus. It can cause mild to severe illness, and at times can lead to death. The influenza viruses that cause disease in people may change every year, so yearly vaccination is needed to reduce the chances of getting sick.

Common side effects: Soreness at the injection site, low-grade fever, and aches. The influenza vaccine is made from killed or inactivated influenza viruses, so your child can't get the flu from the flu shot.

Tell your health care provider beforehand if: Your child is moderately or severely ill, has ever had an allergic reaction to eggs or to a previous dose of the flu vaccine, or has ever had Guillain-Barré syndrome (GBS), a serious neurological disorder that can occur either spontaneously or after certain infections. The disorder typically involves weakness in the legs and arms that can be severe.

Influenza (Flu) Vaccine—Live Intranasal

What it's for: FluMist® is sprayed into both nostrils and protects against flu in healthy children and adolescents ages five to seventeen. In September 2007, the Food and Drug Administration (FDA) approved FluMist for use in children between the ages of two and five.

Common side effects: Runny nose, headache, vomiting, muscle aches, low-grade fever. This vaccine, which contains weakened viruses, usually doesn't cause illness, because the viruses have lost their disease-causing properties.

Tell your health care provider beforehand if: Your child is pregnant, moderately or severely ill, has a weakened immune system, has ever had an allergic reaction to eggs or to a previous dose of the flu vaccine, has a history of asthma or any other history of coughing, wheezing, or shortness of breath, or has a history of Guillain-Barré syndrome (GBS).

Measles, Mumps, Rubella (MMR) Vaccine

What it's for: Protects against measles, mumps, and rubella in children ages twelve months and up. Measles is a respiratory infection that causes skin rash and flu-like symptoms. It can cause severe disease leading to ear infection, pneumonia, seizures, and brain damage. Mumps causes fever, headache, and swollen glands, especially salivary glands. It can also lead to deafness, meningitis (infection of the brain and spinal cord covering), and painful swelling of the testicles or ovaries. Rubella, also called German measles, is an infection of the skin and lymph nodes and can cause arthritis. Rubella infection during pregnancy can lead to birth defects.

Common side effects: Fever and mild rash. In rare cases, swelling of the glands in the cheeks or neck.

Tell your health care provider beforehand if: Your child is ill or has ever had an allergic reaction to gelatin, the antibiotic neomycin, or a previous dose of the MMR vaccine.

Meningococcal Disease Vaccine

What it's for: Menactra® is licensed for use in people ages eleven years and older, up to age fifty-five. In October 2007, FDA approved expanding the age range for Menactra to include children ages two to ten years. Menomune® is licensed for use in children two years and older. These vaccines protect against meningococcal disease, a serious illness caused by a bacteria. It is a leading cause of bacterial meningitis in children two to eighteen years old in the United States. Meningitis is an infection of fluid surrounding the brain and the spinal cord.

Common side effects: Sore arm, headache, fatigue.

Tell your health care provider beforehand if: Your child has had a severe allergic reaction to a previous dose of meningococcal vaccine, has a known sensitivity to vaccine components or latex, which is used in the vial stopper, or has bleeding disorders or a history of Guillain-Barré syndrome (GBS), a serious neurological disorder that can occur either spontaneously or after certain infections. The disorder typically involves weakness in the legs and arms that can be severe.

Recommended Childhood Vaccinations

Pneumococcal Conjugate Vaccine

What it's for: Prevnar® (Pneumococcal 7-valent Conjugate Vaccine) protects infants and toddlers against serious pneumococcal disease, such as meningitis and blood infections, and some ear infections.

Common side effects: Redness, tenderness, swelling at injection site, fever, fussiness, drowsiness, loss of appetite.

Tell your health care provider beforehand if: Your child is moderately or severely ill, or has ever had an allergic reaction to a previous dose.

Pneumococcal Vaccine Polyvalent

What it's for: Pneumovax 23® is licensed for use in children with certain health conditions who are two years or older for the prevention of the twenty-three most prevalent types of pneumococcal bacteria. Pneumococcal disease can lead to serious infections of the blood, the lungs, such as pneumonia, and the covering of the brain (meningitis).

Common side effects: Soreness, warmth, redness, swelling at the site of injection.

Tell your health care provider beforehand if: Your child is allergic to any component of the vaccine, has a respiratory illness or other active infection, or has severely compromised cardiovascular and/or pulmonary function.

Polio Vaccine

What it's for: The inactivated poliovirus vaccine (IPV) protects against the virus that causes polio, an illness that can cause paralysis or death. For children at least two months old.

Common side effects: Soreness at injection site, muscle aches, low-grade fever.

Tell your health care provider beforehand if: Your child has ever had a severe allergic reaction to a previous shot or an allergic reaction to the antibiotics neomycin, streptomycin, or polymyxin B.

Rotavirus Vaccine

What it's for: RotaTeq® is a live vaccine given by mouth to prevent rotavirus gastroenteritis in infants. This viral infection of the stomach and intestines can cause severe diarrhea, vomiting, and fever, which may lead to serious dehydration. For children who are at least six weeks old, but younger than thirty-two weeks.

Common side effects: Mild, temporary diarrhea or vomiting.

Tell your health care provider beforehand if: Your child has a known or weakened immune system, is allergic to any of the ingredients of the vaccine, or has ever had an allergic reaction after getting a dose of the vaccine.

Varicella (Chicken Pox) Vaccine

What it's for: Varivax® (varicella virus vaccine live) protects against chicken pox in people one year and older. Chicken pox, which is caused by the varicella-zoster virus, causes itchy blisters and fever. Complications of chicken pox can include skin infection, scarring, brain swelling, and pneumonia.

Common side effects: Soreness or swelling at the injection site, fever, mild rash.

Tell your health care provider beforehand if: Your child is moderately or severely ill, or has ever had a life-threatening allergic reaction to gelatin, the antibiotic neomycin, or a previous dose of chicken pox vaccine.

Chapter 5

Promoting Wellness

Chapter Contents

Section 5.1—Nutrition for the School-Aged Child 28
Section 5.2—Physical Fitness and Health 33
Section 5.3—Healthy Sleep Habits 35
Section 5.4—The Importance of Handwashing 37

Section 5.1

Nutrition for the School-Aged Child

"Nutrition for the School-Aged Child" (G1086), by Linda Boeckner, Extension Nutrition Specialist, and Karen Schledewitz, Extension Assistant, Copyright © 2006 by the University of Nebraska Board of Regents on behalf of University of Nebraska-Lincoln Extension. Used with permission.

When you send your child off to school, your job related to healthful meals for your child isn't over. During the school years, many nutrition lessons still need to be taught. Your children will likely face new choices about what to eat during and after school. Schoolmates will have a greater influence on these choices.

Nutrients for the Growing Years

Carbohydrates and fats provide energy for growing and physical activity. Through the school years children will have periods of rapid growth and big appetites. When growth slows, appetites will decrease and children may want less food at meals and snacks.

Protein builds, maintains, and repairs body tissue. It is especially important for growth. In the United States, most children do not suffer from lack of dietary protein. It is important, however, to encourage children to eat recommended amounts of protein-rich food each day. Milk and other dairy products, poultry, fish, pork, and beef are examples of good protein sources.

A variety of vitamins and minerals support growth and development during childhood. Calcium from milk and dairy products and some dark green, leafy vegetables is usually sufficient in young children's diets. As children approach their teen years, dietary calcium intakes don't always keep up with recommendations. Calcium is particularly important in building strong bones and teeth. Osteoporosis, a brittle bone disease that affects older adults, begins in childhood if diets do not provide calcium-rich foods.

Iron deficiency anemia can be a problem for some children. Iron is an oxygen-carrying component of blood. Children need iron because of rapidly expanding blood volume during growth. For girls, the beginning

Promoting Wellness

of menstruation in late childhood adds an extra demand for iron due to the regular loss of iron in menstrual blood. Meats, fish, poultry, and enriched breads and cereals are the best sources of dietary iron.

Vitamins A and C come from many different fruits and vegetables. They are important for healthy skin, growth, and fighting infections. The B vitamins (thiamin, niacin, riboflavin, and other B vitamins) come from a variety of foods including grain products, meat and meat substitutes, and dairy products. They promote healthy growth in a variety of ways.

Parents should provide a variety of foods and establish regular meal and snack times and encourage physical activity for their children. In most cases, nutrient and energy needs will be adequately met. If parents are concerned about their children's poor nutrient intakes or their weights, they should consult with a physician or trained nutrition professional, such as a registered dietitian.

Table 5.1 provides guidance for planning general daily food intakes for children. For more information about food selections for your child's specific age, sex, and activity level, go to www.MyPyramid.gov. Look for the section titled, "For Kids."

Snacks

Growing and physically active children need snacks, but poor snack choices lead to too many calories and not enough nutrients. Parents and other caretakers can help children make nutritious snack choices by keeping foods on hand from the food groups shown in Table 5.1.

Safe food handling and preparation is an important part of snacking. Young school children ages five to eight should have snacks that are ready-to-eat or partly prepared. Older children enjoy preparing their own snacks. Review safety rules for using kitchen equipment and set limits for the amount of food preparation that can be done. Demonstrate how to use a microwave oven. Sharp, electrically powered equipment should be off limits unless a child has adult supervision. Encourage children to be responsible for their own kitchen activities by expecting them to clean up after themselves.

Children—Overweight and Physically Unfit?

U.S. children today are more overweight and less fit compared to children of the 1960s. A variety of factors affect this trend but a primary reason is lack of physical activity. Today's average school-aged child spends several hours each week watching television and working on the computer. The result is less time to be physically active. Added to the problem is the decline of physical education as children advance through the grade levels. The 2005 Dietary Guidelines for Americans recommend that children engage in at least sixty minutes of physical activity on most days of the week.

Table 5.1. A Pattern for Daily Food Choices for School-Aged Children

Food Groups	Suggested Daily Amount (exercising 30 to 60 min/day)				Measurement Equivalents	Tip
	5 yr. olds	10 yr. olds	14 yr. old girl	14 yr. old boy		
Grains (includes foods made from whole grains)	5 oz	6 oz	6 oz	8 oz	1 oz. = 1 slice bread, 1 cup ready-to-eat cereal or ½ cup cooked cereal, pasta, or rice	Make at least ½ of your grains whole grains
Vegetables (includes all fresh, frozen, and canned vegetables)	1.5 cups	2.5 cups	2.5 cups	3 cups	1 cup = 1 cup raw or cooked vegetables or 100% juice, 2 cups of raw, leafy greens	Choose a variety of colorful veggies
Fruits (includes all fresh, frozen canned, and dried fruit)	1.5 cups	1.5 cups	2 cups	2 cups	1 cup = 1 cup fruit or 100% juice, ½ cup dried fruit	Eat more fruits than fruit juices
Milk (includes milk, cheese, and yogurt)	2 cups	3 cups	3 cups	3 cups	1 cup = 1 cup milk or yogurt, 1 ½ oz. natural cheese, 2 oz. processed cheese	Eat low-fat or fat-free milk products
Meat and Beans (includes beans, eggs, and nuts)	4 oz.	5 oz.	5.5 oz.	6.5 oz.	1 oz. = 1 oz. lean meat, poultry, or fish, 1 egg, 1 tablespoon peanut butter, ¼ cup cooked dry beans, ½ oz. nuts	Eat lean meat and vary your choices

Promoting Wellness

Parents can become positive examples for their children by joining them in physical activity. Outdoor activities such as playing tag, swinging, walking, bicycling, flying a kite, swimming, building a snow fort, and others will boost energy requirements for a child and help to build healthy weights. Family outings which include hiking, picnicking, trips to the park playground, bicycle trips, and bowling are more ideas.

Diets of school-aged children can also affect their weights. Use caution when dealing with an overweight child. Children should not be pushed to lose weight. Instead, focus on dietary variety within the guidelines found in Table 5.1. Do not isolate children from family

Table 5.2. Food Choices by Level of Fat

Higher Fat Choices	Lower Fat Choices

Grain Food Group (For whole grains, look for whole grain as the first item on ingredient list)

Donuts	Whole Grain Cereal (oatmeal, whole grain corn, whole wheat)
Danish	Variety of whole grain or enriched bread (whole wheat, whole
Croissants	oats, whole rye)
	Pasta (whole wheat)
	Rice (brown rice, wild rice)

Vegetables (eat more dark green and orange vegetables)

Sauteed or deep-fried	Lightly steamed vegetables with herb seasonings or lemon
French fries	Plain potatoes with low-fat yogurt or cottage cheese or light
Au gratin potatoes	amounts of margarine and sour cream
Creamy salads	Raw vegetables
	Salads that use low fat dressing/vinegar/oil

Meat and Beans (vary your protein sources—choose more fish, beans, peas, nuts, and seeds)

Fried eggs and meats	Select lean meat cuts; trim fat
Heavy sauces or gravy	Select lean ham, chicken, turkey to replace luncheon meats
High-fat meat cuts	Hard cooked eggs
Luncheon meats	Roasted or baked chicken
Hot dogs	

Milk and Milk Products (If you can't drink milk, choose lactose-free products)

Whole milk	Select low-fat or nonfat milk, milk products, and yogurt
Regular cheeses	Use low-fat cheeses, such as mozzarella, ricotta, and farmer's
Ice cream	cheese
	Select sherbet or frozen yogurt to replace ice cream

Snack Items (use snacks only to supplement daily meals—not to replace them)

Chips	Unbuttered popcorn
Buttered popcorn	Fruit and fruit shakes with low-fat milk
Candy bars	Low-fat crackers and bread sticks
Cookies	Graham or whole wheat crackers

meals by preparing separate food. The family menus should be appropriate for all family members, including an overweight child.

Keeping fat intake at moderate levels without being too extreme is important. Parents who are too restrictive with fat intake will limit a child's ability to eat sufficient calories to maintain growth. No foods should be forbidden in a child's diet. The key to achieving low to moderate fat levels is offering appropriate choices, balancing high-fat choices with low-fat choices and providing a variety of foods. Look over Table 5.2 to learn about available choices.

Summary

Nutrition for school-aged children should promote growth and meet energy and nutrient needs without promoting fatness. During the school years, children will experience increased opportunities to make choices about their food intakes. Parents can help their children make positive food choices by planning family mealtimes, keeping a variety of foods in supply, and setting positive examples. Habits formed in childhood are likely to carry into adult years.

References

Cavadini, C, Siega-Riz, AM, and Popkin, BM. US adolescent food intake trends from 1965 to 1996. *Arch Dis Child* 83:13–24, 2000.

Ogden, CL, Flegal, KM, Carroll, MD, Johnson, CL. Prevalence and trends in overweight among US children and adolescents, 1999–2000. *JAMA* 288:1728–32, 2000.

Robinson, TN. Reducing children's television viewing to prevent obesity: a randomized controlled trial. *JAMA* 282(16):1561–67, 1999.

United States Department of Health and Human Services and United States Department of Agriculture. *Dietary Guidelines for Americans 2005*. Sixth edition. Washington, D.C.: U.S. Government Printing Office, January 2005.

U.S. Department of Health and Human Services. *Physical Activity and Health: A Report of the Surgeon General*. Atlanta, GA: U.S. Department of Health and Human Services, Centers for Disease Control and Prevention, National Center for Chronic Disease Prevention and Health Promotion, 1996.

Section 5.2

Physical Fitness and Health

Reprinted from "Physical Activity for Everyone: Are There Special Recommendations for Young People?" Centers for Disease Control and Prevention, May 22, 2007.

It is recommended that children and adolescents participate in at least sixty minutes of moderate intensity physical activity most days of the week, preferably daily.[1]

Children and adolescents can choose any type of moderate or higher intensity physical activity, such as brisk walking, playing tag, jumping rope, or swimming, as long as it is adds up to at least one hour a day.

For children and adolescents, regular physical activity has beneficial effects on the following aspects of health:

- Weight
- Muscular strength
- Cardiorespiratory (aerobic) fitness
- Bone mass (through weight-bearing physical activities)
- Blood pressure (for hypertensive youth)
- Anxiety and stress
- Self-esteem

Children and adolescents who are just beginning to be physically active should start out slowly and gradually build to higher levels in order to prevent the risk of injury or feeling defeated from unrealistic goals. It is important that children and adolescents are encouraged to be physically active by doing things that interest them. This will help them establish an active lifestyle early on.

Tips for Parents

As a parent, you have an important role in shaping your children's physical activity attitudes and behaviors. Here are some tips to encourage your children to be more physically active:

- Set a positive example by leading an active lifestyle yourself, and make physical activity part of your family's daily routine such as designating time for family walks or playing active games together.
- Provide opportunities for children to be active by playing with them. Give them active toys and equipment, and take them to places where they can be active.
- Offer positive reinforcement for the physical activities in which your children participate and encourage them as they express interest in new activities.
- Make physical activity fun. Fun activities can be anything the child enjoys, either structured or nonstructured. They may range from team sports, to individual sports, and/or recreational activities such as walking, running, skating, bicycling, swimming, playground activities, and free-time play.
- Ensure that the activity is age appropriate and, to ensure safety, provide protective equipment such as helmets, wrist pads, and knee pads.
- Find a convenient place to be active regularly.
- Limit the time your children watch television or play video games to no more than two hours per day. Instead, encourage your children to find fun activities to do with family members or on their own that simply involve more activity (walking, playing chase, dancing).

References

1. This physical activity recommendation is from the Dietary Guidelines for Americans 2005.

Section 5.3

Healthy Sleep Habits

Excerpted from "Children's Sleep Habits," © 2007 National Sleep Foundation (www.sleepfoundation.org). All rights reserved. Reprinted with permission. For additional information, visit www.sleepfoundation.org.

Every living creature needs to sleep. It is the primary activity of the brain during early development. Circadian rhythms, or the sleep-wake cycle, are regulated by light and dark and these rhythms take time to develop, resulting in the irregular sleep schedules of newborns. The rhythms begin to develop at about six weeks, and by three to six months most infants have a regular sleep-wake cycle.

By the age of two, most children have spent more time asleep than awake and overall, a child will spend 40 percent of his or her childhood asleep. Sleep is especially important for children as it directly impacts mental and physical development.

There are two alternating types or states of sleep:

- **Non-rapid eye movement (NREM) or "quiet" sleep:** During the deep states of NREM sleep, blood supply to the muscles is increased, energy is restored, tissue growth and repair occur, and important hormones are released for growth and development.

- **Rapid eye movement (REM) or "active" sleep:** During REM sleep, our brains are active and dreaming occurs. Our bodies become immobile, breathing and heart rates are irregular.

Babies spend 50 percent of their time in each of these states and the sleep cycle is about fifty minutes. At about six months of age, REM sleep comprises about 30 percent of sleep. By the time children reach preschool age, the sleep cycle is about every ninety minutes.

Sleep and Preschoolers (Three to Five Years)

Preschoolers typically sleep eleven to thirteen hours each night and most do not nap after five years of age. As with toddlers, difficulty falling asleep and waking up during the night are common. With further development of imagination, preschoolers commonly experience nighttime fears and nightmares. In addition, sleepwalking and sleep terrors peak during preschool years.

Sleep Tips for Preschoolers

- Maintain a regular and consistent sleep schedule.
- Have a relaxing bedtime routine that ends in the room where the child sleeps.
- Child should sleep in the same sleeping environment every night, in a room that is cool, quiet, and dark—and without a TV.

Sleep and School-Aged Children (Five to Twelve Years)

Children aged five to twelve need ten to eleven hours of sleep. At the same time, there is an increasing demand on their time from school (e.g., homework), sports, and other extracurricular and social activities. In addition, school-aged children become more interested in TV, computers, the media and internet, as well as caffeine products—all of which can lead to difficulty falling asleep, nightmares, and disruptions to their sleep. In particular, watching TV close to bedtime has been associated with bedtime resistance, difficulty falling asleep, anxiety around sleep, and sleeping fewer hours.

Sleep problems and disorders are prevalent at this age. Poor or inadequate sleep can lead to mood swings, behavioral problems such as hyperactivity, and cognitive problems that impact on their ability to learn in school.

Sleep Tips for School-Aged Children

- Teach school-aged children about healthy sleep habits.
- Continue to emphasize need for regular and consistent sleep schedule and bedtime routine.
- Make child's bedroom conducive to sleep—dark, cool, and quiet.
- Keep TV and computers out of the bedroom.
- Avoid caffeine.

Promoting Wellness

Section 5.4

The Importance of Handwashing

"Quick Facts About . . . Handwashing," April 2007, is reprinted with permission from the Indiana State Department of Health, http://www.in.gov/isdh.

Why is handwashing important?

Handwashing is the single most effective means of preventing the spread of infections. Many diseases, such as the common cold, influenza (flu), ear infections, strep throat, and diarrheal illnesses, can be spread by unwashed or improperly washed hands.

How are diseases spread?

Bacteria and viruses that cause disease can get on your hands in many ways, for example, handling food or animals, touching doorknobs, shaking hands, using phone receivers or computer keyboards, and using the toilet. You can help reduce the spread of many bacteria and viruses by properly washing your hands with soap and water. Always wash your hands before you touch your eyes, nose, mouth, or ears.

When should I wash my hands?

Always wash your hands:

- after using the toilet;
- after helping someone else use the toilet;
- after changing a diaper;
- after helping someone who is ill;
- after blowing your nose, sneezing, or coughing;
- before, during, and after food preparation, especially raw foods;
- before eating;
- after handling soiled utensils and equipment;

- after handling garbage;
- after handling money;
- after handling animals, especially reptiles, (e.g., iguanas, turtles, or snakes) or livestock (e.g., cattle, pigs, or sheep).

What is the proper way to wash my hands?

Wet hands with running water. Lather hands with soap. Wash the palms, back of hands, between fingers, and under fingernails for at least fifteen seconds (about the time it takes to sing "Happy Birthday" twice). Rinse hands with running water. Pat hands dry, beginning at the wrist and moving downward. Cover the faucet handle(s) with a paper towel to turn off the water.

How can handwashing protect me and my family?

Keeping your hands clean is one of the most important ways you can avoid getting sick and spreading germs to others. Foodborne illness outbreaks often happen when a food handler touches food with unwashed or improperly washed hands. Many diarrheal illnesses (such as salmonellosis, hepatitis A, and shigellosis) can be spread from person to person by individuals who fail to wash their hands after using the toilet and then pass the bacteria or virus by handling food, shaking hands, or touching other objects. If the bacteria or virus gets into another person's mouth and is swallowed, that person then becomes sick. Proper handwashing is everyone's responsibility:

- Parents should teach their children the proper way to wash their hands.
- Children should see their parents and other care providers washing their hands properly and frequently.
- Consumers should let restaurants, daycare providers, doctors, health care workers, long-term care facilities, etc., know they are concerned about personal hygiene and the proper use of handwashing to help control infections.

Chapter 6

Preventing Childhood Injuries

Chapter Contents

Section 6.1—Preventing Burns 40
Section 6.2—Preventing Drowning 42
Section 6.3—Preventing Falls 44
Section 6.4—Preventing Poisoning 46
Section 6.5—Preventing Airway Obstruction Injuries 48
Section 6.6—Preventing Bicycle Injuries 50
Section 6.7—Preventing Motor Vehicle Injuries 51

Section 6.1

Preventing Burns

"Preventing Childhood Burns," © 2008 Safe Kids Worldwide.
Reprinted with permission.

Because young children may not perceive danger as readily or may lack the ability to escape a life-threatening burn situation, make sure they are not exposed to open flames or other burn risks:

- Keep matches, candles, gasoline, lighters, and all other flammable materials locked away and out of children's reach.
- Never leave a burning candle unattended. Place candles in safe locations, away from combustible materials and where children or pets cannot tip them over.
- Keep children away from cooking and heating appliances (e.g., space heaters, irons, hair styling tools). Never leave the kitchen while you are cooking. If you must leave the room, take the child with you.

Children's skin burns at lower temperatures and more deeply than that of older children and adults. A child exposed to 140-degree Fahrenheit liquid for three seconds will sustain a third-degree burn:

- Set your water heater thermostat to 120 degrees Fahrenheit or below. Consider installing water faucets and shower heads containing anti-scald technology.
- Use back burners and turn pot handles to the back of the stove when cooking.
- Keep hot foods and liquids away from table and counter edges. Never carry or hold children and hot foods or liquids at the same time.
- Keep appliance cords out of children's reach, especially if the appliances contain hot foods or liquids.

Preventing Childhood Injuries

Precautions to avoid fire in the home can also reduce a child's risk of burn injury:

- Install smoke alarms in your home on every level and in every sleeping area. Test them once a month. Replace the batteries at least two times a year, such as when daylight savings time starts and ends. Ten-year lithium alarms do not require battery changes. Replace all alarms every ten years. For the best protection against different types of fires, consider installing both ionization alarms (better at sensing flaming fires) and photoelectric alarms (better at sensing slow, smoky fires).

- Avoid plugging several appliance cords into the same electrical socket. Replace old or frayed electrical wires and appliance cords, and keep all cords on top of rugs. Cover unused electrical outlets with safety devices.

- Place space heaters at least three feet from curtains, papers, furniture, and other flammable materials. Make sure heaters are stable, and use protective coverings.

- Never smoke in bed. Extinguish all cigarettes before leaving home or going to bed.

Section 6.2

Preventing Drowning

"Preventing Childhood Drowning," © 2008 Safe Kids Worldwide.
Reprinted with permission.

Always actively supervise children in and around water. Don't leave, even for a moment:

- Stay where you can see, hear, and reach kids in water. Avoid talking on the phone, preparing a meal, reading, and other distractions.
- Children should swim only in designated and supervised swimming areas.
- Teach children never to swim alone.

Use barriers to keep kids away from water when you're not around:

- Four-sided isolation fencing, at least five feet high and equipped with self-closing and self-latching gates, should be installed around all pools (including inflatable pools) and spas. Fencing should completely enclose the pool or spa and prevent direct access from a house or yard.
- Install barriers of protection around your home pool or spa in addition to the fencing, such as pool alarms, pool covers, door alarms, or locks.
- Never prop open the gate to a pool barrier. Don't leave toys that could attract children in or around a pool.
- Empty buckets, wading pools, and other containers immediately after use, and store upside down and out of reach.
- Keep toilet lids down and locked and doors to bathrooms and utility rooms closed when not in use.

Pool drains are an often-overlooked drowning hazard:

Preventing Childhood Injuries

- Teach children never to go near a pool drain, with or without a cover, and to pin up long hair when in water.
- Install multiple drains in all pools, spas, whirlpools, and hot tubs. This minimizes the suction of any one drain, reducing risk of death or injury.
- Regularly check to make sure drain covers are secure and have no cracks. Replace flat drain covers with dome-shaped ones.
- Know where the manual cut-off switch for the pump is in case of emergency. Consider installing an approved "safety vacuum release system" (SVRS), a tool that quickly and automatically turns off the pump (and stops the suction) when something is trapped in or blocks the drain.

Use life jackets and other safety gear, but know that any child can get in trouble in the water, even if he is wearing a life jacket or has taken swimming lessons:

- Always wear U.S. Coast Guard–approved personal flotation devices while on boats, in or near open bodies of water, or participating in water sports. A personal flotation device (PFD) should fit snugly and not allow the child's chin or ears to slip through the neck opening.
- Air-filled swimming aids, such as "water wings" and inner tubes, are not safety devices and should never be substituted for PFDs.
- Learn CPR and keep rescue equipment (like a lifesaving ring), a telephone, and emergency phone numbers poolside.

Everyone should know the water safety rules:

- Make sure children take swimming lessons when they're ready, usually after age four. Check with the local department of parks and recreation or Red Cross chapter to find a certified instructor, and look for classes that include emergency water survival techniques training.
- Forty-four states have laws that require children to wear PFDs while participating in recreational boating. The U.S. Coast Guard has also issued a rule requiring children under thirteen to wear PFDs onboard recreational vessels on Coast Guard waters. The rule applies to states without PFD laws. Recreational boats must

carry one properly sized, U.S. Coast Guard–approved PFD, accessible and in good condition, for each person onboard.

- Teach kids the safe way to help someone in trouble in the water: call for help and throw the person something that floats.
- Don't let children dive into water less than nine feet deep, and no one should dive into a river, lake, or ocean.
- Children ages sixteen and under should never operate personal watercraft.

Section 6.3

Preventing Falls

"Preventing Childhood Falls," © 2008 Safe Kids Worldwide.
Reprinted with permission.

All windows above the first floor should be equipped with window guards—preferably guards with emergency release devices in case of fire. Children can fall from windows open as little as four inches:

- Open windows without guards at the top only, or use window stops so they open only a few inches.
- Never rely on window screens to prevent falls.
- Supervise children at all times around open windows.
- Move furniture away from windows, and keep them locked when they're closed.

Never let children play on fire escapes or high porches, decks, or balconies:

- Make sure all railing slats are secure and no more than 3½ inches apart. Securely attach mesh or plastic barriers to cover openings greater than 3½ inches.

Any house with a baby or toddler in it should have safety gates at the top and bottom of every staircase:

Preventing Childhood Injuries

- Safety gates at the tops of stairs must be attached to the wall, as these are more secure than the kind held in place by outward pressure.
- Keep hallways and stairs well-lit and clear of clutter, and don't let children play on stairs.

Keep young children safe by strapping them into seats and carriers and avoiding baby walkers:

- Never leave young children alone on changing tables, beds, couches, or other furniture. Always strap them into high chairs, infant carriers, swings, and strollers.
- Never use baby walkers on wheels. Stationary play centers give your baby a chance to practice standing and moving in an upright position without going anywhere and getting into hazardous situations.
- Always put a baby in a carrier on the floor, not on top of a table or other furniture.

Keep children at play safe with the right safety gear and adult supervision:

- If you have playground equipment, the ground beneath it should be cushioned with shredded rubber, hardwood fiber mulch or chips, or fine sand. Grass and soil are not as good at preventing serious injuries. The material should be twelve inches deep and extend at least six feet in all directions. This won't prevent falls, but it can reduce the risk and severity of injuries.
- Insist that children wear their helmets correctly every time they ride their bikes, scooters, skateboards, or inline skates. Helmets should be centered on top of their heads, with straps snugly fastened under their chins. Make sure their helmets carry stickers indicating they meet safety standards.
- Make sure children wear knee pads, elbow pads, and wrist guards while inline skating or skateboarding. Skaters should take lessons, avoid skating at night and skate on smooth, paved surfaces free of traffic.
- Children under age eight should not ride scooters without close adult supervision. Make sure children riding scooters wear knee pads and elbow pads in addition to helmets.

Section 6.4

Preventing Poisoning

"Preventing Childhood Poisoning," © 2008 Safe Kids Worldwide.
Reprinted with permission.

Store potentially poisonous household products and medications locked out of children's sight and reach:

- Read labels to find out what is poisonous. Potential hazards include makeup, medicine, plants, cleaning products, pesticides, art supplies, and beer, wine, and liquor.
- Never leave potentially poisonous household products unattended while in use.
- Be aware of poisons that may be in your handbag. Store handbags out of the reach of young children.
- Never mix cleaning products.
- Buy child-resistant packages when available. Keep products in their original packages to avoid confusion.

Keep the toll-free nationwide poison control center number (800-222-1222) and local emergency numbers near every telephone. If you suspect poisoning and a child is choking, collapses, can't breathe, or is having a seizure, call 911. Otherwise, take the product to the phone and call the poison control hotline:

- Follow the operator's instructions.
- Don't make the child vomit or give him anything unless directed.
- Keep activated charcoal on hand to be used only on the advice of a poison control center or a physician. Ipecac syrup should no longer be used as a home treatment strategy.

Be safe when taking or administering medication:

Preventing Childhood Injuries

- Always read labels, follow directions, and give medicines to children based on their weights and ages. Only use the dispensers packaged with children's medications.
- Don't take medicine or vitamins in front of kids, and don't call them "candy."
- Throw away old medicine by flushing it down a toilet.
- Tell grandparents and friends about avoiding medication poisoning when your family visits their homes.

Take precautions to avoid other poisons that may be present in the home:

- Test children for lead exposure, and test homes built before 1978 for lead-based paint. If it is found, cover the lead paint with a sealant or hire a professional abatement company to remove the paint. Frequently wash children's hands and faces, as well as their toys and pacifiers, to reduce the risk of ingesting lead-contaminated dust.
- Install carbon monoxide (CO) detectors in every sleeping area and on all levels of your home. Check the batteries every month. If the alarm sounds, leave the home immediately and call for help from a neighbor's home or a cell phone outside the home.
- Ensure that space heaters, furnaces, fireplaces, and wood-burning stoves are vented properly and inspected annually.
- Remove a vehicle from the garage to warm it up, even if the garage door is kept open.

Section 6.5

Preventing Airway Obstruction Injuries

"Preventing Childhood Airway Obstruction Injuries,"
© 2008 Safe Kids Worldwide. Reprinted with permission.

Because most infant suffocation occurs in the sleeping environment, infants should sleep only in properly equipped cribs. They should never sleep on couches, chairs, regular beds or other soft surfaces:

- Place an infant on his or her back on a firm, flat crib mattress in a crib with a Juvenile Products Manufacturers Association (JPMA) label indicating that it meets national safety standards. The mattress should be covered with a fitted sheet.

- Remove pillows, comforters, stuffed toys, and other soft products from the crib.

- Use a sleep sack or swaddle to keep the child warm, or tuck in a light blanket that goes no higher than the chest.

To avoid choking, always supervise young children while they are eating, and keep small objects that are potential choking hazards out of their reach:

- Do not allow children under age three to eat small, round, or hard foods, including hot dogs, hard candy, nuts, grapes, and popcorn.

- Get on the floor on your hands and knees, so that you are at your child's eye level. Look for and remove small items such as jewelry, coins, buttons, pins, nails and stones. Be sure to keep all plastic bags out of reach.

Keep cords and strings that could be strangulation hazards (those that are seven inches or longer) away from children:

- Never hang anything on or above a crib with string or ribbon longer than seven inches.

Preventing Childhood Injuries

- Never put a long cord like a necklace, ribbon, or bib with ties on an infant.
- Clip pacifiers to clothing with short leashes, not long cords.
- Remove hood and neck drawstrings from all children's clothing.
- Remove hood and neck drawstrings from all children's outerwear. Never allow children to wear helmets, necklaces, purses, scarves, or clothing with drawstrings while on playgrounds.
- Tie up all window blind and drapery cords, or cut the ends and retrofit with safety tassels. The inner cords of blinds should be fitted with cord stops.
- Don't use toys with cords longer than seven inches.

Make sure toys and other items children play with do not pose choking or suffocation hazards:

- Ensure that children play with age-appropriate toys, as indicated by choking hazard safety labels. Inspect old and new toys regularly for damage that may cause small pieces to break off. Consider purchasing a small parts tester to determine whether toys and objects in your home may present a choking hazard to young children.
- Make sure toy chests have no lids or have safety hinges. Do not permit children access to household appliances where they could become trapped, such as refrigerators or dryers.
- Don't let children under age eight blow up balloons. Use Mylar balloons instead of latex balloons. If you must use latex balloons, store them out of reach of children, and deflate and discard balloons and balloon pieces after use.

Sleeping environment safety remains important for children up to age eight:

- Children under age eight should not be allowed to sleep on the top bunk of a bunk bed. Ensure that all spaces between the guardrail and bed frame, and all spaces in the head and footboards, are less than 3.5 inches.

Learn CPR for infants and children and the Heimlich maneuver for choking.

Section 6.6

Preventing Bicycle Injuries

"Preventing Injuries to Children Riding Bicycles,"
© 2008 Safe Kids Worldwide. Reprinted with permission.

The single most effective safety device available to reduce head injury and death from bicycle crashes is a helmet:

- Make it a rule—every time you or your child ride a bike, you must wear a bicycle helmet that meets or exceeds the safety standards developed by the U.S. Consumer Product Safety Commission.
- Helmet fit is important. The helmet should be comfortable and snug, but not too tight. It should sit centered on top of your head in a level position, and it should not rock forward and backward or side to side. The helmet straps must always be buckled snugly against your chin.
- If your child is reluctant to wear a helmet, try letting him or her choose his own.

Proper bicycle fit and maintenance are also important for safety:

- Ensure proper bike fit by bringing the child along when shopping for a bike. Buy a bicycle that is the right size for the child, not one he will grow into. When sitting on the seat, the child's feet should touch the ground.
- Make sure the reflectors are secure, the brakes work properly, gears shift smoothly, and tires are tightly secured and properly inflated.

Always model and teach proper bicyclist behavior. Learn the rules of the road, and obey all traffic laws:

- Ride on the right side of the road, with traffic, not against. Stay as far to the right as possible.
- Use appropriate hand signals.

Preventing Childhood Injuries

- Respect traffic signals, stopping at all stop signs and stop lights.
- Stop and look left, right, and left again before entering a street or crossing an intersection. Look back and yield to traffic coming from behind before turning left.

Adult supervision of child cyclists is essential until you are sure a child has good traffic skills and judgment:

- Cycling should be restricted to sidewalks and paths until a child is age ten.
- Children should be able to demonstrate riding competence and knowledge of the rules of the road before they cycle with traffic.

Children should not ride a bicycle when it's dark, in the fog, or in other low-visibility conditions:

- If riding at dusk, dawn, or in the evening is unavoidable, use a light on the bike and make sure it has reflectors as well.
- Wear clothes and accessories that incorporate retroreflective materials to improve your visibility to motorists.

Section 6.7

Preventing Motor Vehicle Injuries

"Preventing Injuries to Children in Motor Vehicle Crashes,"
© 2008 Safe Kids Worldwide. Reprinted with permission.

All children ages twelve and under should be properly restrained in a back seat on every ride.

Choose and use correctly the right restraint for your child:

- Infants should ride in rear-facing car seats as long as possible, until they are at least twelve months old and weigh at least twenty pounds. Keep children rear facing to thirty to thirty-five pounds if your car seat allows it.

- Children who are at least one year old, weigh twenty to forty pounds, and can no longer ride rear-facing should ride in forward-facing car seats secured with harnesses.
- Children more than forty pounds should be correctly secured in belt-positioning booster seats or other appropriate child restraints until the adult lap and shoulder belts fit correctly (usually around age eight and when the child is about 4 feet 9 inches tall).

Any car seat must be installed and used according to the manufacturer's instructions and vehicle owner's manual:

- Check www.recalls.gov for car seat recalls.
- Return the product registration forms for all new car seats to the manufacturer to ensure you will be notified of any recalls.
- Only use a seat with all parts, instructions, and labels.
- Check www.nhtsa.dot.gov to see if a car seat that has been in a crash passes the National Highway Traffic Safety Administration's (NHTSA) test for continued use.

Obey all traffic laws, including those for child restraint use:

- All fifty states and the District of Columbia have child occupant protection laws, which vary widely in their age requirements, exemptions, enforcement procedures, and penalties. Many states have improved their laws to require some older children to ride in booster seats, and some require children of certain ages to ride in the rear seat of a motor vehicle. Check www.safekids.org to find out about the laws currently in effect for your state.

Chapter 7

Fever in Children

What Is a Fever?

Normally, the body temperature is around 98.6°F (37°C). The body temperature varies throughout the day and with the person's level of activity. A slight rise in temperature (below 100.4°F [38°C]) may occur after exercise/physical exertion or when infants and children are overdressed.

A temperature above 100.4°F (38°C) is considered a fever. It is a symptom, rather than a disease. Keep in mind the following facts about fever:

- Harmful effects from fever are rare.

- Fever is one of the body's normal methods for fighting against infections.

- A fever actually helps to fight an infection.

- The degree of the temperature may not indicate how sick the child is.

- In some children fever can be associated with a seizure or dehydration but fever will not lead to brain damage or death.

"Fever" is reprinted with permission from the Cincinnati Children's Hospital Medical Center website, http://www.cincinnatichildrens.org. © 2005 Cincinnati Children's Hospital Medical Center. All rights reserved.

A child with a fever may have warm or hot skin, but it is better to use a thermometer to find out the exact temperature. There are many ways to measure a temperature.

Call Your Child's Doctor

- If your child has a temperature of 100.4°F (38°C) or greater and is younger than three months.
- If your child has a fever that lasts for more than forty-eight hours and your child is older than three months.
- If your child is crying or whimpering and cannot be comforted.
- If your child has a change from the usual type of cry (more shrill than usual).
- If there is less urine than usual or if your child wets fewer diapers than usual (Infants usually have six to eight diapers per day).
- If there are purple spots on the skin or bruising.
- If your child cannot move his or her neck or has a stiff neck.
- If your child has difficulty breathing.
- If your child is difficult to arouse or wake up.
- If your child is not drinking or eating normally.
- Any time you feel uncomfortable with how your child appears or acts.
- If your child has symptoms such as sore throat, ear pain, stomach pain, or pain when urinating.

Treatment

For premature infants or infants less than three months old, call your child's doctor for instructions. For older children, some doctors believe that "fever is your friend" and does not require any treatment such as giving fever reducing medicines until the fever is 102°F (38.8°C) or if the child is fussy and uncomfortable. There is evidence that fevers help to fight an infection.

In general, the main reason for treating a fever is to keep the child as comfortable as possible rather than getting the temperature back to normal. If your child's temperature is more than 102°F (38.8°C), you may give your child a fever medicine such as acetaminophen or

Fever in Children

ibuprofen. Ibuprofen is not recommended in children under six months of age. Acetaminophen is preferred because this medicine is shorter acting. Use ibuprofen or acetaminophen. Do not alternate ibuprofen and acetaminophen to treat fever.

Aspirin should never be given to a child. The use of aspirin has been linked with a rare disorder called Reye syndrome, which can be fatal.

Remember that all medicines can be poisonous if too much is taken. Follow instructions on the label. Be sure to keep all medicines out of the reach of children at all times.

Medication

How much fever medicine do I give? Acetaminophen comes in different preparations and strengths specially made for infants and children such as infant drops or children's elixir. Each type of medicine requires a different amount be given. Read the directions on the label about how much to give your child and be sure to measure the dose correctly. If you are not sure how much to give, or your child is under two years old, call the doctor or pharmacist; they may ask for your child's weight to compute the correct dose for your child. Always use medicine made for children. Never give an infant or child a portion of the adult version of the medication.

How do I measure the correct amount of medicine? If you are using a medicine dropper, hold it at eye level to make sure you are giving the correct amount. Use only the dropper that came with the medicine.

If you are measuring the medicine with a spoon, use a kitchen measuring spoon, because teaspoons come in different sizes and measure different amounts.

If you are using a medicine cup, be sure to fill it to the right mark at eye level.

Tips for Treating a Child with a Fever

Take your child's temperature before giving any more fever medication. It is important to know if the fever has gone up or if the temperature is back to normal. This way, you can track a rising fever or avoid giving medication that is not needed.

Do not wake up your child to give medication or to take a temperature. Sleep is more important.

Dress your child in light clothes.

Give your child more to drink when he or she has a fever. This will help to prevent dehydration.

Allow your child to rest in a cool room.

Chapter 8

Medical Emergencies

Chapter Contents
Section 8.1—Is It a Medical Emergency? 58
Section 8.2—First Aid for Common Emergencies 61

Section 8.1

Is It a Medical Emergency?

"Is It a Medical Emergency?," April 2006, reprinted with permission from www.kidshealth.org. Copyright © 2006 The Nemours Foundation. This information was provided by KidsHealth, one of the largest resources online for medically reviewed health information written for parents, kids, and teens. For more articles like this one, visit www.KidsHealth.org, or www.TeensHealth.org.

Even healthy kids get hurt and sick sometimes. In some cases, you may panic and want to head straight to the emergency room at the nearest hospital. In other cases, it's more difficult to determine whether an injury or an illness needs the attention of a medical professional, or whether you can take care of it at home.

Ultimately, different problems require different levels of care. And when your child needs some sort of medical help, you have lots of options:

- **Handle the problem at home:** Many minor injuries and illnesses, including some cuts, poison ivy rashes, coughs, colds, scrapes, and bruises, can be handled with home care and over-the-counter (OTC) treatments.

- **Call your doctor:** This is a good option in most cases. If you're unsure of the level of medical care your child needs, your child's doctor—or a nurse who works in the office—can help you determine what steps to take and how to take them.

- **Visit an urgent care center:** An urgent care center can be a good option at night and on weekends when your child's doctor may not be in the office, but it's not necessarily a medical emergency. At these clinics, you can usually get things like x-rays, stitches, and care for other minor injuries that aren't life threatening yet require medical attention on the same day.

- **Visit a hospital emergency room (ER):** An ER—also called an emergency department (ED)—can handle a wide variety of serious problems, such as severe bleeding, head trauma, seizures, meningitis, breathing difficulties, dehydration, and bacterial infections.

Medical Emergencies

- **Call 911 for an ambulance:** Some situations are so serious that you need the help of trained medical personnel on the way to the hospital. These might include if your child has been in a car accident, has a head or neck injury, has ingested too much medication and is now hard to arouse, or is not breathing or is turning blue. In these cases it's best to dial 911 for an ambulance.

As a parent, it's hard to make these judgment calls if you don't have a medical degree. You don't want to rush to the ER if it's really not an emergency and can wait until a doctor's appointment. On the other hand, you don't want to hesitate to get medical attention if your child needs treatment right away. If you have questions, the best thing you can do is call your child's doctor. As your child grows—and inevitably runs into more sickness and calamities—you'll learn to trust yourself to decide when it's an emergency.

Remember that in cases when you know the problem is minor, it's best to go to an urgent care center, see your doctor, or handle it at home because the more people who show up at the ER with non-emergencies, the longer everyone has to wait for care. When you can't determine whether it's an emergency or not, call your child's doctor.

Should I Go to the ER?

Here are some examples of when to go the ER:

- Your child has some difficulty breathing or shortness of breath.
- There's a change in your child's mental status, such as suddenly becoming unusually sleepy or difficult to arouse, disoriented, confused, not making sense.
- Your child has a cut or break in the skin that is bleeding and won't stop.
- Your child has a stiff neck along with a fever.
- Your child has a rapid heartbeat that doesn't slow down.
- Your child accidentally ingests a poisonous substance or too much medication.
- Your child has severe bleeding or head trauma.

Other situations may seem alarming, but don't require a trip to the ER. Call your child's doctor if your child has any of these symptoms:

- High fever (above 104° Fahrenheit, 40° Celsius)
- Ear pain
- Pain in the abdomen
- Headache
- Rash
- Mild wheezing
- Persistent cough

When in doubt, call your child's doctor. Even if the doctor isn't available, the office nurse should be able to talk with you and determine whether you should take your child to the ER. Even on weekends and evenings, doctors typically have answering services that allow them to get in touch with you once you leave a message.

Urgent Care Centers

There may be times when your child has an injury or an illness that's not life threatening, but needs medical attention on the same day. If that's the case, consider going to an urgent care center in your area.

Urgent care centers, also known as fast tracks, usually allow you to walk in without an appointment, just as you would to an emergency room. But they are equipped and staffed to treat minor, non-life-threatening issues. Typically, your child will be seen by a doctor, and also may be able to get x-rays or blood drawn.

Most of these clinics offer extended hours on evenings and on weekends for patients to receive treatment when the family doctor is not available. Some are open twenty-four hours a day every day. Cases where you might take your child to an urgent care center include:

- cuts;
- minor injuries;
- vomiting or diarrhea;
- severe ear pain;
- sore throat;
- infected bug bites;
- mild allergic reactions;
- suspected sprain or broken bone;
- minor animal bites.

Medical Emergencies

The doctors who work at freestanding urgent care centers often are ER doctors or family physicians who focus on treating adult and pediatric diseases. Some urgent care centers are also staffed by nurse practitioners and physician assistants. In many children's hospitals, the emergency rooms have special sections for treatment of minor injuries and illnesses that might be treated at an urgent care center.

Find out about the urgent care centers near you before a situation comes up where you need to go to one. Your child's doctor may be able to recommend facilities in the area. In general, you want to find a clinic that meets any state licensing requirements and is staffed by doctors who are board certified in their specialties, such as pediatrics, family medicine, or emergency medicine. Some of these clinics, in addition to accepting walk-in patients, allow you to call ahead to be seen. You might also want to ask if the center accepts your family's insurance plan.

Talk with your child's doctor before your child gets sick about how to handle emergencies and the doctor's policy on addressing medical needs outside of office hours. Having that information ahead of time will mean one less thing to worry about when your child is sick!

Section 8.2

First Aid for Common Emergencies

"Basic First Aid Procedures," © 2008 City of Miami, Department of Fire-Rescue (http://ci.miami.fl.us/Fire). Reprinted with permission.

First Aid Treatments

Nosebleeds: Pinch nose and tilt head forward.

Animal bites: Wash wound, identify animal, and report the bite.

Serious falls: Do *not* move the victim; call 9-1-1.

Severe wounds: Have the victim sit or lie down, apply direct pressure to stop the bleeding, call 9-1-1.

Small wounds: Wash the wound, apply dressing, and bandage.

Bruises: Apply a cold compress.

Burns: For first- and second-degree burns, put burn in cold water, pat dry, and cover with clean bandage. Do not break blisters. For third-degree burns, do not put water on an open wound, do not remove burned-on clothing. Cover the burn lightly and get medical help! A first-degree burn is red, sore, and covers a small area. A second-degree burn is blistered and painful. A third-degree burn causes the skin to be white or charred and there is a loss of skin layers.

For all severe wounds and burns, dial 911.

First Aid Kit

Your basic first aid kit should contain the following items:

- An antiseptic (Betadine®)
- Antibiotic spray or ointment
- Adhesive bandages (various sizes)
- Adhesive tape (1 ½" to 1" wide)
- Sterile gauze pads
- Hydrocortisone cream or Calamine lotion (to relieve minor itching)
- Ice bag or cold pack
- Scissors with rounded ends
- Tweezers
- Thermometer
- Aspirin
- Syrup of Ipecac (for swallowed poisons; use as directed by the Poison Control Center)

Caution: Be sure that all supplies are kept out of the reach of young children.

Part Two

Common Childhood Infections and Related Concerns

Chapter 9

Foodborne Illness

What is foodborne disease?

Foodborne disease is caused by consuming contaminated foods or beverages. Many different disease-causing microbes, or pathogens, can contaminate foods, so there are many different foodborne infections. In addition, poisonous chemicals, or other harmful substances, can cause foodborne diseases if they are present in food.

More than 250 different foodborne diseases have been described. Most of these diseases are infections, caused by a variety of bacteria, viruses, and parasites that can be foodborne. Other diseases are poisonings, caused by harmful toxins or chemicals that have contaminated the food, for example, poisonous mushrooms. These different diseases have many different symptoms, so there is no one "syndrome" that is foodborne illness. However, the microbe or toxin enters the body through the gastrointestinal tract, and often causes the first symptoms there, so nausea, vomiting, abdominal cramps, and diarrhea are common symptoms in many foodborne diseases.

Many microbes can spread in more than one way, so we cannot always know that a disease is foodborne. The distinction matters, because public health authorities need to know how a particular disease is spreading to take the appropriate steps to stop it. For example, *Escherichia coli* O157:H7 infections can spread through contaminated food, contaminated drinking water, contaminated swimming water,

---

Excerpted from "Foodborne Illness," Centers for Disease Control and Prevention, October 25, 2005.

and from toddler to toddler at a day care center. Depending on which means of spread caused a case, the measures to stop other cases from occurring could range from removing contaminated food from stores, chlorinating a swimming pool, or closing a child day care center.

What are the most common foodborne diseases?

The most commonly recognized foodborne infections are those caused by the bacteria *Campylobacter*, *Salmonella*, and *E. coli* O157:H7, and by a group of viruses called calicivirus, also known as the Norwalk and Norwalk-like viruses.

Campylobacter is a bacterial pathogen that causes fever, diarrhea, and abdominal cramps. It is the most commonly identified bacterial cause of diarrheal illness in the world. These bacteria live in the intestines of healthy birds, and most raw poultry meat has *Campylobacter* on it. Eating undercooked chicken, or other food that has been contaminated with juices dripping from raw chicken, is the most frequent source of this infection.

Salmonella is also a bacterium that is widespread in the intestines of birds, reptiles, and mammals. It can spread to humans via a variety of different foods of animal origin. The illness it causes, salmonellosis, typically includes fever, diarrhea, and abdominal cramps. In persons with poor underlying health or weakened immune systems, it can invade the bloodstream and cause life-threatening infections.

E. coli O157:H7 is a bacterial pathogen that has a reservoir in cattle and other similar animals. Human illness typically follows consumption of food or water that has been contaminated with microscopic amounts of cow feces. The illness it causes is often a severe and bloody diarrhea and painful abdominal cramps, without much fever. In 3 to 5 percent of cases, a complication called hemolytic uremic syndrome (HUS) can occur several weeks after the initial symptoms. This severe complication includes temporary anemia, profuse bleeding, and kidney failure.

Calicivirus, or Norwalk-like virus, is an extremely common cause of foodborne illness, though it is rarely diagnosed, because the laboratory test is not widely available. It causes an acute gastrointestinal illness, usually with more vomiting than diarrhea, that resolves within two days. Unlike many foodborne pathogens that have animal reservoirs, it is believed that Norwalk-like viruses spread primarily from one infected person to another. Infected kitchen workers can contaminate a salad or sandwich as they prepare it, if they have the virus on their hands. Infected fishermen have contaminated oysters as they harvested them.

Foodborne Illness

Some common diseases are occasionally foodborne, even though they are usually transmitted by other routes. These include infections caused by *Shigella*, hepatitis A, and the parasites *Giardia lamblia* and *Cryptosporidia*. Even strep throats have been transmitted occasionally through food.

In addition to disease caused by direct infection, some foodborne diseases are caused by the presence of a toxin in the food that was produced by a microbe in the food. For example, the bacterium *Staphylococcus aureus* can grow in some foods and produce a toxin that causes intense vomiting. The rare but deadly disease botulism occurs when the bacterium *Clostridium botulinum* grows and produces a powerful paralytic toxin in foods. These toxins can produce illness even if the microbes that produced them are no longer there.

Other toxins and poisonous chemicals can cause foodborne illness. People can become ill if a pesticide is inadvertently added to a food, or if naturally poisonous substances are used to prepare a meal. Every year, people become ill after mistaking poisonous mushrooms for safe species, or after eating poisonous reef fishes.

Are the types of foodborne diseases changing?

The spectrum of foodborne diseases is constantly changing. A century ago, typhoid fever, tuberculosis, and cholera were common foodborne diseases. Improvements in food safety, such as pasteurization of milk, safe canning, and disinfection of water supplies have conquered those diseases. Today other foodborne infections have taken their place, including some that have only recently been discovered. For example, in 1996, the parasite Cyclospora suddenly appeared as a cause of diarrheal illness related to Guatemalan raspberries. These berries had just started to be grown commercially in Guatemala, and somehow became contaminated in the field there with this unusual parasite. In 1998, a new strain of the bacterium *Vibrio parahaemolyticus* contaminated oyster beds in Galveston Bay and caused an epidemic of diarrheal illness in persons eating the oysters raw. The affected oyster beds were near the shipping lanes, which suggested that the bacterium arrived in the ballast water of freighters and tankers coming into the harbor from distant ports. Newly recognized microbes emerge as public health problems for several reasons: microbes can easily spread around the world, new microbes can evolve, the environment and ecology are changing, food production practices and consumption habits change, and because better laboratory tests can now identify microbes that were previously unrecognized.

In the last fifteen years, several important diseases of unknown cause have turned out to be complications of foodborne infections. For example, we now know that the Guillain-Barré syndrome can be caused by *Campylobacter* infection, and that the most common cause of acute kidney failure in children, hemolytic uremic syndrome, is caused by infection with *E. coli* O157:H7 and related bacteria. In the future, other diseases whose origins are currently unknown may turn out be related to foodborne infections.

What happens in the body after the microbes that produce illness are swallowed?

After they are swallowed, there is a delay, called the incubation period, before the symptoms of illness begin. This delay may range from hours to days, depending on the organism, and on how many of them were swallowed. During the incubation period, the microbes pass through the stomach into the intestine, attach to the cells lining the intestinal walls, and begin to multiply there. Some types of microbes stay in the intestine, some produce a toxin that is absorbed into the bloodstream, and some can directly invade the deeper body tissues. The symptoms produced depend greatly on the type of microbe. Numerous organisms cause similar symptoms, especially diarrhea, abdominal cramps, and nausea. There is so much overlap that it is rarely possible to say which microbe is likely to be causing a given illness unless laboratory tests are done to identify the microbe, or unless the illness is part of a recognized outbreak.

How are foodborne diseases diagnosed?

The infection is usually diagnosed by specific laboratory tests that identify the causative organism. Bacteria such as *Campylobacter*, *Salmonella*, and *E. coli* O157 are found by culturing stool samples in the laboratory and identifying the bacteria that grow on the agar or other culture medium. Parasites can be identified by examining stools under the microscope. Viruses are more difficult to identify, as they are too small to see under a light microscope and are difficult to culture. Viruses are usually identified by testing stool samples for genetic markers that indicate a specific virus is present.

Many foodborne infections are not identified by routine laboratory procedures and require specialized, experimental, and/or expensive tests that are not generally available. If the diagnosis is to be made, the patient has to seek medical attention, the physician must decide

Foodborne Illness

to order diagnostic tests, and the laboratory must use the appropriate procedures. Because many ill persons to not seek attention, and of those that do, many are not tested, many cases of foodborne illness go undiagnosed. For example, the Centers for Disease Control and Prevention (CDC) estimates that thirty-eight cases of salmonellosis actually occur for every case that is actually diagnosed and reported to public health authorities.

How are foodborne diseases treated?

There are many different kinds of foodborne diseases and they may require different treatments, depending on the symptoms they cause. Illnesses that are primarily diarrhea or vomiting can lead to dehydration if the person loses more body fluids and salts (electrolytes) than he or she takes in. Replacing the lost fluids and electrolytes and keeping up with fluid intake are important. If diarrhea is severe, oral rehydration solution such as CeraLyte®, Pedialyte®, or Oralyte® should be drunk to replace the fluid losses and prevent dehydration. Sports drinks such as Gatorade do not replace the losses correctly and should not be used for the treatment of diarrheal illness. Preparations of bismuth subsalicylate (e.g., Pepto-Bismol®) can reduce the duration and severity of simple diarrhea. If diarrhea and cramps occur, without bloody stools or fever, taking an antidiarrheal medication may provide symptomatic relief, but these medications should be avoided if there is high fever or blood in the stools because they may make the illness worse.

When should I consult my doctor about a diarrheal illness?

A health care provider should be consulted for a diarrheal illness that is accompanied by any of the following:

- High fever (temperature over 101.5 F, measured orally)
- Blood in the stools
- Prolonged vomiting that prevents keeping liquids down (which can lead to dehydration)
- Signs of dehydration, including a decrease in urination, a dry mouth and throat, and feeling dizzy when standing up
- Diarrheal illness that lasts more than three days

Do not be surprised if your doctor does not prescribe an antibiotic. Many diarrheal illnesses are caused by viruses and will improve in two or three days without antibiotic therapy. In fact, antibiotics have no effect on viruses, and using an antibiotic to treat a viral infection could cause more harm than good It is often not necessary to take an antibiotic even in the case of a mild bacterial infection. Other treatments can help the symptoms, and careful hand washing can prevent the spread of infection to other people. Overuse of antibiotics is the principal reason many bacteria are becoming resistant. Resistant bacteria are no longer killed by the antibiotic. This means that it is important to use antibiotics only when they are really needed. Partial treatment can also cause bacteria to become resistant. If an antibiotic is prescribed, it is important to take all of the medication as prescribed, and not stop early just because the symptoms seem to be improving.

How does food become contaminated?

We live in a microbial world, and there are many opportunities for food to become contaminated as it is produced and prepared. Many foodborne microbes are present in healthy animals (usually in their intestines) raised for food. Meat and poultry carcasses can become contaminated during slaughter by contact with small amounts of intestinal contents. Similarly, fresh fruits and vegetables can be contaminated if they are washed or irrigated with water that is contaminated with animal manure or human sewage. Some types of *Salmonella* can infect a hen's ovary so that the internal contents of a normal looking egg can be contaminated with *Salmonella* even before the shell is formed. Oysters and other filter feeding shellfish can concentrate *Vibrio* bacteria that are naturally present in seawater, or other microbes that are present in human sewage dumped into the sea.

Later in food processing, other foodborne microbes can be introduced from infected humans who handle the food, or by cross-contamination from some other raw agricultural product. For example, *Shigella* bacteria, hepatitis A virus, and Norwalk virus can be introduced by the unwashed hands of food handlers who are themselves infected. In the kitchen, microbes can be transferred from one food to another food by using the same knife, cutting board, or other utensil to prepare both without washing the surface or utensil in between. A food that is fully cooked can become recontaminated if it touches other raw foods or drippings from raw foods that contain pathogens.

The way that food is handled after it is contaminated can also make a difference in whether or not an outbreak occurs. Many bacterial microbes need to multiply to a larger number before enough are present in food to cause disease. Given warm moist conditions and an ample

Foodborne Illness

supply of nutrients, one bacterium that reproduces by dividing itself every half hour can produce seventeen million progeny in twelve hours. As a result, lightly contaminated food left out overnight can be highly infectious by the next day. If the food were refrigerated promptly, the bacteria would not multiply at all. In general, refrigeration or freezing prevents virtually all bacteria from growing but generally preserves them in a state of suspended animation. This general rule has a few surprising exceptions. Two foodborne bacteria, *Listeria monocytogenes* and *Yersinia enterocolitica*, can actually grow at refrigerator temperatures. High salt, high sugar, or high acid levels keep bacteria from growing, which is why salted meats, jam, and pickled vegetables are traditional preserved foods.

Microbes are killed by heat. If food is heated to an internal temperature above 160°F, or 78°C, for even a few seconds this is sufficient to kill parasites, viruses, or bacteria, except for the *Clostridium* bacteria, which produce a heat-resistant form called a spore. *Clostridium* spores are killed only at temperatures above boiling. This is why canned foods must be cooked to a high temperature under pressure as part of the canning process.

The toxins produced by bacteria vary in their sensitivity to heat. The staphylococcal toxin that causes vomiting is not inactivated even if it is boiled. Fortunately, the potent toxin that causes botulism is completely inactivated by boiling.

What foods are most associated with foodborne illness?

Raw foods of animal origin are the most likely to be contaminated; that is, raw meat and poultry, raw eggs, unpasteurized milk, and raw shellfish. Because filter-feeding shellfish strain microbes from the sea over many months, they are particularly likely to be contaminated if there are any pathogens in the seawater. Foods that mingle the products of many individual animals, such as bulk raw milk, pooled raw eggs, or ground beef, are particularly hazardous because a pathogen present in any one of the animals may contaminate the whole batch. A single hamburger may contain meat from hundreds of animals. A single restaurant omelet may contain eggs from hundreds of chickens. A glass of raw milk may contain milk from hundreds of cows. A broiler chicken carcass can be exposed to the drippings and juices of many thousands of other birds that went through the same coldwater tank after slaughter.

Fruits and vegetables consumed raw are a particular concern. Washing can decrease but not eliminate contamination, so the consumers can do little to protect themselves. Recently, a number of outbreaks have been traced to fresh fruits and vegetables that were processed under less than sanitary conditions. These outbreaks show that the quality of the water used for washing and chilling the produce after it is harvested is critical. Using water that is not clean can contaminate many boxes of produce. Fresh manure used to fertilize vegetables can also contaminate them. Alfalfa sprouts and other raw sprouts pose a particular challenge, as the conditions under which they are sprouted are ideal for growing microbes as well as sprouts, and because they are eaten without further cooking. That means that a few bacteria present on the seeds can grow to high numbers of pathogens on the sprouts. Unpasteurized fruit juice can also be contaminated if there are pathogens in or on the fruit that is used to make it.

What can consumers do to protect themselves from foodborne illness?

A few simple precautions can reduce the risk of foodborne diseases:

- **Cook:** Cook meat, poultry, and eggs thoroughly. Using a thermometer to measure the internal temperature of meat is a good way to be sure that it is cooked sufficiently to kill bacteria. For example, ground beef should be cooked to an internal temperature of 160°F. Eggs should be cooked until the yolk is firm.

- **Separate:** Don't cross-contaminate one food with another. Avoid cross-contaminating foods by washing hands, utensils, and cutting boards after they have been in contact with raw meat or poultry and before they touch another food. Put cooked meat on a clean platter, rather than back on one that held the raw meat.

- **Chill:** Refrigerate leftovers promptly. Bacteria can grow quickly at room temperature, so refrigerate leftover foods if they are not going to be eaten within four hours. Large volumes of food will cool more quickly if they are divided into several shallow containers for refrigeration.

- **Clean:** Wash produce. Rinse fresh fruits and vegetables in running tap water to remove visible dirt and grime. Remove and discard the outermost leaves of a head of lettuce or cabbage. Because bacteria can grow well on the cut surface of fruit or vegetable, be careful not to contaminate these foods while slicing them up on the cutting board, and avoid leaving cut produce at room temperature for many hours. Don't be a source of foodborne illness yourself.

Foodborne Illness

Wash your hands with soap and water before preparing food. Avoid preparing food for others if you yourself have a diarrheal illness. Changing a baby's diaper while preparing food is a bad idea that can easily spread illness.

- **Report:** Report suspected foodborne illnesses to your local health department. The local public health department is an important part of the food safety system. Often calls from concerned citizens are how outbreaks are first detected. If a public health official contacts you to find our more about an illness you had, your cooperation is important. In public health investigations, it can be as important to talk to healthy people as to ill people. Your cooperation may be needed even if you are not ill.

Chapter 10

Streptococcal Bacterial Infections

Chapter Contents

Section 10.1—Group A Streptococcal Infections 76
Section 10.2—Pneumococcal Disease 79
Section 10.3—Rheumatic Fever 83
Section 10.4—Scarlet Fever 86
Section 10.5—Strep Throat 88
Section 10.6—Impetigo 90

Section 10.1

Group A Streptococcal Infections

Excerpted from "Group A Streptococcal (GAS) Disease," Centers for Disease Control and Prevention, April 3, 2008.

What is group A streptococcus (GAS)?

Group A Streptococcus is a bacterium often found in the throat and on the skin. People may carry group A streptococci in the throat or on the skin and have no symptoms of illness. Most GAS infections are relatively mild illnesses such as "strep throat," or impetigo. Occasionally these bacteria can cause severe and even life-threatening diseases.

How are group A streptococci spread?

These bacteria are spread through direct contact with mucus from the nose or throat of persons who are infected or through contact with infected wounds or sores on the skin. Ill persons, such as those who have strep throat or skin infections, are most likely to spread the infection. Persons who carry the bacteria but have no symptoms are much less contagious. Treating an infected person with an antibiotic for twenty-four hours or longer generally eliminates their ability to spread the bacteria. However, it is important to complete the entire course of antibiotics as prescribed. It is not likely that household items like plates, cups, or toys spread these bacteria.

What kind of illnesses are caused by group A streptococcal infection?

Infection with GAS can result in a range of symptoms:

- No illness
- Mild illness (strep throat or a skin infection such as impetigo)
- Severe illness (necrotizing fasciitis, streptococcal toxic shock syndrome)

Streptococcal Bacterial Infections

Severe, sometimes life-threatening, GAS disease may occur when bacteria get into parts of the body where bacteria usually are not found, such as the blood, muscle, or the lungs. These infections are termed "invasive GAS disease." Two of the most severe, but least common, forms of invasive GAS disease are necrotizing fasciitis and streptococcal toxic shock syndrome. Necrotizing fasciitis (occasionally described by the media as "the flesh-eating bacteria") destroys muscles, fat, and skin tissue. Streptococcal toxic shock syndrome (STSS), causes blood pressure to drop rapidly and organs (e.g., kidney, liver, lungs) to fail. STSS is not the same as the "toxic shock syndrome" frequently associated with tampon usage. About 20 percent of patients with necrotizing fasciitis and more than half with STSS die. About 10 to 15 percent of patients with other forms of invasive group A streptococcal disease die.

How common is invasive group A streptococcal disease?

About 9,000 to 11,500 cases of invasive GAS disease occur each year in the United States, resulting in 1,000 to 1,800 deaths annually. STSS and necrotizing fasciitis each comprise an average of about 6 to 7 percent of these invasive cases. In contrast, there are several million cases of strep throat and impetigo each year.

Why does invasive group A streptococcal disease occur?

Invasive GAS infections occur when the bacteria get past the defenses of the person who is infected. This may occur when a person has sores or other breaks in the skin that allow the bacteria to get into the tissue, or when the person's ability to fight off the infection is decreased because of chronic illness or an illness that affects the immune system. Also, some virulent strains of GAS are more likely to cause severe disease than others.

Who is most at risk of getting invasive group A streptococcal disease?

Few people who come in contact with GAS will develop invasive GAS disease. Most people will have a throat or skin infection, and some may have no symptoms at all. Although healthy people can get invasive GAS disease, people with chronic illnesses like cancer, diabetes, and chronic heart or lung disease, and those who use medications such as steroids have a higher risk. Persons with skin lesions (such as cuts, chicken pox, surgical wounds), the elderly, and adults with a history of alcohol abuse or injection drug use also have a higher risk for disease.

What are the early signs and symptoms of necrotizing fasciitis and streptococcal toxic shock syndrome?

Early signs and symptoms of necrotizing fasciitis are as follows:

- Severe pain and swelling, often rapidly increasing
- Fever
- Redness at a wound site

Early signs and symptoms of STSS include the following:

- Fever
- Abrupt onset of generalized or localized severe pain, often in an arm or leg
- Dizziness
- Influenza-like syndrome
- Confusion
- A flat red rash over large areas of the body (only occurs in 10 percent of cases)

How is invasive group A streptococcal disease treated?

GAS infections can be treated with many different antibiotics. For STSS and necrotizing fasciitis, high-dose penicillin and clindamycin are recommended. For those with very severe illness, supportive care in an intensive care unit may also be needed. For persons with necrotizing fasciitis, early and aggressive surgery is often needed to remove damaged tissue and stop disease spread. Early treatment may reduce the risk of death from invasive group A streptococcal disease. However, even the best medical care does not prevent death in every case.

What can be done to help prevent group A streptococcal infections?

The spread of all types of GAS infection can be reduced by good hand washing, especially after coughing and sneezing and before preparing foods or eating. Persons with sore throats should be seen by a doctor who can perform tests to find out whether the illness is strep

Streptococcal Bacterial Infections

throat. If the test result shows strep throat, the person should stay home from work, school, or day care until twenty-four hours after taking an antibiotic. All wounds should be kept clean and watched for possible signs of infection such as redness, swelling, drainage, and pain at the wound site. A person with signs of an infected wound, especially if fever occurs, should immediately seek medical care. It is not necessary for all persons exposed to someone with an invasive group A strep infection (i.e. necrotizing fasciitis or strep toxic shock syndrome) to receive antibiotic therapy to prevent infection. However, in certain circumstances, antibiotic therapy may be appropriate. That decision should be made after consulting with your doctor.

Section 10.2

Pneumococcal Disease

Excerpted from "Pneumococcal Disease in Children: Q&A,"
Centers for Disease Control and Prevention, September 5, 2007.

What is pneumococcal disease?

Pneumococcal disease is defined as infections that are caused by the bacteria *Streptococcus pneumoniae*, also known as pneumococcus. The most common types of infections caused by this bacteria include middle ear infections, pneumonia, blood stream infections (bacteremia), sinus infections, and meningitis.

Which children are most likely to get pneumococcal disease?

Young children are much more likely than older children and adults to get pneumococcal disease. Children under two, children in group child care, and children who have certain illnesses (for example sickle cell disease, human immunodeficiency virus [HIV] infection, chronic heart or lung conditions) are at higher risk than other children to get pneumococcal disease. In addition, pneumococcal disease is more common among children of certain racial or ethnic groups, such as Alaska natives, Native Americans, and African Americans, than among other groups.

How prevalent is pneumococcal disease?

Each year in the United States *Streptococcus pneumoniae* causes approximately 480 cases of meningitis and 4,000 cases of bacteremia or other invasive disease in children under the age of five. Children under two average more than one middle ear infection each year, many of which are caused by pneumococcal infections. *Streptococcus pneumoniae* is the most common cause of bacteremia, pneumonia, meningitis, and otitis media in young children.

What are the symptoms of pneumococcal disease?

Meningitis: High fever, headache, and stiff neck are common symptoms of meningitis in anyone over the age of two years. These symptoms can develop over several hours, or they may take one to two days. Other symptoms may include nausea, vomiting, discomfort looking into bright lights, confusion, and sleepiness. In newborns and small infants, the classic symptoms of fever, headache, and neck stiffness may be absent or difficult to detect, and the infant may only appear slow or inactive, or be irritable, have vomiting, or be feeding poorly.

Pneumonia: In adults, pneumococcal pneumonia is often characterized by sudden onset of illness with symptoms including shaking chills, fever, shortness of breath or rapid breathing, pain in the chest that is worsened by breathing deeply, and a productive cough. In infants and young children, signs and symptoms may not be specific, and may include fever, cough, rapid breathing, or grunting.

Otitis media: Children who have otitis media (middle ear infection) typically have a painful ear, and the eardrum is often red and swollen. Other symptoms that may accompany otitis media include sleeplessness, fever, and irritability.

Blood stream infections: Infants and young children with blood stream infections—also known as bacteremia—typically have nonspecific symptoms including fevers and irritability.

How serious is pneumococcal disease?

Pneumococcal disease is a very serious illness in young children. Pneumococcal infections are now the most common cause of invasive bacterial infection in U. S. children. In the United States it is estimated that pneumococcal infections cause 100 deaths, 450 cases

Streptococcal Bacterial Infections

of meningitis, 4,000 cases of bacteremia or other invasive disease, and 3.1 million cases of otitis media (ear infections) annually in children under five years of age.

Meningitis is the most severe type of pneumococcal disease. Of children less than five years of age with pneumococcal meningitis, about 5 percent will die of their infection and others may have long-term problems such as hearing loss. Many children with pneumococcal pneumonia or blood stream infections will be ill enough to be hospitalized; about 1 percent of children with blood stream infections or pneumonia with a blood stream infection will die of their illness. Nearly all children with ear infections recover, although children with recurrent infections can suffer hearing loss.

How is pneumococcal disease spread?

The bacteria are spread through contact between persons who are ill or who carry the bacteria in their throat. Transmission is mostly through the spread of respiratory droplets from the nose or mouth of a person with a pneumococcal infection. It is common for people, especially children, to carry the bacteria in their throats without being ill from it.

How is pneumococcal disease treated/cured?

Pneumococcal disease is treated with antibiotics. Over the last decade, many pneumococci have become resistant to some of the antibiotics used to treat pneumococcal infections; high levels of resistance to penicillin are common.

Can pneumococcal disease in children be prevented?

In late 2000, the U.S. Food and Drug Administration (FDA) licensed a new vaccine for the prevention of pneumococcal disease in children. The new pneumococcal vaccine, Prevnar® (manufactured by Wyeth-Lederle Vaccines), is a vaccine in which the serotypes are conjugated (or linked) to a protein. This new pneumococcal conjugate vaccine has been shown to be highly effective in preventing invasive pneumococcal disease such as in young children. In a study of the new vaccine among 37,000 infants in California, the vaccine was over 90 percent effective in preventing invasive disease among the children studied. The children who received the new vaccine also had 7 percent fewer episodes of otitis media and a 20 percent decrease in the number of tympanostomy tubes (ear tubes) placed. The vaccine was also shown to decrease the number of episodes of pneumonia.

The Centers for Disease Control and Prevention (CDC) conducted a study soon after the vaccine was licensed and found that the vaccine was highly effective in preventing disease in children under five years of age. The investigators found that the vaccine was 96 percent effective against pneumococcal disease in healthy children who received one dose or more and 81 percent effective in children with medical conditions that put them at risk of pneumococcal disease. The vaccine was also highly effective at preventing pneumococcal disease caused by antibiotic-resistant strains.

Prevnar® is indicated for use in infants and toddlers. The vaccine should be given to all infants younger than twenty-four months of age at two, four, and six months of age, followed by a booster dose at twelve to fifteen months of age. Children who are unvaccinated and are seven to eleven months of age should be given a total of three doses (two months apart) and children age twelve to twenty-three months should be given a total of two doses at least two months apart. Most children who are twenty-four months of age or older only need one dose of the vaccine.

The Advisory Committee on Immunization Practices (ACIP) also recommends the new pneumococcal childhood vaccine be given to children age twenty-four to fifty-nine months at highest risk of infection, including those with certain illness (sickle cell anemia, HIV infection, chronic lung or heart disease). Vaccine should be considered for all children aged twenty-four to thirty-five months and other children through fifty-nine months of age with a priority for those at higher risk, which includes Alaska natives, American Indians, or African Americans and those children who attend out-of-home day care for more than four hours per week.

The recently licensed pneumococcal conjugate vaccine, Prevnar®, is the first pneumococcal vaccine that can be used in children under the age of two years. However, pneumococcal vaccines for the prevention of disease among children and adults who are two years and older have been in use since 1977. Pneumovax® and Pnu-Immune® are 23-valent polysaccharide vaccines that are currently recommended for use in all adults who are older than sixty-five years of age and for persons who are two years and older and at high risk for disease such as persons with sickle cell disease, HIV infection, or other immunocompromising conditions.

Campaigns for judicious use of antibiotics may also slow or reverse emerging drug resistance found among pneumococcal infection.

Section 10.3

Rheumatic Fever

Copyright 2008 A.D.A.M., Inc. Excerpted with permission.

Rheumatic fever is an inflammatory disease that may develop after an infection with Streptococcus bacteria (such as strep throat or scarlet fever). The disease can affect the heart, joints, skin, and brain.

Causes

Rheumatic fever is common worldwide and is responsible for many cases of damaged heart valves. Although it has become far less common in the U.S. since the beginning of the twentieth century, there have been a few outbreaks since the 1980s.

Rheumatic fever mainly affects children ages six to fifteen, and occurs approximately twenty days after strep throat or scarlet fever. In up to a third of cases, the strep infection that caused rheumatic fever may not have had any symptoms.

About 3 percent of people with untreated strep infections get rheumatic fever. People who had a case of rheumatic fever are likely to develop flare-ups with repeated strep infections.

Symptoms

- Fever
- Joint pain, arthritis (mainly in the knees, elbows, ankles, and wrists)
- Joint swelling; redness or warmth
- Abdominal pain
- Skin rash (erythema marginatum)
  - Skin eruption on the trunk and upper part of the arms or legs
  - Eruptions that look ring-shaped or snake-like
- Skin nodules

- Sydenham chorea (emotional instability, muscle weakness, and quick, uncoordinated jerky movements that mainly affect the face, feet, and hands)
- Nosebleeds (epistaxis)
- Heart (cardiac) problems, which may not have symptoms, or may result in shortness of breath and chest pain

Exams and Tests

Because this disease has different forms, there is no specific test that can firmly diagnose it. Your doctor will perform a careful exam, which includes checking your heart sounds, skin, and joints.

Your doctor may also do an electrocardiogram while testing your heart.

You may have blood samples taken to test for recurrent strep infection (such as an antistreptolysin-O [ASO] test), complete blood counts, and erythrocyte sedimentation rate (ESR).

Several major and minor criteria have been developed to help standardize rheumatic fever diagnosis. Meeting these criteria, as well as having evidence of a recent streptococcal infection, can help confirm that you have rheumatic fever.

The major diagnostic criteria include:

- heart inflammation (carditis);
- arthritis in several joints (polyarthritis);
- nodules under the skin (subcutaneous skin nodules);
- rapid, jerky movements (chorea, Sydenham chorea);
- skin rash (erythema marginatum).

The minor criteria include fever, joint pain, high ESR, and other laboratory findings.

You'll likely be diagnosed with rheumatic fever if you meet two major criteria, or one major and two minor criteria, and signs that you've had a previous strep infection.

Treatment

Anti-inflammatory medications such as aspirin or corticosteroids reduce inflammation to help manage acute rheumatic fever.

People who test positive for strep throat should also be treated with antibiotics. You may have to take low doses of antibiotics (such as

Streptococcal Bacterial Infections

penicillin, sulfadiazine, or erythromycin) over the long term to prevent the disease from returning.

Outlook (Prognosis)

Rheumatic fever is likely to come back in people who don't take low-dose antibiotics continually, especially during the first three to five years after the first episode of the disease. Heart complications may be severe, particularly if the heart valves are involved.

Possible Complications

- Damage to heart valves (in particular, mitral stenosis and aortic stenosis)
- Endocarditis
- Heart failure
- Arrhythmias
- Pericarditis
- Sydenham chorea

When to Contact a Medical Professional

Call your health care provider if you develop symptoms of rheumatic fever. Because several other conditions have similar symptoms, you will need careful medical evaluation.

If you have symptoms of strep throat, tell your health care provider. You will need to be evaluated and treated if you do have strep throat, to decrease your risk of developing rheumatic fever.

Prevention

The most important way to prevent rheumatic fever is by getting quick treatment for strep throat and scarlet fever.

Section 10.4

Scarlet Fever

"Scarlet Fever," Centers for Disease Control and Prevention, October 13, 2005.

What is scarlet fever?

Scarlet fever is a disease caused by a bacteria called group A streptococcus, the same bacteria that causes strep throat. Scarlet fever is a rash that sometimes occurs in people that have strep throat. The rash of scarlet fever is usually seen in children under the age of eighteen.

How do you get scarlet fever?

This illness can be caught from other people if you come in contact with the sick person because this germ is carried in the mouth and nasal fluids. If you touch your mouth, nose, or eyes after touching something that has these fluids on them, you may become ill. Also, if you drink from the same glass or eat from the same plate as the sick person, you could also become ill. The best way to keep from getting sick is to wash your hands often and avoid sharing eating utensils.

What are the symptoms of scarlet fever?

The most common symptoms of scarlet fever are as follows:

- A rash first appears as tiny red bumps on the chest and abdomen. This rash may then spread all over the body. It looks like a sunburn and feels like a rough piece of sandpaper. It is usually redder in the arm pits and groin areas. The rash lasts about two to five days. After the rash is gone, often the skin on the tips of the fingers and toes begins to peel.
- The face is flushed with a pale area around the lips.
- The throat is very red and sore. It can have white or yellow patches.

Streptococcal Bacterial Infections

- A fever of 101 degrees Fahrenheit (38.3 degrees Celsius) or higher is common. Chills are often seen with the fever.
- Glands in the neck are often swollen.
- A whitish coating can appear on the surface of the tongue. The tongue itself looks like a strawberry because the normal bumps on the tongue look bigger.

Other less common symptoms include the following:

- Nausea and vomiting
- Headache
- Body aches

How is scarlet fever diagnosed?

Your doctor or health care provider will examine your child and swab the back of the throat with a cotton swab to see if there is a streptococcus infection.

What is the treatment for scarlet fever?

If the swab test (throat culture) shows that there is streptococcus, you will be given an antibiotic prescription for your child. Give this medicine exactly as you are told. It is very important to finish all of the medicine. Never share any of this medicine with family or friends. Ask your doctor or health care provider about over-the-counter medicine to lessen sore throat pain.

Is there anything else I can do to make my child feel better?

Warm liquids like soup or cold foods like popsicles or milkshakes help to ease the pain of the sore throat. Offer these to your child often, especially when he or she has a fever, since the body needs a lot of fluid when it is sick with a fever. A cool mist humidifier will help to keep the air in your child's room moist, which will keep the throat from getting too dry and more sore. Rest is important.

What should I do if I think my child has scarlet fever?

The best thing to do if you think your child may be ill is to call your doctor or health care provider.

Section 10.5

Strep Throat

National Institute of Allergy and Infectious Diseases, November 23, 2007.

Overview

Strep throat is the most common throat infection caused by bacteria.

It is found most often in children between the ages of five and fifteen, although it can occur in younger children and adults. Children younger than three years old can get strep infections, but these usually don't affect the throat.

Strep throat infections usually occur in the late fall, winter, and early spring.

Cause

Strep throat is usually caused by group A streptococcus bacteria. Your healthcare provider may call the infection "acute streptococcal pharyngitis."

Transmission

You can get strep throat by direct contact with saliva or nasal discharge from an infected person. Most people do not get group A strep infections from casual contact with others. A crowded environment like a dormitory, school, or nursing home, however, can make it easier for the bacteria to spread. There have also been reports of contaminated food, especially milk and milk products, causing infection.

Symptoms

If you have strep throat infection, you will have a red and painful sore throat and may have white patches on your tonsils. You also may have swollen lymph nodes in your neck, run a fever, and have a headache.

Streptococcal Bacterial Infections

Nausea, vomiting, and abdominal pain can occur but are more common in children than in adults.

You can get sick within three days after being exposed to the germ. Once infected, you can pass the infection to others for up to two to three weeks even if you don't have symptoms. After twenty-four hours of taking antibiotics, you will no longer spread the bacteria to others.

Diagnosis

Your healthcare provider will take a throat swab to find out if you have strep throat infection. This will be used for a culture (a type of laboratory test) or a rapid strep test, which only takes ten to twenty minutes. If the result of the rapid test is negative, you may get a follow-up culture, which takes twenty-four to forty-eight hours, to confirm the results. If the culture test is also negative, your healthcare provider may suspect you do not have strep, but rather another type of infection.

The results of these throat cultures will help your healthcare provider decide on the best treatment. Most sore throats are caused by viruses, and antibiotics are useless against viruses.

Treatment

If you have strep throat, your healthcare provider will prescribe an antibiotic. This will help lessen symptoms. After twenty-four hours of taking the medicine, you will no longer be able to spread the infection to others. Treatment will also reduce the chance of complications.

Current guidelines by expert groups recommend penicillin as the medicine of choice for treating strep throat because penicillin has been proven to be effective, safe, and inexpensive. Your healthcare provider may instruct you to the take pills for ten days or give you a shot. If you are allergic to penicillin there are other antibiotics your healthcare provider can give you to clear up the illness.

During treatment, you may start to feel better within four days. This can happen even without treatment. Still, it is very important to finish all your medicine to prevent complications.

Section 10.6

Impetigo

"Impetigo," ©2008 Wisconsin Department of Health and Family Services (www.dhfs.wisconsin.gov). Reprinted with permission.

What is impetigo?

Impetigo is an infection of the skin caused primarily by the bacterium *Streptococcus pyogenes*, also known as Group A beta-hemolytic streptococci (GABS). Sometimes another bacterium, *Staphylococcus aureus*, can also be isolated from impetigo lesions.

What are the symptoms of impetigo?

Impetigo begins as a cluster of small blisters that expand and rupture within the first twenty-four hours. The thin yellow fluid that drains from the ruptured blisters quickly dries, forming a honey-colored crust. Impetigo develops most frequently on the legs, but may also be found on the arms, face, and trunk. There is usually no fever.

How does a person get impetigo?

Impetigo may develop after the skin is infected with GABS. The bacterium is usually acquired from skin-to-skin contact with another person with impetigo. Less commonly, impetigo may develop when open skin lesions (such as insect bites or burns) are infected following exposure to a person with streptococcal pharyngitis ("strep throat").

Who gets impetigo?

The infection is most common in settings where there is crowding or activities leading to close person-to-person contact such as in schools and military installations. Impetigo occurs more commonly during the summer and early fall.

Streptococcal Bacterial Infections

How long does it take to develop impetigo following exposure?

Impetigo may develop up to ten days after the skin becomes infected with GABS.

How is impetigo treated?

Impetigo may be treated with an antibiotic taken by mouth or by application of an antibiotic ointment to the affected areas.

How long is a person considered infectious?

A person with impetigo is probably no longer infectious after twenty-four hours of adequate antibiotic treatment. Without treatment, a person may be infectious for several weeks.

What are the complications of impetigo?

Rarely, GABS may invade beyond the skin of a person with impetigo and cause more serious illnesses. Persons with impetigo may also develop post-streptococcal scarlet fever, or glomerulonephritis, a condition that may result in temporary kidney failure. Post-streptococcal glomerulonephritis follows roughly ten days after the onset of streptococcal infection. However, the long-term prognosis is excellent. Scarlet fever is caused by a toxin produced by certain strains of GABS and is characterized by high fever, chills, sore throat, headache, vomiting, and a fine red rash.

What can be done to prevent impetigo?

Simple cleanliness and prompt attention to minor wounds will do much to prevent impetigo. Persons with impetigo or symptoms of GABS infections should seek medical care and if necessary begin antibiotic treatment as soon as possible to prevent spread to others. Individuals with impetigo should be excluded from school, day care, or other situations where close person-to-person contact is likely to occur until at least twenty-four hours after beginning appropriate antibiotic therapy. Sharing of towels, clothing, and other personal articles should be discouraged.

Chapter 11

Other Bacterial Infections

Chapter Contents

Section 11.1—Cat Scratch Disease 94
Section 11.2—Diphtheria 98
Section 11.3—*Haemophilus Influenzae* Type B 100
Section 11.4—Lyme Disease 102
Section 11.5—Methicillin Resistant *Staphylococcus
	Aureus* (MRSA)/Oxacillin Resistant Staph 107
Section 11.6—Mycoplasma Infection 110
Section 11.7—Tetanus 112
Section 11.8—Tuberculosis 115
Section 11.9—Whooping Cough (Pertussis) 118

Section 11.1

Cat Scratch Disease

"Cat Scratch Disease," July 2006, reprinted with permission from www.kidshealth.org. Copyright © 2006 The Nemours Foundation. This information was provided by KidsHealth, one of the largest resources online for medically reviewed health information written for parents, kids, and teens. For more articles like this one, visit www.KidsHealth.org, or www.TeensHealth.org.

Cat scratch disease is a bacterial infection that typically causes swelling of the lymph nodes. It usually results from the scratch, lick, or bite of a cat—more than 90 percent of people with the illness have had some kind of contact with cats, often with kittens.

Bartonella henselae is the bacterium that causes cat scratch disease, and it's found in all parts of the world. Cat scratch disease occurs more often in the fall and winter. In the United States, about twenty-two thousand cases are diagnosed annually, most of them in people under the age of twenty-one. This may be because children are more likely to play with cats and be bitten or scratched.

Fleas spread the bacteria between cats, although currently there is no evidence that fleas can transmit the disease to humans. Once a cat is infected, the bacteria live in the animal's saliva. *Bartonella henselae* does not make a cat sick, and kittens or cats may carry the bacteria for months. Experts believe that almost half of all cats have a *Bartonella henselae* infection at some time in their lives, and cats less than one year old are more likely to be infected.

Signs and Symptoms

Most people with cat scratch disease remember being around a cat, but often cannot recall receiving a scratch or a bite. A blister or a small bump develops several days after the scratch or bite and may be mistaken for an insect bite. This blister or bump is called an inoculation lesion (a wound at the site where the bacteria enter the body), and it is most commonly found on the arms and hands, head, or scalp. These lesions are generally not painful.

Other Bacterial Infections

Usually within a couple of weeks of a scratch or bite, one or more lymph nodes close to the area of the inoculation lesion will swell and become tender. (Lymph nodes are round or oval-shaped organs of the immune system that are often called glands.) For example, if the inoculation lesion is on the arm, the lymph nodes in the elbow or armpit will swell.

These swollen lymph nodes appear most often in the underarm or neck areas, although if the inoculation lesion is on the leg, then the nodes in the groin will be affected. They range in size from about one-half inch to two inches (1 to 5 centimeters) in diameter and may be surrounded by a larger area of swelling under the skin. The skin over these swollen lymph nodes may become warm and red, and occasionally the lymph nodes drain pus.

In most children and adolescents, swollen lymph nodes are the main symptom of the disease, and the illness often is mild. About one-third of people with cat scratch disease have other general symptoms. These include fever (usually less than 101° Fahrenheit or 38.3° Celsius), fatigue, loss of appetite, headache, rash, sore throat, and an overall ill feeling.

Atypical cases of cat scratch disease do occur, but they are much less common. In such cases, a person may have infections of the liver, spleen, bones, joints, or lungs, or a lingering high fever without any other symptoms. Some people get an eye infection known as Parinaud oculoglandular syndrome, with symptoms including: a small sore on the conjunctiva (the membrane lining the eye or inner eyelid), redness of the eye, and swollen lymph nodes in front of the ear. Others may develop inflammation of the brain or seizures, although this is rare. All of these complications of cat scratch disease usually resolve without any lasting illness.

Contagiousness

Cat scratch disease is not contagious from person to person. The bacteria are spread by the scratch or bite of an infected animal, most often a kitten. They can also be transmitted if the animal's saliva comes in contact with broken skin or an eye. Sometimes multiple cases of the illness occur in the same family, but these likely result from contact with the same infected animal.

Having one episode of cat scratch disease usually makes people immune for the rest of their lives.

Prevention

If you are concerned about cat scratch disease, you do not need to get rid of the family pet. The illness is relatively rare and usually mild, and a few steps can go a long way toward limiting your child's chances of contracting the disease.

Teaching children to avoid stray or unfamiliar cats can reduce their exposure to sources of the bacteria. To lower the risk of getting the disease from a family pet or familiar cat, children should avoid rough play with any pets so they can avoid being scratched or bitten. It is also a good idea for people to wash their hands after handling or playing with a cat. If your child is scratched by a pet, wash the injured area thoroughly with soap and water. Keeping the house and your pet free of fleas will reduce the risk that your cat could become infected with the bacteria in the first place.

If you suspect that someone in your family has caught cat scratch disease from your family pet, you don't need to worry that the animal will have to be put to sleep. Talk with your veterinarian about the problem.

Incubation

It typically takes three to ten days for a blister or small bump to appear at the site of a scratch or bite. Lymph node swelling usually begins about one to four weeks later.

Duration

The inoculation lesion where the bacteria entered the body usually takes days to heal. The swollen lymph nodes typically disappear within two to four months, although they occasionally last much longer.

Professional Treatment

Doctors usually diagnose cat scratch disease based on a child's history of exposure to a cat or kitten and a physical examination. During the exam, a doctor will look for signs of a cat scratch or bite and swollen lymph nodes. In some cases, doctors use laboratory tests to help make the diagnosis, including:

- skin tests, blood tests, and cultures to rule out other causes of swollen lymph nodes;
- a blood test that is positive for cat scratch disease;
- a microscopic examination of a removed lymph node that shows signs of cat scratch disease.

Other Bacterial Infections

Most cases of cat scratch disease resolve without any treatment at all. Rarely, a swollen lymph node becomes so large and painful that the doctor may recommend removing fluid from the node with a needle and syringe. Antibiotics can be used to treat the disease. If your child's doctor has prescribed antibiotics, give the medication to your child on schedule for as many days as the doctor has advised.

Home Treatment

A child who has cat scratch disease does not need to be isolated from other family members. Bed rest is not necessary, but it may help if your child tires easily. If your child feels like playing, encourage quiet play while being careful to avoid injuring swollen lymph nodes. To ease the soreness of these nodes, try warm, moist compresses or give your child nonprescription medicines like acetaminophen (such as Tylenol® or ibuprofen (such as Advil® or Motrin®).

When to Call Your Child's Doctor

Call your child's doctor whenever your child has swollen or painful lymph nodes in any area of the body, or if your child is ever bitten by an animal. You should call if your child has been bitten or scratched by a cat and the wound does not seem to be healing, an area of redness around the wound keeps expanding for several days, or your child develops a fever that lasts for a few days after receiving the scratch or bite.

If your child has already been diagnosed with cat scratch disease, call the doctor if your child has a high fever, has lots of pain in a lymph node, seems very sick, or develops any new symptoms.

Section 11.2

Diphtheria

"Diphtheria," © 2008 Virginia Department of Health.
Reprinted with permission.

What is diphtheria?

Diphtheria is a disease caused by bacteria that usually affect the tonsils, throat, nose, or skin.

Who gets diphtheria?

Diphtheria is a rare disease that is most likely to occur where people who have not been vaccinated live in crowded conditions.

How is diphtheria spread?

Diphtheria is transmitted to others through close contact with discharge from an infected person's nose, throat, skin, and eyes.

What are the symptoms of diphtheria?

There are two types of diphtheria. One type involves the nose and throat, and the other involves the skin. Symptoms include sore throat, low-grade fever, and enlarged lymph nodes located in the neck. A membrane may form across the throat. Skin lesions may be painful, swollen and reddened. A person with diphtheria may have no symptoms.

How soon do symptoms appear?

Symptoms usually appear two to five days after exposure, with a range of one to six days.

When and for how long is a person able to spread diphtheria?

Untreated people who are infected with the diphtheria bacteria are usually contagious for up to two weeks, and seldom more than four

Other Bacterial Infections

weeks. If treated with appropriate antibiotics, the contagious period can be limited to less than four days.

Does past infection with diphtheria make a person immune?

Recovery from diphtheria is not always followed by lasting immunity.

Is there a vaccine for diphtheria?

Diphtheria toxoid is usually combined with tetanus toxoid and pertussis vaccine to form a triple vaccine known as DTP. This vaccine should be given at two, four, six, and fifteen months of age, and between four and six years of age. To maintain immunity, a person needs to receive a booster vaccine containing diphtheria toxoid every ten years.

What is the treatment for diphtheria?

Certain antibiotics, such as penicillin and erythromycin, can be prescribed for the treatment of diphtheria.

What can be the effect of not being treated for diphtheria?

If diphtheria goes untreated, serious complications such as heart failure and nerve disorders may occur. Death occurs in about 5 to 10 percent of all cases.

How can diphtheria be prevented?

The single most effective control measure is maintaining the highest possible level of immunization in the community. Other methods of control include prompt treatment of cases and a community surveillance program. Anyone who has close contact with a person with diphtheria will be tested for the disease, given an antibiotic and an immunization, and possibly kept away from school or work until it is clear that they are free of the disease.

Section 11.3

Haemophilus Influenzae *Type B*

"Haemophilus Influenzae Type B (HIB Disease)," © 2008 Wisconsin Department of Health and Family Services (www.dhfs.wisconsin.gov). Reprinted with permission.

What is Haemophilus influenzae *type B (Hib)*?

Hib are bacteria that may cause a variety of diseases including blood infection and meningitis (inflammation of the lining of the brain).

How common is Hib disease?

Since the introduction of the Hib vaccine in 1988, Hib cases have declined by 95 percent in infants and young children. Before the use of an effective vaccine, Hib was the most common cause of bacterial meningitis in children.

Who gets Hib infection?

Anyone can get Hib infection, but it is most common in children between the ages of three months and three years. The elderly and persons with weakened immune systems are also at a higher risk of developing the disease.

How is Hib infection spread?

Hib infection is spread by inhalation of droplets that contain the bacteria from the nose and throat. Although not common, some individuals may carry Hib in their nose and throat without becoming ill and potentially spread the bacteria to others.

What are the symptoms of Hib infection?

Fever is present in all forms of Hib infection. Other symptoms of Hib infection depend on the part of the body affected. Hib can result

Other Bacterial Infections

in sinus infections, earaches, and skin infections. Hib may also cause serious illnesses like meningitis (characterized by the usually sudden onset of fever, lethargy, vomiting, and a stiff and/or rigid neck and back), pneumonia, epiglottitis (inflammation of upper airway), and blood stream infections.

How soon do the symptoms appear?

The period between exposure to Hib and the beginning of symptoms is unknown, but is probably short (two to four days).

Does past infection with Hib make a person immune?

Children who develop Hib infection before twenty-four months of age may not develop immunity and should still be immunized with the Hib vaccine. If Hib infection occurs in an unimmunized child after twenty-four months of age, the child generally develops future immunity and vaccination is not necessary.

What is the treatment for Hib infection?

Hib infections are treated with antibiotics. Patients are no longer infectious twenty-four to forty-eight hours after receiving effective antimicrobial therapy.

What can be done to prevent the spread of Hib infection?

All children should be immunized with Hib conjugate vaccine beginning at approximately two months of age. Close contacts of a person infected with Hib may require immediate preventative antibiotics depending on circumstances.

Section 11.4

Lyme Disease

"Lyme Disease," January 2007, reprinted with permission from www.kidshealth.org. Copyright © 2007 The Nemours Foundation. This information was provided by KidsHealth, one of the largest resources online for medically reviewed health information written for parents, kids, and teens. For more articles like this one, visit www.KidsHealth.org, or www.TeensHealth.org.

Lyme disease is an infection caused by the bacterium *Borrelia burgdorferi*. This bacterium is usually found in animals such as mice and deer. Ixodes ticks can pick up the bacteria when they bite an infected animal, then transmit it to a person, which can lead to Lyme disease.

Ticks live in grass and shrubs and attach themselves to a suitable host as it passes by. Ticks are small and can be hard to see. Immature ticks, or nymphs, are about the size of a poppy seed.

The majority of reported Lyme disease cases occur in the Northeast, upper Midwest, and Pacific coastal areas of the United States because these regions are where ticks tend to live. Though Lyme disease cases have been reported from all over, in 2005 the majority of cases were reported in:

- Connecticut;
- Delaware;
- Maine;
- Maryland;
- Massachusetts;
- Minnesota;
- New Hampshire;
- New York;
- New Jersey;
- Pennsylvania;
- Wisconsin.

Other Bacterial Infections

Some cases of Lyme disease have also been reported in Asia, Europe, and parts of Canada.

Signs and Symptoms

Lyme disease can affect the skin, joints, nervous system, and other organ systems. Symptoms, and their severity, can vary from person to person.

The symptoms of Lyme disease are often described as occurring in three stages, though not everyone experiences all stages:

1. The first sign of infection usually is a circular rash, called erythema migrans, that appears within one to two weeks of infection but may develop up to thirty days after the tick bite. This rash often has a characteristic "bull's-eye" appearance, with a central red spot surrounded by clear skin that is ringed by an expanding red rash. It may also appear as an expanding ring of solid redness. It may be warm to the touch and is usually not painful or itchy. The bull's-eye rash may be more difficult to see on people with darker skin tones, where it may take on a bruise-like appearance. The rash usually resolves in about a month. Although this rash is considered typical of Lyme disease, many patients never develop it.

2. Along with the rash, a person may experience flu-like symptoms such as swollen lymph nodes, fatigue, headache, and muscle aches. Left untreated, symptoms of the initial illness may go away on their own. But in some people, the infection can spread to other parts of the body. Symptoms of this stage of Lyme disease usually appear within several weeks after the tick bite, even in someone who has not developed the initial rash. The person may feel very tired and unwell, or may have more areas of rash that aren't at the site of the bite. Lyme disease can affect the heart, leading to an irregular heart rhythm or chest pain. It can spread to the nervous system, causing facial paralysis (Bell's palsy) or tingling and numbness in the arms and legs. It can start to cause headaches and neck stiffness, which may be a sign of meningitis. Swelling and pain in the large joints can also occur.

3. The last stage of Lyme disease may occur if early disease was not detected or appropriately treated. Symptoms of late Lyme disease can appear any time from weeks to years after an

infectious tick bite and include arthritis, particularly in the knees, and, mainly in adults, cognitive deterioration.

Contagiousness

Lyme disease is not transmitted from person to person. The risk of developing Lyme disease depends on an individual's exposure to ticks. Kids and adults who spend a lot of time outdoors—particularly in or near wooded areas—are more likely to contract Lyme disease.

In rare cases, Lyme disease contracted during pregnancy may infect the fetus. If you are pregnant and are concerned about this, talk with your doctor.

Domestic animals, such as dogs and cats, may become infected with Lyme disease bacteria and may carry infected ticks into areas where humans live. If you have a dog or a cat, talk with your veterinarian about what kinds of tick-control products and other protective measures you can take for your pet.

Diagnosis

The most telling symptom of Lyme disease is the circular bull's-eye rash. Usually, because the rash is very distinct, a person with the rash can be immediately diagnosed with Lyme disease and blood tests are not necessary. Because the rash can rapidly disappear, consider taking a picture of any suspicious rash on your child if you are unable to see the doctor immediately.

In some cases, the bull's-eye rash never forms. In the absence of the rash, doctors must rely on other symptoms combined with an assessment of someone's likelihood of exposure to an infected tick. Blood tests can help diagnose Lyme disease by detecting the presence of antibodies to *Borrelia burgdorferi* in the patient's blood. However, blood tests can give inaccurate results if done within a month after initial infection, since it takes time for the antibodies to develop. Lyme disease can be difficult to diagnose because it may resemble many other medical conditions. Your doctor can help to decide whether your child needs a blood test for Lyme disease.

Treating Lyme Disease

Treatment of early localized Lyme disease typically involves a course of antibiotics administered for three to four weeks.

If diagnosed quickly and treated with antibiotics, Lyme disease in children is almost always treatable. The skin rash usually goes away

Other Bacterial Infections

within several days after starting treatment, but other signs and symptoms may persist for several weeks.

Prevention

Ticks frequently live in shady, moist ground cover and also cling to tall grass, brush, shrubs, and low tree branches. Lawns and gardens may harbor ticks, especially at the edges of woods and forests and around old stone walls (areas where deer and mice, the primary hosts of the deer tick, thrive).

To prevent Lyme disease, avoid contact with soil, leaves, and vegetation as much as possible, especially during May, June, and July, when ticks have not yet matured and are harder to detect.

When you do venture into the great outdoors, follow these tips:

- Wear enclosed shoes and boots, long-sleeved shirts, and long pants. Tuck pants into boots or shoes to prevent ticks from crawling up legs.
- Wear light-colored clothing to help you see ticks easily.
- Keep long hair pulled back or placed in a cap for added protection.
- When outside, don't sit on the ground.
- While outdoors, check yourself and your child frequently for ticks.
- Wash all clothes after leaving tick-infested areas, and bathe and shampoo your child thoroughly to eliminate any unseen ticks.

Insect repellents containing DEET (look for N,N-diethyl-meta-toluamide) can help to repel ticks. Choose one with a 10 to 30 percent concentration of DEET. Generally, DEET should not be applied more than once a day, and is not recommended for babies younger than two months. DEET can be used on exposed skin, as well as clothing, socks, and shoes, but should not be used on the face, under clothing, or on the hands of young children.

Ticks can bite anywhere, but they prefer certain areas of the body, such as:

- behind the ears;
- the back of the neck;
- armpits;

- the groin;
- behind the knees.

If you find a tick on your child, call your doctor, who may want you to save the tick after removal (you can put it in a jar of alcohol to kill it). Use tweezers to grasp the tick firmly at its head or mouth, next to your child's skin. Pull firmly and steadily on the tick until it lets go, then swab the bite site with alcohol.

Myths abound about ways to kill ticks (such as using petroleum jelly or a lit match), but don't try them—these methods don't work.

You can help keep ticks away from your house by keeping lawns mowed and trimmed; clearing brush, leaf litter, and tall grass; and stacking woodpiles off the ground. In addition, you can have a licensed professional spray your yard with insecticide in May and September to prevent ticks from multiplying.

There is no vaccine for Lyme disease currently on the market in the United States.

When to Call the Doctor

If your child has a bull's-eye rash or other symptoms that can occur in Lyme disease—such as swollen lymph glands near a tick bite, general achiness, headache, or fever—call your doctor right away.

Other Bacterial Infections

Section 11.5

Methicillin Resistant Staphylococcus Aureus *(MRSA)/Oxacillin Resistant Staph*

"Oxacillin Resistant *Staph aureus* (ORSA) / Methicillin Resistant *Staph aureus* (MRSA)" is reprinted with permission from the Cincinnati Children's Hospital Medical Center website, http://www.cincinnatichildrens.org. © 2006 Cincinnati Children's Hospital Medical Center. All rights reserved.

What is Staph aureus?

"*Staph*," or *Staphylococcus aureus*, is a bacteria commonly found on the skin.

What is ORSA or MRSA?

ORSA stands for oxacillin resistant *Staph aureus*. MRSA stands for methicillin resistant *Staph aureus*. ORSA and MRSA are different names for the same bacteria.

Oxacillin and methicillin are in the penicillin drug family, and some strains of *Staph* have become resistant to both of these antibiotics as well as other related antibiotics. Other drugs can be used to treat infections caused by this bacteria.

Where are ORSA, MRSA and Staph *found?*

Anywhere on your skin and commonly, in your nose and other moist locations.

Who gets ORSA/MRSA?

Anyone can carry ORSA/MRSA on their skin (or be "colonized" with it) along with many other bacteria.

What causes an ORSA/MRSA infection?

Any break in the skin (whether an insect bite or trauma) can increase the likelihood of an infection by allowing the bacteria to enter.

Some people may first notice a bump or a pimple under the skin with redness or pain.

Who is more likely to get ORSA/MRSA infections?

- People who live with or are in contact with others who have ORSA/MRSA
- People with a history of dry skin, eczema, or other skin conditions
- Children with frequent bug bites or scrapes
- Children in diapers
- People who have been on antibiotics frequently or hospitalized
- Health care workers

However, many people who get ORSA/MRSA infections have no risk factors.

Is ORSA/MRSA more serious than regular Staph?

No. However, it is important to tell medical providers if you have a history of ORSA/MRSA:

- So that the best antibiotics for you or your child can be given
- So appropriate measures can be taken to prevent spread to others

Does having ORSA/MRSA mean something is wrong with my child's immune system?

No. ORSA/MRSA infection can occur in anyone. Being diagnosed with an ORSA/MRSA infection is not a sign of an immune deficiency. ORSA/MRSA infections are being seen in many people with no other medical conditions or risks.

However, if in addition to this infection there are other reasons to be concerned, your doctor may choose to evaluate your child's immune system.

What can I do to decrease the risk of infection with ORSA/MRSA?

Keep your skin healthy:

Other Bacterial Infections

- If you or your child has a skin condition (such as eczema), use the creams and moisturizers that your doctor has instructed you to use.
- Avoid bug bites by using insect repellant.
- Avoid sunburn by using sunscreen.

Prevent spread in your family (if one person is infected or "colonized"):

- Encourage showers instead of baths.
- If your child is too young for a shower, have her or him bathe separately from other family members.
- Periodically clean any bath toys with bleach and water or run them through the dishwasher. Avoid bath toys that cannot be thoroughly cleaned such as those with squeakers.
- All members of the household should routinely practice good hand washing with soap and water.
- Use separate towels and washcloths for each person in your family.
- Avoid contact with persons who have draining sores. If you help care for someone with sores, wash your hands before and after caring for the skin sores.

Generally, regular soap is fine for hand washing. Rubbing your hands with soap and water loosens bacteria, while rinsing with running water removes bacteria from your hands. Your doctor may:

- recommend a special soap (like Hibiclens® or pHisoHex®) to be used once a week for four or more weeks for bathing;
- recommend you use a hypoallergenic moisturizer or Vaseline® on the skin after bathing in order to limit dry skin;
- prescribe mupirocin cream or ointment (like Bactroban® or Centany®) to apply at the first break in the skin or sight of a pimple to try to prevent more serious infections;
- recommend that you and your family use a mupirocin ointment in the nose two to three times a day for five to seven days for all household members to decrease the risk of having ORSA/MRSA;
- prescribe an oral antibiotic early in an effort to prevent serious infections.

Section 11.6

Mycoplasma Infection

"*Mycoplasma pneumonia*," © 2007. Used with permission of the New Hampshire Department of Health and Human Services.

What is Mycoplasma pneumoniae?

Mycoplasma pneumoniae is a bacteria that can cause several kinds of illnesses, most common of which is an illness of the lungs.

What are the usual symptoms of mycoplasma infection?

Usually, mycoplasma infection is a mild illness characterized by fever, cough, bronchitis, sore throat, and headache. Mycoplasma infection may cause a mild form of pneumonia, which is sometimes called "walking pneumonia." In very rare cases, mycoplasma can cause serious illness such as encephalitis (an inflammation of the brain) or meningitis (inflammation of the lining of the brain and spinal cord).

How does someone get mycoplasma infection?

Mycoplasma pneumoniae is spread from person to person from respiratory droplets, such as when someone coughs or sneezes. Someone can also touch something that has the bacteria on it, such as a door handle, and then touch their eye, nose, or mouth and be infected.

Who is at risk for mycoplasma infection?

Each year an estimated two million cases with one hundred thousand pneumonia-related hospitalizations occur in the United States due to *Mycoplasma pneumoniae*. People of all ages are at risk for mycoplasma infection but children under age five rarely become ill. Mycoplasma infection is the leading cause of pneumonia in school-age children and young adults.

Other Bacterial Infections

What is the incubation period for mycoplasma infection?

From the time someone is infected with the bacteria until they become ill can range from one to four weeks.

How is mycoplasma infection diagnosed?

Diagnosis of acute infections is difficult. Mycoplasma infection is usually diagnosed on the basis of typical symptoms. There is a blood test that can be helpful toward diagnosis, but is not always accurate. More specific laboratory tests are sometimes used in special outbreak investigations.

How long is someone infectious after they become infected?

The contagious period is about ten days.

Does past infection with **Mycoplasma pneumoniae** *make a person immune?*

Immunity after mycoplasma infection does occur. However, a person can get mycoplasma more than once (generally milder than the first episode). The duration of immunity is unknown.

What is the treatment for mycoplasma infection?

Antibiotics can treat mycoplasma infection. However, because mycoplasma infection usually resolves on its own, antibiotic treatment of mild symptoms is usually not necessary.

Is there a way to prevent mycoplasma infection?

There are no vaccines against mycoplasma infection. Similar to prevention methods for many respiratory infections, everyone should cover their mouth and nose with a tissue or their arm when coughing or sneezing, then throw away the tissue and wash their hands; stay home from work or school if they are ill; and not share utensils, cups, or toothbrushes.

What do I do if I think I might have mycoplasma infection?

Call your health care provider.

Childhood Diseases and Disorders Sourcebook, Second Edition

Section 11.7

Tetanus

"Tetanus Disease: Questions and Answers," reprinted with permission from the Immunization Action Coalition, www.immunize.org, © 2007.

What causes tetanus?

Tetanus is caused by a toxin (poison) produced by a bacterium, *Clostridium tetani*. The *C. tetani* bacteria cannot grow in the presence of oxygen. They produce spores that are very difficult to kill as they are resistant to heat and many chemical agents.

How does tetanus spread?

C. tetani spores can be found in the soil and in the intestines and feces of many household and farm animals and humans. The bacteria usually enter the human body through a puncture (in the presence of anaerobic [low oxygen] conditions, the spores will germinate).

Tetanus is not spread from person to person.

How long does it take to show signs of tetanus after being exposed?

The incubation period varies from three to twenty-one days, with an average of eight days. The further the injury site is from the central nervous system, the longer the incubation period. The shorter the incubation period, the higher the risk of death.

What are the symptoms of tetanus?

The symptoms of tetanus are caused by the tetanus toxin acting on the central nervous system. In the most common form of tetanus, the first sign is spasm of the jaw muscles, followed by stiffness of the neck, difficulty in swallowing, and stiffness of the abdominal muscles.

Other signs include fever, sweating, elevated blood pressure, and rapid heart rate. Spasms often occur, which may last for several minutes and

Other Bacterial Infections

continue for three to four weeks. Complete recovery, if it occurs, may take months.

How serious is tetanus?

Tetanus has a high fatality rate; during 1998–2000, the case-fatality rate for reported tetanus in the United States was 18 percent.

What are possible complications from tetanus?

Laryngospasm (spasm of the vocal cords) is a complication that can lead to interference with breathing. Patients can also break their spine or long bones from convulsions. Other possible complications include hypertension, abnormal heart rhythm, and secondary infections, which are common because of prolonged hospital stays.

Obviously, the high possibility of death is a major complication.

How is tetanus diagnosed?

The diagnosis of tetanus is based on the clinical signs and symptoms only. Laboratory diagnosis is not useful as the *C. tetani* bacteria often cannot be recovered from the wound of an individual who has tetanus, and conversely, can be isolated from the skin of an individual who does not have tetanus.

What kind of injuries might allow tetanus to enter the body?

Tetanus bacilli live in the soil, so the most dangerous kind of injury involves possible contamination with dirt, animal feces, and manure. Although we have traditionally worried about deep puncture wounds, in reality many types of injuries can allow tetanus bacilli to enter the body. In recent years, a higher proportion of cases had minor wounds than had major ones, probably because severe wounds were more likely to be properly managed. People have become infected with tetanus following surgery, burns, lacerations, abrasions, crush wounds, ear infections, dental infections, animal bites, abortion, pregnancy, body piercing and tattooing, and injection drug use. People can also get tetanus from splinters.

I stepped on a nail in our yard. What should I do?

Any wound that may involve contamination with tetanus bacilli should be attended to as soon as possible. Treatment depends on your vaccination status and the nature of the wound. In all cases, the wound should be cleaned. Seek treatment immediately and bring your immunization record with you.

With wounds that involve the possibility of tetanus contamination, a patient with an unknown or incomplete history of tetanus vaccination needs a tetanus- and diphtheria-containing shot (Td or Tdap) and a dose of tetanus immune globulin (TIG) as soon as possible.

A person with a documented series of three tetanus- and diphtheria-containing shots (Td or Tdap) who has received a booster dose within the last ten years should be protected. However, to ensure adequate protection, a booster dose of vaccine may still be given if it has been more than five years since the last dose and the wound is other than clean and minor.

Is there a treatment for tetanus?

There is no "cure" for tetanus once a person develops symptoms, just supportive treatment and management of complications. The best "treatment" is prevention through immunization.

How common is tetanus in the United States?

Tetanus first became a reportable disease in the late 1940s. At that time, there were 500 to 600 cases reported per year. After the introduction of the tetanus vaccine in the mid-1940s, reported cases of tetanus dropped steadily.

During 1990–2001, a total of 534 cases of tetanus were reported. Most (56%) of these cases occurred among adults age nineteen to sixty-four years and 38 percent were among persons age sixty-five years or older.

Almost all cases of tetanus are in persons who have never been vaccinated, or who completed their childhood series, but did not have a booster dose in the preceding ten years.

What is neonatal tetanus?

Neonatal tetanus is a form of tetanus that occurs in newborn infants, most often through the use of an unsterile cutting instrument on the unhealed umbilical stump. These babies usually have no temporary immunity passed on from their mother because their mother hasn't been vaccinated and therefore has no immunity.

Other Bacterial Infections

Neonatal tetanus is very rare in the United States (three cases reported during 1990–2004), but is common in some developing countries. It causes more than 215,000 deaths worldwide per year.

Can you get tetanus more than once?

Yes! Tetanus disease does not cause immunity because so little of the potent toxin is required to cause the disease. Persons recovering from tetanus should begin or complete the vaccination series.

Section 11.8

Tuberculosis

"Tuberculosis: General Information,"
Centers for Disease Control and Prevention, July 2007.

What is tuberculosis?

Tuberculosis (TB) is a disease caused by germs that are spread from person to person through the air. TB usually affects the lungs, but it can also affect other parts of the body, such as the brain, the kidneys, or the spine. A person with TB can die if they do not get treatment.

What are the symptoms of TB?

The general symptoms of TB disease include feelings of sickness or weakness, weight loss, fever, and night sweats. The symptoms of TB disease of the lungs also include coughing, chest pain, and the coughing up of blood. Symptoms of TB disease in other parts of the body depend on the area affected.

How is TB spread?

TB germs are put into the air when a person with TB disease of the lungs or throat coughs, sneezes, speaks, or sings. These germs can stay in the air for several hours, depending on the environment. Persons who breathe in the air containing these TB germs can become infected; this is called latent TB infection.

What is the difference between latent TB infection and TB disease?

People with latent TB infection have TB germs in their bodies, but they are not sick because the germs are not active. These people do not have symptoms of TB disease, and they cannot spread the germs to others. However, they may develop TB disease in the future. They are often prescribed treatment to prevent them from developing TB disease.

People with TB disease are sick from TB germs that are active, meaning that they are multiplying and destroying tissue in their body. They usually have symptoms of TB disease. People with TB disease of the lungs or throat are capable of spreading germs to others. They are prescribed drugs that can treat TB disease.

What should I do if I have spent time with someone with latent TB infection?

A person with latent TB infection cannot spread germs to other people. You do not need to be tested if you have spent time with someone with latent TB infection. However, if you have spent time with someone with TB disease or someone with symptoms of TB, you should be tested.

What should I do if I have been exposed to someone with TB disease?

People with TB disease are most likely to spread the germs to people they spend time with every day, such as family members or coworkers. If you have been around someone who has TB disease, you should go to your doctor or your local health department for tests.

How do you get tested for TB?

There are two tests that can be used to help detect TB infection. The Mantoux tuberculin skin test is performed by injecting a small amount of fluid (called tuberculin) into the skin in the lower part of the arm. A person given the tuberculin skin test must return within forty-eight to seventy-two hours to have a trained health care worker look for a reaction on the arm. A second test is the QuantiFERON®-TB Gold test. The QuantiFERON®-TB Gold test is a blood test that

Other Bacterial Infections

measures how the patient's immune system reacts to the germs that cause TB.

What does a positive tuberculin skin test or QuantiFERON®-TB Gold test mean?

A positive tuberculin skin test or QuantiFERON®-TB Gold test only tells that a person has been infected with TB germs. It does not tell whether or not the person has progressed to TB disease. Other tests, such as a chest x-ray and a sample of sputum, are needed to see whether the person has TB disease.

What is Bacille Calmette-Guérin (BCG)?

BCG is a vaccine for TB disease. BCG is used in many countries, but it is not generally recommended in the United States. BCG vaccination does not completely prevent people from getting TB. It may also cause a false positive tuberculin skin test. However, persons who have been vaccinated with BCG can be given a tuberculin skin test or QuantiFERON®-TB Gold test.

Why is latent TB infection treated?

If you have latent TB infection but not TB disease, your doctor may want you to take a drug to kill the TB germs and prevent you from developing TB disease. The decision about taking treatment for latent infection will be based on your chances of developing TB disease. Some people are more likely than others to develop TB disease once they have TB infection. This includes people with human immunodeficiency virus (HIV) infection, people who were recently exposed to someone with TB disease, and people with certain medical conditions.

How is TB disease treated?

TB disease can be treated by taking several drugs for six to twelve months. It is very important that people who have TB disease finish the medicine, and take the drugs exactly as prescribed. If they stop taking the drugs too soon, they can become sick again; if they do not take the drugs correctly, the germs that are still alive may become resistant to those drugs. TB that is resistant to drugs is harder and more expensive to treat. In some situations, staff of the local health department meet regularly with patients who have TB to watch them take their medications. This is called directly observed therapy (DOT). DOT helps the patient complete treatment in the least amount of time.

Section 11.9

Whooping Cough (Pertussis)

"Pertussis (Whooping Cough)," © 2008 Wisconsin Department of Health and Family Services (www.dhfs.wisconsin.gov). Reprinted with permission.

What is pertussis?

Pertussis is a contagious bacterial disease that affects the respiratory tract.

Who gets pertussis?

Pertussis can infect persons of all ages, but is most serious in infants and young children.

How is pertussis spread?

The bacteria are spread by contact with the respiratory droplets from an infected person through coughing. Exposure usually occurs after repeated indoor face-to face contact. Household spread is common.

What are the signs and symptoms of pertussis?

In infants and young children, the disease begins much like a cold with a runny nose, possible low-grade fever, and a mild but irritating cough for one to two weeks. The illness progresses to spells of explosive coughing that can interrupt breathing, eating, and sleeping and is commonly followed by vomiting and exhaustion. Following the cough, the patients may make a loud crowing or "whooping" sound as they struggle to inhale air (hence the common name "whooping cough"). The severe coughing spells can last for several weeks to two months or longer. In older children, adolescents, and adults the symptoms are usually milder and without the typical whoop.

What are the complications associated with pertussis?

In infants less than six months of age, the most common complication is bacterial pneumonia (17%) followed by neurologic complications

Other Bacterial Infections

such as seizures (2.1%) and encephalopathy (0.2 %). Loss of weight from nutritional disturbance and dehydration is also a complication from the disease. More than half of the infants with confirmed pertussis require hospitalization.

How soon do symptoms appear after exposure?

Usually in seven to twenty days.

When and for how long is a person able to spread pertussis?

Pertussis is most contagious in the early stage of the illness before the onset of the explosive coughing spell. The spread of pertussis may be up to three weeks or more after cough onset. The spread period can be reduced to five days after the initiation of an appropriate course of antibiotics administered in the early stages of illness.

Is there treatment for pertussis?

There are four antibiotics recommended for the treatment of pertussis that will shorten the period of communicability. Your doctor may chose one of these antibiotics for treatment. The appropriate antibiotics include either a five-day course of azithromycin, a seven-day course of clarithromycin or a fourteen-day course of either erythromycin or trimethoprim/sulfamethoxazole (TMP/SMX). Persons with pertussis should be isolated from school, work, or similar activities until they have completed at least the first five days of an appropriate antibiotic therapy. The remaining doses of antibiotics need to be taken as prescribed.

How can the spread of pertussis be prevented?

Treatment is recommended for well persons who are close contacts (especially household contacts) of the case to prevent or reduce the severity of illness. Any untreated contacts of a case that develop a persistent cough should be tested for pertussis. Confirmed or suspected cases of pertussis that do not receive appropriate antibiotics should be isolated for three weeks.

How is pertussis confirmed?

Confirmation is by polymerase chain reaction (PCR) assay or by laboratory culture of a nasal swab specimen obtained during the early stage of illness. PCR is the test of choice for laboratory diagnosis of pertussis.

How can pertussis be prevented?

Routine immunization of infants and children with acellular pertussis (aP) vaccine is recommended at two, four, six, and fifteen to eighteen months of age with a booster dose at four to six years of age. It is given in a combination with diphtheria and tetanus vaccines called DTaP. The effectiveness of the vaccine in children who have received at least three doses is estimated to be 80 percent; and protection is even greater against severe disease. Protection will begin to diminish after about three years. Persons who experience pertussis after immunization usually have a milder case. DTaP vaccine is currently recommended for children two months through six years of age. A safe and effective acellular pertussis vaccine for adolescents and adults was licensed in 2005. Called Tdap, the vaccine is routinely recommended as a one-time booster for children eleven to twelve years of age. It is also recommended as a one-time booster for adults.

Does past infection with pertussis make a person immune?

Confirmed pertussis is likely to confer immunity. However, the duration of immunity from past infection is unknown.

Chapter 12

Viral Infections

Chapter Contents

Section 12.1—Chickenpox 122
Section 12.2—Common Cold 124
Section 12.3—Croup 131
Section 12.4—Fifth Disease 133
Section 12.5—Hand, Foot, and Mouth Disease 136
Section 12.6—Infectious Mononucleosis 140
Section 12.7—Influenza 142
Section 12.8—Measles 145
Section 12.9—Mumps 147
Section 12.10—Rabies 149
Section 12.11—Rubella (German Measles) 152
Section 12.12—Warts 155

Section 12.1

Chickenpox

"Chickenpox (Varicella)," © 2008 Wisconsin Department of Health and Family Services (www.dhfs.wisconsin.gov). Reprinted with permission.

What is chickenpox?

Chickenpox is a highly communicable disease caused by the Varicella virus, a member of the herpes virus family.

Who gets chickenpox?

Almost everyone gets chickenpox. In metropolitan communities, about 75 percent of the population has had chickenpox by age fifteen and at least 90 percent by young adulthood. In temperate climates, chickenpox occurs most frequently in winter and early spring.

How is chickenpox spread?

Chickenpox is highly contagious. Chickenpox is transmitted to others by direct person-to-person contact, by droplet or airborne spread of discharges from an infected person's nose and throat, or indirectly through articles freshly soiled by discharges from the infected person's lesions. The scabs themselves are not considered infectious.

What are the symptoms of chickenpox?

Initial symptoms include sudden onset of slight fever and feeling tired and weak. An itchy blister-like rash soon follows. The blisters (vesicles) eventually dry, crust over, and form scabs. The blisters tend to be more common on covered than on exposed parts of the body. They may appear on the scalp, armpits, trunk, and even on the eyelids and in the mouth. Mild or unapparent infections occasionally occur in children. The disease is usually more serious in adults than in children.

Viral Infections

How soon do symptoms appear?

Symptoms commonly appear thirteen to seventeen days after exposure with a range of eleven to twenty-one days after exposure.

When and for how long is a person able to spread chickenpox?

A person is usually able to transmit chickenpox from one to two days before the onset of the rash to six days after the appearance of the first lesion. Contagiousness may be prolonged in people with altered immunity.

Does past infection with chickenpox make a person immune?

Chickenpox generally results in lifelong immunity. However, this infection may remain hidden and recur years later as herpes zoster (shingles) in a proportion of older adults and sometimes in children.

What are the complications associated with chickenpox?

Reye syndrome has been a potentially serious complication associated with clinical chickenpox. For this reason, children with chickenpox should not be treated with aspirin, which may increase the risk of Reye syndrome. Newborn children (less than one month old) whose mothers are not immune and patients with leukemia may suffer severe, prolonged, or fatal chickenpox.

Is there a vaccine for chickenpox?

Yes, a chickenpox vaccine was licensed in the United States in 1995 and is recommended for children twelve to eighteen months of age and older children who have not had chickenpox. Recipients of the vaccine should not receive aspirin for six weeks after the vaccination.

To protect high-risk newborns and persons with weakened immune systems following exposure, a shot of varicella zoster immune globulin (VZIG) is effective in modifying or preventing disease if given within ninety-six hours after exposure to a case of chickenpox.

What can a person or community do to prevent the spread of chickenpox?

The best method to prevent further spread of chickenpox is for people infected with the disease to remain home and avoid exposing others who are susceptible. If they develop symptoms, they should remain home until one week after the skin eruption began or until the lesions become dry.

Avoiding exposure of non-immune newborns and patients with weakened immune systems to chickenpox is important.

Section 12.2

Common Cold

National Institute of Allergy and Infectious Diseases, December 10, 2007.

Overview

Sneezing, scratchy throat, runny nose—everyone knows the first signs of a cold, probably the most common illness known. Although the common cold is usually mild, with symptoms lasting one to two weeks, it is a leading cause of doctor visits and missed days from school and work. People in the United States suffer one billion colds each year, according to some estimates. According to the Centers for Disease Control and Prevention (CDC), twenty-two million school days are lost annually in the United States due to the common cold.

Children have about six to ten colds a year. One important reason why colds are so common in children is because they are often in close contact with each other in daycare centers and schools. In families with children in school, the number of colds per child can be as high as twelve a year. Adults average about two to four colds a year, although the range varies widely. Women, especially those aged twenty to thirty years, have more colds than men, possibly because of their closer contact with children. On average, people older than sixty have fewer than one cold a year.

The Cold Season

In the United States, most colds occur during the fall and winter. Beginning in late August or early September, the rate of colds increases slowly for a few weeks and remains high until March or April, when it

Viral Infections

declines. The seasonal variation may relate to the opening of schools and to cold weather, which prompt people to spend more time indoors and increase the chances that viruses will spread to you from someone else.

Seasonal changes in relative humidity also may affect the prevalence of colds. The most common cold-causing viruses survive better when humidity is low—the colder months of the year. Cold weather also may make the inside lining of your nose drier and more vulnerable to viral infection.

Cause

The Viruses

More than two hundred different viruses are known to cause the symptoms of the common cold. Some, such as the rhinoviruses, seldom produce serious illnesses. Others, such as parainfluenza and respiratory syncytial virus, produce mild infections in adults but can lead to severe lower respiratory tract infections in young children.

Rhinoviruses (from the Greek *rhin*, meaning "nose") cause an estimated 30 to 35 percent of all adult colds, and are most active in early fall, spring, and summer. Scientists have identified more than 110 distinct rhinovirus types. These agents grow best at temperatures of about 91 degrees Fahrenheit, the temperature inside the human nose.

Scientists think coronaviruses cause a large percentage of all adult colds. They bring on colds primarily in the winter and early spring. Of the more than thirty kinds, three or four infect humans.

The importance of coronaviruses as a cause of colds is hard to assess because, unlike rhinoviruses, they are difficult to grow in the laboratory.

Approximately 10 to 15 percent of adult colds are caused by viruses also responsible for other, more severe illnesses: adenoviruses, coxsackieviruses, echoviruses, orthomyxoviruses (including influenza A and B viruses, which cause flu), paramyxoviruses (including several parainfluenza viruses), respiratory syncytial virus, and enteroviruses.

The causes of 30 to 50 percent of adult colds, presumed to be viral, remain unidentified. The same viruses that produce colds in adults appear to cause colds in children. The relative importance of various viruses in pediatric colds, however, is unclear because it's difficult to isolate the precise cause of symptoms in research studies of children with colds.

The Weather

There is no evidence that you can get a cold from exposure to cold weather or from getting chilled or overheated.

Other Factors

There is also no evidence that your chances of getting a cold are related to factors such as exercise, diet, or enlarged tonsils or adenoids. On the other hand, research suggests that psychological stress and allergic diseases affecting your nose or throat may have an impact on your chances of getting infected by cold viruses.

Transmission

You can get infected by cold viruses by either of these methods:

- Touching your skin or environmental surfaces, such as telephones and stair rails, that have cold germs on them and then touching your eyes or nose.
- Inhaling drops of mucus full of cold germs from the air.

Symptoms

Symptoms of the common cold usually begin two to three days after infection and often include the following:

- Mucus buildup in your nose
- Difficulty breathing through your nose
- Swelling of your sinuses
- Sneezing
- Sore throat
- Cough
- Headache

Fever is usually slight but can climb to 102 degrees Fahrenheit in infants and young children. Cold symptoms can last from two to fourteen days, but like most people, you'll probably recover in a week. If symptoms recur often or last much longer than two weeks, you might have an allergy rather than a cold.

Colds occasionally can lead to bacterial infections of your middle ear or sinuses, requiring treatment with antibiotics. High fever, significantly swollen glands, severe sinus pain, and a cough that produces mucus may indicate a complication or more serious illness requiring a visit to your healthcare provider.

Treatment

There is no cure for the common cold, but you can get relief from your cold symptoms by doing any of the following:

- Resting in bed
- Drinking plenty of fluids
- Gargling with warm saltwater or using throat sprays or lozenges for a scratchy or sore throat
- Using petroleum jelly for a raw nose
- Taking aspirin or acetaminophen—Tylenol, for example—for headache or fever

A word of caution: Several studies have linked aspirin use to the development of Reye syndrome in children recovering from flu or chickenpox. Reye syndrome is a rare but serious illness that usually occurs in children between the ages of three and twelve years. It can affect all organs of the body but most often the brain and liver. While most children who survive an episode of Reye syndrome do not suffer any lasting consequences, the illness can lead to permanent brain damage or death. The American Academy of Pediatrics recommends children and teenagers not be given aspirin or medicine containing aspirin when they have any viral illness such as the common cold.

Over-the-Counter Cold Medicines

Nonprescription cold remedies, including decongestants and cough suppressants, may relieve some of your cold symptoms but will not prevent or even shorten the length of your cold. Moreover, because most of these medicines have some side effects, such as drowsiness, dizziness, insomnia, or upset stomach, you should take them with care.

Questions have been raised about the safety of nonprescription cold medicines in children and whether the benefits justify any potential risks from the use of these products in children, especially in those under two years of age. Recently, a Food and Drug Administration panel recommended that nonprescription cold medicines not be given to children under the age of six, because cold medicines do not appear to be effective for these children and may not be safe.

Over-the Counter Antihistamines

Nonprescription antihistamines may give you some relief from symptoms such as runny nose and watery eyes, which are symptoms commonly associated with colds.

Antibiotics

Never take antibiotics to treat a cold because antibiotics do not kill viruses. You should use these prescription medicines only if you have a rare bacterial complication, such as sinusitis or ear infection. In addition, you should not use antibiotics "just in case," because they will not prevent bacterial infections.

Steam

Although inhaling steam may temporarily relieve symptoms of congestion, health experts have found that this approach is not an effective treatment.

Prevention

There are several ways you can keep yourself from getting a cold or passing one on to others:

- Because cold germs on your hands can easily enter through your eyes and nose, keep your hands away from those areas of your body.
- If possible, avoid being close to people who have colds.
- If you have a cold, avoid being close to people.
- If you sneeze or cough, cover your nose or mouth, and sneeze or cough into your elbow rather than your hand.

Hand Washing

Hand washing with soap and water is the simplest and one of the most effective ways to keep from getting colds or giving them to others. During cold season, you should wash your hands often and teach your children to do the same. When water isn't available, the Centers for Disease Control and Prevention (CDC) recommends using alcohol-based products made for disinfecting your hands.

Viral Infections

Disinfecting

Rhinoviruses can live up to three hours on your skin. They also can survive up to three hours on objects such as telephones and stair railings. Cleaning environmental surfaces with a virus-killing disinfectant might help prevent spread of infection.

Vaccine

Because so many different viruses can cause the common cold, the outlook for developing a vaccine that will prevent transmission of all of them is dim. Scientists, however, continue to search for a solution to this problem.

Unproven Prevention Methods

Echinacea: Echinacea is a dietary herbal supplement that some people use to treat their colds. Researchers, however, have found that while the herb may help treat your colds if taken in the early stages, it will not help prevent them.

One research study funded by the National Center for Complementary and Alternative Medicine, a part of the National Institutes of Health, found that echinacea is not effective at all in treating children aged two to eleven.

Vitamin C: Many people are convinced that taking large quantities of vitamin C will prevent colds or relieve symptoms. To test this theory, several large-scale, controlled studies involving children and adults have been conducted. To date, no conclusive data has shown that large doses of vitamin C prevent colds. The vitamin may reduce the severity or duration of symptoms, but there is no clear evidence of this effect.

Taking vitamin C over long periods of time in large amounts may be harmful. Too much vitamin C can cause severe diarrhea, a particular danger for elderly people and small children.

Honey: Honey has been considered to be a treatment for coughs and to soothe a sore throat. A recent study conducted at the Penn State College of Medicine compared the effectiveness of a little bit of buckwheat honey before bedtime versus either no treatment or dextromethorphan (DM), the cough suppressant found in many over-the-counter cold medicines. The results of this study suggest that honey may be useful to relieve coughing, but researchers need to do additional studies.

You should never give honey to children under the age of one because of the risk of infantile botulism, a serious disease.

Zinc: Zinc lozenges and zinc lollipops are available over the counter as a treatment for the common cold; however, results from studies designed to test the efficacy of zinc are inconclusive. Although several studies have shown zinc to be effective for reducing the symptoms of the common cold, an equal number of studies have shown zinc is not effective. This may be due to flaws in the way these studies were conducted, or the particular form of zinc used in each case. Therefore, additional studies are needed.

Research

Thanks to basic research, scientists know more about the rhinovirus than almost any other virus, and have powerful new tools for developing antiviral drugs. Although the common cold may never be uncommon, further investigations offer the hope of reducing the huge burden of this universal problem.

Viral Infections

Section 12.3

Croup

"Croup" is reprinted with permission from the Cincinnati Children's Hospital Medical Center website, http://www.cincinnatichildrens.org. © 2005 Cincinnati Children's Hospital Medical Center. All rights reserved.

What Is Croup?

Croup is an infection causing a partial blockage of air as it flows through the larynx (voice box). The noise can be very frightening, and your child's cough may sound like a seal barking. When your child breathes in you may hear a harsh, rasping sound, which is called stridor. The child's voice may be hoarse, too.

Croup may appear after your child has had a cold for several days. Croup is usually caused by a virus and may last several days. Sometimes croup comes on suddenly in the middle of the night. It may disappear in as little as a few hours. It may occur more than one time in a child's life.

Symptoms

Because your child cannot move air in and out of his or her lungs easily, you may see some of the following symptoms:

- The hollow area beneath the child's Adam's apple in the neck may pull in.
- Your child's chest may pull in when he or she breathes in.
- Your child's face may be pale.
- Your child may look frightened.

Stay calm. Croup is frightening to the child and parents. A crying, upset child tends to make the croup worse. Parents can help to relieve croup by being calm themselves, which helps to quiet the child. This relieves the tightness around the larynx and allows the child to breathe more easily.

Treatment

- Take your child into the bathroom and shut the door.
- Turn on the shower and hot water faucets to make steam. Be careful to keep away from the hot water. Cool mist will work, too, and is safer. If the mist seems to upset the child, stop and calm the child. You may also take the child outside to breathe in the cool night air.
- Sit with your child and let him or her breathe in the steam.
- Do not leave your child alone.
- Have someone start a vaporizer or a humidifier in the child's room. Continue to keep your child's room humidified, especially if the air is dry.
- When breathing is easier (ten to fifteen minutes), give your child a popsicle. Later give him or her more clear fluids to drink. This will help keep the throat and airway moist.

Seek Emergency Care

- If your child's breathing does not improve after trying the home treatments for fifteen to thirty minutes
- If your child's breathing problem gets worse
- If your child begins drooling
- If your child has trouble swallowing
- If your child becomes restless and cannot sleep
- If a bluish color is seen around your child's lips

Your observations of your child are important. Tell the doctor what you have seen and what you have done. This information will help the doctor care for your child.

Diet

Avoid milk and thick liquids. These will make your child's phlegm (mucus) thicker and make him or her cough more.

Give warm fluids—such as warm apple juice or lemonade—for coughing spasms, in children over four months of age. These warm fluids may relax vocal cords and loosen sticky mucus.

Activity

Activities such as coloring and looking at books together will help your child stay calm and quiet so he or she may breathe more easily.

Section 12.4

Fifth Disease

"Parvovirus B19 (Fifth Disease)," Centers for Disease Control and Prevention, January 21, 2005.

What is "fifth disease?"

Fifth disease is a mild rash illness that occurs most commonly in children. The ill child typically has a "slapped-cheek" rash on the face and a lacy red rash on the trunk and limbs. Occasionally, the rash may itch. An ill child may have a low-grade fever, malaise, or a "cold" a few days before the rash breaks out. The child is usually not very ill, and the rash resolves in seven to ten days.

What causes fifth disease?

Fifth disease is caused by infection with human parvovirus B19. This virus infects only humans. Pet dogs or cats may be immunized against "parvovirus," but these are animal parvoviruses that do not infect humans. Therefore, a child cannot "catch" parvovirus from a pet dog or cat, and a pet cat or dog cannot catch human parvovirus B19 from an ill child.

Can adults get fifth disease?

Yes, they can. An adult who is not immune can be infected with parvovirus B19 and either have no symptoms or develop the typical rash of fifth disease, joint pain or swelling, or both. Usually, joints on both sides of the body are affected. The joints most frequently affected are the hands, wrists, and knees. The joint pain and swelling usually resolve in a week or two, but they may last several months. About 50 percent of adults, however, have been previously infected with parvovirus B19, have developed immunity to the virus, and cannot get fifth disease.

Is fifth disease contagious?

Yes. A person infected with parvovirus B19 is contagious during the early part of the illness, before the rash appears. By the time a child has the characteristic "slapped cheek" rash of fifth disease, for example, he or she is probably no longer contagious and may return to school or child care center. This contagious period is different than that for many other rash illnesses, such as measles, for which the child is contagious while he or she has the rash.

How does someone get infected with parvovirus B19?

Parvovirus B19 has been found in the respiratory secretions (e.g., saliva, sputum, or nasal mucus) of infected persons before the onset of rash, when they appear to "just have a cold." The virus is probably spread from person to person by direct contact with those secretions, such as sharing drinking cups or utensils. In a household, as many as 50 percent of susceptible persons exposed to a family member who has fifth disease may become infected. During school outbreaks, 10 to 60 percent of students may get fifth disease.

How soon after infection with parvovirus B19 does a person become ill?

A susceptible person usually becomes ill four to fourteen days after being infected with the virus, but may become ill as long as twenty days after infection.

Does everyone who is infected with parvovirus B19 become ill?

No. During outbreaks of fifth disease, about 20 percent of adults and children who are infected with parvovirus B19 do not develop any symptoms. Furthermore, other persons infected with the virus will have a nonspecific illness that is not characteristic of fifth disease. Persons infected with the virus, however, do develop lasting immunity that protects them against infection in the future.

How is fifth disease diagnosed?

A physician can often diagnose fifth disease by seeing the typical rash during a physical examination. In cases in which it is important to confirm the diagnosis, a blood test may be done to look for antibodies

Viral Infections

to parvovirus. Antibodies are proteins produced by the immune system in response to parvovirus B19 and other germs. If immunoglobulin M (IgM) antibody to parvovirus B19 is detected, the test result suggests that the person has had a recent infection.

Is fifth disease serious?

Fifth disease is usually a mild illness that resolves on its own among children and adults who are otherwise healthy. Joint pain and swelling in adults usually resolve without long-term disability.

Parvovirus B19 infection may cause a serious illness in persons with sickle-cell disease or similar types of chronic anemia. In such persons, parvovirus B19 can cause an acute, severe anemia. The ill person may be pale, weak, and tired, and should see his or her physician for treatment. (The typical rash of fifth disease is rarely seen in these persons.) Once the infection is controlled, the anemia resolves. Furthermore, persons who have problems with their immune systems may also develop a chronic anemia with parvovirus B19 infection that requires medical treatment. People who have leukemia or cancer, who are born with immune deficiencies, who have received an organ transplant, or who have human immunodeficiency virus (HIV) infection are at risk for serious illness due to parvovirus B19 infection.

Occasionally, serious complications may develop from parvovirus B19 infection during pregnancy.

How are parvovirus B19 infections treated?

Treatment of symptoms such as fever, pain, or itching is usually all that is needed for fifth disease. Adults with joint pain and swelling may need to rest, restrict their activities, and take medicines such as aspirin or ibuprofen to relieve symptoms. The few people who have severe anemia caused by parvovirus B19 infection may need to be hospitalized and receive blood transfusions. Persons with immune problems may need special medical care, including treatment with immune globulin (antibodies), to help their bodies get rid of the infection.

Can parvovirus B19 infection be prevented?

There is no vaccine or medicine that prevents parvovirus B19 infection. Frequent hand washing is recommended as a practical and probably effective method to decrease the chance of becoming infected.

Excluding persons with fifth disease from work, child care centers, or schools is not likely to prevent the spread of the virus, since people are contagious before they develop the rash.

Section 12.5

Hand, Foot, and Mouth Disease

Centers for Disease Control and Prevention, September 5, 2006.

What is hand, foot, and mouth disease?

Hand, foot, and mouth disease (HFMD) is a common illness of infants and children. It is characterized by fever, sores in the mouth, and a rash with blisters. HFMD begins with a mild fever, poor appetite, malaise ("feeling sick"), and frequently a sore throat. One or two days after the fever begins, painful sores develop in the mouth. They begin as small red spots that blister and then often become ulcers. They are usually located on the tongue, gums, and inside of the cheeks. The skin rash develops over one to two days with flat or raised red spots, some with blisters. The rash does not itch, and it is usually located on the palms of the hands and soles of the feet. It may also appear on the buttocks. A person with HFMD may have only the rash or the mouth ulcers.

Is HFMD the same as foot-and-mouth disease?

No. HFMD is often confused with foot-and-mouth disease of cattle, sheep, and swine. Although the names are similar, the two diseases are not related at all and are caused by different viruses.

What causes HFMD?

Viruses from the group called enteroviruses cause HFMD. The most common cause is coxsackievirus A16; sometimes, HFMD is caused by enterovirus 71 or other enteroviruses. The enterovirus group includes polioviruses, coxsackieviruses, echoviruses, and other enteroviruses.

Viral Infections

Is HFMD serious?

Usually not. HFMD caused by coxsackievirus A16 infection is a mild disease and nearly all patients recover without medical treatment in seven to ten days. Complications are uncommon. Rarely, the patient with coxsackievirus A16 infection may also develop "aseptic" or viral meningitis, in which the person has fever, headache, stiff neck, or back pain, and may need to be hospitalized for a few days. Another cause of HFMD, EV71 may also cause viral meningitis and, rarely, more serious diseases, such as encephalitis, or a poliomyelitis-like paralysis. EV71 encephalitis may be fatal. Cases of fatal encephalitis occurred during outbreaks of HFMD in Malaysia in 1997 and in Taiwan in 1998.

Is HFMD contagious?

Yes, HFMD is moderately contagious. Infection is spread from person to person by direct contact with nose and throat discharges, saliva, fluid from blisters, or the stool of infected persons. A person is most contagious during the first week of the illness. HFMD is not transmitted to or from pets or other animals.

How soon will someone become ill after getting infected?

The usual period from infection to onset of symptoms ("incubation period") is three to seven days. Fever is often the first symptom of HFMD.

Who is at risk for HFMD?

HFMD occurs mainly in children under ten years old, but may also occur in adults too. Everyone is at risk of infection, but not everyone who is infected becomes ill. Infants, children, and adolescents are more likely to be susceptible to infection and illness from these viruses, because they are less likely than adults to have antibodies and be immune from previous exposures to them. Infection results in immunity to the specific virus, but a second episode may occur following infection with a different member of the enterovirus group.

What are the risks to pregnant women exposed to children with HFMD?

Because enteroviruses, including those causing HFMD, are very common, pregnant women are frequently exposed to them, especially during summer and fall months. As for any other adults, the risk of infection is higher for pregnant women who do not have antibodies from earlier exposures to these viruses, and who are exposed to young children—the primary spreaders of enteroviruses.

Most enterovirus infections during pregnancy cause mild or no illness in the mother. Although the available information is limited, currently there is no clear evidence that maternal enteroviral infection causes adverse outcomes of pregnancy such as abortion, stillbirth, or congenital defects. However, mothers infected shortly before delivery may pass the virus to the newborn. Babies born to mothers who have symptoms of enteroviral illness around the time of delivery are more likely to be infected. Most newborns infected with an enterovirus have mild illness, but, in rare cases, they may develop an overwhelming infection of many organs, including liver and heart, and die from the infection. The risk of this severe illness in newborns is higher during the first two weeks of life.

Strict adherence to generally recommended good hygienic practices by the pregnant woman may help to decrease the risk of infection during pregnancy and around the time of delivery.

When and where does HFMD occur?

Individual cases and outbreaks of HFMD occur worldwide, more frequently in summer and early autumn. In the recent past, major outbreaks of HFMD attributable to enterovirus 71 have been reported in some South East Asian countries (Malaysia, 1997; Taiwan, 1998).

How is HFMD diagnosed?

HFMD is one of many infections that result in mouth sores. Another common cause is oral herpesvirus infection, which produces an inflammation of the mouth and gums (sometimes called stomatitis). Usually, the physician can distinguish between HFMD and other causes of mouth sores based on the age of the patient, the pattern of symptoms reported by the patient or parent, and the appearance of the rash and sores on examination. A throat swab or stool specimen may be sent to a laboratory to determine which enterovirus caused the illness. Since the testing often takes two to four weeks to obtain a final answer, the physician usually does not order these tests.

How is HFMD treated?

No specific treatment is available for this or other enterovirus infections. Symptomatic treatment is given to provide relief from fever, aches, or pain from the mouth ulcers.

Viral Infections

Can HFMD be prevented?

Specific prevention for HFMD or other non-polio enterovirus infections is not available, but the risk of infection can be lowered by good hygienic practices. Preventive measures include frequent hand washing, especially after diaper changes, cleaning of contaminated surfaces and soiled items first with soap and water, and then disinfecting them by diluted solution of chlorine-containing bleach (made by mixing approximately one quarter cup of bleach with one gallon of water. Avoidance of close contact (kissing, hugging, sharing utensils, etc.) with children with HFMD may also help to reduce the risk of infection to caregivers.

What about HFMD in the child care setting?

HFMD outbreaks in child care facilities occur most often in the summer and fall months, and usually coincide with an increased number of cases in the community.

The Centers for Disease Control and Prevention (CDC) has no specific recommendations regarding the exclusion of children with HFMD from child care programs, schools, or other group settings. Children are often excluded from group settings during the first few days of the illness, which may reduce the spread of infection, but will not completely interrupt it. Exclusion of ill persons may not prevent additional cases since the virus may be excreted for weeks after the symptoms have disappeared. Also, some persons excreting the virus, including most adults, may have no symptoms. Some benefit may be gained, however, by excluding children who have blisters in their mouths and drool or who have weeping lesions on their hands.

If an outbreak occurs in the child care setting:

- Make sure that all children and adults use good hand washing technique, especially after diaper changes.

- Thoroughly wash and disinfect contaminated items and surfaces using diluted solution of chlorine-containing bleach.

Section 12.6

Infectious Mononucleosis

Excerpted from "Epstein-Barr Virus and Infectious Mononucleosis,"
Centers for Disease Control and Prevention, January 10, 2008.

Epstein-Barr virus, frequently referred to as EBV, is a member of the herpesvirus family and one of the most common human viruses. The virus occurs worldwide, and most people become infected with EBV sometime during their lives. In the United States, as many as 95 percent of adults between thirty-five and forty years of age have been infected. Infants become susceptible to EBV as soon as maternal antibody protection (present at birth) disappears. Many children become infected with EBV, and these infections usually cause no symptoms or are indistinguishable from the other mild, brief illnesses of childhood. In the United States and in other developed countries, many persons are not infected with EBV in their childhood years. When infection with EBV occurs during adolescence or young adulthood, it causes infectious mononucleosis 35 to 50 percent of the time.

Symptoms of infectious mononucleosis are fever, sore throat, and swollen lymph glands. Sometimes, a swollen spleen or liver involvement may develop. Heart problems or involvement of the central nervous system occurs only rarely, and infectious mononucleosis is almost never fatal. There are no known associations between active EBV infection and problems during pregnancy, such as miscarriages or birth defects. Although the symptoms of infectious mononucleosis usually resolve in one or two months, EBV remains dormant or latent in a few cells in the throat and blood for the rest of the person's life. Periodically, the virus can reactivate and is commonly found in the saliva of infected persons. This reactivation usually occurs without symptoms of illness.

EBV also establishes a lifelong dormant infection in some cells of the body's immune system. A late event in a very few carriers of this virus is the emergence of Burkitt lymphoma and nasopharyngeal carcinoma, two rare cancers that are not normally found in the United States. EBV appears to play an important role in these malignancies, but is probably not the sole cause of disease.

Viral Infections

Most individuals exposed to people with infectious mononucleosis have previously been infected with EBV and are not at risk for infectious mononucleosis. In addition, transmission of EBV requires intimate contact with the saliva (found in the mouth) of an infected person. Transmission of this virus through the air or blood does not normally occur. The incubation period, or the time from infection to appearance of symptoms, ranges from four to six weeks. Persons with infectious mononucleosis may be able to spread the infection to others for a period of weeks. However, no special precautions or isolation procedures are recommended, since the virus is also found frequently in the saliva of healthy people. In fact, many healthy people can carry and spread the virus intermittently for life. These people are usually the primary reservoir for person-to-person transmission. For this reason, transmission of the virus is almost impossible to prevent.

The clinical diagnosis of infectious mononucleosis is suggested on the basis of the symptoms of fever, sore throat, swollen lymph glands, and the age of the patient. Usually, laboratory tests are needed for confirmation. Serologic results for persons with infectious mononucleosis include an elevated white blood cell count, an increased percentage of certain atypical white blood cells, and a positive reaction to a "mono spot" test.

There is no specific treatment for infectious mononucleosis, other than treating the symptoms. No antiviral drugs or vaccines are available. Some physicians have prescribed a five-day course of steroids to control the swelling of the throat and tonsils. The use of steroids has also been reported to decrease the overall length and severity of illness, but these reports have not been published.

It is important to note that symptoms related to infectious mononucleosis caused by EBV infection seldom last for more than four months. When such an illness lasts more than six months, it is frequently called chronic EBV infection. However, valid laboratory evidence for continued active EBV infection is seldom found in these patients. The illness should be investigated further to determine if it meets the criteria for chronic fatigue syndrome, or CFS. This process includes ruling out other causes of chronic illness or fatigue.

Section 12.7

Influenza

"The Flu: A Guide for Parents,"
Centers for Disease Control and Prevention, 2007–2008.

What is the flu?

The flu (influenza) is an infection of the nose, throat, and lungs that is caused by influenza virus. The flu can spread from person to person. Most people with flu are sick for about a week, but then feel better. However, some people (especially young children, pregnant women, older people, and people with chronic health problems) can get very sick and some can die.

What are the symptoms of the flu?

Most people with the flu feel tired and have fever, headache, dry cough, sore throat, runny or stuffy nose, and sore muscles. Some people, especially children, may also have stomach problems and diarrhea. Cough can last two or more weeks.

How does the flu spread?

People that have the flu usually cough, sneeze, and have a runny nose. This makes droplets with virus in them. Other people can get the flu by breathing in these droplets or getting them in their nose or mouth.

How long can a sick person spread the flu to others?

Most healthy adults may be able to spread the flu from one day before getting sick to up to five days after getting sick. This can be longer in children and in people who don't fight disease as well (people with weakened immune systems).

How can I protect my child from the flu?

A flu vaccine is the best way to protect against the flu. The Centers for Disease Control and Prevention (CDC) recommends that all

Viral Infections

children from the ages of six months up to their fifth birthday get a flu vaccine every fall or winter (children getting a vaccine for the first time need two doses).

Flu shots can be given to children six months and older.

A nasal-spray vaccine can be given to healthy children two years and older (children under five years old who have had wheezing in the past year or any child with chronic health problems should get the flu shot).

You can protect your child by getting a flu vaccine for yourself too. Also encourage your child's close contacts to get a flu vaccine. This is very important if your child is younger than five or has a chronic health problem like asthma (breathing disease) or diabetes (high blood sugar levels).

Is there medicine to treat the flu?

There are antiviral drugs for children one year and older that can make your child feel better, be less contagious, and get better sooner. But these drugs need to be approved by a doctor. They should be started during the first two days that your child is sick for them to work. Your doctor can discuss with you if these drugs are right for your child.

How else can I protect my child against flu?

Take time to get a flu vaccine and get your child vaccinated too.

Take everyday steps to prevent the spread of germs. This includes the following:

- Clean your hands often and cover your coughs and sneezes.
- Tell your child to:
   - stay away from people who are sick;
   - clean hands often;
   - keep hands away from face;
   - cover coughs and sneezes to protect others (it's best to use a tissue, then throw it away).

What should I use for hand cleaning?

Washing hands with soap and water (for as long as it takes to sing the Happy Birthday song twice) will help protect your child from germs. When soap and water are not available, wipes or gels with alcohol in them can be used (the gels should be rubbed into your hands until they are dry).

What can I do if my child gets sick?

Consult your doctor and make sure your child gets plenty of rest and drinks a lot of fluids. If your child is older than two years, you can buy medicine (over-the-counter) without a prescription that might make your child feel better. Be careful with these medicines and follow the instructions on the package. But never give aspirin or medicine that has aspirin in it to children or teenagers who may have the flu.

What if my child seems very sick?

Call or take your child to a doctor right away if your child:

- has a high fever or fever that lasts a long time;
- has trouble breathing or breathes fast;
- has skin that looks blue;
- is not drinking enough;
- seems confused, will not wake up, does not want to be held, or has seizures (uncontrolled shaking);
- gets better but then worse again;
- has other conditions (like heart or lung disease, diabetes) that get worse.

Can my child go to school if he or she is sick?

No. Your child should stay home to rest and to avoid giving the flu to other children.

Should my child go to school if other children are sick?

It is not unusual for some children in school to get sick during the winter months. If many children get sick, it is up to you to decide whether to send your child to school. You might want to check with your doctor, especially if your child has other health problems.

When can my child go back to school after having the flu?

Keep your child home from school until his or her temperature has been normal for twenty-four hours. Remind your child to cover his or her mouth when coughing or sneezing, to protect others (you may want to send some tissue and wipes or gels with alcohol in them to school with your child).

Section 12.8

Measles

"Measles Disease In-Short,"
Centers for Disease Control and Prevention, October 2006.

Description

A respiratory disease caused by a virus.

The virus normally grows in the cells that line the back of the throat and in the cells that line the lungs.

Symptoms

Rash, high fever, cough, runny nose, and red, watery eyes (lasts about a week).

Complications

Diarrhea, ear infections, pneumonia, encephalitis, seizures, and death.

Approximately 20 percent of reported measles cases experience one or more complications. These complications are more common among children under five years of age and adults over twenty years old.

Measles causes ear infections in nearly one out of every ten children who get it. As many as one out of twenty children with measles gets pneumonia, and about one child in every one thousand who get measles will develop encephalitis. (This is an inflammation of the brain that can lead to convulsions, and can leave your child deaf or mentally retarded.) For every one thousand children who get measles, one or two will die from it. Measles can also make a pregnant woman have a miscarriage, give birth prematurely, or have a low-birth-weight baby.

In developing countries, where malnutrition and vitamin A deficiency are prevalent, measles has been known to kill as many as one out of four people. It is the leading cause of blindness among African children. Measles kills almost one million children in the world each year.

Transmission

Spread by contact with an infected person, through coughing and sneezing (highly contagious).

The disease is highly contagious, and can be transmitted from four days prior to the onset of the rash to four days after the onset. If one person has it, 90 percent of their susceptible close contacts will also become infected with the measles virus.

The virus resides in the mucus in the nose and throat of the infected person. When that person sneezes or coughs, droplets spray into the air. The infected mucus can land in other people's noses or throats when they breathe or put their fingers in their mouth or nose after handling an infected surface. The virus remains active and contagious on infected surfaces for up to two hours. Measles spreads so easily that anyone who is not immunized will probably get it, eventually.

Vaccine

Measles vaccine (contained in measles, mumps, and rubella [MMR], measles and rubella [MR], and measles vaccines) can prevent this disease.

The MMR vaccine is a live, attenuated (weakened), combination vaccine that protects against the measles, mumps, and rubella viruses. It was first licensed in the combined form in 1971 and contains the safest and most effective forms of each vaccine.

It is made by taking the measles virus from the throat of an infected person and adapting it to grow in chick embryo cells in a laboratory. As the virus becomes better able to grow in the chick embryo cells, it becomes less able to grow in a child's skin or lungs. When this vaccine virus is given to a child it replicates only a little before it is eliminated from the body. This replication causes the body to develop an immunity that, in 95 percent of children, lasts for a lifetime.

A second dose of the vaccine is recommended to protect those 5 percent who did not develop immunity in the first dose and to give "booster" effect to those who did develop an immune response.

Section 12.9

Mumps

"Mumps: Q&A about the Disease,"
Centers for Disease Control and Prevention, October 16, 2006.

What is mumps?

It is an infection caused by the mumps virus.

Who can get mumps?

Anyone who is not immune from either previous mumps infection or from vaccination can get mumps. Before the routine vaccination program was introduced in the United States, mumps was a common illness in infants, children, and young adults. Because most people have now been vaccinated, mumps is now a rare disease in the United States. Of those people who do get mumps, up to half have very mild, or no symptoms, and therefore do not know they were infected with mumps.

What are the symptoms of mumps?

The most common symptoms are fever, headache, muscle aches, tiredness, and loss of appetite followed by onset of parotitis (swollen and tender salivary glands under the ears—on one or both sides).

Are there complications of mumps?

The most common complication is the inflammation of the testicles (orchitis) in males who have reached puberty, but rarely does this lead to fertility problems.

Other rare complications include the following:

- Inflammation of the brain and/or tissue covering the brain and spinal cord (encephalitis/meningitis)
- Inflammation of the ovaries (oophoritis) and/or breasts (mastitis) in females who have reached puberty

- Spontaneous abortion particularly in early pregnancy (miscarriage)
- Deafness, usually permanent

How soon do symptoms appear?

Symptoms typically appear sixteen to eighteen days after infection, but this period can range from twelve to twenty-five days after infection.

How is mumps spread?

Mumps is spread by mucus or droplets from the nose or throat of an infected person, usually when a person coughs or sneezes. Surfaces of items (e.g. toys) can also spread the virus if someone who is sick touches them without washing their hands, and someone else then touches the same surface and then rubs their eyes, mouth, nose, etc. (this is called fomite transmission).

How long is an infected person able to spread the disease?

Mumps virus has been found in respiratory secretions three days before the start of symptoms until nine days after onset. Although mumps virus has been detected on rare occasions for up to nine days after symptom onset, the patient is most infectious within the first five days. Therefore, the Centers for Disease Control and Prevention (CDC) now recommends isolating mumps patients for five days following onset of symptoms (parotitis).

What is the treatment for mumps?

There is no specific treatment. Supportive care should be given as needed. If someone becomes very ill, they should seek medical attention. If someone seeks medical attention, they should call their doctor in advance so that they don't have to sit in the waiting room for a long time and possibly infect other patients.

How do I protect myself (my kids/my family)?

Mumps vaccine (usually measles, mumps, and rubella [MMR]), is the best way to prevent mumps. Other things people can do to prevent mumps and other infections is to wash hands well and often with soap, and to teach children to wash their hands too. Eating utensils should not be shared, and surfaces that are frequently touched (toys,

Viral Infections

doorknobs, tables, counters, etc.) should also be regularly cleaned with soap and water, or with cleaning wipes.

Section 12.10

Rabies

"Rabies," © 2008 Wisconsin Department of Health and Family Services (www.dhfs.wisconsin.gov). Reprinted with permission.

What is rabies?

Rabies is a viral disease affecting the central nervous system. It is transmitted from infected mammals to man and is invariably fatal once symptoms appear. Human rabies is rare in the United States, but still frequently occurs in many developing nations.

Who gets rabies?

All mammals including man are susceptible to rabies. In Wisconsin, skunks and bats are the most likely animals to carry the rabies virus, although rabies also has occurred with some regularity in dogs, cats, foxes, raccoons and livestock.

How is rabies spread to humans?

Rabies is almost always contracted by exposure to a rabid animal. The exposure is nearly always through a bite, but rabies can also be transmitted if a rabid animal scratches a person or if its saliva comes into contact with broken skin.

Because bites and scratches from bats may go unnoticed if a person is sleeping, is very young, or is mentally incapacitated, a physician should be contacted if a bat is found in the same room with a young child, or with a sleeping or mentally incapacitated adult.

What are the symptoms of rabies?

Early symptoms may include irritability, headache, fever, and itching or pain at the exposure site. The disease eventually progresses to

Childhood Diseases and Disorders Sourcebook, Second Edition

spasms of the throat and the muscles used for breathing, convulsions, delirium, paralysis, and death. It is important to note that by the time any symptoms appear, rabies cannot be successfully treated.

How soon after exposure do symptoms appear?

The time between exposure and the onset of symptoms is variable but averages two to twelve weeks in humans. Incubation periods of over one year have been reported.

Is a human able to spread rabies?

Person to person transmission is extremely rare, however, precautions should be taken to prevent exposure to the saliva of the diseased person. Tissues from individuals with rabies must not be used in transplant procedures.

What is the treatment for exposure to rabies?

The most effective rabies prevention is immediate thorough cleansing of animal bite or scratch wounds with liberal amounts of soap and water. If circumstances of the exposure warrant it, a physician may give the bite victim an injection of rabies immune globulin and five injections of a rabies vaccine administered in the arm as a preventive measure.

In most instances, however, observation or testing of the biting animal will rule out the possibility of rabies and will therefore eliminate any need for the bite victim to undergo the series of injections. Because of this, it is important for bite victims to notify their local health department (or local law enforcement when public health staff are unavailable) whenever a bite occurs to ensure that the biting animal is appropriately and legally observed or tested for rabies. The victim's physician should also be notified promptly.

What happens if rabies exposure goes untreated?

Exposure of a human to a rabid animal does not always result in rabies. If preventive treatment is obtained promptly following a rabies exposure, nearly all cases of rabies will be prevented. However, if preventive treatment is not administered and signs of rabies develop, the disease is invariably fatal. All animal bites, regardless of whether the animal is available for rabies observation or testing, should be evaluated by a health professional to determine if treatment is necessary.

Viral Infections

What can be done to prevent the spread of rabies?

Exposure to rabies may be minimized by eliminating stray dogs and cats, having pet dogs, cats, ferrets, and livestock vaccinated against rabies, and staying away from all wild animals, especially those acting abnormally. Do not keep exotic or wild animals as pets, regardless of how young or cute they are. Exclude bats from living quarters by keeping screens in good repair and by closing up any small openings that could allow them to enter.

Persons traveling to developing countries in which rabies is prevalent, or persons who are at ongoing risk of possible rabies exposure (e.g., veterinarians, animal control officers) should ask their doctor about receiving the pre-exposure rabies vaccination.

Persons who are bitten by any mammal should promptly cleanse the bite wound with liberal amounts of soap and water, and contact their physician and their local health department. Persons who have been in close physical proximity to bats and who cannot rule out the possibility of physical contact should likewise contact their physician. If the offending animal can be safely captured without incurring further injury, it is generally advisable to do so, and then hold the animal until the local health department can be consulted.

Section 12.11

Rubella (German Measles)

"Rubella Disease: Questions and Answers,"
reprinted with permission from the Immunization Action Coalition,
www.immunize.org, © 2007.

What causes rubella?

Rubella is caused by a virus.

How does rubella spread?

Rubella spreads from person to person through the air. Rubella is contagious but less so than measles and chickenpox.

How long does it take to show signs of rubella after being exposed?

The incubation period varies from twelve to twenty-three days (average, fourteen days). Symptoms are often mild and may be inapparent up to half of the time.

What are the symptoms of rubella?

Children with rubella usually first break out in a rash, which starts on the face and progresses down the body. Older children and adults usually first suffer from low-grade fever, swollen glands in the neck or behind the ears, and upper respiratory infection before they develop a rash. Adult women often develop pain and stiffness in their finger, wrist, and knee joints, which may last up to a month. Up to half of people infected with rubella virus have no symptoms at all.

How serious is rubella?

Rubella is usually a mild disease in children; adults tend to have more complications. The main concern with rubella disease, however, is the effect it has on an infected pregnant woman. Rubella infection

Viral Infections

in the first trimester of pregnancy can lead to fetal death, premature delivery, and serious birth defects.

What are possible complications from rubella?

Encephalitis (brain infection) occurs in one in six thousand cases, usually in adults. Temporary blood problems, including low platelet levels and hemorrhage, also occur rarely. Up to 70 percent of adult women with rubella have pain and/or swelling of the joints, which is usually temporary.

The most serious complication of rubella infection is congenital rubella syndrome (CRS), the result when the rubella virus attacks a developing fetus. Up to 85 percent of infants infected during the first trimester of pregnancy will be born with some type of birth defect, including deafness, eye defects, heart defects, mental retardation, and more. Infection early in the pregnancy (less than twelve weeks gestation) is the most dangerous; defects are rare when infection occurs after twenty weeks gestation.

Is there a treatment for rubella?

There is no "cure" for rubella, only supportive treatment (e.g., bed rest, fluids, and fever reduction).

How do I know if my child has rubella?

Because the rubella rash looks similar to other rashes, the only sure way to diagnose rubella is by a laboratory test.

How long is a person with rubella contagious?

The disease is most contagious when the rash is erupting, but the virus can be spread from seven days before, to five to seven days after the rash begins.

If I think my child has been exposed to rubella, what should I do?

If your child has not been vaccinated against rubella, receiving the vaccine after exposure to the virus will not help prevent disease if the child has already been infected. However, if the child did not become infected after this particular exposure, the vaccine will help protect him or her against future exposure to rubella.

How common is rubella in the United States?

Due to good immunization coverage, rubella and CRS are rare in the United States at the present time. However, outbreaks continue to occur in groups of susceptible individuals who refuse immunization for religious or philosophic reasons and among some foreign-born immigrants, who come from areas where rubella vaccine is not routinely used. Rubella can be imported into the United States at any time.

Rubella outbreaks are unfortunately followed by an increase in CRS. Two rubella outbreaks in 1990–91, in California and Pennsylvania, resulted in the birth of fifty-eight infants with CRS.

Can you get rubella more than once?

Second cases of rubella are believed to be very rare.

Why do people call rubella "German measles"?

Rubella was first described as a separate disease in the German medical literature in 1814.

Viral Infections

Section 12.12

Warts

"Warts," reprinted with permission from the
American Academy of Dermatology, ©2007. All rights reserved.

What are warts?

Warts are noncancerous skin growths caused by a viral infection in the top layer of the skin. Viruses that cause warts are called human papillomavirus (HPV). Warts are usually skin-colored and feel rough to the touch, but they can be dark, flat, and smooth. The appearance of a wart depends on where it is growing.

How many kinds of warts are there?

There are several different kinds of warts including:

- common warts;
- foot (plantar) warts;
- flat warts.

Common warts usually grow on the fingers, around the nails, and on the backs of the hands. They are more common where skin has been broken, for example where fingernails are bitten or hangnails picked. These are often called "seed" warts because the blood vessels to the wart produce black dots that look like seeds.

Foot warts are usually on the soles (plantar area) of the feet and are called plantar warts. When plantar warts grow in clusters they are known as mosaic warts. Most plantar warts do not stick up above the surface like common warts because the pressure of walking flattens them and pushes them back into the skin. Like common warts, these warts may have black dots. Plantar warts have a bad reputation because they can be painful, feeling like a stone in the shoe.

Flat warts are smaller and smoother than other warts. They tend to grow in large numbers—twenty to one hundred at any one time. They can occur anywhere, but in children they are most common on the face.

In adults they are often found in the beard area in men and on the legs in women. Irritation from shaving probably accounts for this.

How do you get warts?

Warts are passed from person to person, sometimes indirectly. The time from the first contact to the time the warts have grown large enough to be seen is often several months. The risk of catching hand, foot, or flat warts from another person is small.

Why do some people get warts and others don't?

Some people get warts depending on how often they are exposed to the virus. Wart viruses occur more easily if the skin has been damaged in some way, which explains the high frequency of warts in children who bite their nails or pick at hangnails. Some people are just more likely to catch the wart virus than are others, just as some people catch colds very easily. Patients with a weakened immune system also are more prone to a wart virus infection.

Do warts need to be treated?

In children, warts can disappear without treatment over a period of several months to years. However, warts that are bothersome, painful, or rapidly multiplying should be treated. Warts in adults often do not disappear as easily or as quickly as they do in children.

How do dermatologists treat warts?

Dermatologists are trained to use a variety of treatments, depending on the age of the patient and the type of wart.

Common warts: Common warts in young children can be treated at home by their parents on a daily basis by applying salicylic acid gel, solution, or plaster. There is usually little discomfort but it can take many weeks of treatment to obtain favorable results. Treatment should be stopped at least temporarily if the wart becomes sore. Warts may also be treated by "painting" with cantharidin in the dermatologist's office. Cantharidin causes a blister to form under the wart. The dermatologist can then clip away the dead part of the wart in the blister roof in a week or so.

For adults and older children cryotherapy (freezing) is generally preferred. This treatment is not too painful and rarely results in scarring.

Viral Infections

However, repeat treatments at one- to three-week intervals are often necessary. Electrosurgery (burning) is another good alternative treatment. Laser treatment can also be used for resistant warts that have not responded to other therapies.

Foot warts: Foot warts are difficult to treat because the bulk of the wart lies below the skin surface. Treatments include the use of salicylic acid plasters, applying other chemicals to the wart, or one of the surgical treatments including laser surgery, electrosurgery, or cutting. The dermatologist may recommend a change in footwear to reduce pressure on the wart and ways to keep the foot dry since moisture tends to allow warts to spread.

Flat warts: Flat warts are often too numerous to treat with methods mentioned above. As a result, "peeling" methods using daily applications of salicylic acid, tretinoin, glycolic acid, or other surface peeling preparations are often recommended. For some adults, periodic office treatments for surgical treatments are sometimes necessary.

What are some of the other treatments for warts?

There are several different lasers used for the treatment of warts. Laser therapy is used to destroy some types of warts. Lasers are more expensive and require the injection of a local anesthesia to numb the area treated.

Another treatment is to inject each wart with an anti-cancer drug called bleomycin. The injections may be painful and can have other side effects.

Immunotherapy, which attempts to use the body's own rejection system, is another method of treatment. Several methods of immunotherapy are being used. With one method the patient is made allergic to a certain chemical, which is then painted on the wart. A mild allergic reaction occurs around the treated warts, and may result in the disappearance of the warts.

Warts may also be injected with interferon, a treatment to boost the immune reaction and cause rejection of the wart.

Can I treat my own warts without seeing a doctor?

There are some wart remedies available without a prescription. However, you might mistake another kind of skin growth for a wart, and end up treating something more serious as though it were a wart.

If you have any questions about either the diagnosis or the best way to treat a wart, you should seek your dermatologist's advice.

What about the use of hypnosis or "folk" remedies?

Many people, patients and doctors alike, believe folk remedies and hypnosis are effective. Since warts, especially in children, may disappear without treatment, it's hard to know whether it was a folk remedy or just the passage of time that led to the cure. Since warts are generally harmless, there may be times when these treatments are appropriate. Medical treatments can always be used if necessary.

What about the problem of recurrent warts?

Sometimes it seems as if new warts appear as fast as old ones go away. This may happen because the old warts have shed virus into the surrounding skin before they were treated. In reality new "baby" warts are growing up around the original "mother" warts. The best way to limit this is to treat new warts as quickly as they develop so they have little time to shed virus into nearby skin. A check by your dermatologist can help assure the treated wart has resolved completely.

Is there any research going on about warts?

Research is moving along very rapidly. There is great interest in new treatments, as well as the development of a vaccine against warts. We hope there will be a solution to the annoying problem of warts in the not too distant future.

Chapter 13

Encephalitis

Definition

Encephalitis is an inflammation (irritation and swelling) of the brain, usually caused by infections.

Causes

Encephalitis is most often caused by a viral infection, and many types of viruses may cause it. Exposure to viruses can occur through insect bites, food or drink contamination, inhalation of respiratory droplets from an infected person, or skin contact. In rural areas, arboviruses—carried by mosquitoes or ticks, or accidentally ingested, are the most common cause.

In urban areas, enteroviruses are most common, including coxsackievirus, poliovirus, and echovirus. Other causes include herpes simplex infection, varicella (chickenpox or shingles), measles, mumps, rubella, adenovirus, rabies, eastern equine encephalitis virus, West Nile virus, and extremely rarely, allergic reaction to vaccinations.

Once the virus has entered the bloodstream, it may localize in the brain, causing inflammation of brain tissue and surrounding membranes. White blood cells invade the brain tissue as they try to fight off the infection.

© 2008 A.D.A.M., Inc. Reprinted with permission.

The brain tissue swells (cerebral edema), which may cause destruction of nerve cells, bleeding within the brain (intracerebral hemorrhage), and brain damage.

Encephalitis is uncommon. It affects approximately 1,500 people per year in the U.S. The elderly and infants are more vulnerable and may have a more severe course of the disease.

Although most forms of encephalitis are caused by viruses, bacteria can also cause this problem. For example, Lyme disease, syphilis, and tuberculosis, all caused by bacteria, can cause encephalitis. acquired immunodeficiency syndrome (AIDS) patients and various other high-risk individuals throughout the world can develop encephalitis due to parasites such as toxoplasmosis. Autoimmune disease and effects of cancer can also cause encephalitis.

Symptoms

- Fever
- Headache
- Vomiting
- Light sensitivity
- Stiff neck and back (occasionally)
- Confusion, disorientation
- Drowsiness
- Clumsiness, unsteady gait
- Irritability or poor temper control

Emergency symptoms:

- Loss of consciousness, poor responsiveness, stupor, coma
- Seizures
- Muscle weakness or paralysis
- Sudden onset of:
    - Memory loss (amnesia), impaired short-term memory, or impaired long-term memory
- "Flat" mood or lack of discernible mood, or mood inappropriate for the situation
- Diminished interest in daily activities

Encephalitis

- Inflexibility, extreme self-centeredness, indecisiveness, or withdrawal from social interaction
- Impaired judgment

Exams and Tests

Various symptoms resembling meningitis may be present. An examination may show signs of meningeal irritation (especially neck stiffness), increased intracranial pressure, or other neurologic symptoms such as muscle weakness, mental confusion, speech problems, and abnormal reflexes. The patient may have a skin rash, mouth ulcers, and signs of involvement of other organs such as the liver and lungs.

A lumbar puncture test and cerebrospinal fluid (CSF) examination may show clear fluid, high pressure, high white blood cell count, and high protein levels—indications of inflammation. Blood may be present in the CSF.

Sometimes the virus can be detected in CSF, blood, or urine through a laboratory test called viral culture. However, this test is cumbersome and rarely useful. In some cases, viral PCR (polymerase chain reaction, a test able to detect very tiny amounts of viral DNA) may identify the virus. Health care providers also rely on serology tests to provide evidence of viral infection. Serologies detect proteins called antibodies, which are produced in response to a specific virus or other foreign invader.

An electroencephalogram (EEG), a test of the electrical activity of the brain, may provide indirect clues for the diagnosis of encephalitis. Some EEG wave patterns may suggest a seizure disorder, or point to a specific virus as cause of the infection. Certain EEG wave patterns can suggest encephalitis due to herpes, for instance.

A brain magnetic resonance image (MRI), which provides high-quality pictures of the brain, or a computed tomography (CT) scan of the head may be used to determine internal bleeding or specific areas of brain inflammation.

Treatment

The goals of treatment are to provide supportive care and relieve symptoms. Antiviral medications, such as acyclovir (Zovirax®) and foscarnet (Foscavir®) may be prescribed for herpes encephalitis or other severe viral infections. Most of the time, however, no specific antiviral drugs are available to combat the infection.

Antibiotics may be prescribed when the infection is caused by some organisms, such as certain bacteria. Anti-seizure medications (such a phenytoin) are used to suppress seizures. On rare occasions, steroids, which are strong anti-inflammatory drugs (such as dexamethasone) are used to reduce brain swelling.

Sedatives may be needed to treat irritability or restlessness. Other medications, like acetaminophen, may be used for fever and headache.

Supportive care (rest, nutrition, fluids) allows the body to fight the infection. Reorientation and emotional support of confused or delirious persons may be helpful.

If brain function is severely affected, interventions like physical therapy and speech therapy may be necessary after the acute illness is controlled.

Outlook (Prognosis)

The outcome varies. Some cases are mild, short, and relatively harmless, followed by full recovery. Other cases are severe, and permanent impairment or death is possible.

The acute phase normally lasts for one to two weeks, with gradual or sudden disappearance of fever and neurologic symptoms. Neurologic symptoms may require many months before full recovery.

Possible Complications

Permanent brain damage that affects memory, speech, vision, hearing, muscle control, or sensation may occur in people who survive severe cases of encephalitis.

When to Contact a Medical Professional

Go to the emergency room or call the local emergency number (such as 911) if sudden fever, neurologic changes, and other symptoms suggestive of encephalitis occur.

Prevention

Controlling mosquitoes (a mosquito bite can transmit some viruses) may reduce the chance of some infections that can lead to encephalitis.

Animal vaccination is important to prevent encephalitis caused by rabies virus. Vaccination is available to prevent a form of viral encephalitis that often affects people living in dorms or in the military.

Chapter 14

Meningitis

What is meningitis?

Meningitis is an infection of the fluid of a person's spinal cord and the fluid that surrounds the brain. People sometimes refer to it as spinal meningitis. Meningitis is usually caused by a viral or bacterial infection. Knowing whether meningitis is caused by a virus or bacterium is important because the severity of illness and the treatment differ. Viral meningitis is generally less severe and resolves without specific treatment, while bacterial meningitis can be quite severe and may result in brain damage, hearing loss, or learning disability. For bacterial meningitis, it is also important to know which type of bacteria is causing the meningitis because antibiotics can prevent some types from spreading and infecting other people. Before the 1990s, *Haemophilus influenzae* type b (Hib) was the leading cause of bacterial meningitis, but new vaccines being given to all children as part of their routine immunizations have reduced the occurrence of invasive disease due to *H. influenzae*. Today, *Streptococcus pneumoniae* and *Neisseria meningitidis* are the leading causes of bacterial meningitis.

What are the signs and symptoms of meningitis?

High fever, headache, and stiff neck are common symptoms of meningitis in anyone over the age of two years. These symptoms can develop

---

"Meningococcal Disease," Centers for Disease Control and Prevention, October 12, 2005.

over several hours, or they may take one to two days. Other symptoms may include nausea, vomiting, discomfort looking into bright lights, confusion, and sleepiness. In newborns and small infants, the classic symptoms of fever, headache, and neck stiffness may be absent or difficult to detect, and the infant may only appear slow or inactive, be irritable, have vomiting, or be feeding poorly. As the disease progresses, patients of any age may have seizures.

How is meningitis diagnosed?

Early diagnosis and treatment are very important. If symptoms occur, the patient should see a doctor immediately. The diagnosis is usually made by growing bacteria from a sample of spinal fluid. The spinal fluid is obtained by performing a spinal tap, in which a needle is inserted into an area in the lower back where fluid in the spinal canal is readily accessible. Identification of the type of bacteria responsible is important for selection of correct antibiotics.

Can meningitis be treated?

Bacterial meningitis can be treated with a number of effective antibiotics. It is important, however, that treatment be started early in the course of the disease.

Appropriate antibiotic treatment of most common types of bacterial meningitis should reduce the risk of dying from meningitis to below 15 percent, although the risk is higher among the elderly.

Is meningitis contagious?

Yes, some forms of bacterial meningitis are contagious. The bacteria are spread through the exchange of respiratory and throat secretions (i.e., coughing, kissing). Fortunately, none of the bacteria that cause meningitis are as contagious as things like the common cold or the flu, and they are not spread by casual contact or by simply breathing the air where a person with meningitis has been.

However, sometimes the bacteria that cause meningitis have spread to other people who have had close or prolonged contact with a patient with meningitis caused by *Neisseria meningitidis* (also called meningococcal meningitis) or Hib. People in the same household or daycare center, or anyone with direct contact with a patient's oral secretions (such as a boyfriend or girlfriend) would be considered at increased risk of acquiring the infection. People who qualify as close contacts of a person with meningitis caused by *N. meningitidis* should

Meningitis

receive antibiotics to prevent them from getting the disease. Antibiotics for contacts of a person with Hib meningitis disease are no longer recommended if all contacts four years of age or younger are fully vaccinated against Hib disease.

Are there vaccines against meningitis?

Yes, there are vaccines against Hib, against some serogroups of *N. meningitidis*, and against many types of *Streptococcus pneumoniae*. The vaccines against Hib are very safe and highly effective.

There are two vaccines against *N. meningitidis* available in the United States. Meningococcal polysaccharide vaccine (MPSV4 or Menomune®) has been approved by the Food and Drug Administration (FDA) and available since 1981. Meningococcal conjugate vaccine (MCV4 or MenactraT®) was licensed in 2005. Both vaccines can prevent four types of meningococcal disease, including two of the three types most common in the United States (serogroup C, Y, and W-135) and a type that causes epidemics in Africa (serogroup A). Meningococcal vaccines cannot prevent all types of the disease. But they do protect many people who might become sick if they didn't get the vaccine. Meningitis cases should be reported to state or local health departments to assure follow-up of close contacts and recognize outbreaks.

MCV4 is recommended for all children at their routine preadolescent visit (eleven to twelve years of age). For those who have never gotten MCV4 previously, a dose is recommended at high school entry. Other adolescents who want to decrease their risk of meningococcal disease can also get the vaccine. Other people at increased risk for whom routine vaccination is recommended are college freshmen living in dormitories, microbiologists who are routinely exposed to meningococcal bacteria, U.S. military recruits, anyone who has a damaged spleen or whose spleen has been removed; anyone who has terminal complement component deficiency (an immune system disorder), anyone who is traveling to the countries which have an outbreak of meningococcal disease, and those who might have been exposed to meningitis during an outbreak. MCV4 is the preferred vaccine for people eleven to fifty-five years of age in these risk groups, but MPSV4 can be used if MCV4 is not available. MPSV4 should be used for children two to ten years old, and adults over fifty-five, who are at risk.

Although large epidemics of meningococcal meningitis do not occur in the United States, some countries experience large, periodic epidemics. Overseas travelers should check to see if meningococcal vaccine is recommended for their destination. Travelers should receive the vaccine at least one week before departure, if possible. Information on areas for which meningococcal vaccine is recommended can be obtained by calling the Centers for Disease Control and Prevention.

There are vaccines to prevent meningitis due to *S. pneumoniae* (also called pneumococcal meningitis) which can also prevent other forms of infection due to *S. pneumoniae*. The pneumococcal polysaccharide vaccine is recommended for all persons over sixty-five years of age and younger persons at least two years old with certain chronic medical problems. There is a newly licensed vaccine (pneumococcal conjugate vaccine) that appears to be effective in infants for the prevention of pneumococcal infections and is routinely recommended for all children greater than two years of age.

Chapter 15

Pneumonia

Pneumonia is a potentially fatal infection that causes inflammation (redness and swelling) inside the lungs, resulting in breathing difficulty.

Among the most vital organs, the lungs pump air in and out of the body so that blood can exchange carbon dioxide for the oxygen that it circulates through the body. When breathing in, air flows through the trachea (windpipe) and then into two branches called bronchi inside the lungs. In turn the bronchi subdivide almost twenty times into smaller and smaller passages creating numerous bronchioles (smaller airways). Each of these airways ends in a cluster of tiny air sacs called alveoli. This creates a vast amount of surface where the blood can collect oxygen inside a small space, the chest cavity.

When certain foreign materials, bacteria, fungi, or viruses enter the body through the lungs and penetrate the natural defenses in the lungs, pneumonia can develop. What is commonly referred to as pneumonia is actually more than fifty variations of the condition, ranging from mild (such as "walking pneumonia") to life threatening. It may affect only one lung or both lungs (sometimes called double pneumonia). Pneumonia can occur independently, after certain illnesses (e.g., colds or influenza), or along with other illnesses.

More than sixty thousand Americans die each year from pneumonia. It can strike people of any age, but it is of greatest risk to the elderly, infants and very young children, and persons with chronic illnesses.

"Pneumonia," © Cedars-Sinai Medical Center. All rights reserved. Reprinted with permission. The text of this document is available online at http://www.csmc.edu/6038.html; accessed February 6, 2008.

Symptoms

Although early treatment is the best way to recover fully and quickly, pneumonia is challenging to diagnose. It sometimes seems like a simple cold or the flu, and its signs can vary depending on what is causing the pneumonia. Symptoms include:

- a persistent cough;
- an unexplained fever, especially one of 102° F or higher for several days in a row;
- chest pain that changes with breathing;
- chills and sweats;
- shortness of breath;
- suddenly feeling worse after a cold or influenza.

Anyone with these symptoms should not hesitate to call a doctor. People who should be especially concerned with these symptoms include older adults and individuals who are undergoing chemotherapy, have a suppressed immune system, are taking drugs that suppress the immune system (e.g., prednisone), are affected by alcoholism, have been injured, are confined to bed, or have heart conditions or other conditions that affect the ability to breathe.

Pneumonia can turn fatal within twenty-four hours under certain conditions. Seeking early treatment is important to ensure that the condition does not become life threatening. Some complications that can occur with pneumonia are as follows:

- The lungs may swell because the disease can fill up the air spaces inside the lungs, making breathing difficult.
- The infection that causes the pneumonia can spread into the bloodstream and then to other organs.
- Fluid can collect between the lining (pleurae) of the lungs and the lining of the inside of the chest. When fluid collects inside it is called pleural effusion. This fluid can become infected (a condition known as empyema) and may need to be drained through a tube inserted between the ribs.

Causes

Some of the organisms that cause pneumonia are commonly found in the air. The lung's natural defenses normally protect against infection

Pneumonia

from these organisms, but they sometimes break through these defenses. Pneumonia may be caused by any of the following:

- **Bacteria:** The most common cause of pneumonia is bacterial infection, and many different bacteria can cause the condition, producing mild to severe cases. Bacterial pneumonia can occur independently or following illnesses, such as colds, flu, or upper respiratory infections.

- **Fungi:** Certain types of fungus can cause pneumonia. When the fungus is inhaled, some people develop symptoms of acute pneumonia, others develop a form that lasts for months, although most people experience few if any symptoms. *Pneumocystis carinii*, a yeast-like fungi that is known as an opportunistic infection because it usually affects individuals with compromised immune systems, such as those with acquired immunodeficiency syndrome (AIDS) or undergoing chemotherapy.

- **Viruses:** Several different viruses can cause pneumonia, including some of the same viruses that cause influenza. This type of pneumonia usually hits in the fall and winter and is more serious in people with heart or lung disease. People who have viral pneumonia can also develop bacterial pneumonia.

- **Other microorganisms:** In rare cases, other living organisms may be responsible for pneumonia. These organisms include amoebas and mycoplasmas (which have characteristics of both bacteria and virus).

- **Other foreign materials:** Pneumonia can occur when food, mucus, vomit, chemicals, or other substances enter the lungs. Called aspiration pneumonia, this condition can develop from accidentally inhaling substances during a seizure, unconsciousness, or stroke.

Risk Factors

Persons who are at greater risk of developing pneumonia include those who:

- abuse alcohol (alcohol interferes with the action of the white blood cells, which fight infections);
- abuse drugs (injection of illegal drugs can put you at greater risk of getting infections that can affect your lungs);

- are age sixty-five or older;
- are smokers (smoke damages the air passages inside the lungs);
- are very young children (whose immune systems are not fully developed);
- have an impaired immune system due to chemotherapy, immunosuppressant drugs, or illness;
- have been exposed to certain chemicals or pollutants;
- have certain diseases, such as human immunodeficiency virus (HIV)/AIDS, heart disease, emphysema, or diabetes;
- have had the spleen removed;
- live in areas where exposure to types of fungus is greater (An example is valley fever, which is widespread throughout Southern California and the desert of the Southwest. This fungus does not affect everyone who is exposed to it, but a few develop severe pneumonia.)

Diagnosis

To diagnose pneumonia, doctors usually begin with a medical history and a physical examination. Often the medical history may indicate a risk of having pneumonia. During the examination, the doctor uses a stethoscope to listen for abnormal bubbling, crackling, or rumbling sounds that may indicate thick liquid in the lungs or inflammation (swelling) from an infection.

The doctor may recommend a blood test to check the white blood cell count and to detect viruses, bacteria, or other organisms. A phlegm sample may be tested to help determine the cause of the pneumonia.

The doctor may also recommend a chest x-ray to confirm the diagnosis and to note the location and spread of the infection. If the x-ray does not confirm pneumonia, more sophisticated imaging may be needed, such as computed tomography (CT) scan.

Treatment

Because pneumonia has different causes and different degrees of seriousness, treatment will vary according to the type of pneumonia a person has. Prescribed treatment may include the following:

- **Antibiotics:** Normally given for bacterial infections, antibiotics may also be prescribed for other types of pneumonia. Antibiotics

Pneumonia

should be taken for the complete period prescribed to prevent the infection from returning and to reduce the formation of antibiotic-resistant bacteria.

- **Bed rest:** Stress and fatigue can weaken the immune system, which could allow a relapse.
- **Fluids:** Drinking plenty of fluids, especially water, helps prevent dehydration and break up phlegm in the lungs.
- **Over-the-counter medications:** These medications may be recommended to alleviate aches, pains, coughing, and fever.
- **Oxygen:** In severe cases involving breathing difficulty, oxygen may be administered for several days.

About four to six weeks after treatment for pneumonia, the doctor will probably schedule a follow-up visit. Because the lungs may still be infected, the doctor will track the patient's progress to prevent a relapse or complications. Patients who are not feeling better by that time may need more tests to find out why.

Prevention

Pneumonia usually is not something that a person "catches" from other people. People with pneumonia, however, may want to stay away from those with compromised immune systems. People can develop pneumonia due to weakened resistance. The following may be helpful in avoiding pneumonia, especially for those at greater risk of developing it:

- Do not smoke. Smoking damages the lungs' ability to protect against infections.
- Get enough rest and moderate exercise, and eat a die rich in fruits, vegetables, and whole grains. These measures boost strength and help protect against serious illnesses and infections.
- Get vaccinated against pneumococcal pneumonia at least once after the age of sixty-five. People with chronic lung or heart disease, diabetes, or sickle cell anemia and those with the spleen removed, on chemotherapy, or who have a lowered immune system may want to discuss a pneumonia vaccination with their doctor. Prevnar®, a pneumonia vaccine, can help protect young children under the age of two or those who are older and have a special risk of getting pneumonia.

Childhood Diseases and Disorders Sourcebook, Second Edition

- Get vaccinated against the flu every year because pneumonia can be a complication of having the flu.
- Regularly wash hands, which come in contact every day with many germs, including those that cause pneumonia. Hand washing also helps reduce chances of getting colds and flu.

Chapter 16

Reye Syndrome

What is Reye syndrome?

Reye syndrome is a rare illness that affects all bodily organs but is most harmful to the brain and the liver. It occurs primarily among children who are recovering from a viral infection, such as chicken pox or the flu. It usually develops a week after the onset of the viral illness but can also occur a few days after onset. Liver-related complications of Reye syndrome include fatty deposits, abnormal liver function tests, and poor blood clotting and bleeding caused by liver failure.

What are the symptoms of Reye syndrome?

Reye syndrome is often misdiagnosed as encephalitis, meningitis, diabetes, drug overdose, poisoning, sudden infant death syndrome, or psychiatric illness.

Symptoms include persistent or recurrent vomiting, listlessness, personality changes such as irritability or combativeness, disorientation, delirium, convulsions, and loss of consciousness. If these symptoms are present during or soon after a viral illness, medical attention should be sought immediately. The symptoms of Reye syndrome in infants do not follow a typical pattern; for example, vomiting does not

"Reye Syndrome," © 2007 American Liver Foundation (www.liverfoundation.org). All rights reserved. Reprinted with permission.

always occur. The onset of Reye syndrome can be rapid, and signs and symptoms may worsen within hours.

What causes Reye syndrome?

The cause of Reye syndrome remains a mystery. However studies have shown that using aspirin to treat viral illnesses increases the risk of developing Reye syndrome. A physician should be consulted before giving a child any aspirin or anti-nausea medicines during a viral illness, which could hide the symptoms of the condition.

How is Reye syndrome diagnosed?

If your child becomes sick with a possible case of Reye syndrome, doctors will want blood tests to evaluate his or her liver function. They may also evaluate other possible causes of liver problems and make sure your child does not have one of the rare inherited disorders that mimic Reye syndrome. In addition to blood and urine tests, diagnostic procedures may include spinal taps or liver biopsy.

How is Reye syndrome treated?

There is no cure for Reye syndrome. Successful management, which relies on early diagnosis, is aimed primarily at protecting the brain from irreversible damage by reducing brain swelling, preventing complications in the lungs, and anticipating cardiac arrest.

If my child has been diagnosed with Reye syndrome, what should I ask our doctor?

Speak to your doctor about possible long-term complications connected with Reye syndrome. Though rare, Reye syndrome can result in permanent liver or nervous system damage.

Who is at risk for Reye syndrome?

Reye syndrome occurs most commonly in children between the ages of four and twelve, although it can occur at any age. It usually develops about a week after common viral infections such as influenza or chickenpox. Reye syndrome can also develop after an ordinary upper respiratory infection such as a cold. The precise reason is unknown, but using aspirin to treat a viral illness or infection may trigger the condition in children.

Reye Syndrome

Reye syndrome may be a metabolic condition—one without symptoms (asymptomatic)—that is unmasked by viral illnesses.

What is the best way to prevent Reye syndrome?

To reduce the risk of Reye syndrome, avoid giving aspirin or medications that contain aspirin to your child to treat viral illnesses. Other names for aspirin include: acetylsalicylic acid, acetylsalicylate, salicylic acid, and salicylate. Unless specifically instructed to do so by your child's doctor, do not give aspirin to anyone younger than nineteen.

If your child or teenager has the flu or chickenpox, use other medications such as acetaminophen, ibuprofen, or naproxen sodium to reduce fever or relieve pain. Check the label on any medication to make sure it does not include aspirin before giving it your child, and be sure to give the correct dose.

Chapter 17

Parasitic and Fungal Infections

Chapter Contents

Section 17.1—Ascariasis 178
Section 17.2—*Baylisascaris* Infection 180
Section 17.3—Cryptosporidiosis 182
Section 17.4—Giardiasis 188
Section 17.5—*Hymenolepis* (Dwarf Tapeworm) Infection 193
Section 17.6—Pediculosis (Head Lice) 195
Section 17.7—Pinworm Infection 202
Section 17.8—Scabies 204
Section 17.9—Swimmer's Itch 207
Section 17.10—Tinea 209
Section 17.11—Toxocariasis 212

Section 17.1

Ascariasis

National Institute of Allergy and Infectious Diseases,
September 13, 2007.

Overview

Ascariasis, or roundworm infection of the intestines, is common throughout the world in both temperate and tropical areas where sanitation and hygiene are poor. In those areas, everyone may be harboring the parasite.

Ascariasis is one of the most common human parasitic infections. An estimated 1.4 billion people worldwide have ascariasis, and the disease is most common in children between the ages of three and eight. According to the World Health Organization, ascariasis causes approximately sixty thousand deaths annually worldwide.

Cause

Ascaris infection is caused by a parasitic roundworm called *Ascaris lumbricoides*. This worm resembles the common earthworm. Ranging in length from six to thirteen inches, the female worm may grow to be as thick as a pencil. Up to one hundred worms could potentially infect the human body.

Transmission

Almost more than any other parasitic disease, inadequate personal hygiene leads to *Ascaris* infection. Human feces found in fields, streets, and backyards are a major source of infective eggs in heavily populated areas.

The eggs do not infect humans when first excreted by the roundworm. They usually are transmitted by hand to mouth. The use of human feces as fertilizer may also permit transmission of infective eggs through food that is grown in the soil and eaten without being thoroughly washed. The eggs are resistant to extremes of temperature and humidity.

Parasitic and Fungal Infections

The eggs require several weeks to develop and become infective. If you swallow infective eggs, they pass into your intestines, where they hatch into larvae and then begin their journey through your body. Once through your intestinal wall, the eggs reach your lungs by means of the bloodstream or lymphatic system.

In your lungs, they pass through the air sacs and are carried up the bronchial tree with respiratory secretions and into your throat.

When in your throat, you re-swallow them, and they return to the small intestine, where they grow, mature, and mate.

The worms become mature in about two months.

Symptoms

If you have only a few roundworms in your intestines, you might not have symptoms. If you do have symptoms, you may have vague or sporadic feelings of abdominal pain.

The first sign of infection may be the presence of a live worm in your vomit or stool. If the larvae have migrated to your lungs, you may have an illness resembling pneumonia with wheezing, cough, and fever. This stage of the disease precedes the intestinal phase by weeks, and the symptoms are difficult for a healthcare provider to diagnose.

If you have a heavy infection of the worms, you may have a partial or complete blockage of the small intestine and experience the following symptoms:

- Severe abdominal pain
- Vomiting
- Restlessness
- Disturbed sleep

The heavier or greater the worm infection, the more severe your symptoms are likely to be. Your pancreas might become inflamed. Serious infections, especially those causing blockages, can be fatal.

Diagnosis

Once mature female roundworms are in your intestines, a healthcare provider can diagnose the infection by finding the eggs (or live worms) in your stool.

Lung infection is more difficult to diagnose, but can be confirmed by finding evidence of the larvae in lung or stomach fluids.

Treatment

Your healthcare provider can treat *Ascaris* infection successfully with mebendazole, albendazole, or pyrantel pamoate.

Section 17.2

Baylisascaris *Infection*

"*Baylisascaris procyonis* (Raccoon Round Worm),"
© 2008 Wisconsin Department of Health and Family Services (www.dhfs.wisconsin.gov). Reprinted with permission.

What is Baylisascaris procyonis?

This is a large roundworm parasite that lives in the intestines of raccoons. The worm does not harm the raccoon, but on rare occasions can cause serious illness in humans.

How is this raccoon roundworm spread?

The adult worms shed microscopic eggs that are passed in the raccoon's feces. Millions of eggs may be passed each day. These eggs can survive for months to years in the environment. The parasite is transmitted when the eggs are ingested by another animal. Humans generally become infected from accidentally ingesting eggs from soil, water, hands, or other objects which are contaminated with raccoon feces.

What are the signs and symptoms of Baylisascaris procyonis *in humans?*

The severity of the disease depends to a large extent on how many eggs are ingested. These eggs hatch into larvae which then cause disease by migrating through the central nervous system, eyes, and other organs. Symptoms include nausea, lethargy, liver enlargement, incoordination, loss of muscle control, coma, and blindness. Fatalities are extremely rare, but have been reported. There have been no human cases ever reported in Wisconsin.

Parasitic and Fungal Infections

How soon after infection do symptoms appear?

In general, symptoms appear one to three weeks post-infection, although they may take as long as two months. This interval depends on the number of eggs ingested.

Who is at greatest risk for Baylisascaris procyonis *infection?*

Because of young children's tendency to put their fingers or objects into their mouths, such children are at risk if they play in areas which are frequented by raccoons. Hunters, trappers, taxidermists, and wildlife rehabilitators are also at increased risk if they handle raccoons or items contaminated with raccoon feces. In general, the risk of acquiring the infection is very low, and requires a fairly substantial exposure to raccoon feces.

How are Baylisascaris procyonis *infections treated in humans?*

There are no consistently effective treatment regimens available at this time.

How can I avoid exposure to this parasite?

Do not keep raccoons as pets; this is not only dangerous, it is also illegal. Baby raccoons are often infected. Discourage raccoons from visiting your home or yard by eliminating access to food sources like garbage cans and bird feeders. Raccoons may nest in (and defecate on) places like woodpiles, attics, chimneys, sheds, and barn lofts. Entrances to these areas can be sealed when the raccoons are away. Accumulated feces and contaminated wood, soil, hay, or straw should be removed and burned or deeply buried in a site remote from houses. It is important to wear disposable gloves, boots, and a dust mask (such as a painter's mask) when disposing of such material. Contaminated surfaces can be decontaminated by flaming with a propane torch (used for concrete and other nonflammable surfaces) or with boiling Lysol.

Childhood Diseases and Disorders Sourcebook, Second Edition

Section 17.3

Cryptosporidiosis

"*Cryptosporidium* Infection," Centers for
Disease Control and Prevention, December 18, 2007.

What is cryptosporidiosis?

Cryptosporidiosis is a diarrheal disease caused by microscopic parasites of the genus *Cryptosporidium*. Once an animal or person is infected, the parasite lives in the intestine and passes in the stool. The parasite is protected by an outer shell that allows it to survive outside the body for long periods of time and makes it very resistant to chlorine-based disinfectants. Both the disease and the parasite are commonly known as "Crypto."

During the past two decades, Crypto has become recognized as one of the most common causes of waterborne disease (recreational water and drinking water) in humans in the United States. The parasite is found in every region of the United States and throughout the world.

How is cryptosporidiosis spread?

Cryptosporidium lives in the intestine of infected humans or animals. Millions of crypto parasites can be released in a bowel movement from an infected human or animal. Consequently, *Cryptosporidium* is found in soil, food, water, or surfaces that have been contaminated with infected human or animal feces. A person becomes infected by swallowing *Cryptosporidium* parasites. You cannot become infected through contact with blood. Crypto can be spread in the following ways:

- By putting something in your mouth or accidentally swallowing something that has come in contact with the stool of a person or animal infected with Crypto.

- By swallowing recreational water contaminated with Crypto. Recreational water is water in swimming pools, hot tubs, Jacuzzis, fountains, lakes, rivers, springs, ponds, or streams that can be contaminated with sewage or feces from humans or animals.

Parasitic and Fungal Infections

- By swallowing water or beverages contaminated by stool from infected humans or animals.
- By eating uncooked food contaminated with Crypto. Thoroughly wash with uncontaminated water all vegetables and fruits you plan to eat raw. See below for information on making water safe.
- By touching your mouth with contaminated hands. Hands can become contaminated through a variety of activities, such as touching surfaces (e.g., toys, bathroom fixtures, changing tables, diaper pails) that have been contaminated by stool from an infected person, changing diapers, caring for an infected person, and handling an infected cow or calf.

What are the symptoms of cryptosporidiosis?

The most common symptom of cryptosporidiosis is watery diarrhea. Other symptoms include the following:

- Stomach cramps or pain
- Dehydration
- Nausea
- Vomiting
- Fever
- Weight loss

Some people with Crypto will have no symptoms at all. While the small intestine is the site most commonly affected, *Cryptosporidium* infections could possibly affect other areas of the digestive tract or the respiratory tract.

How long after infection do symptoms appear?

Symptoms of cryptosporidiosis generally begin two to ten days (average seven days) after becoming infected with the parasite.

How long will symptoms last?

In persons with healthy immune systems, symptoms usually last about one to two weeks. The symptoms may go in cycles in which you may seem to get better for a few days, then feel worse again before the illness ends.

Who is most at risk for cryptosporidiosis?

People who are most likely to become infected with *Cryptosporidium* include the following:

- Children who attend daycare centers, including diaper-aged children
- Child care workers
- Parents of infected children
- People who take care of other people with cryptosporidiosis
- International travelers
- Backpackers, hikers, and campers who drink unfiltered, untreated water
- People, including swimmers, who swallow water from contaminated sources
- People who handle infected cattle
- People exposed to human feces through sexual contact

Contaminated water may include water that has not been boiled or filtered, as well as contaminated recreational water sources (e.g., swimming pools, lakes, rivers, ponds, and streams). Several community-wide outbreaks of cryptosporidiosis have been linked to drinking municipal water or recreational water contaminated with *Cryptosporidium*.

Who is most at risk for getting seriously ill with cryptosporidiosis?

Although Crypto can infect all people, some groups are more likely to develop more serious illness.

Young children and pregnant women may be more susceptible to the dehydration resulting from diarrhea and should drink plenty of fluids while ill.

If you have a severely weakened immune system, you are at risk for more serious disease. Your symptoms may be more severe and could lead to serious or life-threatening illness. Examples of persons with weakened immune systems include those with acquired immunodeficiency syndrome (AIDS); cancer and transplant patients who are taking certain immunosuppressive drugs; and those with inherited diseases that affect the immune system.

Parasitic and Fungal Infections

What should I do if I think I may have cryptosporidiosis?

If you suspect that you have cryptosporidiosis, see your health care provider.

How is a cryptosporidiosis diagnosed?

Your health care provider will ask you to submit stool samples to see if you are infected. Because testing for Crypto can be difficult, you may be asked to submit several stool specimens over several days. Tests for Crypto are not routinely done in most laboratories. Therefore, your health care provider should specifically request testing for the parasite.

What is the treatment for cryptosporidiosis?

Nitazoxanide has been approved for treatment of diarrhea caused by *Cryptosporidium* in people with healthy immune systems. Consult with your health care provider for more information. Most people who have healthy immune systems will recover without treatment. Diarrhea can be managed by drinking plenty of fluids to prevent dehydration. Young children and pregnant women may be more susceptible to dehydration. Rapid loss of fluids from diarrhea may be especially life threatening to babies; therefore, parents should talk to their health care provider about fluid replacement therapy options for infants. Antidiarrheal medicine may help slow down diarrhea, but talk to your health care provider before taking it.

People who are in poor health or who have a weakened immune system are at higher risk for more severe and more prolonged illness. The effectiveness of nitazoxanide in immunosuppressed individuals is unclear. For persons with AIDS, anti-retroviral therapy that improves immune status will also decrease or eliminate symptoms of Crypto. However, even if symptoms disappear, cryptosporidiosis is often not curable and the symptoms may return if the immune status worsens. See your health care provider to discuss anti-retroviral therapy used to improve your immune status.

If I have been diagnosed with Cryptosporidium, should I worry about spreading the infection to others?

Yes, *Cryptosporidium* can be very contagious. Infected individuals should follow these guidelines to avoid spreading the disease to others:

- Wash your hands frequently with soap and water, especially after using the toilet, after changing diapers, and before eating or preparing food.

- Do not swim in recreational water (pools, hot tubs, lakes rivers, the ocean, etc.) if you have cryptosporidiosis and for at least two weeks after the diarrhea and/or symptoms stop. You can pass *Cryptosporidium* in your stool and contaminate water for several weeks after your symptoms have ended. You do not even need to have an accident in the water. Immersion in the water may be enough for contamination to occur. This has resulted in outbreaks of cryptosporidiosis among recreational water users. Note: You may not be protected in a chlorinated pool because *Cryptosporidium* is chlorine-resistant and can live for days in chlorine-treated swimming pools.

- Avoid sexual practices that might result in oral exposure to stool (e.g., oral-anal contact).

- Avoid close contact with anyone who has a weakened immune system.

How can I protect myself from cryptosporidiosis?

Practice good hygiene: Wash hands thoroughly and frequently with soap and water. Wash hands after using the toilet and before handling or eating food (especially for persons with diarrhea). Wash hands after every diaper change, especially if you work with diaper-aged children, even if you are wearing gloves. Protect others by not swimming if you are experiencing diarrhea (this is essential for children in diapers).

Avoid water that might be contaminated: Do not swallow recreational water. Do not drink untreated water from shallow wells, lakes, rivers, springs, ponds, and streams. Do not drink untreated water during community-wide outbreaks of disease caused by contaminated drinking water. Do not use or consume untreated ice or tap water when traveling in countries where the water supply might be unsafe.

In the United States, nationally distributed brands of bottled or canned carbonated soft drinks are safe to drink. Commercially packaged noncarbonated soft drinks and fruit juices that do not require refrigeration until after they are opened (those that are stored unrefrigerated on grocery shelves) also are safe.

Parasitic and Fungal Infections

If you are unable to avoid using or drinking water that might be contaminated, then you can treat the water for *Cryptosporidium* by heating the water to a rolling boil for at least one minute, or using a filter that has an absolute pore size of 1 micron or smaller, or one that has been National Science Foundation—rated for "cyst removal."

Do not rely on chemicals to kill *Cryptosporidium*. Because it has a thick outer shell, this particular parasite is highly resistant to disinfectants such as chlorine and iodine.

Avoid food that might be contaminated: Use safe, uncontaminated water to wash all food that is to be eaten raw. After washing vegetables and fruit in safe, uncontaminated water, peel them if you plan to eat them raw. Avoid eating uncooked foods when traveling in countries with minimal water treatment and sanitation systems.

Take extra care when traveling: If you travel to developing nations, you may be at a greater risk for *Cryptosporidium* infection because of poorer water treatment and food sanitation. Warnings about food, drinks, and swimming are even more important when visiting developing countries. Avoid foods and drinks, in particular raw fruits and vegetables, tap water, or ice made from tap water, unpasteurized milk or dairy products, and items purchased from street vendors. These items may be contaminated with *Cryptosporidium*. Steaming-hot foods, fruits you peel yourself, bottled and canned processed drinks, and hot coffee or hot tea are probably safe. Talk with your health care provider about other guidelines for travel abroad.

Section 17.4

Giardiasis

Centers for Disease Control and Prevention,
September 17, 2004. Reviewed by David A. Cooke, M.D., July 2008.

What is giardiasis?

Giardiasis is a diarrheal illness caused by a one-celled, microscopic parasite, *Giardia intestinalis* (also known as *Giardia lamblia*). Once an animal or person has been infected with *Giardia intestinalis*, the parasite lives in the intestine and is passed in the stool. Because the parasite is protected by an outer shell, it can survive outside the body and in the environment for long periods of time.

During the past two decades, *Giardia* infection has become recognized as one of the most common causes of waterborne disease (found in both drinking and recreational water) in humans in the United States. *Giardia* are found worldwide and within every region of the United States.

How do you get giardiasis and how is it spread?

The *Giardia* parasite lives in the intestine of infected humans or animals. Millions of germs can be released in a bowel movement from an infected human or animal. *Giardia* is found in soil, food, water, or surfaces that have been contaminated with the feces from infected humans or animals. You can become infected after accidentally swallowing the parasite; you cannot become infected through contact with blood. *Giardia* can be spread by any of the following:

- Accidentally putting something into your mouth or swallowing something that has come into contact with feces of a person or animal infected with *Giardia*.

- Swallowing recreational water contaminated with *Giardia*. Recreational water includes water in swimming pools, hot tubs, Jacuzzis, fountains, lakes, rivers, springs, ponds, or streams that can be contaminated with sewage or feces from humans or animals.

Parasitic and Fungal Infections

- Eating uncooked food contaminated with *Giardia*.
- Accidentally swallowing *Giardia* picked up from surfaces (such as bathroom fixtures, changing tables, diaper pails, or toys) contaminated with feces from an infected person.

What are the symptoms of giardiasis?

Giardia infection can cause a variety of intestinal symptoms, which include the following:

- Diarrhea
- Gas or flatulence
- Greasy stools that tend to float
- Stomach cramps
- Upset stomach or nausea

These symptoms may lead to weight loss and dehydration. Some people with giardiasis have no symptoms at all.

How long after infection do symptoms appear?

Symptoms of giardiasis normally begin one to two weeks (average seven days) after becoming infected.

How long will symptoms last?

In otherwise healthy persons, symptoms of giardiasis may last two to six weeks. Occasionally, symptoms last longer.

Who is most likely to get giardiasis?

Anyone can get giardiasis. Persons more likely to become infected include the following:

- Children who attend daycare centers, including diaper-aged children
- Child care workers
- Parents of infected children
- International travelers
- People who swallow water from contaminated sources

- Backpackers, hikers, and campers who drink unfiltered, untreated water
- Swimmers who swallow water while swimming in lakes, rivers, ponds, and streams
- People who drink from shallow wells

Contaminated water includes water that has not been boiled, filtered, or disinfected with chemicals. Several community-wide outbreaks of giardiasis have been linked to drinking municipal water or recreational water contaminated with *Giardia*.

What should I do if I think I may have giardiasis?

See your health care provider.

How is a Giardia *infection diagnosed?*

Your health care provider will likely ask you to submit stool samples to check for the parasite. Because *Giardia* can be difficult to diagnose, your provider may ask you to submit several stool specimens over several days.

What is the treatment for giardiasis?

Several prescription drugs are available to treat *Giardia*. Although *Giardia* can infect all people, young children and pregnant women may be more susceptible to dehydration resulting from diarrhea and should, therefore, drink plenty of fluids while ill.

My child does not have diarrhea, but was recently diagnosed as having giardiasis. My health care provider says treatment is not necessary. Is this true?

Treatment is not necessary when the child has no symptoms. However, there are a few exceptions. If your child does not have diarrhea, but is having nausea, fatigue (very tired), weight loss, or a poor appetite, you and your health care provider may wish to consider treatment. If your child attends a daycare center where an outbreak is continuing to occur despite efforts to control it, screening and treating children who have no obvious symptoms may be a good idea. The same is true if several family members are ill, or if a family member is pregnant and therefore not able to take the most effective anti-*Giardia* medications.

If I have been diagnosed with giardiasis, should I worry about spreading the infection to others?

Yes, a *Giardia* infection can be very contagious. Follow these guidelines to avoid spreading giardiasis to others:

- Wash your hands with soap and water after using the toilet, changing diapers, and before eating or preparing food.
- Do not swim in recreational water (pools, hot tubs, lakes or rivers, the ocean, etc.) if you have *Giardia* and for at least two weeks after diarrhea stops. You can pass *Giardia* in your stool and contaminate water for several weeks after your symptoms have ended. This has resulted in outbreaks of *Giardia* among recreational water users.
- Avoid fecal exposure during sexual activity.

How can I prevent a **Giardia** *infection?*

Practice good hygiene: Wash hands thoroughly with soap and water. Wash hands after using the toilet and before handling or eating food (especially for persons with diarrhea). Wash hands after every diaper change, especially if you work with diaper-aged children, even if you are wearing gloves. Protect others by not swimming if you are experiencing diarrhea (essential for children in diapers).

Avoid water that might be contaminated: Do not swallow recreational water. Do not drink untreated water from shallow wells, lakes, rivers, springs, ponds, and streams. Do not drink untreated water during community-wide outbreaks of disease caused by contaminated drinking water. Do not use untreated ice or drinking water when traveling in countries where the water supply might be unsafe.

In the United States, nationally distributed brands of bottled or canned carbonated soft drinks are safe to drink. Commercially packaged noncarbonated soft drinks and fruit juices that do not require refrigeration until after they are opened (those that are stored unrefrigerated on grocery shelves) also are safe.

If you are unable to avoid using or drinking water that might be contaminated, then you can make the water safe to drink by heating the water to a rolling boil for at least one minute or using a filter that has an absolute pore size of 1 micron or smaller, or one that has been National Science Foundation–rated for "cyst removal."

If you cannot heat the water to a rolling boil or use a recommended filter, then try chemically treating the water by chlorination or iodination. Using chemicals may be less effective than boiling or filtering because the amount of chemical required to make the water safe is highly dependent on the temperature, pH, and cloudiness of the water.

Avoid food that might be contaminated: Wash and/or peel all raw vegetables and fruits before eating. Use safe, uncontaminated water to wash all food that is to be eaten raw. Avoid eating uncooked foods when traveling in countries with minimal water treatment and sanitation systems.

If my water comes from a well, should I have my well water tested?

It depends. You should consider having your well water tested if you can answer "yes" to any of the following questions:

- Are members of your family or others who use your well water becoming ill? If yes, your well may be the source of infection.

- Is your well located at the bottom of a hill or is it considered shallow? If so, runoff from rain or floodwater may be draining directly into your well, causing contamination.

- Is your well in a rural area where animals graze? Well water can become contaminated with feces if animal waste seepage contaminates the ground water. This can occur if your well has cracked casings, is poorly constructed, or is too shallow.

Tests used to specifically identify *Giardia* are often expensive, difficult, and usually require hundreds of gallons of water to be pumped through a filter. If you answered "yes" to the above questions, consider generally testing your well for fecal contamination by testing it for the presence of coliforms or *E. coli* instead of *Giardia*. Although tests for fecal coliforms or *E. coli* do not specifically tell you whether *Giardia* is present, these tests will show whether your well water has been contaminated by fecal matter.

These tests are only useful if your well is not routinely disinfected with chlorine, since chlorine kills fecal coliforms and *E. coli*. If the tests are positive, it is possible that the water may also be contaminated with *Giardia* or other harmful bacteria and viruses. Contact your county health department, your county cooperative extension service, or a local laboratory to find out who offers water testing in your area.

Parasitic and Fungal Infections

If the fecal coliform test comes back positive, indicating that your well is fecally contaminated, stop drinking the well water and contact your local water authority for instructions on how to disinfect your well.

Section 17.5

Hymenolepis *(Dwarf Tapeworm)* Infection

"Hymenolepis Infection," Centers for Disease Control and Prevention, September 21, 2004. Reviewed by David A. Cooke, M.D., July 2008.

What is the most common kind of tapeworm infection?

The dwarf tapeworm or *Hymenolepis nana* is the most common tapeworm infection diagnosed in the in the United States and throughout the world. Infection is diagnosed in children, in persons living in institutional settings, and in people who live in areas where sanitation and personal hygiene is inadequate.

How did I get infected?

One can get infected by accidentally ingesting tapeworm eggs. This can happen by ingesting fecally contaminated foods and water, by touching your mouth with contaminated fingers, or by ingesting contaminated soil.

Adult tapeworms are very small in comparison with other tapeworms and may reach 15–40 mm (up to two inches) in length. The adult tapeworm is made up of many small segments, called proglottids. As the tapeworm matures inside the intestines, these segments break off and pass into the stool. An adult tapeworm can live for four to six weeks. However, once you are infected, the dwarf tapeworm may cause auto infection (the tapeworm may reproduce inside the body) and continue the infection.

What are the symptoms of a tapeworm infection?

Most people who are infected do not have any symptoms. Those who have symptoms may experience nausea, weakness, loss of appetite, diarrhea, and abdominal pain. Young children, especially those with a heavy infection, may develop a headache, itchy bottom, or have difficulty sleeping. Sometimes infection is misdiagnosed as a pinworm infection.

Contrary to popular belief, a tapeworm infection does not generally cause weight loss. You cannot feel the tapeworm inside your body.

How is tapeworm infection diagnosed?

Diagnosis is made by identifying tapeworm eggs in stool. Your health care provider will ask you to submit stool specimens collected over several days to see if you are infected.

Is a tapeworm infection serious?

No. Infection with the dwarf tapeworm is generally not serious. However, prolonged infection can lead to more severe symptoms; therefore, medical attention is needed to eliminate the tapeworm.

How is a tapeworm infection treated?

Treatment is available. A prescription drug called praziquantel is given. The medication causes the tapeworm to dissolve within the intestines. Praziquantel is generally well tolerated. Sometimes more than one treatment is necessary.

Can infection be spread to other family members?

Yes. Eggs are infectious (meaning they can re-infect you or infect others) immediately after being shed in feces.

What should I do if I think I have a tapeworm infection?

See your health care provider for diagnosis and treatment.

How can dwarf tapeworm infection be prevented?

Wash hands with soap and water after using the toilet, and before handling food.

If you work in a childcare center where you change diapers, be sure to wash your hands thoroughly with plenty of soap and warm water after every diaper change, even if you wear gloves.

When traveling in countries where food is likely to be contaminated, wash, peel, or cook all raw vegetables and fruits with safe water before eating.

Parasitic and Fungal Infections

Section 17.6
Pediculosis (Head Lice)

"Head Lice Infestation" and "Treating Head Lice Infestation," Centers for Disease Control and Prevention, August 19, 2006.

Head Lice Infestation

What are head lice?

Also called *Pediculus humanus capitis,* head lice are parasitic insects found on the heads of people. Having head lice is very common. However, there are no reliable data on how many people get head lice in the United States each year.

Who is at risk for getting head lice?

Anyone who comes in close contact (especially head-to-head contact) with someone who already has head lice is at greatest risk. Occasionally, head lice may be acquired from contact with clothing (such as hats, scarves, coats) or other personal items (such as brushes or towels) that belong to an infested person. Preschool and elementary-age children, three to eleven, and their families are infested most often. Girls get head lice more often than boys, women more than men. In the United States, African Americans rarely get head lice. Personal hygiene or cleanliness in the home or school has nothing to do with getting head lice.

What do head lice look like?

There are three forms of lice: the egg (also called a nit), the nymph, and the adult.

Egg/Nit: Nits are head lice eggs. They are very small, about the size of a knot in thread, hard to see, and are often confused for dandruff or hair spray droplets. Nits are laid by the adult female at the base of the hair shaft nearest the scalp. They are firmly attached to the hair shaft. They are oval and usually yellow to white. Nits take about one week to hatch. Eggs that are likely to hatch are usually located within one-quarter inch of the scalp.

Nymph: The nit hatches into a baby louse called a nymph. It looks like an adult head louse, but is smaller. Nymphs mature into adults about seven days after hatching. To live, the nymph must feed on blood.

Adult: The adult louse is about the size of a sesame seed, has six legs, and is tan to grayish-white. In persons with dark hair, the adult louse will look darker. Females, which are usually larger than the males, lay eggs. Adult lice can live up to thirty days on a person's head. To live, adult lice need to feed on blood. If the louse falls off a person, it dies within two days.

Where are head lice most commonly found?

They are most commonly found on the scalp, behind the ears, and near the neckline at the back of the neck. Head lice hold on to hair with hook-like claws found at the end of each of their six legs. Head lice are rarely found on the body, eyelashes, or eyebrows.

What are the signs and symptoms of head lice infestation?

- Tickling feeling of something moving in the hair.
- Itching, caused by an allergic reaction to the bites.
- Irritability.
- Sores on the head caused by scratching. These sores can sometimes become infected.

How did my child get head lice?

Contact with an already infested person is the most common way to get head lice. Head-to-head contact is common during play at school and at home (sports activities, on a playground, slumber parties, at camp).

Less commonly, head lice can be transmitted in the following ways:

- Wearing clothing, such as hats, scarves, coats, sports uniforms, or hair ribbons, recently worn by an infested person.
- Using infested combs, brushes, or towels.
- Lying on a bed, couch, pillow, carpet, or stuffed animal that has recently been in contact with an infested person.

Parasitic and Fungal Infections

How is head lice infestation diagnosed?

An infestation is diagnosed by looking closely through the hair and scalp for nits, nymphs, or adults. Finding a nymph or adult may be difficult; there are usually few of them and they can move quickly from searching fingers. If crawling lice are not seen, finding nits within one-quarter inch of the scalp confirms that a person is infested and should be treated. If you only find nits more than one-quarter inch from the scalp (and don't see a nymph or adult louse), the infestation is probably an old one and does not need to be treated. If you are not sure if a person has head lice, the diagnosis should be made by your health care provider, school nurse, or a professional from the local health department or agricultural extension service.

Treating Head Lice Infestation

How can I treat a head lice infestation?

The most important step in treating a head lice infestation is to treat the person and other family members with head lice with medication to kill the lice. Wash clothing and bedding worn or used by the infested person in the two-day period just before treatment is started.

Treat the infested person: Requires using an over-the-counter (OTC) or prescription medication. Follow these treatment steps: Before applying treatment, remove all clothing from the waist up. Apply lice medicine, also called pediculicide, according to label instructions. If your child has extra long hair (longer than shoulder length), you may need to use a second bottle. Pay special attention to instructions on the bottle regarding how long the medication should be left on and whether rinsing the hair is recommended after treatment. Warning: Do not use a cream rinse or combination shampoo/conditioner before using lice medicine. Do not re-wash hair for one to two days after treatment. Have the infested person put on clean clothing after treatment. If a few live lice are still found eight to twelve hours after treatment, but are moving more slowly than before, do not retreat. Comb dead and remaining live lice out of the hair. The medicine may take longer to kill lice.

If, after eight to twelve hours of treatment, no dead lice are found and lice seem as active as before, the medicine may not be working. See your health care provider for a different medication; follow treatment directions. Nit (head lice egg) combs, often found in lice medicine packages, should be used to comb nits and lice from the hair shaft. Many flea combs made for cats and dogs are also effective. After treatment, check hair and comb with a nit comb to remove nits and lice every two to three days. Continue to check for two to three weeks until you are sure all lice and nits are gone.

If using OTC pediculicides, retreat in seven to ten days. If using the prescription drug malathion, retreat in seven to ten days *only* if crawling bugs are found.

Treat the household: Head lice do not survive long if they fall off a person and cannot feed. You don't need to spend a lot of time or money on housecleaning activities. Follow these steps to help avoid re-infestation by lice that have recently fallen off the hair or crawled onto clothing or furniture.

To kill lice and nits, machine wash all washable clothing and bed linens that the infested person wore or used during the two days before treatment. Use the hot water (130°F) cycle. Dry laundry using high heat for at least twenty minutes.

Dry clean clothing that is not washable, (coats, hats, scarves, etc.), or store all clothing, stuffed animals, comforters, etc., that cannot be washed or dry-cleaned in a plastic bag; seal for two weeks.

Soak combs and brushes for one hour in rubbing alcohol or Lysol, or wash with soap and hot (130°F) water.

Vacuum the floor and furniture. The risk of getting re-infested from a louse that has fallen onto a carpet or sofa is very small. Don't spend a lot of time on this. Just vacuum the places where the infested person usually sits or lays. Do not use fumigant sprays; they can be toxic if inhaled or absorbed through the skin.

Prevent reinfestation: Lice are most commonly spread directly by head-to-head contact and much less frequently by lice that have crawled onto clothing or belongings. As a short-term measure to control a head lice outbreak in a community, school, or camp, you can teach children to avoid playtime and other activities that are likely to spread lice. Avoid head-to-head contact common during play at school and at home (sports activities, on a playground, slumber parties, at camp). Do not share clothing, such as hats, scarves, coats, sports uniforms, or hair ribbons. Do not share infested combs, brushes, or towels. Do not lie on beds, couches, pillows, carpets, or stuffed animals that have recently been in contact with an infested person.

Parasitic and Fungal Infections

My child has head lice. I don't. Should I treat myself to prevent being infested?

No, although anyone living with an infested person can get head lice. Check household contacts for lice and nits every two to three days. Treat only if crawling lice or nits (eggs) within one-quarter inch of the scalp are found.

I have heard that head lice medications don't work, or that head lice are resistant to medication. Is this true?

Like germs that are resistant to antibiotics, some lice also develop resistance to the medicine used to kill them. Resistance tends to be scattered. It may be present in one neighborhood, but not another. However, there are many reasons why medications may seem not to work.

Misdiagnosis of a head lice infestation: A diagnosis can be made if a person has crawling bugs on the head or many lice eggs within one-quarter inch (about the width of your little finger) of the scalp. Nits found on the hair shaft further than one-quarter inch from the scalp have already hatched. Treatment is not recommended for people who only have nits further than one-quarter inch away from the scalp.

Not following treatment instructions fully: Common problems include making the hair too wet with water before applying a pediculicide (this dilutes the pediculicide); using a cream rinse or conditioner shampoo before applying a pediculicide (this interferes with the medication); failing to leave the pediculicide on long enough (be sure to follow drug label instructions); re-shampooing the hair again immediately after applying the pediculicide (don't rewash hair for one to two days after treatment); using an inadequate amount of medication (extra long hair may require two bottles of pediculicide to fully wet the hair); or not combing. Using medication alone may not be enough to cure a head lice infestation. Combing the hair to remove lice and eggs has been shown to help.

Medication not working at all (resistance): If head lice medication does not kill any crawling bugs within twenty-four hours, then resistance is likely. If the medication kills some of the bugs or the bugs are twitching twenty-four hours after treatment then resistance to medication is probably not occurring.

Medication kills crawling bugs, but is not able to penetrate the eggs: It is very difficult for head lice medication to penetrate the nit shell. Medication may effectively kill crawling bugs, but may not treat the nits. This is why follow-up treatment is recommended.

New infection: You can get infested more than once with head lice. Children often get reinfested from a playmate. If your child is infested, discuss it with parents of the children your child plays with. Treating all infested children at the same time will help prevent reinfestation.

Should my pets be treated for head lice?

No. Head lice do not live on pets.

My child is under two years old and has been diagnosed with head lice. Can I treat him or her with prescription or OTC drugs?

For children under two years old, remove crawling bugs and nits using a nit comb. If this does not work, ask your child's health care provider for treatment recommendations. The safety of head lice medications has not been tested in children two years of age and under.

What OTC medications are available to treat head lice?

Many head lice medications are available at your local drug store. Each OTC product contains one of the following active ingredients.

Pyrethrins, often combined with piperonyl butoxide: Brand name products include A-200®, Pronto®, R&C®, Rid®, and Triple X®.

Pyrethrins are natural extracts from the chrysanthemum flower. Though safe and effective, pyrethrins only kill crawling lice, not unhatched nits. A second treatment is recommended in seven to ten days to kill any newly hatched lice. Treatment failures are common.

Permethrin: Brand name product Nix®.

Permethrins are similar to natural pyrethrins. Permethrins are safe and effective and may continue to kill newly hatched lice for several days after treatment. A second treatment may be necessary in seven to ten days to kill any newly hatched lice that may have hatched after residual medication from the first treatment was no longer active. Treatment failures are common.

Parasitic and Fungal Infections

What are the prescription drugs used to treat head lice?

Malathion (Ovide®): When used as directed, malathion is effective in treating lice. Some medication remains on the hair and can kill newly hatched lice for seven days after treatment. Malathion is intended for use on people six years of age and older. Few side effects have been reported. Malathion may sting if applied to open sores caused by scratching. The medication is flammable.

Lindane (Kwell®): When used as directed, the drug is probably safe. Overuse, misuse, or accidentally swallowing lindane can be toxic to the brain and other parts of the nervous system. For those reasons lindane is generally used only if other medications have failed. Lindane should not be used if excessive scratching has caused open sores on the head. It should be used with caution in persons who weigh less than 110 pounds.

Which head lice medicine is best for me?

If you aren't sure, ask your pharmacist or health care provider. When using the medicine, always follow the instructions on the package insert unless the physician directs otherwise.

When treating head lice:

- Do not use extra amounts of the lice medication unless instructed. These drugs are insecticides and can be dangerous when misused or overused.
- Do not treat the infested person more than three times with the same medication if it does not seem to work. See your health care provider for alternative medication.
- Do not mix head lice drugs.

Should household sprays be used to kill adult lice?

No. Spraying the house is not recommended. Fumigants and room sprays can be toxic if inhaled or absorbed through the skin.

Should I have a pest control company spray my house?

No. Vacuuming floors and furniture is enough to treat the household.

Section 17.7

Pinworm Infection

National Institute of Allergy and Infectious Diseases,
November 23, 2007.

Overview

In the United States, pinworm infection, or enterobiasis, is the most common of all parasitic roundworm infections. It primarily affects school-age children. Due to the fact that pinworm infection is spread mainly by children, it is found most often in family groups, daycare centers, schools, and camp settings.

Cause

Pinworm infection is caused by an intestinal roundworm called *Enterobius vermicularis*.

Pinworms are small, threadlike roundworms found primarily in the colon and rectum. The life cycle of the pinworm—egg, larva (immature stage), and mature worm—takes place inside the human body and requires from three to six weeks to complete.

The pinworm is the most common roundworm parasite in temperate climates—even in areas that adhere to good sanitation practices.

Transmission

Pinworms enter your body when you swallow their eggs. One female pinworm may expel thousands of eggs into the environment. As the eggs are moist and rather resistant to drying, they can infect humans even after being distributed in dust for several days.

The female pinworm deposits her eggs in the area around your anus. You can expose yourself to the infective eggs by scratching the contaminated area. The eggs then attach to your fingertips and from there go into your mouth. When you swallow, the eggs travel to your intestines.

The eggs also may be scattered into the air from bed linen and articles of clothing. They are capable of clinging to surfaces such as

Parasitic and Fungal Infections

bedding, clothing, toys, doorknobs, furniture, and faucets for up to two weeks.

Symptoms

Folklore is filled with fantastic descriptions of symptoms and abnormal behavior attributed to pinworm infection. In fact, many people have no symptoms at all. Of those who do, the symptoms are usually mild and barely noticeable.

The movement of egg-laden female worms from your anus to deposit their eggs will often produce itching around the anus or vagina. This itching may become very intense, interfere with sleep, and make you irritable.

Diagnosis

Your healthcare provider can diagnose pinworm infection by simply finding the eggs. The most common way to collect the eggs involves swabbing the anal area with the sticky side of a piece of transparent cellophane tape. The tape is then transferred to a slide and your healthcare provider will look for the eggs under a microscope.

Treatment

In the event that your healthcare provider prescribes medicine for this condition, all members of your household should take it, regardless of whether they have symptoms. Medicines, such as mebendazole or pyrantel pamoate, are the most useful in treating pinworm infection.

To relieve the intense itching that often accompanies pinworm infection, your healthcare provider may also prescribe a soothing ointment or cream.

Because of the strong probability that children will be reinfected outside the home, in a daycare setting, for example, strenuous efforts to eliminate the eggs from the home are of little help.

Prevention

Some of the ways that you and your children can prevent becoming infected or reinfected with pinworms include the following:

- Bathing after waking up
- Washing night clothes and bed sheets frequently

- Washing your hands routinely, particularly after using the bathroom or changing diapers
- Changing underwear every day
- Avoiding nail biting and scratching the anal area

Research

Researchers supported by the National Institute of Allergy and Infectious Diseases are conducting basic and clinical research on the prevention, control, and treatment of a variety of parasitic diseases, including some caused by parasitic roundworms.

Section 17.8

Scabies

Centers for Disease Control and Prevention, February 10, 2005.

What is scabies?

Scabies is an infestation of the skin with the microscopic mite *Sarcoptes scabei*. Infestation is common, found worldwide, and affects people of all races and social classes. Scabies spreads rapidly under crowded conditions where there is frequent skin-to-skin contact between people, such as in hospitals, institutions, child-care facilities, and nursing homes.

What are the signs and symptoms of scabies infestation?

- Pimple-like irritations, burrows, or rash of the skin, especially the webbing between the fingers; the skin folds on the wrist, elbow, or knee; the penis, the breast, or the shoulder blades.
- Intense itching, especially at night and over most of the body.
- Sores on the body caused by scratching. These sores can sometimes become infected with bacteria.

Parasitic and Fungal Infections

How did I get scabies?

By direct, prolonged, skin-to-skin contact with a person already infested with scabies. Contact must be prolonged (a quick handshake or hug will usually not spread infestation). Infestation is easily spread to sexual partners and household members. Infestation may also occur by sharing clothing, towels, and bedding.

Who is at risk for severe infestation?

People with weakened immune systems and the elderly are at risk for a more severe form of scabies, called Norwegian or crusted scabies.

How long will mites live?

Once away from the human body, mites do not survive more than forty-eight to seventy-two hours. When living on a person, an adult female mite can live up to a month.

Did my pet spread scabies to me?

No. Pets become infested with a different kind of scabies mite. If your pet is infested with scabies (also called mange) and they have close contact with you, the mite can get under your skin and cause itching and skin irritation. However, the mite dies in a couple of days and does not reproduce. The mites may cause you to itch for several days, but you do not need to be treated with special medication to kill the mites. Until your pet is successfully treated, mites can continue to burrow into your skin and cause you to have symptoms.

How soon after infestation will symptoms begin?

For a person who has never been infested with scabies, symptoms may take four to six weeks to begin. For a person who has had scabies, symptoms appear within several days. You do not become immune to an infestation.

How is scabies infestation diagnosed?

Diagnosis is most commonly made by looking at the burrows or rash. A skin scraping may be taken to look for mites, eggs, or mite fecal matter to confirm the diagnosis. If a skin scraping or biopsy is taken and returns negative, it is possible that you may still be infested.

Typically, there are fewer than ten mites on the entire body of an infested person; this makes it easy for an infestation to be missed.

Can scabies be treated?

Yes. Several lotions are available to treat scabies. Always follow the directions provided by your physician or the directions on the package insert. Apply lotion to a clean body from the neck down to the toes and left overnight (eight hours). After eight hours, take a bath or shower to wash off the lotion. Put on clean clothes. All clothes, bedding, and towels used by the infested person two days before treatment should be washed in hot water; dry in a hot dryer. A second treatment of the body with the same lotion may be necessary seven to ten days later. Pregnant women and children are often treated with milder scabies medications.

Who should be treated for scabies?

Anyone who is diagnosed with scabies, as well as his or her sexual partners and persons who have close, prolonged contact to the infested person should also be treated. If your health care provider has instructed family members to be treated, everyone should receive treatment at the same time to prevent reinfestation.

How soon after treatment will I feel better?

Itching may continue for two to three weeks, and does not mean that you are still infested. Your health care provider may prescribe additional medication to relieve itching if it is severe. No new burrows or rashes should appear twenty-four to forty-eight hours after effective treatment.

Parasitic and Fungal Infections

Section 17.9

Swimmer's Itch

"Swimmer's Itch," ©2008 Wisconsin Department of Health and Family Services (www.dhfs.wisconsin.gov). Reprinted with permission.

What is swimmer's itch?

Swimmer's itch is a skin rash caused by a parasite (schistosomes) which ordinarily infect birds, semi-aquatic mammals, and snails. Common grackles, red-winged blackbirds, ducks, geese, swans, muskrats, and moles have been found to carry the parasite. As part of their developmental life cycle, these parasites are released from infected snails, migrate through the water, and are capable of penetrating the skin of man. After penetration, these parasites remain in the skin and die but can cause an allergic reaction in some people. The parasite in man does not mature, reproduce, or cause any permanent infection.

Who gets swimmer's itch?

Only about one-third of the people who come in contact with the parasite develop swimmer's itch. People who swim or wade in infested water may experience this itchy rash. All age groups and both sexes can be involved, but children are most often infected due to their habits of swimming or wading in shallow water and playing on the beach as the water evaporates from the skin. Swimmer's itch may be prevalent among bathers in lakes in many parts of the world, including the Great Lakes region of North America and certain coastal beaches.

How is swimmer's itch spread?

An individual may get the infection by swimming or wading in infested water and then allowing water to evaporate off the skin rather than drying the skin with a towel. Person-to-person spread does not occur.

What are the symptoms of swimmer's itch?

Whenever infested water is allowed to evaporate off the skin, an initial tingling sensation may be felt associated with the penetration of the parasite into the skin. The irritated spot reaches its maximum size after about twenty-four hours; the itching may continue for several days. The symptoms should disappear within a week.

How soon do the symptoms begin?

A person's first exposure to infested water may not result in the itchy rash. Repeated exposure increases a person's allergic sensitivity to the parasite and increases the likelihood of rash development. Symptoms may appear within one to two hours of exposure.

What is the treatment for swimmer's itch?

There is no treatment necessary for swimmer's itch. Some people may get relief from the itching by applying skin lotions or creams to the infected site.

What can be done to reduce the chances of getting swimmer's itch?

- Toweling off immediately after swimming or wading in infested water can be very helpful in preventing rash development.
- Swim in water away from the shore.
- Avoid swimming in areas where snails have accumulated.

Don't encourage birds to stay near swimming areas by feeding them.

Section 17.10

Tinea

Reprinted with permission from "Tinea Infections: Athlete's Foot, Jock Itch and Ringworm," May 2007, http://familydoctor.org/online/famdocen/home/common/infections/common/fungal/316.html. Copyright © 2007 American Academy of Family Physicians. All rights reserved.

What is tinea?

Tinea is a fungus that can grow on your skin, hair, or nails. As it grows, it spreads out in a circle, leaving normal-looking skin in the middle. This makes it look like a ring. At the edge of the ring, the skin is lifted up by the irritation and looks red and scaly. To some people, the infection looks like a worm is under the skin. Because of the way it looks, tinea infection is often called "ringworm." However, there really isn't a worm under the skin.

How did I get a fungal infection?

You can get a fungal infection by touching a person who has one. Some kinds of fungi live on damp surfaces, like the floors in public showers or locker rooms. You can easily pick up a fungus there. You can even catch a fungal infection from your pets. Dogs and cats, as well as farm animals, can be infected with a fungus. Often this infection looks like a patch of skin where fur is missing.

What areas of the body are affected by tinea infections?

Fungal infections are named for the part of the body they infect. Tinea corporis is a fungal infection of the skin on the body. ("Corporis" is the Latin word for body.) If you have this infection, you may see small, red spots that grow into large rings almost anywhere on your arms, legs, or chest.

Tinea pedis is usually called "athlete's foot." ("Pedis" is the Latin word for foot.) The moist skin between your toes is a perfect place for a fungus to grow. The skin may become itchy and red, with a white, wet surface. The infection may spread to the toenails. (This is called tinea unguium — "unguium" comes from the Latin word for nail.) Here it causes the toenails to become thick and crumbly. It can also spread to your hands and fingernails.

When a fungus grows in the moist, warm area of the groin, the rash is called tinea cruris. ("Cruris" comes from the Latin for leg.) The common name for this infection is "jock itch." Tinea cruris generally occurs in men, especially if they often wear athletic equipment.

Tinea capitis, which is called "ringworm," causes itchy, red areas, usually on the head. ("Capitis" comes from the Latin for head.) The hair is destroyed, leaving bald patches. This tinea infection is most common in children.

How do I know if I have a fungal infection?

The best way to know for sure is to ask your doctor. Other skin problems can look just like a fungal infection but have very different treatments. To find out what is causing your rash, your doctor may scrape a small amount of the irritated skin onto a glass slide (or clip off a piece of nail or hair). Then he or she will look at the skin, nail, or hair under a microscope. After doing this, your doctor will usually be able to tell if your skin problem is caused by a fungus.

Sometimes a piece of your skin, hair, or nail will be sent to a lab to grow the fungus in a test tube. This is another way the lab can tell if your skin problem is caused by a fungus. They can also find out the exact type of fungus. This process takes a while because a fungus grows slowly.

How do I get rid of a tinea infection?

Once your doctor decides that you have a tinea infection, medicine can be used to get rid of it. You may only need to put a special cream on the rash for a few weeks. This is especially true for jock itch.

It can be harder to get rid of fungal infections on other parts of the body. Sometimes you have to take medicine by mouth. This medicine usually has to be taken for a long time, maybe even for months. Irritated skin takes time to heal. New hair or nails will have to grow back.

Some medicines can have unpleasant effects on the rest of your body, especially if you're also taking other medicines. There are some newer medicines that seem to work better with fewer side effects. You may need to have blood tests to make sure that your body is not having a bad reaction to the medicine.

Parasitic and Fungal Infections

What can I do to prevent tinea infections?

Skin that is kept clean and dry is your best defense. However, you're also less likely to get a tinea infection if you do the following things:

- When you're at home, take your shoes off and expose your feet to the air.
- Change your socks and underwear every day, especially in warm weather.
- Dry your feet carefully (especially between the toes) after using a locker room or public shower.
- Avoid walking barefoot in public areas. Instead, wear "flip-flops," sandals, or water shoes.
- Don't wear thick clothing for long periods of time in warm weather. It will make you sweat more.
- Throw away worn-out exercise shoes. Never borrow other people's shoes.
- Check your pets for areas of hair loss. Ask your veterinarian to check them too. It's important to check pets carefully, because if you don't find out whether they're causing your fungal infection, you may get it again from them, even after treatment.

Can tinea cause serious illness?

A fungus rarely spreads below the surface of the body to cause serious illness. Your body usually prevents this. However, people with weak immune systems, such as people with acquired immunodeficiency syndrome (AIDS), may have a hard time getting well from a fungal infection.

Tinea infections usually don't leave scars after the fungus is gone. Sometimes, people don't even know they have a fungal infection and get better without any treatment.

Section 17.11

Toxocariasis

Centers for Disease Control and Prevention, November 5, 2007.

What is toxocariasis?

Toxocariasis is a zoonotic (animal to human) infection caused by the parasitic roundworms commonly found in the intestine of dogs (*Toxocara canis*) and cats (*T. cati*).

What are the symptoms of toxocariasis?

There are two major forms of toxocariasis:

- **Ocular larva migrans (OLM):** *Toxocara* infections can cause OLM, an eye disease that can cause blindness. OLM occurs when a microscopic worm enters the eye; it may cause inflammation and formation of a scar on the retina. Each year more than seven hundred people infected with *Toxocara* experience permanent partial loss of vision.

- **Visceral larva migrans (VLM):** Heavier, or repeated *Toxocara* infections, while rare, can cause VLM, a disease that causes swelling of the body's organs or central nervous system. Symptoms of VLM, which are caused by the movement of the worms through the body, include fever, coughing, asthma, or pneumonia.

How serious is infection with Toxocara?

In most cases, *Toxocara* infections are not serious, and many people, especially adults infected by a small number of larvae (immature worms), may not notice any symptoms. The most severe cases are rare, but are more likely to occur in young children, who often play in dirt, or eat dirt (pica) contaminated by dog or cat stool.

How is toxocariasis spread?

The most common *Toxocara* parasite of concern to humans is *T. canis*, which puppies usually contract from the mother before birth

Parasitic and Fungal Infections

or from her milk. The larvae mature rapidly in the puppy's intestines; when the pup is three or four weeks old, they begin to produce large numbers of eggs that contaminate the environment through the animal's stool. The eggs soon develop into infective larvae.

How can I get toxocariasis?

You or your children can become infected after accidentally ingesting (swallowing) infective *Toxocara* eggs in soil or other contaminated surfaces.

What should I do if I think I have toxocariasis?

See your health care provider to discuss the possibility of infection and, if necessary, to be examined. A blood test is available for diagnosis.

What is the treatment for toxocariasis?

VLM is treated with antiparasitic drugs, usually in combination with anti-inflammatory medications. Treatment of OLM is more difficult and usually consists of measures to prevent progressive damage to the eye.

Who is at risk for toxocariasis?

Young children; owners of dogs and cats.

How can you prevent toxocariasis?

- Have your veterinarian treat your dogs and cats, especially young animals, regularly for worms.
- Wash your hands well with soap and water after playing with your pets and after outdoor activities, especially before you eat. Teach children to always wash their hands after playing with dogs and cats and after playing outdoors.
- Do not allow children to play in areas that are soiled with pet or other animal stool.
- Clean your pet's living area at least once a week. Feces should be either buried or bagged and disposed of in the trash.
- Teach children that it is dangerous to eat dirt or soil.

Part Three

Common Childhood Medical Conditions

Chapter 18

Allergies

Chapter Contents
Section 18.1—Allergic Reactions in Kids 218
Section 18.2—Food Allergies 228

Section 18.1

Allergic Reactions in Kids

Reprinted from "What Are Allergies?" "What Causes Allergies?" "Diagnosis," "Treatment," and "Prevention" with permission from the Asthma and Allergy Foundation of America, © 2005. All rights reserved.

What Are Allergies?

Allergies reflect an overreaction of the immune system to substances that usually cause no reaction in most individuals. These substances can trigger sneezing, wheezing, coughing, and itching. Allergies are not only bothersome, but many have been linked to a variety of common and serious chronic respiratory illnesses (such as sinusitis and asthma). Additionally, allergic reactions can be severe and even fatal. However, with proper management and patient education, allergic diseases can be controlled, and people with allergies can lead normal and productive lives.

Common Allergic Diseases

Allergic rhinitis (hay fever or "indoor/outdoor," "seasonal," "perennial," or "nasal" allergies): Characterized by nasal stuffiness, sneezing, nasal itching, clear nasal discharge, and itching of the roof of the mouth and/or ears.

Allergic asthma (asthma symptoms triggered by an allergic reaction): Characterized by airway obstruction that is at least partially reversible with medication and is always associated with allergy. Symptoms include coughing, wheezing, shortness of breath or rapid breathing, chest tightness, and occasional fatigue and slight chest pain.

Food allergy: Most prevalent in very young children and frequently outgrown, food allergies are characterized by a broad range of allergic reactions. Symptoms may include itching or swelling of lips or tongue; tightness of the throat with hoarseness; nausea and vomiting; diarrhea; occasionally chest tightness and wheezing; itching of the eyes; decreased blood pressure; or loss of consciousness and anaphylaxis.

Allergies

Drug allergy: Is characterized by a variety of allergic responses affecting any tissue or organ. Drug allergies can cause anaphylaxis; even those patients who do not have life-threatening symptoms initially may progress to a life-threatening reaction.

Anaphylaxis (extreme response to a food or drug allergy): Characterized by life-threatening symptoms. This is a medical emergency and the most severe form of allergic reaction. Symptoms include a sense of impending doom; generalized warmth or flush; tingling of palms, soles of feet, or lips; light-headedness; bloating; and chest tightness. These can progress into seizures, cardiac arrhythmia, shock, and respiratory distress. Possible causes can be medications, vaccines, food, latex, and insect stings and bites.

Latex allergy: An allergic response to the proteins in natural, latex rubber characterized by a range of allergic reactions. Persons at risk include healthcare workers, patients having multiple surgeries, and rubber-industry workers. Symptoms include hand dermatitis, eczema, and urticaria; sneezing and other respiratory distress; and lower respiratory problems including coughing, wheezing, and shortness of breath.

Insect sting/bite allergy: Characterized by a variety of allergic reactions; stings cannot always be avoided and can happen to anyone. Symptoms include pain, itching, and swelling at the sting site or over a larger area and can cause anaphylaxis. Insects that sting include bees, hornets, wasps, yellow jackets, and fire and harvest ants.

Urticaria (hives, skin allergy): A reaction of the skin, or a skin condition commonly known as hives. Characterized by the development of itchy, raised white bumps on the skin surrounded by an area of red inflammation. Acute urticaria is often caused by an allergy to foods or medication.

Atopic dermatitis (eczema, skin allergy): A chronic or recurrent inflammatory skin disease characterized by lesions, scaling, and flaking; it is sometimes called eczema. In children, it may be aggravated by an allergy or irritant.

Contact dermatitis (skin allergy): Characterized by skin inflammation; this is the most common occupational disease representing up to 40 percent of all occupational illnesses. Contact dermatitis is one of the most common skin diseases in adults. It results from the direct contact with an outside substance with the skin. There are currently about three thousand known contact allergens.

Allergic conjunctivitis (eye allergy): Characterized by inflammation of the eyes; it is the most common form of allergic eye disease. Symptoms can include itchy and watery eyes and lid distress. Allergic conjunctivitis is also commonly associated with the presence of other allergic diseases such as atopic dermatitis, allergic rhinitis, and asthma.

What Causes Allergies?

The substances that cause allergic disease in people are known as allergens. "Antigens," or protein particles like pollen, food, or dander enter our bodies through a variety of ways. If the antigen causes an allergic reaction, that particle is considered an "allergen"—an antigen that triggers an allergic reaction. These allergens can get into our body in several ways:

- **Inhaled into the nose and the lungs:** Examples are airborne pollens of certain trees, grasses, and weeds; house dust that includes dust mite particles, mold spores, cat and dog dander, and latex dust.

- **Ingested by mouth:** Frequent culprits include shrimp, peanuts, and other nuts.

- **Injected:** Such as medications delivered by needle like penicillin or other injectable drugs, and venom from insect stings and bites.

- **Absorbed through the skin:** Plants such as poison ivy, sumac, and oak and latex are examples.

What Makes Some Pollen Cause Allergies, and Not Others?

Plant pollens that are carried by the wind cause most allergies of the nose, eyes, and lungs. These plants (including certain weeds, trees, and grasses) are natural pollutants produced at various times of the year when their small, inconspicuous flowers discharge literally billions of pollen particles.

Because the particles can be carried significant distances, it is important for you not only to understand local environmental conditions, but also conditions over the broader area of the state or region in which you live. Unlike the wind-pollinated plants, conspicuous wildflowers or flowers used in most residential gardens are pollinated by bees, wasps, and other insects and therefore are not widely capable of producing allergic disease.

What Is the Role of Heredity in Allergy?

Like baldness, height, and eye color, the capacity to become allergic is an inherited characteristic. Yet, although you may be born with the genetic capability to become allergic, you are not automatically allergic to specific allergens. Several factors must be present for allergic sensitivity to be developed:

- The specific genes acquired from parents
- The exposure to one or more allergens to which you have a genetically programmed response
- The degree and length of exposure

A baby born with the tendency to become allergic to cow's milk, for example, may show allergic symptoms several months after birth. A genetic capability to become allergic to cat dander may take three to four years of cat exposure before the person shows symptoms. These people may also become allergic to other environmental substances with age.

On the other hand, poison ivy allergy (contact dermatitis) is an example of an allergy in which hereditary background does not play a part. The person with poison ivy allergy first has to be exposed to the oil from the plant. This usually occurs during youth, when a rash does not always appear. However, the first exposure may sensitize or cause the person to become allergic and, when subsequent exposure takes place, a contact dermatitis rash appears and can be quite severe. Many plants are capable of producing this type of rash. Substances other than plants, such as dyes, metals, and chemicals in deodorants and cosmetics, can also cause a similar dermatitis.

Diagnosis

If you break out in hives when a bee stings you, or you sneeze every time you pet a cat, you know what some of your allergens are. But if the pattern is not so obvious, try keeping a record of when, where, and under what circumstances your reactions occur. This can be as easy as jotting down notes on a calendar. If the pattern still isn't clear, make an appointment with your doctor for help.

Doctors diagnose allergies in three steps:

- **Personal and medical history:** Your doctor will ask you questions to get a complete understanding of your symptoms and their possible causes. Bring your notes to help jog your memory. Be ready to answer questions about your family history, the kinds of medicines you take, and your lifestyle at home, school, and work.

- **Physical examination:** If your doctor suspects an allergy, he/she will pay special attention to your ears, eyes, nose, throat, chest, and skin during the physical examination. This exam may include a pulmonary function test to detect how well you exhale air from your lungs. You may also need an x-ray of your lungs or sinuses.

- **Tests to determine your allergens:** Your doctor may do a skin test, patch test, or blood test.

Skin test: For most people, skin tests are the most accurate and least expensive way to confirm suspected allergens. There are two types of allergen skin tests. In prick/scratch testing, a small drop of the possible allergen is placed on the skin, followed by lightly pricking or scratching with a needle through the drop. In intra-dermal (under the skin) testing, a very small amount of allergen is injected into the outer layer of skin.

With either test, if you are allergic to the substance, you will develop redness, swelling, and itching at the test site within twenty minutes. You may also see a "wheal" or raised, round area that looks like a hive. Usually, the larger the wheal, the more sensitive you are to the allergen.

Patch test: This test determines if you have contact dermatitis. Your doctor will place a small amount of a possible allergen on your skin, cover it with a bandage, and check your reaction after forty-eight hours. If you are allergic to the substance, you should develop a rash.

Blood tests: Allergen blood tests (also called radioallergosorbent tests [RAST], enzyme-linked immunosorbent assays [ELISA], fluorescent allergosorbent tests [FAST], multiple radioallergosorbent tests [MAST], or radioimmunosorbent tests [RIST]) are sometimes used when people have a skin condition or are taking medicines which interfere with skin testing. Your doctor will take a blood sample and send

Allergies

it to a laboratory. The lab adds the allergen to your blood sample, and then measures the amount of antibodies your blood produces to attack the allergens.

Treatment

Good allergy treatment is based on the results of your allergy tests, your medical history, and the severity of your symptoms. It can include three different treatment strategies: avoidance of allergens, medication options, and/or immunotherapy (allergy shots).

Avoiding Your Allergens

The best way to prevent allergy symptoms and minimize your need for allergy medicine is to avoid your allergens as much as possible and to eliminate the source of allergens from your home and other environments. For important tips, talk to your doctor.

Medication

Some people don't take allergy medicines because they don't take their symptoms seriously ("Oh, it's only my allergies.") The result may be painful complications such as sinus or ear infections. Don't take the risk. There are so many safe prescription and nonprescription medicines to relieve allergy symptoms! Following is a brief list of medications taken for allergies. They are available in nonprescription and prescription form:

- Antihistamines and decongestants are the most common medicines used for allergies. Antihistamines help relieve rashes and hives, as well as sneezing, itching, and runny nose. Prescription antihistamines are similar to their nonprescription counterparts, but many of them do not cause drowsiness. Decongestant pills, sprays, and nose drops reduce stuffiness by shrinking swollen membranes in the nose. It is important to remember that using a nonprescription nasal decongestant spray more than three days in a row may cause the swelling and stuffiness in your nose to become worse, even after you stop using the medicine. This is called a "rebound" reaction. Some nonprescription "cold" medicines combine an antihistamine, a pain reliever like aspirin or acetaminophen, and a decongestant. Aspirin can cause asthma attacks in some people. Don't take a chance: if you have asthma, talk with your doctor before taking any nonprescription allergy medicine.

- Eye drops may provide temporary relief from burning or bloodshot eyes. However, only prescription allergy eye drops contain antihistamines that can reduce itching, tearing and swelling.

- Corticosteroid creams or ointments relieve itchiness and halt the spread of rashes. Corticosteroids are not the same as anabolic steroids that are used illegally by some athletes to build muscles. If your rash does not go away after using a nonprescription corticosteroid for a week, see your doctor.

- Corticosteroid nasal sprays help reduce the inflammation that causes nasal congestion without the chance of the "rebound" effect found in nonprescription nose sprays.

- Cromolyn sodium prevents the inflammation which causes nasal congestion. Because it has few, if any, side effects, cromolyn can be safely used over long periods of time.

- Oral corticosteroids may be prescribed to reduce swelling and stop severe allergic reactions. Because these medications can cause serious side effects, you should expect your doctor to carefully monitor you.

- Epinephrine comes in pre-measured, self-injectable containers, and is the only medication which can help during a life-threatening anaphylactic attack. To be effective, epinephrine must be given within minutes of the first sign of serious allergic reaction.

New prescription and nonprescription drugs are approved periodically. If the prescription you are taking is not on this list, ask your doctor which category it falls into, so that you can refer to this chart.

Immunotherapy (Allergy Shots)

When it is not possible to avoid your allergens and treatment with medications alone does not solve the problem, immunotherapy can often prevent allergy symptoms. It involves giving a person increasingly higher doses of their allergen over time. For reasons that we do not completely understand, the person gradually becomes less sensitive to that allergen. This can be effective for some people with hay fever, certain animal allergies, and insect stings. It is usually not effective for allergies to food, drugs, or feathers, nor is it effective for hives or eczema.

Allergies

Prevention

There are some simple things you can do to prevent allergies at home, work school, outside, and when you travel.

At Home

- Dust to control mites. By dusting surfaces and washing bedding often, you can control the amount of dust mites in your home.

- Vacuum often. Although cleaning can sometimes trigger allergic reactions, with dust in the air, vacuuming once or twice a week will reduce the surface dust mites. Wear a mask when doing housework and consider leaving for a few hours after you clean to avoid allergens in the air. You can also make sure your vacuum has an air filter to capture dust.

- Reduce pet dander. If you have allergies, you should avoid pets with feathers or fur like birds, dogs, and cats. Animal saliva and dead skin, or pet dander, can cause allergic reactions. If you can't bear to part with your pet, you should at least keep it out of the bedroom.

- Shut out pollen. When you clean your windows, do you see a film of pollen on the frame or sill? One easy way to prevent pollen from entering your home is to keep windows and doors closed. Use an air filter and clean it regularly or run the air conditioner and change the filter often.

- Avoid mold spores. Mold spores grow in moist areas. If you reduce the moisture in the bathroom and kitchen, you will reduce the mold. Fix any leaks inside and outside of your home and clean moldy surfaces. Plants can carry pollen and mold too, so limit the number of houseplants. Dehumidifiers will also help reduce mold.

At Work

Allergies at home and work are similar and affect millions of people each year. Allergy symptoms, like sneezing, nasal congestion, and headache, may make it difficult to concentrate. Every work environment will have specific allergy problems so talk to your health care provider or pharmacist about how you can prevent allergies at your specific workplace.

At School

Children may face allergens in the classroom and playground. In fact, children in the United States miss about two million school days each year because of allergy symptoms. Parents, teachers, and health care providers can work together to help prevent and treat childhood allergies. Monitor the classroom for plants, pets, or other items that may carry allergens. Encourage your child to wash his/her hands after playing outside. Many of the allergens in the home will also be found at school. Although it may not be an option to vacuum or dust the classroom, there may be treatment options to help a child manage his/her symptoms during the school day.

Outside

There are certain times during the year when plants and trees release pollen into the air. The timing of these pollen seasons depends on your geographic location. Different regions have different types of plants that pollinate at different times. Depending on where you live, allergy seasons may be mild or severe. Experts estimate that thirty-five million Americans suffer from allergies because of airborne pollen!

Tiny particles that are released from trees, weeds, and grasses are known as pollen. These particles are carried by the wind from tall treetops all the way to your nose. But before you shrug off fancy flowers in fear of sniffles, remember that the types of pollen that most commonly cause your allergies are from plain-looking plants, such as trees, grasses, and weeds. These plants produce small and light pollen, perfect for catching a ride on a gentle breeze.

Similar to pollen, mold spores are a seasonal pest. If you are sensitive to mold spores, you may have symptoms from spring to late fall. Yet, even after the first frost of winter, some mold spores can continue to grow in freezing temperatures. The severity of your mold spore allergies can depend on the climate that you live in. In the warmest areas of the United States, mold spores grow all year! But before you move to Antarctica, remember that mold spores also grow indoors, making it a year-round problem.

Traveling

We are all on the go and there are a few things to keep in mind to prevent outdoor allergies during peak season, when the pollen count is high:

Allergies

- Stay inside during peak pollen times, usually between 10:00 a.m. and 4:00 p.m.
- Keep your car windows closed when traveling.
- Stay indoors when humidity is high and on days with high wind, when dust and pollen are more likely to be in the air.
- Wear a facemask if you are outside to limit the amount of pollen you inhale.
- Shower after spending time outside to wash away pollen that collects on your skin and hair.

Planes, Trains, and Automobiles

If you suffer from allergies, there may be other concerns when you travel. The allergy climate may be different than the one where you live. When you travel by car, bus, or train, you may find dust mites, mold spores, and pollen bothersome. Turn on the air conditioner or heater before getting in your car and travel with the windows closed to avoid allergens from outside. Travel early in the morning or late in the evening when the air quality is better.

When flying to your favorite vacation spot, remember that air quality and dryness on planes can affect you if you have allergies. If a cruise is your next vacation, be aware of the season and temperature at your destination(s). In tropical, damp climates there are allergens like dust mites, mold spores, and pollen. In cold, damp climates, you may be exposed to dust mites and mold spores. Once you arrive at your hotel, there may be dust mites and mold spores lurking. If you are staying with family or friends, the same types of allergens that you find at home may be present.

Section 18.2

Food Allergies

"Understanding Food Allergy," © 2007 International Food Information Council Foundation (www.ific.org). All rights reserved. Reprinted with permission.

Allergies affect the lives of millions of people around the world. Fresh spring flowers, a friend's cat or dog, even the presence of dust can make people itch, sneeze, and scratch almost uncontrollably. But what about that seemingly innocent peanut butter sandwich, glass of milk, or fish fillet?

A growing number of Americans have an allergy to these or other foods. Food allergies can be life threatening. Knowledge about food allergies can help save a life.

What is a food allergy?

Food allergy is a reaction of the body's immune system to something in a food or an ingredient in a food—usually a protein. It can be a serious condition and should be diagnosed by a board-certified allergist. A true food allergy (also called "food hypersensitivity") and its symptoms can take many forms.

Which foods cause food allergy?

The eight most common food allergens—milk, eggs, peanuts, tree nuts, soy, wheat, fish, and crustacean shellfish—cause most food allergic reactions. However, many other foods have been identified as allergens for some people, such as certain fruits or vegetables and seeds. Most children with food allergies to milk, eggs, soy, and wheat will outgrow their allergy. However, allergy to peanuts, tree nuts, and fish usually persists. Shellfish allergies often develop during later childhood or adulthood, and the most common food allergy among adults is shellfish. Peanuts and tree nuts account for most of the severe cases of food allergy.

What are the symptoms of food allergy?

Symptoms of food allergy differ greatly among individuals. They can also differ in the same person during different exposures. Allergic reactions to food can vary in severity, time of onset, and may be affected by when the food was eaten. Exercise can also be a factor.

Some food allergies affect only the gastrointestinal tract (stomach and intestines). These are often infant or early childhood conditions, but some can persist. Celiac disease is sometimes considered a food allergy because it is the result of an adverse immune response to gluten, a protein in wheat, barley, and certain other grains. However, unlike some childhood food allergies, which are sometimes outgrown, Celiac disease stays with you through your lifetime. This condition is also diagnosed in adults—in fact, the most common age at diagnosis now is about forty, and most patients have had at least ten years of symptoms before diagnosis.

Common symptoms of food allergy include skin irritations such as rashes, hives, and eczema, and gastrointestinal symptoms such as nausea, diarrhea, and vomiting. Sneezing, runny nose, and shortness of breath can also result from food allergy, but such symptoms are usually seen at the same time as symptoms in other areas of the body in a more severe reaction. In other words, isolated sneezing and runny nose, or isolated shortness of breath is not common with food allergy. Some individuals may experience a more severe reaction called anaphylaxis.

What is anaphylaxis?

According to the American Academy of Allergy, Asthma and Immunology (AAAAI), anaphylaxis is a life threatening allergic reaction. It is a condition which affects several different parts of the body which may include the skin: flushing, itching, or hives; the airway: swelling of the throat, difficulty talking or breathing; the intestines: nausea, vomiting, or diarrhea; and the ability of the heart to pump blood: low blood pressure or unconsciousness.

Symptoms usually appear rapidly, sometimes within minutes of exposure to the allergen, and can be life threatening. Immediate medical attention is necessary when anaphylaxis occurs. Standard emergency treatment often includes an injection of epinephrine (adrenaline) to open up the airway and help reverse the reaction.

Do I have a food allergy?

Of all the individuals who have any type of food sensitivity, most have food intolerances. Fewer people have true food allergy involving the immune system. According to recent studies, approximately eleven million Americans—2 percent of adults and 6 to 8 percent of children under the age of three—have a true food allergy.

What are other reactions or sensitivities to foods called?

Other reactions to foods that don't involve the immune system are commonly called food intolerance. Such reactions can be divided into "toxic" or "nontoxic" non-immunologic reactions to foods. Toxic reactions to foods include bacterial food poisoning, which can cause diarrhea. A nontoxic reaction is caused by a variety of naturally occurring components in food, resulting in a chemical or "drug-like" reaction when consumed at high enough doses. An example would be the "burning" sensation experienced when eating foods like chili peppers.

Nontoxic types of food intolerance can also include adverse reactions to a food substance that involves digestion or metabolism (breakdown of food by the body). Lactose intolerance is an example of the most common type of food intolerance. It occurs when a person lacks an enzyme needed to digest milk sugar. If a person who is lactose-intolerant eats too much of a milk product, they may experience symptoms such as gas, bloating, and abdominal pain.

Other suspected adverse reactions such as fatigue, behavior problems, and many other symptoms attributed to foods such as corn, high fructose corn syrup, and sugar, for example, have not been proven.

Am I allergic to food additives?

Probably not. Misconceptions abound regarding allergy to food additives and preservatives. Although some food additives, like sulfites, have been shown to trigger asthma or hives in certain people, most studies performed on additives with modern methods have been negative. Sulfite sensitivity or sulfite-induced asthma is an exception though. It affects about 6 percent of people with asthma. When they eat food or beverages with a high enough concentration of sulfite, it can cause a severe asthma attack that could be life-threatening.

Aspartame, monosodium glutamate, and several food dyes have been studied extensively. Scientific evidence shows that they do not cause allergic reactions.

What should I do if I believe I have had an adverse reaction to a certain food?

You should see a board-certified allergist to get a diagnosis. An allergist and dietitian can best help the food-allergic patient manage dietary issues with little sacrifice to nutrition or the pleasure of eating.

Making a diagnosis may include:

- a thorough medical history;
- the analysis of a food diary; and
- several tests including skin-prick tests, radioallergosorbent (RAST) tests (blood test), and food challenges (using different foods to test for allergic reactions).

Once a diagnosis is complete, an allergist will help set up an action plan to manage allergic reactions that may occur. An action plan may include taking medication by injection to control allergic reactions. Information on how to avoid the food(s) should also be provided.

Reading food labels for all foods is important to effectively manage true food allergies.

What important information should I know and share with my family and friends?

Because food allergy can be life threatening, the allergy-producing food must be completely avoided. If you, or someone else, are experiencing a severe food-allergic reaction, call 911 (or an ambulance) immediately.

Most life-threatening allergic reactions to foods occur when eating away from the home. It is important to explain your situation and needs clearly to your host or food server. If necessary, ask to speak with the chef or manager. Some foods have been reported to cause reactions when inhaled, as with the steam from poached fish or boiling crab pots. It is very important to know how cross-contact of foods can occur in a restaurant, bakery, or home, in order to safeguard yourself against an allergic reaction. An allergist and the Food Allergy and Anaphylaxis Network can help you.

The Food Allergen Labeling and Consumer Protection Act (FALCPA), an FDA (U.S. Food and Drug Administration) law implemented in January 2006, requires allergens to be listed on food labels in easily understood language. Always look at the listings on labels to determine the presence of the eight major allergens. Since food and beverage manufacturers are continually making improvements, food-allergic persons should read the food label for every product purchased, each time it is purchased.

Many different foods can cause food-allergic reactions. However, most reactions to foods are not true food allergies, but some type of food intolerance.

Food sensitivities may be a food allergy or a food intolerance.

The eight most common food allergens are milk, eggs, peanuts, tree nuts, soy, wheat, fish, and crustacean shellfish.

If you, or someone else, are having a serious allergic reaction to a food, call 911 (or an ambulance) immediately!

Chapter 19

Blood and Circulatory Disorders

Chapter Contents

Section 19.1—Anemia 234
Section 19.2—Sickle Cell Anemia 239
Section 19.3—Thalassemia 242
Section 19.4—Hemophilia 244
Section 19.5—Thrombocytopenia 247
Section 19.6—Thrombophilia 256
Section 19.7—von Willebrand Disease 259

Section 19.1

Anemia

"The Facts about Anemia," © 2005 Medical College of Wisconsin.
Reprinted with permission of Medical College of Wisconsin HealthLink,
www.healthlink.mcw.edu.

Anemia is the most common disorder of the blood. It occurs when the amount of red blood cells or hemoglobin (oxygen-carrying protein) in the blood becomes low. Hemoglobin helps red blood cells carry oxygen from the lungs to all parts of the body. When it is low, the tissues of the body don't receive enough oxygen-rich blood and can't produce the energy they need to function properly.

There are many types of anemia, all with different causes.

Iron deficiency anemia: Iron deficiency anemia (IDA) is the most common type of anemia. IDA occurs when you don't have enough iron in your body. You need iron to make hemoglobin. This can happen when you lose blood from problems like heavy periods, ulcers, colon polyps, or colon cancer. A diet that doesn't have enough iron in it can also cause IDA. Pregnancy can cause IDA if there's not enough iron for the mother and fetus. You can get iron from foods like ground beef, clams, spinach, lentils, baked potato with skin, sunflower seeds, and cashews.

Megaloblastic anemia: Megaloblastic (or vitamin deficiency) anemia most often occurs when the body doesn't get enough folic acid or vitamin B_{12}. These vitamins help the body maintain healthy blood and a healthy nervous system. With this type of anemia, the body makes red blood cells that can't deliver oxygen properly. Folic acid supplement pills can treat this type of anemia. You can also get folic acid in beans and legumes; citrus fruits and juices; wheat bran and other whole grains; dark green leafy vegetables; and poultry, pork, shellfish, and liver. Sometimes, with this disease, your health care provider may not realize you're not getting enough B_{12}. This usually happens to someone with pernicious anemia, a type of autoimmune disease. B_{12} deficiency may also be more common in people with other autoimmune diseases, like Crohn disease. Not getting enough B_{12} can

Blood and Circulatory Disorders

cause numbness in the legs and feet, problems walking, memory loss, and problems seeing. The treatment depends on the cause, but you may need to get B_{12} shots or take special B_{12} pills.

Anemia from underlying diseases: Certain diseases can hurt the body's ability to make red blood cells. For example, people with kidney disease, especially those getting dialysis (which takes out wastes from the blood if the kidneys can't), are at higher risk for developing anemia. Their kidneys can't create enough hormones to make blood cells, and iron is lost in dialysis.

Anemia from inherited blood diseases: If you have a blood disease in your family, there is a higher risk that you will also have this disease. One type of inherited blood disease is sickle cell anemia. Instead of having normal red blood cells that move through blood vessels easily, sickle cells are hard and have a curved edge. These cells cannot squeeze through small blood vessels and block the organs from getting blood. Your body destroys sickle red cells quickly, but it can't make new red blood cells fast enough. This causes anemia. Another inherited blood disease is thalassemia. It happens when the body is missing certain genes or when variant (different from normal) genes are passed down from parents that affect how the body makes hemoglobin.

Aplastic anemia: Aplastic anemia is a rare problem that happens when the body doesn't make enough red blood cells. Since this affects the white blood cells too, there is a higher risk for infections and bleeding that can't be stopped. This can be caused by many things: cancer treatments (radiation or chemotherapy), exposure to toxic chemicals (like those used in some insecticides, paint, and household cleaners), some drugs (like those that treat rheumatoid arthritis), autoimmune diseases (like lupus), viral infection that affects bone marrow, or bone marrow diseases.

The treatment depends on how serious the anemia is. It can be treated with blood transfusions, medicines, or a bone marrow transplant.

Signs and Symptoms of Anemia

Anemia takes some time to develop. In the beginning, you may not have any signs or they may be mild. But as it gets worse, you may have these symptoms:

- Fatigue

- Weakness
- Not doing well in work or school
- Low body temperature
- Pale skin
- Rapid heartbeat
- Shortness of breath
- Chest pain
- Dizziness
- Irritability
- Numbness or coldness in your hands and feet
- Headache

Diagnosis and Treatment

Anemia is diagnosed by a blood test. If you have anemia, your health care provider may want to do other tests to find out what's causing it, like stomach ulcers or polyps.

Treatment depends on the cause of the anemia. For example, treatment for sickle cell anemia is different than treatment for a diet low in iron or folic acid. Talk to your health care provider about the best treatment for the cause of your anemia.

Prevention

These steps can help prevent some types of anemia:

- Eat foods high in iron: red meat; fish; chicken; liver; eggs; dried fruits like apricots, prunes, and raisins; lentils and beans; green, leafy vegetables like spinach and broccoli; tofu; cereal with iron in it (iron-fortified).
- Eat/drink foods that help your body absorb iron, like orange juice, strawberries, broccoli, or other fruits and vegetables with vitamin C.
- Don't drink coffee or tea with meals. These drinks make it harder for your body to absorb iron.
- Calcium can hurt your absorption of iron. If you have a hard time getting enough iron, talk to your health care provider about the best way to get enough calcium too.

Blood and Circulatory Disorders

- Make sure you get enough folic acid and vitamin B_{12} in your diet.
- Talk to your health care provider about taking iron supplement pills. Do not take these pills without talking to your health care provider first. These pills come in two forms: ferrous and ferric. The ferrous form is better absorbed by your body. But taking iron pills can cause side effects like nausea, vomiting, constipation, and diarrhea. Reduce these side effects by taking these steps:
  - Start with half of the recommended dose. Gradually increase to the full dose.
  - Take the pill in divided doses.
  - Take the pill with food.
  - If one type of iron pill is causing problems, ask your health care provider for another brand.
- If you are a nonpregnant woman of childbearing age, get tested for anemia every five to ten years. This can be done during a regular health exam. Testing should start in adolescence.
- If you are a nonpregnant woman of childbearing age with these risk factors for iron deficiency, get tested every year:
  - Heavy periods
  - Low iron intake
  - Previous diagnosis of anemia

How Much Iron?

Most people get enough iron through a regular healthy diet that has iron-rich foods. But some groups of people often don't get enough iron:

- Teenage girls/women of childbearing age (especially those who have heavy menstrual losses, who have had more than one child, or use an intrauterine device [IUD])
- Older infants and toddlers
- Pregnant women

Many pregnant women have a hard time getting enough iron. During pregnancy, your body demands more iron because of the growing needs from the fetus, the higher volume of blood, and blood loss during delivery. Not getting enough iron can cause preterm labor and delivering a low-birthweight baby. If you're pregnant, make sure you get 27 mg of iron every day. Take an iron supplement pill to be sure. This dosage might be part of your prenatal vitamin. Get tested for anemia at your first prenatal visit.

These groups of people should be screened periodically for iron deficiency. If the tests show that the body isn't getting enough iron, iron supplements may be prescribed. Many health care providers prescribe iron supplements during pregnancy because many pregnant women don't get enough. They can help when diet alone can't restore the iron level back to normal. Talk with your healthcare provider to find out if you are getting enough iron through your diet or if you or your child needs to be taking iron supplements.

Milligrams (mg) of iron per day for special groups:

- Infants and children:
    - 7 to 12 months: 11 mg
    - 1 to 3 years: 7 mg
    - 4 to 8 years: 10 mg
- Females:
    - 9 to 13 years: 8 mg
    - 14 to 18 years: 15 mg
    - 19 to 50 years: 18 mg
    - 51+ years: 8 mg
- Pregnant:
    - 9 to 50 years: 27 mg
- Breastfeeding:
    - 9 to 18 years: 10 mg
    - 19 to 50 years: 9 mg

Blood and Circulatory Disorders

Section 19.2

Sickle Cell Anemia

"Learning About Sickle Cell Disease," National Human Genome Research Institute, National Institutes of Health, November 28, 2007.

What Do We Know about Heredity and Sickle Cell Disease?

Sickle cell disease is the most common inherited blood disorder in the United States. Approximately eighty thousand Americans have the disease.

In the United States, sickle cell disease is most prevalent among African Americans. About one in twelve African Americans and about one in one hundred Hispanic Americans carry the sickle cell trait, which means they are carriers of the disease.

Sickle cell disease is caused by a mutation in the hemoglobin-beta gene found on chromosome 11. Hemoglobin transports oxygen from the lungs to other parts of the body. Red blood cells with normal hemoglobin (hemoglobin-A) are smooth and round and glide through blood vessels.

In people with sickle cell disease, abnormal hemoglobin molecules—hemoglobin S—stick to one another and form long, rod-like structures. These structures cause red blood cells to become stiff, assuming a sickle shape. Their shape causes these red blood cells to pile up, causing blockages and damaging vital organs and tissue.

Sickle cells are destroyed rapidly in the bodies of people with the disease, causing anemia. This anemia is what gives the disease its commonly known name—sickle cell anemia.

The sickle cells also block the flow of blood through vessels, resulting in lung tissue damage that causes acute chest syndrome, pain episodes, stroke, and priapism (painful, prolonged erection). It also causes damage to the spleen, kidneys, and liver. The damage to the spleen makes patients—especially young children—easily overwhelmed by bacterial infections.

A baby born with sickle cell disease inherits a gene for the disorder from both parents. When both parents have the genetic defect, there's a 25 percent chance that each child will be born with sickle cell disease.

If a child inherits only one copy of the defective gene (from either parent), there is a 50 percent chance that the child will carry the sickle cell trait. People who only carry the sickle cell trait typically don't get the disease, but can pass the defective gene on to their children.

New Treatments Prolong Life

Until recently, people with sickle cell disease were not expected to survive childhood. But today, due to preventive drug treatment, improved medical care, and aggressive research, half of sickle cell patients live beyond fifty years.

Treatments for sickle cell include antibiotics, pain management, and blood transfusions. A new drug treatment, hydroxyurea, which is an anti-tumor drug, appears to stimulate the production of fetal hemoglobin, a type of hemoglobin usually found only in newborns. Fetal hemoglobin helps prevent the "sickling" of red blood cells. Patients treated with hydroxyurea also have fewer attacks of acute chest syndrome and need fewer blood transfusions.

Bone Marrow Transplantation: The Only Cure

Currently the only cure for sickle cell disease is bone marrow transplantation. In this procedure a sick patient is transplanted with bone marrow from healthy, genetically compatible sibling donors. However only about 18 percent of children with sickle cell disease have a healthy, matched sibling donor. Bone marrow transplantation is a risky procedure with many complications.

Gene Therapy Offers Promise of a Cure

Researchers are experimenting with attempts to cure sickle cell disease by correcting the defective gene and inserting it into the bone marrow of those with sickle cell to stimulate production of normal hemoglobin. Recent experiments show promise. In December 2001, scientists at Harvard Medical School and MIT, supported by the National Institutes of Health (NIH), announced that they had corrected sickle cell disease in mice using gene therapy.

Researchers used bioengineering to create mice with a human gene that produces the defective hemoglobin causing sickle cell disease. Bone marrow containing the defective hemoglobin gene was removed from the mice and genetically "corrected" by the addition of the anti-sickling

Blood and Circulatory Disorders

human beta-hemoglobin gene. The corrected marrow was then transplanted into other mice with sickle cell disease. The genetically corrected mice began producing high levels of normal red blood cells and showed a dramatic reduction in sickled cells. Scientists are hopeful that the techniques can be applied to human gene transplantation using autologous transplantation, in which some of the patient's own bone marrow cells would be removed and genetically corrected.

Is There a Test for Sickle Cell Disease?

Doctors diagnosis sickle cell through a blood test that checks for hemoglobin S—the defective form of hemoglobin. To confirm the diagnosis, a sample of blood is examined under a microscope to check for large numbers of sickled red blood cells—the hallmark trait of the disease.

In more than forty states, testing for the defective sickle cell gene is routinely performed on newborns.

Sickle cell disease can also be detected in an unborn baby. Amniocentesis, a procedure in which a needle is used to take fluid from around the baby for testing, can show whether the fetus has sickle cell disease or carries the sickle cell gene. If the test shows that the child will have sickle cell disease, some parents may choose not to continue the pregnancy. Genetic counselors can help parents make these difficult decisions.

A new technique used in conjunction with in vitro fertilization, called pre-implantation genetic diagnosis (PGD), enables parents who carry the sickle cell trait to test embryos for the defective gene before implantation, and to choose to implant only those embryos free of the sickle cell gene.

Section 19.3

Thalassemia

"Learning About Thalassemia,"
National Human Genome Research Center,
National Institutes of Health, November 25, 2007.

What Do We Know about Heredity and Thalassemia?

Thalassemia is actually a group of inherited diseases of the blood that affect a person's ability to produce hemoglobin, resulting in anemia. Hemoglobin is a protein in red blood cells that carries oxygen and nutrients to cells in the body. About one hundred thousand babies worldwide are born with severe forms of thalassemia each year. Thalassemia occurs most frequently in people of Italian, Greek, Middle Eastern, Southern Asian, and African ancestry.

The two main types of thalassemia are called "alpha" and "beta," depending on which part of an oxygen-carrying protein in the red blood cells is lacking. Both types of thalassemia are inherited in the same manner. The disease is passed to children by parents who carry the mutated thalassemia gene. A child who inherits one mutated gene is a carrier, which is sometimes called "thalassemia trait." Most carriers lead completely normal, healthy lives.

A child who inherits two thalassemia trait genes—one from each parent—will have the disease. A child of two carriers has a 25 percent chance of receiving two trait genes and developing the disease, and a 50 percent chance of being a thalassemia trait carrier.

Most individuals with alpha thalassemia have milder forms of the disease, with varying degrees of anemia. The most severe form of alpha thalassemia, which affects mainly individuals of Southeast Asian, Chinese, and Filipino ancestry, results in fetal or newborn death.

A child who inherits two copies of the mutated gene for beta thalassemia will have beta thalassemia disease. The child can have a mild form of the disease, known as thalassemia intermedia, which causes milder anemia that rarely requires transfusions.

Thalassemia Major: A Serious Disorder

The more severe form of the disease is thalassemia major, also called Cooley Anemia. It is a serious disease that requires regular blood transfusions and extensive medical care.

Those with thalassemia major usually show symptoms within the first two years of life. They become pale and listless and have poor appetites. They grow slowly and often develop jaundice. Without treatment, the spleen, liver, and heart soon become greatly enlarged. Bones become thin and brittle. Heart failure and infection are the leading causes of death among children with untreated thalassemia major.

The use of frequent blood transfusions and antibiotics has improved the outlook for children with thalassemia major. Frequent transfusions keep their hemoglobin levels near normal and prevent many of the complications of the disease. But repeated blood transfusions lead to iron overload—a buildup of iron in the body—that can damage the heart, liver, and other organs. Drugs known as "iron chelators" can help rid the body of excess iron, preventing or delaying problems related to iron overload.

Thalassemia has been cured using bone marrow transplants. However, this treatment is possible only for a small minority of patients who have a suitable bone marrow donor. The transplant procedure itself is still risky and can result in death.

Gene Therapy Offers Hope for a Cure

Scientists are working to develop a gene therapy that may offer a cure for thalassemia. Such a treatment might involve inserting a normal beta globin gene (the gene that is abnormal in this disease) into the patient's stem cells, the immature bone marrow cells that are the precursors of all other cells in the blood.

Another form of gene therapy could involve using drugs or other methods to reactivate the patient's genes that produce fetal hemoglobin—the form of hemoglobin found in fetuses and newborns. Scientists hope that spurring production of fetal hemoglobin will compensate for the patient's deficiency of adult hemoglobin.

Is There a Test for Thalassemia?

Blood tests and family genetic studies can show whether an individual has thalassemia or is a carrier. If both parents are carriers, they may want to consult with a genetic counselor for help in deciding whether to conceive or whether to have a fetus tested for thalassemia.

Prenatal testing can be done around the eleventh week of pregnancy using chorionic villi sampling (CVS). This involves removing a tiny piece of the placenta. Or, the fetus can be tested with amniocentesis around the sixteenth week of pregnancy. In this procedure, a needle is used to take a sample of the fluid surrounding the baby for testing.

Assisted reproductive therapy is also an option for carriers who don't want to risk giving birth to a child with thalassemia. A new technique, pre-implantation genetic diagnosis (PGD), used in conjunction with in vitro fertilization, may enable parents who have thalassemia or carry the trait to give birth to healthy babies. Embryos created in vitro are tested for the thalassemia gene before being implanted into the mother, allowing only healthy embryos to be selected.

Section 19.4

Hemophilia

"Learning about Hemophilia," National Human Genome Research Institute, National Institutes of Health, November 26, 2007.

What is hemophilia?

Hemophilia is a bleeding disorder that slows down the blood clotting process. People who have hemophilia often have longer bleeding after an injury or surgery. People who have severe hemophilia have spontaneous bleeding into the joints and muscles. Hemophilia occurs more commonly in males than in females.

The two most common types of hemophilia are hemophilia A (also known as classic hemophilia) and hemophilia B (also known as Christmas disease). People who have hemophilia A have low levels of a blood clotting factor called factor eight (FVIII). People who have hemophilia B have low levels of factor nine (FIX).

The two types of hemophilia are caused by permanent gene changes (mutations) in different genes. Mutations in the FVIII gene cause hemophilia A. Mutations in the FIX gene cause hemophilia B. Proteins made by these genes have an important role in the blood clotting process. Mutations in either gene keep clots from forming when there is an injury, causing too much bleeding that can be difficult to stop.

Blood and Circulatory Disorders

Hemophilia A is the most common type of this condition. One in 5,000 to 10,000 males worldwide have hemophilia A. Hemophilia B is less common, and it affects 1 in 20,000 to 34,500 males worldwide.

What are the symptoms of hemophilia?

Symptoms of hemophilia include prolonged oozing after injuries, tooth extractions, or surgery; renewed bleeding after initial bleeding has stopped; easy or spontaneous bruising; and prolonged bleeding.

In both severe hemophilia A and severe hemophilia B, the most frequent symptom is spontaneous joint bleeding. Other serious sites of bleeding include the bowel, the brain, and soft tissues. These types of bleeding can lead to throwing up blood or passing blood in the stool, stroke, and sudden severe pain in the joints or limbs. Painful bleeding into the soft tissues of the arms and legs can lead to nerve damage.

Individuals who have severe hemophilia are usually diagnosed within the first year of life. People who have moderate hemophilia do not usually have spontaneous bleeding, but they do have longer bleeding and oozing after small injuries. They are usually diagnosed before they reach five or six years.

Individuals who have mild hemophilia do not have spontaneous bleeding. If they are not treated they may have longer bleeding when they have surgery, teeth removed, or major injuries. Individuals with mild hemophilia may not be diagnosed until later in life.

How is hemophilia diagnosed?

Hemophilia A and B are diagnosed by measuring factor clotting activity. Individuals who have hemophilia A have low factor VIII clotting activity. Individuals who have hemophilia B have low factor IX clotting activity.

Genetic testing is also available for the factor VIII gene and the factor IX gene. Genetic testing of the FVIII gene finds a disease-causing mutation in up to 98 percent of individuals who have hemophilia A. Genetic testing of the FIX gene finds disease-causing mutations in more than 99 percent of individuals who have hemophilia B.

Genetic testing is usually used to identify women who are carriers of a FVIII or FIX gene mutation, and to diagnose hemophilia in a fetus during a pregnancy (prenatal diagnosis). It is sometimes used to diagnose individuals who have mild symptoms of hemophilia A or B.

What is the treatment for hemophilia?

There is currently no cure for hemophilia. Treatment depends on the severity of hemophilia.

Treatment may involve slow injection of a medicine called desmopressin (DDAVP) by the doctor into one of the veins. DDAVP helps to release more clotting factor to stop the bleeding. Sometimes, DDAVP is given as a medication that can be breathed in through the nose (nasal spray).

People who have moderate to severe hemophilia A or B may need to have an infusion of clotting factor taken from donated human blood or from genetically engineered products called recombinant clotting factors to stop the bleeding. If the potential for bleeding is serious, a doctor may give infusions of clotting factor to avoid bleeding (preventive infusions) before the bleeding begins. Repeated infusions may be necessary if the internal bleeding is serious.

When bleeding has damaged joints, physical therapy is used to help them function better. Physical therapy helps to keep the joints moving and prevents the joints from becoming frozen or badly deformed. Sometimes the bleeding into joints damages them or destroys them. In this situation, the individual may be given an artificial joint.

When a person who has hemophilia has a small cut or scrape, using pressure and a bandage will take care of the wound. An ice pack can be used when there are small areas of bleeding under the skin.

Researchers have been working to develop a gene replacement treatment (gene therapy) for hemophilia A. Research of gene therapy for hemophilia A is now taking place. The results are encouraging. Researchers continue to evaluate the long-term safety of gene therapies. The hope is that there will be a genetic cure for hemophilia in the future.

Individuals who have hemophilia A and B are living much longer and with less disability than they did thirty years ago. This is because of the use of the intravenous infusion of factor VIII concentrate, home infusion programs, prophylactic treatment, and improved patient education.

Is hemophilia inherited?

Hemophilia is inherited in an X-linked recessive pattern. A condition is considered X-linked when gene mutation that causes it is located on the X chromosome, one of the two sex chromosomes. In males (who have only one X chromosome), one altered copy of the gene in each cell is enough to cause the condition. Since females have two X chromosomes, a mutation must be present in both copies of the gene to cause the hemophilia. Males are affected by X-linked recessive disorders much more frequently than females. A major characteristic of X-linked inheritance is that fathers cannot pass X-linked traits to their sons.

A female who is a carrier has a 1 in 2 (50 percent) chance to pass on her X chromosome with the gene mutation for hemophilia A or B to a boy who will be affected. She has a 1 in 2 (50 percent) chance to pass on her X chromosome with the normally functioning gene to a boy who will not have hemophilia.

Section 19.5

Thrombocytopenia

Excerpted from "Thrombocytopenia," National Heart Lung and Blood Institute, National Institutes of Health, January 2008.

What Is Thrombocytopenia?

Thrombocytopenia is a condition in which your blood has a low number of blood cell fragments called platelets.

Platelets are made in your bone marrow along with other kinds of blood cells. They travel through your blood vessels and stick together (clot) to stop any bleeding that could happen if a blood vessel is damaged. Platelets also are called thrombocytes, because a clot also is called a thrombus.

Overview

When your blood has a low number of platelets, mild to serious bleeding can occur. This bleeding can happen inside the body (internal bleeding) or on the skin.

A normal platelet count is 150,000 to 450,000 platelets per microliter of blood. A count of less than 150,000 platelets per microliter is lower than normal. But the risk for serious bleeding doesn't occur until the count becomes very low—less than 10,000 or 20,000 platelets per microliter. Milder bleeding sometimes occurs when the count is less than 50,000 platelets per microliter.

How long thrombocytopenia lasts depends on its cause. It can range from days to years.

The treatment for this condition also depends on its cause and severity. Mild thrombocytopenia most often doesn't need treatment. If the condition is causing serious bleeding, or if you're at risk for serious bleeding, you may need medicines or blood or platelet transfusions. Rarely, the spleen may need to be removed.

Outlook

Thrombocytopenia can be fatal, especially if the bleeding is severe or occurs in the brain. However, the overall outlook is good, especially if the cause of the low platelet count is found and treated.

What Causes Thrombocytopenia?

A number of factors can cause thrombocytopenia (a low platelet count). The condition can be inherited (passed from parents to children), or it can develop at any age. Sometimes the cause isn't known.

In general, a low platelet count occurs for one of the following reasons:

- The body's bone marrow doesn't make enough platelets.
- The bone marrow makes enough platelets, but the body destroys them or uses them up.
- The spleen holds onto too many platelets.
- A combination of the above factors also may cause a low platelet count.

The Bone Marrow Doesn't Make Enough Platelets

Bone marrow is the sponge-like tissue inside the bones. It contains stem cells that develop into red blood cells, white blood cells, and platelets. When stem cells are damaged, they don't grow into healthy blood cells.

Several conditions or factors can damage stem cells.

Cancer: Cancer, such as leukemia or lymphoma, can damage the bone marrow and destroy blood stem cells. Cancer treatments, such as radiation and chemotherapy, also destroy the stem cells.

Aplastic anemia: Aplastic anemia is a rare, serious blood disorder in which the bone marrow stops making enough new blood cells. This lowers the number of platelets in your blood.

Toxic chemicals: Exposure to toxic chemicals, such as pesticides, arsenic, and benzene, can slow the production of platelets.

Medicines: Some medicines, such as diuretics and chloramphenicol, can slow the production of platelets. Chloramphenicol (an antibiotic) is rarely used in the United States.

Common over-the-counter medicines, such as aspirin or ibuprofen, also can affect platelets.

Alcohol: Alcohol also slows the production of platelets. A temporary drop in platelets is common among heavy drinkers, especially if they're eating foods that are low in iron, vitamin B_{12}, or folate.

Viruses: Chickenpox, mumps, rubella, Epstein-Barr virus, or parvovirus can decrease your platelet count for a while. People who have acquired immunodeficiency syndrome (AIDS) often develop thrombocytopenia.

Genetic conditions: Some genetic conditions, such as Wiskott-Aldrich and May-Hegglin syndromes, can cause low numbers of platelets in the blood.

The Body Destroys Its Own Platelets

A low platelet count can occur even if the bone marrow makes enough platelets. The body may destroy its own platelets due to autoimmune diseases, certain medicines, infections, surgery, pregnancy, and some conditions that cause too much blood clotting.

Autoimmune diseases: With autoimmune diseases, the body's immune system destroys its own platelets. One example of this type of disease is called idiopathic thrombocytopenic purpura, or ITP.

In most cases, the body's immune system is thought to cause ITP. Normally, your immune system helps your body fight off infections and diseases. But if you have ITP, your immune system attacks and destroys its own platelets—for an unknown reason.

Other autoimmune diseases that destroy platelets include lupus and rheumatoid arthritis.

Medicines: A reaction to some medicines can confuse your body and cause it to destroy its platelets. Any medicine can cause this reaction, but it happens most often with quinine, antibiotics that contain sulfa, and some medicines for seizures, such as Dilantin,® vancomycin, and rifampin.

Heparin is a medicine commonly used to prevent blood clots. But an immune reaction may trigger the medicine to cause blood clots and thrombocytopenia. This condition is called heparin-induced thrombocytopenia (HIT). HIT rarely occurs outside of a hospital.

In HIT, the body's immune system attacks a substance formed by heparin and a protein on the surface of the platelets. This attack activates the platelets and they start to form blood clots. Blood clots can form deep in the legs, or a clot can break loose and travel to the lungs.

Infection: A low platelet count can occur after blood poisoning from a widespread bacterial infection. A virus, such as mononucleosis or cytomegalovirus, also can cause a low platelet count.

Surgery: Platelets can be destroyed when they pass through manmade heart valves, blood vessel grafts, or machines and tubing used for blood transfusions or bypass surgery.

Pregnancy: About 5 percent of pregnant women develop mild thrombocytopenia when they're close to delivery. The exact cause isn't known for sure.

Rare and serious conditions that cause blood clots: Some diseases can cause a low platelet count. Two examples are thrombotic thrombocytopenic purpura (TTP) and disseminated intravascular clotting (DIC).

TTP is a rare blood condition. It causes blood clots to form in the body's small blood vessels, including vessels in the brains, kidneys, and heart.

DIC is a rare complication of pregnancy, severe infections, or severe trauma. Tiny blood clots form suddenly throughout the body.

In both conditions, the blood clots use up many of the blood's platelets.

The Spleen Holds On to Too Many Platelets

Usually, one-third of the body's platelets are held in the spleen. If the spleen is enlarged, it will hold on to too many platelets. This means that not enough platelets will circulate in the blood.

Blood and Circulatory Disorders

An enlarged spleen is often due to severe liver disease—such as cirrhosis or cancer. Cirrhosis is a disease in which the liver is scarred. This prevents it from working properly.

An enlarged spleen also may be due to a bone marrow condition, such as myelofibrosis. With this condition, the bone marrow is scarred and isn't able to make blood cells.

Who Is At Risk for Thrombocytopenia?

People who are at highest risk for thrombocytopenia are those affected by one of the conditions or factors discussed above. This includes people who have:

- certain types of cancer, aplastic anemia, or autoimmune diseases;
- been exposed to certain toxic chemicals;
- a reaction to certain medicines;
- certain viruses;
- certain genetic conditions.

People at highest risk also include heavy alcohol drinkers and pregnant women.

What Are the Signs and Symptoms of Thrombocytopenia?

Mild to serious bleeding causes the main signs and symptoms of thrombocytopenia. Bleeding can occur inside the body (internal bleeding) or on the skin.

Signs and symptoms can appear suddenly or over time. Mild thrombocytopenia often has no signs or symptoms. Many times, it's found during a routine blood test.

Check with your doctor if you have any signs of bleeding. Severe thrombocytopenia can cause bleeding in almost any part of the body. This can lead to a medical emergency and should be treated right away.

Bleeding on the skin is usually the first sign of a low platelet count. This may appear as any of the following:

- Small red or purple spots on the skin called petechiae (pe-TEE-key-ay). These spots often occur on the lower legs.

- Purple, brown, and red bruises called purpura. Bruising may happen easily and often.
- Prolonged bleeding, even from minor cuts.
- Bleeding or oozing from the mouth or nose, especially nosebleeds or bleeding from brushing your teeth.

A bleeding problem also can appear as abnormal vaginal bleeding (especially heavy menstrual flow). A lot of bleeding after surgery or dental work also may mean you have a bleeding problem.

Heavy bleeding into the intestines or the brain is serious and can be fatal. Signs and symptoms include the following:

- Blood in the urine or stool or bleeding from the rectum. Blood in the stool can appear as red blood or as a dark, tarry color. (Taking iron supplements also can cause dark, tarry stools.)
- Headaches and other neurological symptoms. These are very rare, but you should discuss them with your doctor.

How Is Thrombocytopenia Diagnosed?

Your doctor will diagnose thrombocytopenia based on your medical history, a physical exam, and test results. A hematologist also may be involved in your care. This is a doctor who treats blood diseases.

Once thrombocytopenia is diagnosed, your doctor will begin looking for its cause.

Diagnostic Tests

Your doctor may order one or more of the following tests to help diagnose a low platelet count.

Complete blood count: A complete blood count (CBC) measures the levels of red blood cells, white blood cells, and platelets in your blood. For this test, a small amount of blood is drawn from a blood vessel, usually in your arm.

If you have thrombocytopenia, the results of this test will show that your platelet count is low.

Blood smear: A blood smear is used to check the appearance of your platelets under a microscope. For this test, a small amount of blood is drawn from a blood vessel, usually in your arm.

Blood and Circulatory Disorders

Bone marrow tests: Bone marrow tests check whether your bone marrow is healthy. Blood cells, including platelets, are made in bone marrow. The two bone marrow tests are aspiration and biopsy.

Bone marrow aspiration may be done to find out why your bone marrow isn't making enough blood cells. For this test, your doctor removes a small amount of fluid bone marrow through a needle. He or she examines the sample under a microscope to check for abnormal cells.

A bone marrow biopsy often is done right after an aspiration. For this test, your doctor removes a small amount of bone marrow tissue through a needle. Your doctor examines the tissue to check the number and types of cells in the bone marrow.

Other tests: If a bleeding problem is suspected, you may need other blood tests as well. For example, tests called prothrombin time (PT) and partial thromboplastin time (PTT) may be done to see whether your blood is clotting properly.

Your doctor may order an ultrasound to check your spleen. An ultrasound uses sound waves to create pictures of your spleen. This will allow your doctor to see whether your spleen is enlarged.

How Is Thrombocytopenia Treated?

Treatment for thrombocytopenia depends on its cause and how severe the condition is. The primary goal of treatment is to prevent death and disability caused by bleeding.

If your condition is mild, you may not need treatment. Your doctor should reassure you that a fully normal platelet count isn't necessary to prevent bleeding, even with severe cuts or accidents.

Thrombocytopenia often improves when its underlying cause is treated. People who inherit the condition usually don't need treatment.

If a reaction to medicine is causing a low platelet count, your doctor may prescribe other medicine. Most people recover after the offending medicine has been stopped. For heparin-induced thrombocytopenia (HIT), stopping the heparin isn't enough. Often, you'll need another medicine to prevent blood clotting.

If your immune system is causing a low platelet count, your doctor may prescribe medicines to suppress the immune system. When the condition is severe, treatments may include the following:

- **Medicines:** You may be given steroids. This medicine can be given through a vein or by mouth. One example of this type of medicine is prednisone. You also may be given immunoglobulin. This medicine is given through a vein.

- **Blood or platelet transfusions:** This type of treatment is reserved for people who have active bleeding or are at a high risk for bleeding.
- **Splenectomy:** This is surgery to remove the spleen. This treatment is most often used for adults who have idiopathic thrombocytopenic purpura.

How Can Thrombocytopenia Be Prevented?

Whether you can prevent thrombocytopenia depends on its specific cause. Most cases of the condition can't be prevented. However, you can take steps to prevent its complications:

- Avoid heavy drinking. Alcohol slows the production of platelets.
- Avoid medicines that have decreased your platelet count in the past.
- Be aware of medicines that may affect your platelets and raise your risk for bleeding. Two examples of such medicines are aspirin and ibuprofen. These medicines may thin your blood too much.
- Talk with your doctor about getting vaccinated for viruses that can affect your platelets. You may need vaccines for mumps, measles, rubella, and chickenpox. You may want to have your child vaccinated for these viruses as well. Talk to you child's doctor about these vaccines.

Living with Thrombocytopenia

You can take steps to avoid complications of thrombocytopenia. Watch what medicines you take, avoid injury, and contact your doctor if you have fever or other signs or symptoms of an infection.

Medicines

Avoid medicines that may affect your platelets and raise your risk for bleeding. Two examples of such medicines are aspirin and ibuprofen. These medicines may thin your blood too much. Be careful when using over-the-counter medicines, because many contain aspirin or ibuprofen.

Blood and Circulatory Disorders

Tell your doctor about all of the medicines you take, including over-the-counter medicines, vitamins, supplements, and herbal remedies.

Injury

Avoid injuries that can cause bruising and bleeding. Don't participate in contact sports such as boxing, football, or karate. These sports are likely to lead to injuries that can cause bleeding.

Other sports, such as skiing or horseback riding, also put you at risk for injuries that can cause bleeding. Ask your doctor about physical activities that are safe for you.

Take safety precautions, such as using seatbelts and wearing gloves when working with knives and other tools.

If your child has thrombocytopenia, try to protect him or her from injuries, especially head injuries that can cause bleeding in the brain. Ask your child's doctor whether you need to restrict your child's activities.

Infection

If you've had your spleen removed, you may be more likely to become ill from certain types of infection. Watch for fever or other signs and symptoms of infection and report them to your doctor promptly. People who have had their spleens removed may need vaccinations to prevent these infections.

Section 19.6

Thrombophilia

"Thrombophilia," © Hemophilia and Thrombosis Center at the University of Colorado Denver (www.uchsc.edu/htc). Reprinted with permission.

What is thrombophilia?

Thrombophilia, also called hypercoagulability or prothrombotic state, means an increased risk for excessive blood clotting in the veins and arteries. Substances in your blood (called proteins) work with tiny particles (called platelets) to form the blood clot. Forming a clot is called "coagulation." Coagulation is a natural, life saving mechanism when you are injured and bleeding because it slows blood loss. However, your blood should not clot when it's just trying to move through your body. If blood clots inside your blood vessels, it is called "thrombosis"—it can either partially or completely block the flow of blood in the vessel. The tendency to clot too much is called hypercoagulation or thrombophilia.

Why is thrombophilia dangerous?

When abnormal clotting occurs inside the blood vessel, it can fully or partially stop the flow of blood to the extremity it normally supplies. A clot inside a blood vessel is called a "thrombus." Sometimes the thrombus can travel through the bloodstream and get stuck in a smaller vessel in your lungs. This kind of a clot is called a "pulmonary embolus," and keeps blood from getting to your lungs. Blood clots can cause at-risk women to have miscarriages. A clot that blocks a blood vessel in the brain can cause a stroke and a clot in a blood vessel in your heart can cause a heart attack.

Am I at risk for a clot?

There are several factors, called risk factors, that increase your chances of developing a dangerous clot. Usually, more than one of the risks factors needs to be present to form a clot. You are more likely to be at risk of deep-vein thrombosis (DVT) if:

- you have injured the deep veins in your arms or legs (for example, a broken bone, severe muscle injury, or have surgery);
- the blood flow through your veins is slowed as with long car, bus, train, or airplane rides or bed rest;
- you have an inherited or acquired risk factor, like Factor V Leiden or protein C deficiency;
- you have a previous history of a blood clot;
- you have a family member who has had a clot in the past.

Some people have a combination of these risk factors and are at a higher risk than those who have fewer factors.

How do I know if I have a clot?

The most common place for a clot is in the leg. You may have swelling, pain, and redness in the calf or behind the knee. A more rare site for clotting is in the lungs, which makes it hard to breathe. In even rarer cases, the clot might occur in the arm or another part of the body. Again, swelling, pain, and/or redness may be present in the area of the clot.

Can thrombophilia be treated?

There are medicines that can thin your blood and make it less likely to clot. Some people with thrombophilia only need to take blood-thinning medications when they have an increased risk such as surgery, trauma, pregnancy, or long plane/car trip. Other people with thrombophilia need to take medicine for the rest of their lives.

The two most common blood-thinning medications are called heparin and Coumadin® (warfarin). Usually, your doctor will give you heparin first, because heparin works right away. Heparin comes in two forms and if you are in the hospital, you may get your heparin through an intravenous (IV) line. You may go home on heparin that must be injected under the skin. After being on heparin for the time suggested by your doctor, you might start taking Coumadin. Coumadin is taken by mouth and takes longer to begin working so you should continue the heparin until the Coumadin is working in your blood.

These medications can cause you to bleed more easily. You might notice that cuts take longer to clot and that you may bruise more easily. If you have any unusual bleeding, call your doctor right away.

What can I do to help avoid a clot?

- Avoid standing or sitting in the same position for long periods of time as in long car or plane rides.
- Avoid oral birth control or hormone therapy (consult physician).
- Consult your physician before becoming pregnant.
- Exercise regularly (walking, jogging, swimming) and keep your weight at a normal level.
- Avoid smoking.
- Avoid alcohol.
- Keep well hydrated.
- Check your cholesterol regularly.
- Consult your physician when you have an infection and are on medications.
- Prevent venous stasis (wear compression stockings, elevate legs).

Section 19.7

von Willebrand Disease

"von Willebrand Disease," © 2006 National Hemophilia Foundation (www.hemophilia.org). Reprinted with permission.

What Is von Willebrand Disease?

Von Willebrand disease (VWD) is a bleeding disorder caused by a defect or deficiency of a blood clotting protein, called von Willebrand factor. The disease is estimated to occur in 1 to 2 percent of the population. The disease was first described by Erik von Willebrand, a Finnish physician who reported a new type of bleeding disorder among island people in Sweden and Finland.

Von Willebrand factor is a protein critical to the initial stages of blood clotting. This glue-like protein, produced by the cells that line the blood vessel walls, interacts with blood cells called platelets to form a plug, which prevents the blood from flowing at the site of injury. People with von Willebrand disease are unable to make this plug because they do not have enough von Willebrand factor or their factor is abnormal.

Researchers have identified many variations of the disease, but most fall into the following classifications:

- **Type I:** This is the most common and mildest form of von Willebrand disease. Levels of von Willebrand factor are lower than normal, and levels of factor VIII may also be reduced.

- **Type II:** In these people, the von Willebrand factor itself has an abnormality. Depending on the abnormality, they may be classified as having type IIa or type IIb. In type IIa, the level of von Willebrand factor is reduced, as is the ability of platelets to clump together. In type IIb, although the factor itself is defective, the ability of platelets to clump together is actually increased.

- **Type III:** This is severe von Willebrand disease. These people may have a total absence of von Willebrand factor, and factor VIII levels are often less than 10 percent.

- **Pseudo (or platelet-type) von Willebrand disease:** This disorder resembles type IIb von Willebrand disease, but the defects appear to be in the platelets, rather than the von Willebrand factor.

Von Willebrand disease is a genetic disease that can be inherited from either parent. It affects males and females equally. A man or woman with VWD has a 50 percent chance of passing the gene on to his or her child. There are no racial or ethnic associations with the disorder. A family history of a bleeding disorder is the primary risk factor.

VWD subtype I and II are usually inherited in what is known as a "dominant" pattern. This means that if even one parent has the gene and passes it to a child, the child will have the disorder.

VWD type III von Willebrand disease, however, is usually inherited in a "recessive" pattern. This type occurs when the child inherits the gene from both parents. Even if both parents have mild or asymptomatic disease, their children are likely to be severely affected.

Diagnosis of von Willebrand disease can be difficult. Blood tests can be performed to determine the amount, structure, and function of von Willebrand factor. Since levels can vary, sometimes tests may need to be repeated. A person suspected of having von Willebrand disease should be referred to a hematologist who specializes in the diagnosis and treatment of bleeding disorders.

Usually, people with VWD bruise easily, have recurrent nosebleeds, or bleed after tooth extraction, tonsillectomy, or other surgery. Recurrent nosebleeds are also a hallmark of VWD. Women can have increased menstrual bleeding.

For minor bleeds, treatment may be unnecessary. There are a range of treatment choices that depend on whether the VWD is mild or severe.

Stimate® or desmopressin acetate (DDAVP), a nasal spray, is the treatment of choice for mild von Willebrand disease. Bleeding is usually controlled in individuals with mild von Willebrand disease by using this nasal spray to boost their own factor VIII and von Willebrand levels. DDAVP may be given to increase the amount of the von Willebrand factor long enough for surgery or dental procedures to be performed. DDAVP is a synthetic product that carries no risk of infectious disease.

For excessive bleeding, infusions of a factor VIII concentrate rich in von Willebrand factor, such as Humate-P®, Alphanate®, or Koate DVI®, may be required. Humate-P, manufactured by ZLB-Behring, is the only FDA-approved Factor VIII concentrate for use in von Willebrand disease.

Blood and Circulatory Disorders

If trauma occurs or surgery is anticipated, desmopressin acetate can be given as a means of raising the von Willebrand factor level.

Aspirin and many of the drugs used for pain can aggravate bleeding because they interfere with platelet function. People who have von Willebrand disease can take acetaminophen for pain relief because it does not inhibit platelet function.

Chapter 20

Cancer

Chapter Contents

Section 20.1—Leukemia 264
Section 20.2—Lymphoma 269
Section 20.3—Neuroblastoma 276
Section 20.4—Sarcoma 279

Section 20.1

Leukemia

"Leukemia," © 2008 The Leukemia & Lymphoma Society.
All rights reserved. Reprinted with permission.

What Is Leukemia?

Leukemia is the general term used to describe four different disease-types called:

- acute myelogenous leukemia (AML);
- acute lymphocytic leukemia (ALL);
- chronic myelogenous leukemia (CML);
- chronic lymphocytic leukemia (CLL).

The terms lymphocytic or lymphoblastic indicate that the cancerous change takes place in a type of marrow cell that forms lymphocytes. The terms myelogenous or myeloid indicate that the cell change takes place in a type of marrow cell that normally goes on to form red cells, some types of white cells, and platelets.

Acute lymphocytic leukemia and acute myelogenous leukemia are each composed of blast cells, known as lymphoblasts or myeloblasts. Acute leukemias progress rapidly without treatment.

Chronic leukemias have few or no blast cells. Chronic lymphocytic leukemia and chronic myelogenous leukemia usually progress slowly compared to acute leukemias.

How Does Leukemia Develop?

The four types of leukemia each begin in a cell in the bone marrow. The cell undergoes a leukemic change and it multiplies into many cells. The leukemia cells grow and survive better than normal cells and, over time, they crowd out normal cells.

Normal stem cells in the marrow form three main cell types: red cells, platelets, and white cells. There are two major types of white

Cancer

cells: germ-ingesting cells (neutrophils and monocytes) and lymphocytes, which are part of the body's immune system and help to fight to infection.

The rate at which leukemia progresses and how the cells replace the normal blood and marrow cells are different with each type of leukemia.

Acute Leukemias

In acute myelogenous leukemia (AML) and acute lymphocytic leukemia (ALL), the original acute leukemia cell goes on to form about a trillion more leukemia cells. These cells are described as "nonfunctional" because they do not work like normal cells. They also crowd out the normal cells in the marrow; in turn, this causes a decrease in the number of new normal cells made in the marrow. This further results in low red cell counts (anemia).

Chronic Leukemias

In chronic myelogenous leukemia (CML), the leukemia cell that starts the disease makes blood cells (red cells, white cells, and platelets) that function almost like normal cells. The number of red cells is usually less than normal, resulting in anemia. But many white cells and sometimes many platelets are still made. Even though the white cells are nearly normal in how they work, their counts are high and continue to rise. This can cause serious problems if the patient does not get treatment. If untreated, the white cell count can rise so high that blood flow slows down and anemia becomes severe.

In chronic lymphocytic leukemia (CLL), the leukemia cell that starts the disease makes too many lymphocytes that do not function. These cells replace normal cells in the marrow and lymph nodes. They interfere with the work of normal lymphocytes, which weakens the patient's immune response. The high number of leukemia cells in the marrow may crowd out normal blood-forming cells and lead to a low red cell count (anemia). A very high number of leukemia cells building up in the marrow also can lead to low neutrophil and platelet counts.

Unlike the other three types of leukemia, some patients with CLL may have disease that does not progress for a long time. Some people with CLL have such slight changes that they remain in good health and do not need treatment for long periods of time. Most patients require treatment at the time of diagnosis or soon after.

Risk Factors

People can get leukemia at any age. In 2007, about and 40,440 adults and 3,800 children were expected to develop leukemia. It is most common in people over age sixty. The most common types in adults are AML and CLL. ALL is the most common form of leukemia in children.

For most types of leukemia, the risk factors and possible causes are not known. Most people who have any of the specific risk factors that have been identified do not get leukemia—and most people with leukemia do not have these risk factors.

Some risk factors for AML are:

- certain chemotherapies used for lymphoma or other types of cancer;
- Down syndrome and some other genetic diseases;
- chronic exposure to benzene (such as in the workplace) that exceeds federally approved safety limits;
- radiation therapy used to treat other types of cancer;
- tobacco smoke.

Exposure to high doses of radiation therapy is also a risk factor for ALL and CML. Other possible risk factors for the four types of leukemia are continually under study.

Leukemia is not contagious (catching).

Signs and Symptoms

Some signs or symptoms of leukemia are similar to other more common and less severe illnesses. Specific blood tests and bone marrow tests are needed to make a diagnosis. Signs and symptoms vary based on the type of leukemia.

For acute leukemia, they include:

- tiredness or no energy;
- shortness of breath during physical activity;
- pale skin;
- mild fever or night sweats;
- slow healing of cuts and excess bleeding;
- black-and-blue marks (bruises) for no clear reason;
- pinhead-size red spots under the skin;

Cancer

- aches in bones or joints (for example, knees, hips, or shoulders);
- low white cell counts, especially monocytes or neutrophils.

People with CLL or CML may not have any symptoms. Some patients learn they have CLL or CML after a blood test as part of a regular checkup. Sometimes, a person with CLL may notice enlarged lymph nodes in the neck, armpit, or groin and go to the doctor. The person may feel tired or short of breath (from anemia) or have frequent infections, if the CLL is more severe. In these cases, a blood test may show an increase in the lymphocyte count.

CML signs and symptoms tend to develop slowly. People with CML may feel tired and short of breath while doing everyday activities; they may also have an enlarged spleen (leading to a "dragging" feeling on the upper left side of the belly), night sweats, and weight loss.

Each type of leukemia may have other symptoms or signs that prompt a person to get a medical checkup.

The best advice for any person troubled by symptoms such as a lasting, low-grade fever, unexplained weight loss, tiredness, or shortness of breath is to see a health care provider.

Diagnosis

A complete blood count (CBC) is used to diagnose leukemia. This blood test may show high or low levels of white cells and show leukemic cells in the blood. Sometimes, platelet counts and red cell counts are low. Bone marrow tests (aspiration and biopsy) are often done to confirm the diagnosis and to look for chromosome abnormalities. These tests identify the leukemia cell type.

A complete blood exam and a number of other tests are used to diagnose the type of leukemia. These tests can be repeated after treatment begins to measure how well the treatment is working.

Treatment

The ways in which patients are affected and how patients are treated are different for each type of leukemia.

Each main type of leukemia has different subtypes. A patient's age, general health, and subtype may play a role in determining the best treatment plan. Blood tests and bone marrow tests are used to identify AML, ALL, CML, or CLL subtypes.

It is important to get medical care at a center where doctors are experienced in treating patients with leukemia. The aim of leukemia treatment is to bring about a complete remission. Today, more and more leukemia patients are in complete remission at least five years after treatment.

Patients with an acute leukemia need to start treatment right away. Usually, they begin induction therapy with chemotherapy in the hospital.

More inpatient treatment is usually needed even after a patient is in remission. This is called consolidation therapy or post induction therapy. This part of treatment may include chemotherapy with or without allogeneic stem cell transplantation (sometimes called "bone marrow transplantation").

Patients with CML need to begin treatment once they are diagnosed. They usually begin treatment with imatinib mesylate (Gleevec®). This drug is taken by mouth. Gleevec® does not cure CML. But it keeps CML under control for many patients for as long as they take it. Other drugs, such as dasatinib (Sprycel®), are used for certain patients instead of Gleevec®.

Allogeneic stem cell transplantation is the only treatment that can cure CML at this time. This treatment is most successful in younger patients. But patients up to sixty years of age who have a matched donor may be considered for this treatment. Allogeneic transplantation can be a high-risk procedure. Studies are under way to see whether CML patients have better long-term outcomes with drug therapy or with transplantation.

Some CLL patients do not need treatment for long periods of time after diagnosis. Patients who need treatment may receive chemotherapy or monoclonal antibody therapy alone or in combination. Allogeneic stem cell transplantation is a treatment option for certain patients.

New Treatment Methods

New cancer treatments are under study in clinical trials to help a growing number of patients achieve remission or be cured of their disease.

Follow-Up

AML, ALL, CML, and CLL patients who are in remission need to see their doctors regularly for exams and blood tests. Bone marrow tests may be needed from time to time. The doctor may recommend longer periods of time between follow-up visits if a patient continues to be disease free.

Patients and caregivers should talk with their healthcare providers about long-term and late effects of cancer treatment. Cancer-related fatigue is one common long-term effect.

Get Support

After diagnosis, many people with leukemia do survive and live many good, quality years. Knowing more about the disease and its treatment may make it easier to cope.

It may be helpful to write down questions to ask your doctor. Then you can write down your doctor's answers and review them later. You may want to bring a family member or friend with you to the doctor. This person can listen, take notes, and offer support. Some patients record information and listen to it at home.

Section 20.2

Lymphoma

"About Lymphoma" and "Lymphoma Treatment," © 2005 Seattle Cancer Care Alliance (www.seattlecca.org). Reprinted with permission.

Lymphoma

What Is Lymphoma?

Lymphoma is cancer of the lymph system. This is part of your child's immune system. It's a network of small vessels that collect a watery fluid called lymph from all around the body. White blood cells called lymphocytes travel in the lymph, fighting infection and disease. Along the network of lymph vessels are lymph nodes—bean-like structures that filter the lymph and serve as activity centers that resist disease.

Other structures play a role in the lymph system, too: the spleen, which helps make lymphocytes; the thymus, where lymphocytes mature and multiply; the tonsils, positioned to resist infections that enter through the nose or mouth; the stomach and intestines, which have patches of lymph tissue; and the bone marrow, where blood cells are made.

The lymph system is virtually everywhere throughout the body, and lymphoma can begin in many places. It can also spread to organs not directly related to the lymph system.

Types of Lymphoma

There are two major types of lymphoma:

- Hodgkin lymphoma, named for the doctor who first diagnosed it. This form is more common in older children or teens. It's rare in children younger than age five.
- Non-Hodgkin lymphoma. This name applies to all other forms of lymphoma. The incidence of non-Hodgkin lymphoma increases throughout childhood into young adulthood.

Both types develop from the lymph system. But they affect the body differently, spread differently, and respond differently to treatment.

Doctors divide Hodgkin and non-Hodgkin lymphoma into subtypes based on the specific type of cell affected, the level of maturity reached by the cells, their appearance under a microscope, or the way they grow. The subtype sometimes helps doctors decide which treatments are most likely to be effective.

Risk Factors

Doctors do not know what causes lymphoma in children. There are several factors that may increase a child's risk. But most children who have lymphoma have none of these risk factors.

Children may be at higher risk for non-Hodgkin lymphoma if any of these is true:

- They have a genetic disorder that interferes with their immune system.
- Their immune system was suppressed using drugs because they had an organ transplant.
- They have human immunodeficiency virus (HIV), which has weakened their immune system.
- They were exposed to radiation such as from a nuclear reactor accident or explosion of an atomic bomb.

For Hodgkin lymphoma, the issues of risk are less straightforward. Doctors hope that ongoing research will help us better understand the risk factors. The following are links that have been noted, but none of these causes the disease:

- Risk is higher in monozygotic twins and siblings.
- Risk for some forms of the disease is linked with exposure to the Epstein-Barr virus or a history of mononucleosis.
- For older adolescents and young adults, higher socioeconomic status is a risk factor. For children under age ten, lower socioeconomic status is a risk factor.
- For older adolescents, having fewer siblings and childhood playmates is a risk factor.

Symptoms

The symptoms of lymphoma can be caused by other noncancerous conditions. So it's important to see a doctor if your child has symptoms that concern you.

These are possible symptoms of lymphoma:

- Shortness of breath, breathing trouble, wheezing, or high-pitched breathing, caused by an enlarged thymus or lymph nodes in the chest
- Swelling in the head, neck, upper arms, or chest, caused by lymphoma pressing on the major vein that drains blood from these areas
- Trouble swallowing
- Swollen lymph nodes in the neck, underarm, chest, abdomen, pelvis, or groin
- Unexplained fever, weight loss, or night sweats—sometimes called "B symptoms"
- Itchy skin, in the case of Hodgkin lymphoma

Symptoms of non-Hodgkin lymphoma can come on extremely rapidly, sometimes within days to weeks before diagnosis. Some types of non-Hodgkin lymphoma can come on slowly over several months. For Hodgkin lymphoma, there is usually a longer, slower onset of lymph node symptoms. Swelling and symptoms can be present for as long as a year before diagnosis. However, B symptoms generally come on more rapidly and are present for less than a few months before the disease is diagnosed.

Diagnosis

Your child's doctor will do a physical exam first to look for signs of lymphoma. The doctor will also ask about your child's health history.

If the doctor thinks that your child may have lymphoma, the doctor will probably perform a biopsy next to confirm the diagnosis. To perform a biopsy, a doctor removes a small sample of tissue to examine under a microscope. This may mean removing part or all of a lymph node or some tissue by surgery.

Another method is to take a sample of fluid or tissue using a needle, called needle biopsy or fine needle aspiration. This type of biopsy may be done to check the bone marrow or the fluid around the lungs (pleural fluid) or in the membrane around the abdominal organs (peritoneal fluid). Usually this is not enough to diagnose lymphoma in children.

Your child's doctor may also want your child to have imaging studies, such as a chest x-ray, computed tomography (CT) scan, gallium scan, or positron emission tomography (PET) scan, to see pictures of the inside of the child's body. This allows the doctor to look for enlarged lymph nodes, tumors, or areas of cancer activity.

Doctors may do further tests to detect whether the cancer has spread around the lymph system or to other areas. This helps your child's doctor determine the stage of your child's cancer, which will be important when it's time to make decisions about your child's treatment. The additional tests may include these or other tests:

- **Complete blood count, or CBC:** to determine how many cells of each type are circulating in the blood stream

- **Blood chemistry analysis:** to look for chemicals in the blood that indicate disease in certain organs or tissues

- **Lumbar puncture, or spinal tap:** to remove cerebrospinal fluid (CFS) from the spinal column and check it for cancer cells; used in non-Hodgkin lymphoma only

- **Bone marrow test:** to see if the lymphoma has spread to the bone marrow

Staging

Staging refers to the way doctors classify lymphoma based on where it is in the body. Staging systems are different for non-Hodgkin to be at one of these stages:

- **Stage I:** This stage applies to children who have lymphoma in only one area or lymph node, and that structure is not in the abdomen or chest.
- **Stage II:** This stage applies to children who have any one of these:
  - Lymphoma in only one area, including the lymph nodes in that area.
  - Lymphoma in two or more areas or lymph nodes, with all the cancer on the same side of the diaphragm. (The diaphragm muscle controls breathing and separates the chest and abdomen.)
  - Lymphoma that started in the stomach or intestines and that was completely removed through surgery.
- **Stage III:** This stage applies to children who have any one of these:
  - Lymphoma on both sides of the diaphragm
  - Lymphoma that started in the chest
  - Lymphoma in two or more areas in the abdomen
  - Lymphoma around the spine
- **Stage IV:** This stage applies to children who have lymphoma in their bone marrow, brain, spine, or spinal fluid.

Children who have Hodgkin lymphoma are considered to be at one of these stages:

- **Stage I:** This stage applies to children who have lymphoma in one group of lymph nodes. Doctors will add the letter "E" after "Stage I" if the lymphoma has spread to a structure nearby that isn't part of the lymph system.
- **Stage II:** This stage applies to children who have lymphoma in two or more groups of lymph nodes on the same side of the diaphragm (the muscle that controls breathing and separates the chest and abdomen). Doctors will add the letter "E" after "Stage II" if the lymphoma has spread to a structure nearby that isn't part of the lymph system.
- **Stage III:** This stage applies to children who have lymphoma on both sides of the diaphragm. Doctors will add the letter "E" after "Stage III" if the lymphoma has spread to a structure

nearby that isn't part of the lymph system. They will add the letter "S" if the only area of disease below the diaphragm is the spleen. (The disease may be stage III, IIIE, IIIS, or IIIE+S.)

- **Stage IV:** This stage applies to children who have either of these:
  - Lymphoma throughout one nonlymph organ and in lymph nodes distant from that organ.
  - Lymphoma throughout one or more organs that aren't in the lymph system. (In children it's rare not to have at least one structure affected in the lymph system.)

Doctors may further classify Hodgkin lymphoma based on whether your child has the B symptoms—fever, weight loss, or night sweats.

Lymphoma Treatment

Most children who have either Hodgkin or non-Hodgkin lymphoma are cured. The success of treatment depends on many factors, some of which are described below. As doctors find more successful treatments through clinical trials, the prognosis for children with lymphoma will continue to improve.

Your child's doctor and health care team will recommend a treatment plan for your child based on the type of lymphoma your child has, the stage of the disease, whether and how many places it has spread, and your child's overall health. Here is a summary of the most common treatments for childhood lymphoma.

Non-Hodgkin Lymphoma

Standard treatment for non-Hodgkin lymphoma is combination chemotherapy (using multiple drugs). Radiation therapy is rarely used to treat non-Hodgkin lymphoma except when the disease has spread to the central nervous system (brain and spinal cord) or testes. If the child's cancer recurs, doctors may recommend other treatments, such as a high-dose chemotherapy along with a stem cell transplant, radiation, or one of the new treatments that is being studied in clinical trials.

More than two-thirds of children diagnosed with non-Hodgkin lymphoma survive more than five years after their diagnosis. Many live much longer. The cure rate for non-Hodgkin lymphoma ranges from 65 to 100 percent of patients depending on the type of non-Hodgkin lymphoma, the extent of disease at the time of diagnosis, and how quickly the lymphoma responds to initial therapy. Initial treatment lasts from several months to a couple of years, depending on the type and extent of the disease.

Most children with non-Hodgkin lymphoma have disease that has spread to other places in the body at the time of diagnosis (stage III or IV disease).

Hodgkin Lymphoma

After the diagnosis is confirmed by a biopsy (surgery), standard treatment for Hodgkin lymphoma is combination chemotherapy (using multiple drugs) along with radiation therapy. Also, researchers are studying the use of high-dose chemotherapy along with a stem cell transplants in children who have Hodgkin lymphoma that has recurred after initial treatment.

Overall, 80 to 98 percent of children and adolescents with Hodgkin lymphoma are cured of their disease. The cure rate depends on the stage of the lymphoma, associated symptoms, the size of any tumors, and other factors about the child's disease. For those with the most mild disease, over 95 percent are cured.

Section 20.3

Neuroblastoma

"Neuroblastoma," © 2008 Children's Healthcare of Atlanta (www.choa.org). Reprinted with permission.

Neuroblastoma is a cancer which develops from branches of nerves from the spinal cord. These branches may reach many areas of the body and tumors can be found in many different places. In half of the cases of children with neuroblastoma, the tumors are found in the abdomen and usually involve the adrenal gland, which sits on top of the kidney. Neuroblastoma is sometimes (but less frequently) found in the chest, neck, pelvis, or head.

What are some of the signs and symptoms of neuroblastoma?

The symptoms of neuroblastoma depend upon where the cancer is. For example, if the tumor is in the abdomen, the child's belly may look enlarged or bloated. If there is bone involvement with the tumor, there may be bone pain resulting in a limp or the child's refusal to walk or to use a certain arm or leg. Other general signs may be loss of appetite, failure to gain weight, unexplained fevers, a tired feeling, pale skin, and minor aches and pains.

What causes neuroblastoma?

The cause of neuroblastoma is not known at this time. We do know that it cannot be spread to others. We also know that some infants are born with it, suggesting that it can occur while the unborn child's nervous system cells are growing and maturing.

Who gets neuroblastoma?

Although neuroblastoma is the third most common type of cancer in children, it is still rare. There are about five hundred newly diagnosed cases of neuroblastoma each year in the United States. In most cases, it is a disease of early childhood. Fifty percent of these children are under two years old when diagnosed. Overall, 75 percent of all children with neuroblastoma are under five years old.

Is neuroblastoma inherited?

There is no information to support this. It does not tend to run in families or to occur in other family members.

What are metastases?

Metastases refers to the spread of cancer from its original location to other parts of the body. Neuroblastoma can spread, usually to the bones or the bone marrow. Neuroblastoma has often been called a "silent tumor" because 60 percent of children with this tumor already have metastases before any signs of the disease are noticed.

What is staging?

Staging is the process of finding out the extent of disease present at the time of initial diagnosis. Neuroblastoma has been divided into four stages for purposes of better matching the therapy to the disease:

- **Stage 1:** The tumor is confined to the organ and can be completely removed by surgery.

- **Stage 2:** The tumor has not been completely removed or has spread to lymph nodes located on the same side of the body as the tumor.

- **Stage 3:** The tumor has spread from its original site to lymph nodes in the opposite side of the body.

- **Stage 4:** The tumor has spread to distant locations in the body such as the bone marrow, bones, liver, or lymph nodes.

- **Stage 4S:** Same as stage 4 but reserved for infants under one year of age, who have small tumors that have spread to the liver, bone marrow, or skin, but not the bones.

How can neuroblastoma be treated?

The method of treatment proposed for your child will depend upon the stage of disease at the time of diagnosis and on certain features of your child's tumor.

There are three types of therapy commonly used to treat neuroblastoma. They are chemotherapy, surgery, and bone marrow transplantation. The type of therapy chosen will depend upon the age of the child and the extent of the disease. The decision of how to treat the disease is made by both you and your child's doctor.

In a number of newborns with neuroblastoma the tumors disappear without therapy. In general, this is not true for older children with neuroblastoma. Over 60 percent of all children with neuroblastoma are older than one year and have metastases. Most children receive a combination of surgery and chemotherapy to treat their disease; a few children may also need radiation therapy.

Chemotherapy is the use of medications to kill cancer cells. Chemotherapy not only destroys cancer cells, but also affects the growth of normal cells and therefore has side effects which will be explained to you.

Surgery to remove the bulk of the tumor may be done early, during the diagnostic period, or later after the tumor has been shrunk with radiation or chemotherapy drugs. If there is wide spread of the disease, surgery is usually done after chemotherapy to minimize the risk of injury to vital organs that the neuroblastoma may be affecting.

Stem cell transplantation is the use of higher doses of chemotherapy and sometimes radiation therapy, followed by the infusion of stem cells (young cells from the bone marrow) that have been previously collected from the patient. If your child has stage 3 or 4 neuroblastoma, more information will be given to you about this treatment option.

How long will my child's therapy last?

The usual length of treatment is about nine months. It involves one scheduled hospitalization lasting about a week, per month, and follow-up blood tests as an outpatient.

Section 20.4

Sarcoma

"About Bone Cancer and Soft Tissue Sarcoma" and "Sarcoma Treatment," © 2005 Seattle Cancer Care Alliance (www.seattlecca.org). Reprinted with permission.

About Bone Cancer and Soft Tissue Sarcoma

What Is Sarcoma?

Sarcoma is a form of cancer that begins in the bone, soft tissues, or connective tissues. There are many types of sarcoma:

- Osteosarcoma starts in cells that are designed to form new bone. Instead of building bone, these cancerous cells destroy it and weaken the bone's structure. Osteosarcoma can occur in any bone. In children it usually starts around the knee joint. Other common sites are higher in the femur (the thigh bone) or in the humerus (the upper arm bone) near the shoulder. Sometimes it spreads to other bones or the lungs. Rarely osteosarcoma begins in tissue outside the bone. Adolescents and young adults develop osteosarcoma more often than any other age group.

- The Ewing family of tumors makes up another type of sarcoma. Ewing sarcoma usually forms a tumor in the bones of the lower body: the pelvis or the upper or lower leg. Other tumors in the Ewing family can develop in soft tissue. The Ewing family of tumors is most common in adolescents.

- Soft tissue sarcomas can develop in any of the soft tissues that connect or support other structures. These include muscles, tendons, fat, blood vessels, lymph vessels, nerves, and the soft tissues in and around joints (synovial tissues). Soft tissue sarcoma is rare in children. The most common type occurs in skeletal muscles—the muscles that attach to our bones and allow us to bend our joints. This type is called rhabdomyosarcoma. It usually begins in the arms or legs. Other common sites include the head or neck (such as the base of the skull or around the eye) or in the urinary or reproductive organs.

Risk Factors

Doctors do not know what causes sarcoma in children. Depending on the type of sarcoma, there may be factors that increase a child's risk. For instance, children with certain uncommon inherited conditions have greater risk of developing soft tissue sarcoma. But almost all children who have sarcoma have no risk factors.

Symptoms

The symptoms of sarcoma depend on the type of disease, where it is, and how much it has grown or spread. The symptoms listed here can also be caused by other noncancerous conditions. So it's important to see a doctor if your child has symptoms that concern you.

These are possible symptoms of osteosarcoma:

- Bone or joint pain that gets worse
- Unexplained lump or swelling in the arm or leg
- Broken bone for no known reason

Ewing sarcoma may cause these symptoms:

- Unexplained lump with pain and swelling in the area
- Loss of appetite, fever, feeling of illness, fatigue, and weight loss if the disease has spread to other areas

Children with rhabdomyosarcoma usually have a fast-growing lump in their arm or leg. Symptoms of soft tissue sarcoma, including rhabdomyosarcoma, can vary depending the location. For instance, a tumor in or around the urinary tract can interfere with urination, or a tumor at the base of the skull can compress facial nerves, causing weakness or pain there.

Diagnosis

Your child's doctor will do a physical exam first to look for signs of cancer and will ask about your child's health history. Then the doctor may recommend a number of tests to help identify the type of cancer and see whether it has spread.

If the doctor thinks that your child may have sarcoma, the doctor will perform a biopsy next to confirm the diagnosis. To perform a biopsy, a doctor removes a small sample of tissue to examine under a microscope. This may mean removing part or all of the suspicious tissue surgically.

Your child's doctor may also want your child to have imaging studies, such as an x-ray, ultrasound, computed tomography (CT) scan, magnetic resonance imaging (MRI), or positron emission tomography (PET) scan, in order to see pictures of the inside of the child's body. This allows the doctor to look for tumors or areas of cancer activity.

Staging

Staging refers to the way doctors classify cancer based on where it is in the body. This, along with other factors, helps doctors choose a course of treatment. There is no common staging system for all types of sarcoma.

Osteosarcoma and Ewing tumors of the bone are classified as localized (in only one part of the body) or metastatic (spread to another part).

Soft tissue sarcomas, including rhabdomyosarcoma, may be divided into four stages depending on these factors:

- Whether the tumor is more than two inches in diameter

- Whether it has spread to lymph nodes (bean-like structures that filter watery fluid collected from around your body and that serve as activity centers for disease resistance)

- Whether it has spread to other areas of the body

- How much the tumor resembles normal tissue and how fast it is growing

Sarcoma Treatment

Your child's doctor and health care team will recommend a treatment plan for your child based on many factors. These include the type of sarcoma your child has; the location, size, and stage of the disease; your child's age and overall health; and how the cancer responds to the initial treatment. Here is a summary of the most common treatments for childhood sarcoma.

Osteosarcoma: Patients with osteosarcoma have chemotherapy before surgery to remove as much of their cancer as possible.

Ewing sarcoma family of tumors: For Ewing sarcoma, doctors use chemotherapy. Depending on the location of the cancer, many patients also have surgery to remove tumors. Doctors may recommend radiation therapy, too, because this form of cancer is typically very sensitive to radiation.

Soft tissue sarcoma: Soft tissue sarcoma can begin in many different parts of the body, and treatment may vary depending on the location. Most patients with soft tissue sarcoma have surgery to remove areas of cancer. Doctors usually use chemotherapy and radiation therapy to control the cancer or kill cancer cells that remain in the child's body after surgery.

Outlook

More than two-thirds of young patients diagnosed with sarcoma survive without recurrence for more than five years following their diagnosis, and most live much longer. The cure rate ranges from 20 to 90 percent of patients depending on the type of sarcoma, the extent of disease at the time of diagnosis, and how quickly the sarcoma responds to initial therapy.

Chapter 21

Cardiovascular Disorders

Chapter Contents

Section 21.1—Arrhythmia 284
Section 21.2—Heart Murmurs 290
Section 21.3—Hyperlipidemia (High Cholesterol) 292
Section 21.4—Hypertension 297
Section 21.5—Kawasaki Disease 302

Childhood Diseases and Disorders Sourcebook, Second Edition

Section 21.1

Arrhythmia

"Children and Arrhythmia," "Types of Arrhythmia in Children," and "Treating Arrhythmias in Children," reprinted with permission www.americanheart.org. © 2007 American Heart Association, Inc.

Children and Arrhythmia

If your child has been diagnosed with an abnormal heart rate, you're probably alarmed. That's understandable. But by learning more about your child's condition, you'll be less afraid. You'll also be better able to care for your child.

About Heart Rhythms

The heart rate is the number of times the heart beats each minute. In an older child or teenager who's resting, the heart beats about 70 times a minute. In a newborn it beats about 140 times a minute. Usually the heart rhythm is regular. This means the heart beats evenly (at regular intervals). The heart rate changes easily. Exercise makes the heart beat faster. During sleep it slows down.

An irregular heartbeat is an arrhythmia. The most common irregularity occurs during breathing. When a child breathes in, the heart rate normally speeds up for a few beats. When the child breathes out, it slows down again. This variation with breathing is called sinus arrhythmia. It's completely normal.

Sometimes a doctor may find other kinds of arrhythmia. Then he or she may want to perform some tests. The doctor may also recommend that a pediatric cardiologist (a doctor specializing in children's heart problems) examine your child.

Knowing Your Child's History

Arrhythmias (also called dysrhythmias) may occur at any age. Many times they have no symptoms. Often parents and children never suspect an arrhythmia and are surprised when a doctor finds one during a routine physical exam. Rhythm abnormalities are usually evaluated

Cardiovascular Disorders

much like other health problems. Your child's history—or what you and your child report about the problem—is very important. You may be asked questions like:

- Is your child aware of unusual heartbeats?
- Does anything bring on the arrhythmia? Is there anything your child or the family can do to make it stop?
- If it's a fast rate, how fast?
- Does your child feel weak, lightheaded, or dizzy?
- Has your child ever fainted?

Some medicines may make arrhythmias worse. Be sure to tell your doctor about all the prescribed and over-the-counter medications that your child takes. If your child has an arrhythmia, discuss this with the doctor and ask what to look for.

Types of Arrhythmia in Children

There are many different kinds of abnormal heart rhythms. If an abnormal rhythm occurs, it's important to find out what kind it is. Treatment recommendations depend on its type. Arrhythmias can cause the heart rate to be irregular, fast, or slow. Fast rhythms are called tachycardia. Slow ones are called bradycardia.

Premature Atrial Contraction (PAC) and Premature Ventricular Contraction (PVC)

Premature beats or extra beats most often cause irregular heart rhythms. Those that start in the upper chambers (atria) are called premature atrial contractions or PACs. Premature ventricular contractions or PVCs start in the ventricles. If you've ever felt your heart "skip a beat," it was probably from this type of arrhythmia. The heart really doesn't skip a beat. Instead, an extra beat comes sooner than normal. Then there's a pause that causes the next beat to be more forceful. You felt this more-forceful beat.

Premature beats are very common in normal children and teenagers—most people have them at some time. Usually no cause can be found and no special treatment is needed. The premature beats may disappear later. Even if they continue, your child will stay well and won't need any restrictions. Occasionally premature beats may be caused by disease or injury to the heart. Your child's doctor may recommend more tests to make sure your child's heart is OK.

Tachycardia

A fast heart rate is called tachycardia. The definition of "too fast" usually depends on the person's age and physical activity. A newborn has tachycardia if the resting rate is more than 160 beats a minute. A teenager has it if the resting heart rate is more than 100 beats a minute. An exercising teenager may have a normal heart rate of up to 200 beats a minute.

Sinus tachycardia is a normal increase in the heart rate. It occurs with fever, excitement, and exercise. No treatment is needed. Rarely, disease, such as anemia (low blood counts) or increased thyroid activity can cause this fast heart rate. In these cases, when the disease is treated, the tachycardia goes away.

Supraventricular Tachycardia (SVT)

The most common abnormal tachycardia in children is supraventricular tachycardia (SVT). It's also called paroxysmal atrial tachycardia (PAT) or paroxysmal supraventricular tachycardia (PSVT). The fast heart rate involves both the heart's upper and lower chambers. This isn't a life-threatening problem for most children and adolescents. Treatment is only considered if episodes are prolonged or frequent. For many infants, SVT is a time-limited problem. Treatment with medications often stops after six to twelve months.

SVT may occur in very young infants with otherwise-normal hearts. The heart rate is usually more than 220 beats a minute. Infants with an SVT episode may breathe faster than normal and seem fussy or sleepier than usual. This situation must be diagnosed and treated to return the heart rate to normal. Once the rhythm is normal, medication usually can prevent future episodes.

Sometimes SVT can be detected while a baby is still in the womb. Then the mother may take medications to slow her baby's heart rate. If an older infant or child has SVT, the child may be aware of the rapid heart rate. This may be associated with palpitations, dizziness, lightheadedness, chest discomfort, upset stomach, or weakness. Some children can learn ways to slow down their heart rate. Straining—such as closing the nose and mouth and trying to breathe out—may be successful. This is called a Valsalva maneuver.

Older children are more likely to have more episodes of tachycardia. They're more likely to need prolonged treatment. They also may need more diagnostic tests. It's unusual for episodes of SVT to keep a child from enjoying normal activities. Most children who have episodes of tachycardia stay well even though they may need to keep taking medicine. Your child will probably need periodic check-ups but will be able to enjoy unrestricted normal activities.

Treating SVT usually has two parts. The first is stopping a current episode; the second is preventing recurrences. The approach to preventing recurrences depends on the child's age. In some cases—especially those of infants—the child may need to enter the hospital for treatment and special studies.

Sometimes simple procedures can stop a fast heart rhythm. Gagging or putting ice on the face are examples. Your child's doctor can explain this to you in more detail. At other times intravenous medications may be needed to control or stop the tachycardia. Another way to stop SVT is to place a small catheter (a thin, flexible tube) through the nostril into the esophagus. A small amount of electricity is sent through this catheter to stop the SVT. On rare occasions doctors stop SVT by giving a small electrical shock to the chest wall. This is called electrical countershock or cardioversion. A sedative or anesthetic is given before this procedure.

Wolff-Parkinson-White Syndrome

If an abnormal conduction pathway runs between the atria and ventricles, the electrical signal may arrive at the ventricles sooner than normal. This condition is called Wolff-Parkinson-White syndrome (WPW syndrome). It's named after the three people who first described it. WPW syndrome is recognized by certain changes on the electrocardiogram (ECG). Many people with WPW syndrome don't have symptoms or episodes of tachycardia.

Often medication can improve this condition. Sometimes, though, such treatment doesn't work. Then your child will need more tests. Eliminating the abnormal pathway by passing energy through a catheter may be needed. Surgery is another option.

Ventricular Tachycardia (VT)

Ventricular tachycardia (VT) is a fast heart rate that starts in the lower chambers (ventricles). This uncommon but potentially serious condition can threaten a child's life. VT may result from serious heart disease; it usually requires prompt treatment. VT occasionally occurs in children with otherwise normal hearts. Often specialized tests, including an intracardiac electrophysiologic procedure, may be needed to evaluate the tachycardia and the effect of drug treatment. Some forms of VT may not need treatment.

If treatment is required, it includes medicines and addressing the cause, if possible. The type and length of treatment depends on what's causing the problem. In some people radiofrequency ablation or surgery may be needed to control the tachycardia.

Bradycardia

A heart rate that's too slow is called bradycardia. What's "too slow" depends on a person's age and activity. A newborn usually won't have a heart rate of less than 80 beats a minute. An athletically trained teenager may have a normal resting heart rate of 50 beats a minute.

Sick Sinus Syndrome

Sometimes the sinus node doesn't work properly. Some children who've had open-heart surgery have this problem. When the sinus node's work is seriously disturbed, it's called sick sinus syndrome. A child with this syndrome may not have any symptoms or may be tired, dizzy, or faint. Children with sick sinus syndrome have episodes of tachycardia and bradycardia. Fortunately, sick sinus syndrome is unusual in children. If it does occur, an artificial pacemaker, medications, or both may be needed.

Complete Heart Block

Heart block means that the heart's electrical signal can't pass normally from the upper to the lower chambers. The electrical signal within the heart is blocked, not the blood flow. When this occurs, another "natural" pacemaker in the lower chambers takes over, but at a slower rate.

Heart block may be present at—or even before—birth. (This is congenital heart block.) Disease or an injury to the electrical conduction system during heart surgery can also cause it. When the natural pacemaker in the lower chambers isn't fast enough or reliable enough, an artificial pacemaker is put in.

Treating Arrhythmias in Children

Many options are available to treat rhythm abnormalities in children. Most treatment is directed at a specific problem. A detailed discussion of all the options isn't possible here.

Medications

Many rhythm disorders, especially tachycardias, respond to medications. Several drugs are now available and more are being developed.

These drugs can't cure the arrhythmia, but they can improve symptoms. They do this by preventing the episodes from starting, decreasing the heart rate during the episode, or shortening how long the episode lasts.

Sometimes it's hard to find the best medication for a child. Several drugs may need to be tried before the right one is found. Some children must take medication every day; others need medications only when they have a tachycardia episode. It's very important to take the medication as prescribed.

All medications have side effects, including drugs to treat arrhythmias. Most of the side effects aren't serious and disappear when the dose is changed or the medication is stopped. But some side effects are very serious. That's why some children are admitted to the hospital to begin the medication. If your child is prescribed medication, it's very important that your child take the medication just the way the doctor prescribes it.

It's often necessary to monitor how much of a drug is in your child's blood. The goal is to make sure there's enough of the drug to be effective, but not so much that harmful side effects occur. These blood tests require taking a small amount of blood from a vein or the finger. It's a good idea to talk to your child about this before the doctor visit.

Other Treatments

Radiofrequency ablation: Some tachycardias are life-threatening or significantly interfere with a child's normal activities. These problems may warrant more permanent treatment. One procedure, called radiofrequency catheter ablation, is done with several catheters in the heart. One is positioned right over the area that's causing the tachycardia. Then its tip is heated and that small area of the heart is altered so electrical current won't pass through the tissue.

Surgery: Sometimes surgery that interrupts the abnormal connection in the heart is required to permanently stop the tachycardia.

Artificial pacemaker: A variety of rhythm disorders can be controlled with an artificial pacemaker. Slow heart rates, such as heart block, are the most common reason to use a pacemaker. But new technology now lets doctors treat some fast heart rates with a pacemaker, too. An artificial pacemaker is a small device (one to two ounces, 1.5 by 1.5 inches). It's put inside the body and connected to the heart with a thin wire. It works by sending small, painless amounts of electricity to the heart to make it beat.

Inserting a pacemaker is a simple operation. The wires are attached to the heart, and the pacemaker is placed in the abdomen (belly) or under the skin of the chest wall. Sometimes only one wire is attached to the heart. In other cases two wires are used. Many different models and brands of pacemakers exist. Some can sense when your child is active and increase the heart's beating to keep up with exercise.

If your child has a pacemaker, he or she will need regular checkups. It's important to check the pacemaker's battery and make sure the wires are working properly. Pacemaker batteries usually last for years, but the pacemaker will still need to be replaced periodically throughout the user's lifetime. Sometimes the wires also need to be replaced. Regular checkups can show if anything needs replacing.

Most children with pacemakers can engage in normal activities. Your doctor may advise against participating in some contact sports, however. Talk to your child's cardiologist about this.

Section 21.2

Heart Murmurs

"Heart Murmurs in Pediatric Patients," © 2008 Children's Healthcare of Atlanta (www.choa.org). Reprinted with permission.

What is a heart murmur?

Murmurs are sounds made by blood circulating through the heart's chambers or valves, or through blood vessels near the heart.

What causes a heart murmur?

Heart murmurs may be caused by a number of factors or diseases, including the following:

- Defective heart valves
- Holes in the heart walls (atrial septal defect or ventricle septal defect)
- Surgical repair of congenital (present at birth) heart defects

- Fever
- Anemia (a decrease in the red cells in the blood)

What are the different types of murmurs?

Your child's physician will evaluate a murmur based on several factors. Murmurs are analyzed for pitch, loudness, and duration. They also are graded according to their intensity (on a scale of one to six, with one being very faint and six being very loud).

Types of murmurs include the following:

Systolic murmur: A heart murmur that occurs during a heart muscle contraction. Systolic murmurs are divided into ejection murmurs (due to blood flow through a narrowed vessel or irregular valve) and regurgitant murmurs.

Diastolic murmur: A heart murmur that occurs during heart muscle relaxation between beats. Diastolic murmurs are due to a narrowing (stenosis) of the mitral or tricuspid valves, or regurgitation of the aortic or pulmonary valves.

Continuous murmur: A heart murmur that occurs throughout the cardiac cycle. Murmurs related to a congenital (present at birth) heart defect or other problem involving the heart structures will be heard the loudest in the area of the chest where the problem occurs. Some large defects have almost no murmur in the newborn due to normally elevated pressures in the blood vessels in the lungs. Murmurs may be inconsistent and difficult to hear in an infant who is agitated or crying. Thus, murmurs may be missed or not detected.

Do all murmurs signify heart disease?

Not all heart murmurs are symptoms of heart disease. Sometimes, a murmur may be heard in a normal child who has a fever or who is anemic; these murmurs often go away when the underlying problem is treated.

Some children have what is known as an innocent murmur. These murmurs are not related to congenital heart defects, and usually resolve by the time a child reaches adulthood. If your child's physician hears an innocent murmur, he may want to perform additional tests to ensure a heart defect is not present. A child with an innocent murmur can live a normal life and be as active as any other healthy child.

Section 21.3

Hyperlipidemia (High Cholesterol)

"Hyperlipidemia/Cholesterol Problems in Children" is reprinted with permission from the Cincinnati Children's Hospital Medical Center website, http://www.cincinnatichildrens.org. © 2006 Cincinnati Children's Hospital Medical Center. All rights reserved.

What Is Hyperlipidemia?

Hyperlipidemia is a term that means you have a high level of lipids (fats/cholesterol) circulating in the blood. There are different types of hyperlipidemias, all of which are risk factors for developing heart disease.

Other factors such as genetics, environment, habits, and the presence of other diseases such as diabetes and hypertension may also contribute to the development of heart disease. Some of these factors are within our control; others are not.

Studies have shown an association between high blood cholesterol and premature heart attacks. Excess cholesterol in the blood can settle in the arteries and form a plaque (a raised lesion on the inside of an artery).

Over time, this plaque can build up and narrow the arteries, which in turn may clog the flow of blood. This process can begin in early childhood and may eventually result in coronary artery disease, heart attacks, or stroke.

What Is Cholesterol?

Cholesterol is a naturally occurring substance found in all foods derived from animals such as, meat, poultry, seafood, eggs, and dairy products. Cholesterol is not present in foods derived from plants.

Humans also manufacture cholesterol in our bodies. Dietary cholesterol, as well as other fats in the diet, may be absorbed by the body and raise blood cholesterol.

Cholesterol is necessary for life. It is a building block for hormones and a component of cell membranes. The goal of treating patients with elevated blood cholesterol levels is not to eliminate cholesterol from the blood, but to achieve and maintain a safe level.

Cardiovascular Disorders

Doctors generally recommend that total blood cholesterol be below 170 mg/dl for children two to nineteen years.

If an initial blood test shows a high total cholesterol level, the next step is to do a more detailed analysis to determine the balance of low-density lipoproteins (LDLs) and high-density lipoproteins (HDLs). This is called a lipid profile, which is generally done after a ten- to twelve-hour period of fasting, without any food or beverage.

When your doctor obtains a fasting lipid profile, your results are generally presented as total cholesterol, triglyceride, HDL, and LDL cholesterol (in some instances you will get a very low density lipoprotein [VLDL] level as well).

Total cholesterol is a measurement reflecting the presence of three particles in the blood:

- High-density lipoprotein (HDL)
- Low-density lipoprotein (LDL)
- Very low density lipoprotein (VLDL)

HDLs and LDLs are two different kinds of cholesterol particles and VLDLs are rich in triglycerides (or fats). Collectively, cholesterol and triglycerides are known as lipids.

HDL and LDL particles are covered with a protein that allows them to dissolve in the bloodstream. LDL particles, commonly referred to as "bad" cholesterol, carry most of the body's cholesterol, which may be deposited in the blood vessels to begin formation of plaque.

This process is associated with the development of cardiovascular disease. HDLs, referred to as "good" cholesterol, in contrast, seem to offer protection against cardiovascular disease by carrying some of the cholesterol out of the bloodstream and preventing it from being deposited.

Triglycerides are fats circulating in your bloodstream.

Table 21.1. Cholesterol Guidelines for Children 2–19 Years

Total Cholesterol (mg/dl)	LDL cholesterol (mg/dl)	Interpretation
Less than 170	Less than 100	Normal
170–200	100–130	Borderline
Greater than 200	Greater than 130	High (increased risk if male with HDL < 45 or female with HDL < 50)

The Preventive Cholesterol Treatment Center at Cincinnati Children's Hospital Medical Center recommends treatment for all children with an LDL count of 100 or higher with a family history of coronary artery disease. More aggressive criteria may be used if there have been cardiac events.

Why Treat High Cholesterol in Children?

Evidence suggests that children with high cholesterol are likely to have high cholesterol when they are adults. Concern about developing disease is greater if there is a family history of heart disease, since the evidence is strong that heart disease runs in families.

Autopsies of healthy individuals killed in accidents or wars have shown noticeable damage to the arteries of young adults.

The damage appears to be related to cholesterol levels in the blood. This evidence suggests that the process that leads to heart disease and heart attacks begins during childhood and the teenage years.

Behavior is learned. While we cannot change our genetic heritage, we can stop smoking, exercise regularly, and choose to eat a healthful, nutrient-dense, low-fat, low-cholesterol diet. You have the opportunity now to teach your child healthy behavior patterns that will last a lifetime.

Treating High Cholesterol in Kids

The first step in treatment of high cholesterol is to set reasonable, attainable goals for your child and your family and to modify your family's diet to achieve these goals.

The National Cholesterol Education Program (NCEP) recommends dietary modifications as a primary treatment for anyone with elevated cholesterol. Initial dietary guidelines to lower your blood cholesterol are outlined below:

- Total fat in the diet should be reduced to no more than 30 percent of your calories. Total fat consists of all the fats you eat regardless of the type. An average child should take in about 1,500 to 2,400 calories per day, depending on age and activity level, which would translate to approximately 50 to 80 grams of total fat per day. Note: Be careful to look at labels for total fat content. Avoid choosing foods that are simply labeled "cholesterol free" because a product can be cholesterol free and still be very high in fat. Dietary fat can be converted to cholesterol in our bodies.

Cardiovascular Disorders

- Saturated fats have been shown to elevate blood cholesterol levels. They are mainly found in animal products—any meat, poultry, or fish and anything that comes from an animal such as dairy products. Plant oils that are high in saturated fats include coconut, palm, and palm kernel oils. Saturated fats need not be eliminated from the diet but should be limited to less than 10 percent of your calories.

- Dietary cholesterol should be no more than 200–300 mg per day. Cholesterol *only* comes from animal sources and is never found in vegetable products. Remember to look at fat and saturated fat contents as well as cholesterol contents.

- Fiber should be included daily. It is recommended that we get 25–30 grams of fiber per day. Most Americans do not meet this goal. Fiber can act like a sponge in taking some of the fat out of the body without letting it get absorbed into the bloodstream. Including whole grains, beans, high-fiber cereals, and vegetables daily can help increase fiber.

- Simple sugars should be limited, especially if triglyceride levels are high. High-sugary foods have been warned off by dentists for years due to the increased incidence of dental caries. Triglyceride levels may be affected by the sugar content of the diet as well as by the fat content. Regular soft drinks and other sugar-sweetened beverages can be especially troublesome. Did you know one twelve-ounce can of regular soft drink has the equivalent of 10+ teaspoons of sugar in it? Try not to "reward" children with high-fat or high-sugar treats. Stickers, crayons, books, or small toys work well as positive incentives.

Dietary Goals for Children

Special "diet" foods are not necessary to meet these goals. A complete, low-fat diet is safe for children over age two years and can be easily achieved through consumption of "normal" foods.

Providing a well-balanced diet including a variety of foods sounds too simple to be true. In reality, this is the solution.

There are no magical "good" foods or "bad" foods that will change your child's cholesterol. Teaching your children to select a wide variety of foods which are lower in fat and saturated fat can be the first step in dietary modification.

These dietary modifications need to be more than switching high-fat "junk" food to fat-free "junk" food. While it is nice to have so many good-tasting fat-free products out on the market, we need to remember the nutrient content of the foods we are giving our children.

Obesity is a growing concern among American children today and has been recognized by the Centers for Disease Control as an epidemic in the United States. It is important to recognize that even though you may be purchasing all fat-free products this does not mean they are calorie free and they still need to be limited in quantity. New growth charts have been developed incorporating body mass index (BMI) information to allow careful monitoring of weight.

Tips for Keeping Kids' Cholesterol Levels Down

Encourage the whole family to participate in dietary modification. Your child will be much more successful if they are not tempted by high-fat foods brought into the house of other family members.

Set good examples—children live what they learn and learn by example. If parents have poor eating habits, their children are likely to mimic those habits. This goes for exercise, as well as dietary intake.

Use positive terms when referring to dietary modifications. Negative comments regarding low-fat or healthy foods should be kept to yourself. Avoid the term "diet" as this refers to a temporary solution. Make dietary modifications for a lifetime.

Make foods appealing to kids. Use colorful veggies or fruits. Cut things into special shapes kids enjoy.

If you are carefully controlling what your child eats at home, your child will have more flexibility when eating away from home.

Be creative and get kids involved in meal planning and preparation. Teach your children to read labels and what to look for on the label.

Help your child maintain their desirable body weight. Encourage physical activities and limit sedentary activities. Offer a wide variety of tasty low-fat, nutrient-dense foods to your family. Limit intake of "empty calorie" foods.

It is unrealistic to expect anyone to eat only healthy food, but limiting quantity and frequency of high-fat and high-sugar foods along with regular exercise can help kids lower their cholesterol levels and decrease their risk for developing coronary artery disease later in life.

What If Diet Doesn't Work?

If dietary treatment does not lower your child's cholesterol after you and your child make a concentrated effort for a significant length of time—up to a year—drug therapy will be considered.

Section 21.4

Hypertension

"Hypertension in Pediatric Patients," © 2008 Children's
Healthcare of Atlanta (www.choa.org). Reprinted with permission.

What Is Blood Pressure?

Blood pressure, measured with a blood pressure cuff and stethoscope by a nurse or other healthcare provider, is the force of the blood pushing against the artery walls.

Two numbers are recorded when measuring blood pressure:

- The higher number, or systolic pressure, refers to the pressure inside the artery when the heart contracts and pumps blood through the body.

- The lower number, or diastolic pressure, refers to the pressure inside the artery when the heart is at rest and is filling with blood.

Each time the heart beats, it pumps blood into the arteries, resulting in the highest blood pressure as the heart contracts.

Both the systolic and diastolic pressures are recorded as "mm Hg" (millimeters of mercury). This recording represents how high the mercury column is raised by the pressure of the blood.

What Is Hypertension?

Hypertension, or high blood pressure, means that there is higher than normal pressure inside the arteries either during systole (when the heart contracts and pumps blood through the body), or during diastole (when the heart is at rest and is filling with blood).

If the pressure is high during the pumping phase (systole), then the first number recorded with a blood pressure reading (the systolic pressure) will be high.

If the pressure is high during the resting period (diastole), then the second number recorded (the diastolic pressure) will be high.

Is a Blood Pressure Reading Always the Same?

Blood pressure can be affected by many factors, including the following:

- **The time of day:** Blood pressures fluctuate during waking hours, and are lower as we sleep.
- **Physical activity:** Blood pressure is usually higher during and immediately after exercise, and lower at rest.
- **Emotional moods:** Feelings (such as fear, anger, or happiness) can affect blood pressure.
- **Stress:** Physical or emotional stress can elevate blood pressure.
- **Your child's age, height, weight, and gender:** Blood pressure varies for each child.
- **Other illnesses:** Other illnesses your child may have (such as kidney or heart disease) affect blood pressure.

Children (and adults) may be anxious in a physician's office, not knowing what may happen and being afraid of a possibly painful experience ahead of them. Infants, toddlers, and preschoolers may be fearful of being separated from their parent or caregiver. Many emotions related to visiting the clinic can affect blood pressure and may give falsely high readings.

Before determining that a child has high blood pressure, a physician or nurse will take several readings when your child is calm, and you are present to comfort him, if needed. The staff may let some time elapse before retaking a blood pressure reading, to make sure your child has rested and become calm. More meaningful blood pressure readings can be obtained this way.

When Is the Blood Pressure Too High?

Blood pressures vary depending on the age of your child, as well as according to height and weight, and the gender of your child. Generally, blood pressure is low in infancy, and rises slowly as children age. Boys' blood pressures are slightly higher than girls' are, and taller people generally have higher blood pressures than short people do.

For example, an infant may have a quite normal blood pressure of 80/45 mm Hg, while that value in an adult is considered low. A teenager may have an acceptable blood pressure of 110/70 mm Hg, but that value would be of concern in a toddler.

Cardiovascular Disorders

The National High Blood Pressure Education Program (NHBEP) recently prepared tables that help a physician determine when your child's blood pressure is higher than other children's blood pressure. The NHBEP prepared a table for boys and a separate one for girls. A range of blood pressure values is given based on how old and how tall your child is. According to the tables, If your child has a blood pressure that is higher than 90 to 95 percent of other boys or girls his or her age and height, then he or she may have high blood pressure.

Again, many factors, including emotions, can affect blood pressure. Readings that are high compared to the values on the table may need to be investigated further by your child's physician.

Why Is Hypertension a Concern?

High blood pressure, or hypertension, directly increases the risk of coronary heart disease (heart attack) and stroke (brain attack). With high blood pressure, the arteries may have an increased resistance against the flow of blood, causing the heart to pump harder to circulate the blood.

Heart attack and stroke related to high blood pressure are rare in children and adolescents. Yet, studies of young adults with high blood pressure found that many had high blood pressure as a child. By their twenties, studies show that children and adolescents with high blood pressure will exhibit harmful effects on the heart and blood vessels even with mild hypertension.

What Causes Hypertension?

Blood pressure is classified as "primary," or without a definite cause, and "secondary," or related to an illness or behavior.

Factors that seem to contribute to primary hypertension in adults, and possibly in children, include the following:

- High blood cholesterol levels
- Being overweight
- Inactivity
- Smoking

Secondary causes of hypertension in children include the following:

- Illnesses: The kidneys play an important role in regulating blood pressure, and often have diminished ability to perform this vital task when they are diseased. A congenital (present at birth) heart defect called coarctation of the aorta may also cause high blood pressure readings. Head injury may raise the pressure inside the brain, which affects the body's ability to regulate blood pressure normally.

- Use of prescription or illegal recreational drugs (such as steroids taken to decrease inflammation, oral contraceptives, or cocaine).
- Obesity.
- Immobility (such as with a chronic illness).
- Severe pain (such as with cancer or burns).

Who Is at Risk for Developing Hypertension?

Primary hypertension (with an unknown cause) is the most common cause of high blood pressure in adolescents and adults, but is less common in children.

Many children with high blood pressure also have adult relatives with hypertension, so there may be a hereditary aspect to the disease.

There is a higher incidence of high blood pressure in African-American children after the age of twelve and into adulthood.

How Is Hypertension Diagnosed?

Your child's physician may note an elevated blood pressure reading during a routine office visit. Obtaining calm, resting blood pressures on several different occasions (days, weeks, or months apart) will provide better information about whether the blood pressure elevation is consistent or due to fear or stress.

Your child's physician will obtain a medical history, including information about your child's diet, exercise level, home and school activities, and possible stressors. A physical examination may also be performed.

Diagnostic tests may help determine if your child's high blood pressure is related to an illness, or is "essential" or "primary" hypertension, meaning it has no known cause. Diagnostic procedures may include:

- urinalysis;
- blood tests (including those to evaluate kidney function and cholesterol levels).

Other tests may be needed to evaluate the health of other organs (such as the heart or kidneys) which may contribute to hypertension.

Treatment for Hypertension

Specific treatment for high blood pressure will be determined by your child's physician based on:

- your child's age, overall health, and medical history;
- extent of the condition;
- your child's tolerance for specific medications, procedures, or therapies;
- expectations for the course of the condition;
- your opinion or preference.

If a secondary cause has been found, such as kidney disease, the underlying disease will be treated. If no cause has been determined, the first treatment approach is lifestyle therapy, including the following:

- Weight reduction
- Increasing physical activity
- Healthy diet

These interventions can lower systolic and diastolic blood pressure, improve the strength of the heart, and lower blood cholesterol—all important steps in preventing heart disease as an adult.

Medications to control high blood pressure are only needed in about 1 percent of children with the disorder. Consult your child's physician for more information.

Section 21.5

Kawasaki Disease

"Kawasaki Disease," reprinted with permission www.americanheart.org. © 2008 American Heart Association, Inc.

What is Kawasaki disease?

Kawasaki disease is a children's illness. It's also known as Kawasaki syndrome or mucocutaneous (mu"ko-ku-TA'ne-us) lymph node syndrome. It and acute rheumatic (roo-MAT'ik) fever are the two leading causes of acquired heart disease in children in the United States.

Who gets Kawasaki disease?

About 80 percent of the people with Kawasaki disease are under age five. Children over age eight are rarely affected. The disease occurs more often among boys (over 60 percent) and among those of Asian ancestry. But it can occur in every racial and ethnic group. Over four thousand cases of Kawasaki disease are being diagnosed annually in the United States. Less than 1 percent of those who get it die.

What happens to those with Kawasaki disease?

The symptoms of Kawasaki disease include:

- fever;
- rash;
- swollen hands and feet;
- irritation and redness of the whites of the eyes;
- swollen lymph glands in the neck;
- irritation and inflammation of the mouth, lips, and throat.

Doctors don't know what causes Kawasaki disease, but it doesn't seem to be hereditary or contagious. Scientists who've studied it think the evidence strongly suggests it's caused by an infectious agent such

Cardiovascular Disorders

as a virus. It's very rare for more than one child in a family to develop Kawasaki disease. Less than 2 percent of children have another attack of Kawasaki disease.

In as many as 15 to 25 percent of the children with Kawasaki disease, the heart is affected. The coronary arteries or the heart muscle itself can be damaged.

How does Kawasaki disease affect the heart?

The coronary arteries are most often affected. Part of a coronary wall can be weakened and balloon (bulge out) in an aneurysm. A blood clot can form in this weakened area and block the artery, sometimes leading to a heart attack. The aneurysm can also burst, but this rarely happens.

Other changes include inflammation of the heart muscle (myocarditis) or the sac surrounding the heart (pericarditis). Arrhythmias (abnormal heart rhythms) or abnormal functioning of some heart valves also can occur.

Usually all the heart problems go away in five or six weeks, and there's no lasting damage. Sometimes coronary artery damage persists, however.

An arrhythmia or damaged heart muscle can be detected using an electrocardiogram (EKG). An echocardiogram (or "echo") is used to look for possible damage to the heart or coronary arteries.

How is Kawasaki disease treated?

Even though the cause of Kawasaki disease is unknown, certain medicines are known to help. Aspirin is often used to reduce fever, rash, joint inflammation and pain, and to help prevent blood clots from forming. Another medicine, intravenous gamma globulin, can decrease the risk of developing coronary artery abnormalities when given early in the illness.

Chapter 22

Diabetes

What Is Diabetes?

Diabetes is a chronic disease in which the body does not make or properly use insulin, a hormone that is needed to convert glucose and other food into energy. People with diabetes have increased blood glucose levels due to an absence of insulin or failure to respond to insulin's effects (insulin resistance). Inadequate insulin results in high concentrations of glucose that build up in the blood and spill into the urine, causing an obligate urinary excretion of glucose. As a result, the body loses its main source of fuel.

Type 1 Diabetes

Type 1 diabetes is an autoimmune disease in which the immune system destroys the insulin-producing beta cells of the pancreas that regulate blood glucose. Type 1 diabetes has an acute onset, with children and adolescents usually able to pinpoint when symptoms began. Onset can occur at any age, but it most often occurs in children and young adults.

Since the pancreas can no longer produce insulin, people with type 1 diabetes require daily injections of insulin for life. Children with type 1 diabetes are at risk for long-term complications (damage to cardiovascular system, kidneys, eyes, nerves, blood vessels, gums, and teeth).

Excerpted from "Overview of Diabetes in Children and Adolescents," National Diabetes Education Program, National Institutes of Health, August 2006.

Type 1 diabetes accounts for 5 to 10 percent of all diagnosed cases of diabetes, but is the leading cause of diabetes in children. A diabetes management plan for young people includes insulin therapy, self-monitoring of blood glucose, healthy eating, and physical activity. The plan is designed to ensure proper growth and prevention of hypoglycemia. New management strategies are helping children with type 1 diabetes live long and healthy lives.

Symptoms: The symptoms of type 1 diabetes usually develop over a short period of time. They include increased thirst and urination, constant hunger, weight loss, and blurred vision. Children also may feel very tired. If not diagnosed and treated with insulin, the individual with type 1 diabetes can lapse into a life-threatening diabetic coma, known as diabetic ketoacidosis or DKA. Often, children will present with vomiting, a sign of DKA, and mistakenly be diagnosed as having gastroenteritis. New-onset diabetes can be differentiated from a GI infection by the frequent urination that accompanies continued vomiting as opposed to decreased urination due to dehydration if the vomiting is caused by a GI "bug."

Risk factors: A combination of genetic and environmental factors put people at increased risk for type 1 diabetes. Researchers are working to identify these factors and to stop the autoimmune process that destroys the pancreas.

Co-morbidities: Autoimmune diseases such as celiac disease and autoimmune thyroiditis are associated with type 1 diabetes.

Type 2 Diabetes

The first stage in the development of type 2 diabetes is often insulin resistance causing an inadequate response to insulin and requiring increasing amounts of insulin to control blood glucose. Initially, the pancreas responds by producing more insulin, but after several years, insulin production may decrease and diabetes develops. Type 2 diabetes used to occur mainly in adults who were overweight and ages forty and older. Now, as more children and adolescents in the United States become overweight and inactive, type 2 diabetes is occurring more often in young people.

Symptoms: Type 2 diabetes usually develops slowly and insidiously in children. Symptoms may be similar to those of type 1 diabetes. A

Diabetes

child or teen can feel very tired, thirsty, or nauseated and have to urinate often. Other symptoms may include weight loss, blurred vision, frequent infections, and slow healing of wounds or sores. Some children or adolescents with type 2 diabetes may show no symptoms at all when they are diagnosed, and others may present with vaginal yeast infection or burning on urination due to yeast infection. Therefore, it is important for health care providers to identify and test children or teens who are at high risk for the disease.

Signs of diabetes: Physical signs of insulin resistance include acanthosis nigricans, where the skin around the neck or in the armpits appears dark, thick, and feels velvety. High blood pressure and dyslipidemia also are associated with insulin resistance.

Risk factors: Being overweight, having a family member who has type 2 diabetes, being a member of a high-risk ethnic group, having signs of insulin resistance, being older than ten years of age, and experiencing puberty are risk factors for the disease.

Co-morbidities: Children with type 2 diabetes also are at risk for the long-term complications of diabetes and the co-morbidities associated with insulin resistance (lipid abnormalities and hypertension).

The cornerstone of diabetes management for children with type 2 is healthy eating, with portion control, and increased physical activity. To control their diabetes, children with type 2 diabetes also may need to take oral anti-diabetes medication, insulin, or both. Ongoing efforts to prevent and treat type 2 diabetes in children will require the involvement of health care providers, school personnel, community institutions, and government agencies working together.

"Hybrid" or "Mixed" Diabetes

While for the most part it is easy to determine if a child or teenager has type 1 or type 2 diabetes, some children have elements of both kinds of diabetes. This phenomenon may be called "hybrid" or "mixed" diabetes. It is not surprising that some children may have elements of both type 1 and type 2 diabetes, given the fact that more children are becoming overweight. Youth with hybrid diabetes are likely to have both of the following:

- Insulin resistance that is associated with obesity and type 2 diabetes

- Antibodies against the pancreatic islet cells that are associated with autoimmunity and type 1 diabetes

Signs and symptoms: The signs and symptoms are the same as those for type 1 and type 2 diabetes.

Management: At the time of diagnosis, the clinician should attempt to determine which type of diabetes is present. Measuring antibodies against islet cells and assessing insulin production by measuring C-peptide levels help make the distinction. C-peptide levels are best determined about a year after diagnosis. The presence of hybrid diabetes may affect how the child or teen is treated. Insulin injections are likely to be needed (as for type 1), and oral diabetes medications may be used to improve insulin resistance (as for type 2). It is important to counsel the child or teen about healthy eating habits and the need for daily physical activity so he or she can reach a healthy weight.

Maturity-Onset Diabetes of the Young

Maturity-onset diabetes of the young (MODY) is a rare form of diabetes in children that is caused by a single gene defect that results in faulty insulin secretion. MODY is defined by its early onset (usually before age twenty-five), absence of ketosis, and autosomal dominant inheritance.[1] Thus each child of a parent with MODY has a 50 percent chance of inheriting the same type of diabetes. MODY is thought to account for 2 to 5 percent of all cases of diabetes and often goes unrecognized.[1] Treatment of MODY varies. Some children respond to diet therapy, exercise, or oral anti-diabetes medications that enhance insulin release. Others may require insulin therapy.

Secondary Diabetes

Diabetes can occur in children with other diseases such as cystic fibrosis or those needing glucocorticoid drugs. These causes may account for 1 to 5 percent of all diagnosed cases of diabetes.

Treatment Strategies

The basic elements of type 1 diabetes management are insulin administration, nutrition management, physical activity, blood glucose testing, and the avoidance of hypoglycemia. Algorithms are used for insulin dosing based on blood glucose level and food intake.

Diabetes

Children receiving fixed insulin doses of intermediate- and rapid-acting insulins must have food given at the time of peak action of the insulin. Children receiving a long-acting insulin analogue or using an insulin pump receive a rapid-acting insulin analogue just before a meal, with the amount of pre-meal insulin based on carbohydrate content of the meal, using an insulin:carbohydrate ratio and a sliding scale for hyperglycemia. Further adjustment of insulin or food intake may be made based on anticipation of special circumstances such as increased exercise. Children on these regimens are expected to check their blood glucose levels routinely before meals and at bedtime.

Management of type 2 diabetes involves nutrition management, increased physical activity, and blood glucose testing. If this is not sufficient to normalize blood glucose levels, oral anti-diabetes medication or insulin therapy are used as well. The only oral agent approved for use in children and adolescents is metformin. All aspects of the regimen are individualized.

There is no single recipe to manage diabetes that fits all children. Blood glucose targets, frequency of blood glucose testing, type, dose and frequency of insulin, use of insulin injections or a pump, and details of nutrition management all may vary among individuals. The family and diabetes care team determine the regimen that best suits each child's individual characteristics and circumstances.

Blood Glucose Goals

To control diabetes and prevent complications, blood glucose levels must be managed as close to a "normal" range as is safely possible (70 to 100 mg/dl before eating). Families should work with their health care team to set target blood glucose levels appropriate for the child.

Hypoglycemia

Diabetes treatment can sometimes cause blood glucose levels to drop too low, with resultant hypoglycemia. Taking too much insulin, missing a meal or snack, or exercising too much may cause hypoglycemia. A child can become irritable, shaky, and confused. When blood glucose levels fall very low, loss of consciousness or seizures may develop.

When hypoglycemia is recognized, the child should drink or eat a concentrated sugar to raise the blood glucose value to greater than 80 mg/dl. Once the blood glucose is over 80, the child can eat food containing protein to maintain blood glucose levels in the normal range. The concentrated sugar will increase blood glucose levels and cause resolution of symptoms quickly, avoiding over-treatment of "lows." If the child is unable to eat or drink, a glucose gel may be administered to the buccal mucosa of the cheek or glucagon may be injected.

Glycemic goals may need to be modified to take into account the fact that most children younger than six or seven years of age have a form of "hypoglycemic unawareness." They lack the cognitive capacity to recognize and respond to hypoglycemic symptoms and may be at greater risk for hypoglycemia.[2]

Hyperglycemia

Causes of hyperglycemia include forgetting to take medications on time, eating too much, and getting too little exercise. Being ill also can raise blood glucose levels. Over time, hyperglycemia can cause damage to the eyes, kidneys, nerves, blood vessels, gums, and teeth.

Monitoring Complications and Reducing Cardiovascular Disease Risk

The following recommendations are based on the American Diabetes Association's standards of medical care.[2]

Retinopathy: Although retinopathy most commonly occurs after the onset of puberty and after five to ten years of diabetes duration, it has been reported in prepubertal children and with diabetes duration of only one to two years. Referrals should be made to eye care professionals with expertise in diabetic retinopathy, an understanding of the risk for retinopathy in the pediatric population, as well as experience in counseling the pediatric patient and family on the importance of early prevention and intervention. The first ophthalmologic examination should be obtained once the child is ten years of age or older and has had diabetes for three to five years. After the initial examination, annual routine follow-up is generally recommended. Less frequent examinations may be acceptable on the advice of an eye care professional.

Nephropathy: To reduce the risk and/or slow the progression of nephropathy, optimize glucose and blood pressure control. Annual screening for microalbuminuria should be initiated once the child is ten years of age and has had diabetes for five years. Screening may be done with a random spot urine sample analyzed for microalbumin-to-creatinine ratio. Confirmed, persistently elevated microalbumin levels should be treated with an angiotensin-converting enzyme (ACE) inhibitor, titrated to normalization of microalbumin excretion if possible.

Neuropathy: Although it is unclear whether foot examinations are important in children and adolescents, annual foot examinations are painless, inexpensive, and provide an opportunity for education about foot care. The risk for foot complications is increased in people who have had diabetes over ten years.[3]

Lipids: In children older than two years of age with a family history of total cholesterol over 240 mg/dl, or a cardiovascular disease event before age fifty-five, or if family history is unknown, perform a lipid profile after diagnosis of diabetes and when glucose control has been established. If family history is not a concern, then perform a lipid profile at puberty. Based on data obtained from studies in adults, having diabetes is equivalent to having had a heart attack, making diabetes a key risk factor for future cardiovascular disease.

Pubertal children should have a lipid profile at the time of diagnosis after glucose control has been established. If lipid values fall within the accepted risk levels (low-density lipoprotein [LDL] less than 100 mg/dl), repeat lipid profile every five years.

The goal for LDL cholesterol in children and adolescents with diabetes is less than 100 mg/dl (2.60 mmol/l). If the LDL cholesterol is greater than 100 mg/dl, the child should be treated with an exercise plan and a Step 2 American Heart Association diet. If, after six months of diet and exercise, the LDL cholesterol (LDL-C) level remains above 160 mg/dl, pharmacologic agents should be given. If, the LDL-C is between 130 and 160 mg/dl, pharmacologic therapy should be considered. Statins are the agents of choice. Weight loss, increased physical activity, and improvement in glycemic control often result in improvements in lipid levels.

Blood pressure: Careful control of hypertension in children is critical. Hypertension in childhood is defined as an average systolic or diastolic blood pressure greater than the 95th percentile for age, sex, and height measured on at least three separate days.

Helping Children Manage Diabetes

The health care provider team, in partnership with the young person with diabetes and caregivers, can develop a personal diabetes plan for the child that puts a daily schedule in place to keep diabetes under control. The plan shows the child how to follow a healthy meal plan, get regular physical activity, check blood glucose levels, take insulin or oral medication as prescribed, and manage hyperglycemia and hypoglycemia.

Follow a healthy meal plan: Young people with diabetes need to follow a meal plan developed by a registered dietitian, diabetes educator, or physician. For children with type 1 diabetes, the meal plan must ensure proper nutrition for growth. For children with type 2, the meal plan should outline appropriate changes in eating habits that lead to better energy balance and reduce or prevent obesity. A meal plan also helps keep blood glucose levels in the target range.

Children or adolescents and their families can learn how different types of food—especially carbohydrates such as breads, pasta, and rice—can affect blood glucose levels. Portion sizes, the right amount of calories for the child's age, and ideas for healthy food choices at meal and snack time also should be discussed, including reduction in soda and juice consumption. Family support for following the meal plan and setting up regular meal times is a key to success, especially if the child or teen is taking insulin.

Get regular physical activity: Children with diabetes need regular physical activity, ideally a total of sixty minutes each day. Physical activity helps to lower blood glucose levels, especially in children and adolescents with type 2 diabetes. Physical activity is also a good way to help children control their weight. In children with type 1 diabetes, the most common problem encountered during physical activity is hypoglycemia. If possible, a child or a teen should check blood glucose levels before beginning a game or a sport. If blood glucose levels are too low, the child should not be physically active until the low blood glucose level has been treated.

Check blood glucose levels regularly: Young people with diabetes should know the acceptable range for their blood glucose. Children, particularly those using insulin, should check blood glucose values regularly with a blood glucose meter, preferably one with a built-in memory. A health care team member can teach a child how to use a blood glucose meter properly and how often to use it. Children should keep a journal or other record of blood glucose results to discuss with their health care team. This information helps providers make any needed changes to the child's or teen's personal diabetes plan.

Diabetes

Take all diabetes medication as prescribed: Parents, caregivers, school nurses, and others can help a child or teen learn how to take medications as prescribed. For type 1 diabetes, a child or teen takes insulin at prescribed times each day via multiple injections or an insulin pump. Some young people with type 2 diabetes need oral medication or insulin or both. In any case, it is important to stress that all medication should be balanced with food and activity every day.

References

1. Nobre EL, Lopes LO, Miranda A, Pragosa M, de Castro JJ. Mature onset diabetes of the young (MODY). *Acta Med Port* 2002; 15 (6) : 435–39.

2. American Diabetes Association. Clinical Practice Recommendations—Standards of Medical Care in Diabetes. *Diabetes Care* 2005; 28(Suppl. 1): S4–36.

3. American Diabetes Association. Type 2 diabetes in children and adolescents. *Pediatrics* 2000; 105 (3): 671–80.

Chapter 23

Ear, Nose, and Throat Disorders

Chapter Contents

Section 23.1—Enlarged Adenoids 316
Section 23.2—Hearing Loss 319
Section 23.3—Nosebleeds 322
Section 23.4—Obstructive Sleep Apnea 324
Section 23.5—Otitis Media (Ear Infection) 327
Section 23.6—Perforated Eardrum 333
Section 23.7—Sinusitis 335
Section 23.8—Swimmer's Ear 344
Section 23.9—Tonsillitis 347

Section 23.1

Enlarged Adenoids

"Enlarged Adenoids," October 2007, reprinted with permission from www.kidshealth.org. Copyright © 2007 The Nemours Foundation. This information was provided by KidsHealth, one of the largest resources online for medically reviewed health information written for parents, kids, and teens. For more articles like this one, visit www.KidsHealth.org, or www.TeensHealth.org.

Often, tonsils and adenoids are surgically removed at the same time. Although you can see the tonsils by looking in your child's throat, adenoids aren't directly visible. Your child's doctor has to use a small mirror or a special scope to get a peek at your child's adenoids.

So, what are adenoids anyway? They're a mass of tissue, located in the passage that connects the back of the nasal cavity to the throat. Adenoids—which are also called nasopharyngeal tonsils but are separate from the tonsils in the throat—filter out bacteria and viruses entering through the nose and produce antibodies to help the body fight infections.

Some doctors believe that adenoids may not be important at all after kids reach their third birthday. In fact, adenoids usually shrink after about five years of age, and they often practically disappear by the teenage years.

What Are the Symptoms of Enlarged Adenoids?

Because adenoids trap germs that enter a child's body, adenoid tissue sometimes temporarily swells as it tries to fight off an infection. There are several symptoms associated with enlarged adenoids. You may notice that your child:

- complains of difficulty breathing through the nose;
- is breathing through the mouth;
- talks as if his or her nostrils are pinched;
- breathes noisily;
- snores while sleeping;

- stops breathing for a few seconds while sleeping (called sleep apnea).

If enlarged adenoids are suspected, your child's doctor may:

- ask about and then check your child's ears, nose, and throat;
- listen to your child's breathing through a stethoscope;
- feel your child's neck near the jaw.

To get a really close look, the doctor may even want to take one or more x-rays. For a suspected infection, the doctor may prescribe oral antibiotics or maybe an injection of penicillin.

When Is Surgery Necessary?

If enlarged or infected adenoids keep bothering your child and medicine doesn't stop them from coming back, the doctor may recommend surgically removing them with a procedure called an adenoidectomy. This may be recommended if your child experiences one or more of the following:

- Difficulty breathing
- Sleep apnea
- Recurrent infections

Having your child's adenoids removed is especially important when repeated infections lead to sinus and ear infections. Badly swollen adenoids can interfere with ear pressure and fluid movement, which can sometimes lead to hearing loss. Therefore, kids whose infected adenoids cause frequent earaches and fluid buildup may need to get an adenoidectomy as well as ear tube surgery.

And although adenoids can be taken out without the tonsils, if your child is having tonsil problems, they may need to be removed at the same time. A tonsillectomy with an adenoidectomy is the most common operation for children.

What Happens During the Surgery?

Surgery, no matter how common or simple the procedure, is often frightening for both the child and parent. You can help prepare your child for surgery by talking about what to expect. During the adenoidectomy and/or tonsillectomy:

- Your child will receive general anesthesia. This means the surgery will be performed in an operating room so that an anesthesiologist can monitor your child.
- Your child will be asleep for about twenty minutes.
- The surgeon can get to the tonsils and/or the adenoids through your child's open mouth — there's no need to cut through skin.
- The surgeon removes the tonsils and/or the adenoids with a series of incisions and then cauterizes (or seals) the blood vessels.
- Your child will wake up in the recovery area. In most cases, the total time in the hospital is five to ten hours. However, kids who have trouble breathing or show signs of bleeding will return immediately to the operating room. And kids under three years of age and those with chronic disease, such as seizure disorders or cerebral palsy, will usually stay overnight for observation.

The typical recuperation after a tonsillectomy and/or an adenoidectomy often involves a week or more of pain and discomfort due to the exposure of the throat muscles. Because of throat pain, your child will probably prefer eating a lot of soft foods, like ice cream, pudding, and soups.

About a week after surgery, everything should return to normal. The cut area will be left to heal naturally, which means there are no stitches to worry about. There's a small chance any tissue that's left behind can swell, but it rarely causes new problems.

After surgery, a child's symptoms typically disappear immediately, unless there's a lot of swelling that could lead to some temporary symptoms.

Understanding Enlarged Adenoids

Even though some kids may need surgery, it's important to remember that enlarged adenoids are normal in others. If your child's adenoids aren't infected, the doctor may choose to wait to operate because the adenoids may eventually shrink on their own as adolescence approaches.

Section 23.2

Hearing Loss

Excerpted from "Florida Resource Guide for Families of Young Children with Hearing Loss," © 2005 Florida Department of Health Children's Medical Services. Reprinted with permission.

How We Hear

Sound travels through the air in the form of waves of varying frequencies. The frequencies of these waves determines the pitches of the sound we hear. Sound waves enter the outer ear through the external ear canal and are transmitted to the middle ear. Sound is directed to the eardrum. The movement of the sound waves causes the eardrum to vibrate. This vibration causes three tiny bones to move back and forth in the middle ear. This mechanical vibration is then directed into the inner ear, the cochlea. The cochlea is lined with a membrane that has thousands of hair cells on it. The purpose of the hair cells in the cochlea is to code them into an electrical signal that the brain can recognize. The hair cells have nerve fibers from the auditory nerve in them that change the mechanical energy of the sound wave into electrical energy. This electrical energy stimulates the nerve and sends a signal representing the sound wave into the brain. The normally functioning ear responds to a wide range of frequencies (pitches) and intensities (loudness). Hearing loss generally reduces the intensity of a sound and can affect different frequency ranges, depending on the type and degree of hearing loss.

Learning about Hearing Loss

There are different kinds of hearing loss. A child may have a conductive hearing loss, a sensorineural hearing loss, or a mixed hearing loss. All types of hearing loss reduce loudness of some sounds or eliminate the ability to hear different pitches or to hear speech clearly. A child's hearing loss may be categorized in one of the following degrees: mild, moderate, severe, or profound. The hearing loss may be in one ear (unilateral loss) or in both ears (bilateral loss). The loss may be temporary or permanent.

Conductive hearing loss: A conductive hearing loss occurs when there is a problem in the outer or middle ear. The most common cause of conductive hearing loss in young children is a middle ear infection called otitis media. Otitis media is defined as inflammation of the middle ear, usually with fluid, which may or may not be infected. The condition is very common in young children and is the reason for many visits to the pediatrician. It is important that ear infections be treated by a physician as quickly as possible to reduce potential hearing loss. Most children will experience some occurrences of middle ear infection. However, significant problems result from infections that last for several months, despite medical treatment.

When multiple ear infections occur prior to eighteen months of age, there is the possibility that the child will have trouble with listening skill development, some speech sounds, language development, and early reading skills.

There are also other types of conductive hearing loss in young children. Some children are born with a physical abnormality of the outer or middle ear. This may not be surgically treated until the age of six and often into adolescence, leaving these children with a hearing loss until the surgery.

Sensorineural hearing loss: Sensorineural hearing loss occurs when the inner ear (cochlea) or the auditory nerve is malformed or has been damaged. There are many early causes of sensorineural hearing loss including loss of oxygen during birth, extremely low birth weight, inheritance, and maternal viruses or drug use (particularly in the first twelve weeks of pregnancy). A child may be born with normal hearing and acquire a loss due to a viral disease such as meningitis or exposure to certain drugs. There are also some inherited conditions that are associated with progressive sensorineural hearing loss (loss of more hearing over time). Children with sensorineural hearing loss need to receive appropriate amplification and audiological management as soon as the hearing loss is identified. Regardless of the degree of hearing loss, or if the hearing loss is present in only one ear, audiological management should include ongoing auditory testing and follow-up, referral for related medical follow-up, fitting and trial of hearing aids, and monitoring of the effectiveness of amplification.

Ear, Nose, and Throat Disorders

Table 23.1. Degree of Hearing Loss and Potential Effects

Degree of Loss	Potential Effects
Mild 26–40 dB	May have difficulty hearing faint or distant speech. A child with a mild loss may miss up to 10 percent of the speech signal when the speaker is at a distance greater than three feet, or if the environment is noisy. Likely to experience some difficulty in communication and educational settings. Consider need for hearing aids and intervention.
Moderate 41–55 dB	Understands conversational speech at a distance of three to five feet. Amplification may enable listener to hear and discriminate all sounds. Without amplification, 50 to 100 percent of the speech signal may be missed. Intelligibility of speech may be affected unless optimally amplified.
Moderate/Severe 56–70 dB	Conversation must be very loud to be heard without amplification. A 55 dB loss can mean 100 percent of the speech signal is missed in a typical conversational situation. When amplified, may have difficulty in settings requiring verbal communication, especially in large groups. Delays in spoken language and reduced speech intelligibility expected without intervention and amplification.
Severe 71–90 dB	If loss is pre-lingual, spoken language and speech may not develop spontaneously, or could be severely delayed. Without amplification, is aware of loud voices about one foot from the ear and is likely to rely on vision for communication. With consistent use of amplification, parent attention to communication strategies, and an effective communication environment, language development and speech may develop to be normal or near normal.
Profound 91 dB or greater	If loss is pre-lingual, spoken language and speech will not develop spontaneously. Without amplification, relies on vision rather than hearing for communication and learning. Potential candidate for the cochlear implant. With consistent use of cochlear implant or amplification, committed parent, auditory oral or auditory verbal communication techniques, or a communication system like cued speech, language development and speech may develop to be normal or near normal.

Mixed hearing loss: When a child has both a conductive and a sensorineural loss in the same ear, it is called a mixed hearing loss. Children with permanent sensorineural hearing loss are as susceptible to middle ear infections as children with normal hearing and may add a conductive hearing loss to their existing sensorineural hearing loss. A child's pediatric audiologist should regularly test all kinds of hearing loss as part of the child's ongoing audiological management.

Section 23.3

Nosebleeds

"Nosebleeds," © 2005 Allen ENT and Allergy (www.entallen.com). Reprinted with permission.

In the United States, one of every seven people will develop a nosebleed at some time. Nosebleeds tend to occur during winter months and in dry, cold climates. They can occur at any age but are most common in children aged two to ten years and adults aged fifty to eighty years. For unknown reasons, nosebleeds most commonly occur in the morning hours.

What Causes Nosebleeds?

The common site for a nosebleed to start is just inside the entrance of the nostril, on the nasal septum, which is the middle harder part of the nostril. Here the blood vessels are quite fragile and can rupture easily for no apparent reason. This delicate area is also more likely to bleed with the following:

- Picking the nose
- Dry air irritating the nose
- Colds, upper respiratory infections, sinus infections
- Blowing the nose
- Minor injuries to the nose

In the above situations, the bleeding tends to last only a short time and is usually easy to control. The bleeding may be more prolonged and harder to stop in rare circumstances. High blood pressure, heart failure, blood clotting disorders, and taking "blood thinning" drugs

Ear, Nose, and Throat Disorders

(anticoagulants) such as warfarin or aspirin can be associated with more serious nose bleeds.

Bleeding sometimes comes from other areas further back in the nose. It is sometimes due to uncommon disorders of the nose, or to serious injuries to the nose.

What Is the Treatment for Nosebleeds?

For most nosebleeds, simple first aid can usually stop the bleeding:

- If you are not feeling faint, sit up and lean slightly forward.
- With a finger and thumb, pinch the lower fleshy end of the nose, completely blocking the nostrils. It is useless to put pressure over the root of the nose or nose bones. Usually, if you apply light pressure for ten to twenty minutes, the bleeding will stop.
- If available, a cold flannel or compress around the nose and front of face will help. The cold helps the blood vessels to close down (constrict) and stop bleeding.
- Once the nosebleed has stopped, do not pick the nose or try and blow out any of the blood remaining in the nostrils. This may cause another nosebleed.
- Over-the-counter medications such as oxymetazoline (Afrin®) can cause constriction of the blood vessels and may reduce bleeding. These medications should only be used as instructed by a physician.

Seek medical help if bleeding is heavy, or it does not stop within twenty to thirty minutes. Sometimes the nose needs to be packed by a doctor to stop the bleeding. Rarely, a nosebleed is so heavy that a blood transfusion is needed, and surgery may be required to stop it.

Prevention of Nosebleeds

In order to prevent nosebleeds, your physician may recommend different strategies to moisturize and heal the nose. These strategies include:

- humidification of the ambient air;
- nasal saline sprays to moisturize the nose;

- "Ayr" nasal gel or Polysporin applied gently just on the inside septum;
- avoiding trauma or manipulation of the nose.

Recurring Nosebleeds

When nosebleeds become a recurrent problem often one will be referred to an otolaryngologist (ear, nose, and throat specialist). The physician will often examine the nose. The physician may elect to perform nasal endoscopy, which is an office examination of the nose with a small fiberoptic scope. The vessels and the back of the nose are clearly visualized, aiding in accurate diagnosis and treatment. It is often possible to cauterize ("burn") the bleeding point. This is usually a minor procedure which is usually successful in stopping recurrent bleeds.

Section 23.4

Obstructive Sleep Apnea

"Obstructive Sleep Apnea," reviewed by Steven D. Handler, M.D., M.B.E., and Carole L. Marcus, M.B.B.Ch., December 2005. © 2005 Children's Hospital of Philadelphia. Reprinted with permission.

What is obstructive sleep apnea?

Obstructive sleep apnea (OSA) occurs when a child stops breathing during sleep. The cessation of breathing usually occurs because there is a blockage (obstruction) in the airway. It affects many children. Childhood obstructive sleep apnea is most commonly found in children between two and six years of age, but can occur at any age.

What causes obstructive sleep apnea?

In children, the most common cause of obstructive sleep apnea is enlarged tonsils and adenoids. During sleep there is a considerable decrease in muscle tone, which affects the airway and breathing. Many of these children have little difficulty breathing when awake; however, with decreased muscle tone during sleep, the airway becomes smaller, and the tonsils and adenoids block the airway, making the flow of air more difficult and the work of breathing harder.

It is like breathing through a small, flimsy straw with the straw occasionally collapsing and blocking airflow. Many of the short pauses (lasting only a few seconds) cause a brief arousal that increases muscle tone, opens the airway, and allows the child to resume breathing.

Although the actual number of minutes of arousal during the night may be small, the repeated disruptions (a comparable image would be someone poking you fifteen to thirty times a night) can result in a poor night's sleep, which can lead to significant daytime problems in children. The child is usually unaware of waking up, and the parent often describes very restless sleep but usually does not describe the child's waking up completely.

Who is at risk?

Sleep apnea is more common in children who are overweight; however, some children with enlarged tonsils and/or adenoids may even be underweight. Other children who are at high risk for sleep apnea include those with a small jaw, craniofacial syndromes, muscle weakness, or Down syndrome.

What are the symptoms of obstructive sleep apnea?

The following are the most common symptoms of obstructive sleep apnea. However, every child is different and symptoms may vary. Symptoms may include:

- **Snoring:** Loud snoring or noisy breathing during sleep.
- **Periods of not breathing:** Although the chest wall is moving, no air or oxygen is moving through the nose or mouth into the lungs. The duration of these periods is variable and measured in seconds.
- **Mouth breathing:** The passage to the nose may be completely blocked by enlarged tonsils and adenoids leading to the child only being able to breathe through his or her mouth.
- **Restlessness during sleep:** The frequent arousals lead to restless sleeping or "tossing and turning" throughout the night.
- **Sleeping in odd positions:** The child may arch his neck backward (hyperextend) in order to open the airway or sleep sitting up.

- **Behavior problems or sleepiness:** May include irritability, crankiness, frustration, hyperactivity, and difficulty paying attention.
- **School problems:** Children may do poorly in school, even being labeled as "slow" or "lazy."
- **Bed wetting:** Also known as nocturnal enuresis, although there are many causes for bedwetting besides sleep apnea.
- **Frequent infections:** May include a history of chronic problems with tonsils, adenoids, and/or ear infections.

In addition, the symptoms of obstructive sleep apnea may resemble other conditions or medical problems. Be sure to always consult your child's physician.

How is obstructive sleep apnea diagnosed?

Your child's physician should be consulted if you are concerned about your child's breathing during the night. Your child may be referred to a specialist, such as a sleep specialist, an ear, nose, and throat (ENT) physician (otolaryngologist), or a pulmonary doctor for further evaluation.

In addition to a complete medical history and physical examination, diagnostic procedures for obstructive sleep apnea may include an overnight sleep study (also called polysomnography) and an evaluation of the upper airway by visualization and/or x-rays.

What is a sleep study?

Your doctor will discuss the usefulness of a sleep study in the evaluation of obstructive sleep apnea.

How is obstructive sleep apnea treated?

The treatment for obstructive sleep apnea is based on its cause. Since enlarged tonsils and adenoids are the most common cause of obstructive sleep apnea in children, surgical removal of the tonsils (tonsillectomy) and adenoids (adenoidectomy) is usually the recommended treatment. An ear, nose, and throat specialist will make the evaluation for such surgery. Other types of surgery are occasionally needed in children with craniofacial abnormalities. Weight loss and treatment of other medical problems may also be helpful in the management of obstructive sleep apnea.

In cases where surgery is not helpful, another effective treatment is continuous positive airway pressure (CPAP). CPAP involves wearing a mask over the nose during sleep attached to a machine that blows air through the nasal passages and into the airway. This air pressure keeps the airway open and allows the child to breathe normally during sleep.

If left untreated, OSA can cause poor growth ("failure to thrive"), high blood pressure, and heart problems. OSA can also affect behavior and cognition. Therefore, it is important to get it evaluated early.

In all cases, the specific treatment for obstructive sleep apnea depends on many factors and is tailored for each child. Please discuss your child's condition, treatment options, and your preference with your child's physician or health care provider.

Section 23.5

Otitis Media (Ear Infection)

National Institute on Deafness and Other Communication Disorders, July 2002. Revised by David A. Cooke, M.D., July 2008.

What is otitis media?

Otitis media is an infection or inflammation of the middle ear. This inflammation often begins when infections that cause sore throats, colds, or other respiratory or breathing problems spread to the middle ear. These can be viral or bacterial infections. Seventy-five percent of children experience at least one episode of otitis media by their third birthday. Almost half of these children will have three or more ear infections during their first three years. It is estimated that medical costs and lost wages because of otitis media amount to five billion dollars a year in the United States. Although otitis media is primarily a disease of infants and young children, it can also affect adults.

How do we hear?

The ear consists of three major parts: the outer ear, the middle ear, and the inner ear. The outer ear includes the pinna—the visible part of the ear—and the ear canal. The outer ear extends to the tympanic membrane or eardrum, which separates the outer ear from the middle ear. The middle ear is an air-filled space that is located behind the eardrum. The middle ear contains three tiny bones, the malleus, incus, and stapes, which transmit sound from the eardrum to the inner ear. The inner ear contains the hearing and balance organs. The cochlea contains the hearing organ that converts sound into electrical signals which are associated with the origin of impulses carried by nerves to the brain, where their meanings are appreciated.

Why are more children affected by otitis media than adults?

There are many reasons why children are more likely to suffer from otitis media than adults. First, children have more trouble fighting infections. This is because their immune systems are still developing. Another reason has to do with the child's eustachian tube. The eustachian tube is a small passageway that connects the upper part of the throat to the middle ear. It is shorter and straighter in the child than in the adult. It can contribute to otitis media in several ways.

The eustachian tube is usually closed but opens regularly to ventilate or replenish the air in the middle ear. This tube also equalizes middle ear air pressure in response to air pressure changes in the environment. However, a eustachian tube that is blocked by swelling of its lining or plugged with mucus from a cold or for some other reason cannot open to ventilate the middle ear. The lack of ventilation may allow fluid from the tissue that lines the middle ear to accumulate. If the eustachian tube remains plugged, the fluid cannot drain and begins to collect in the normally air-filled middle ear.

One more factor that makes children more susceptible to otitis media is that adenoids in children are larger than they are in adults. Adenoids are composed largely of cells (lymphocytes) that help fight infections. They are positioned in the back of the upper part of the throat near the eustachian tubes. Enlarged adenoids can, because of their size, interfere with the eustachian tube opening. In addition, adenoids may themselves become infected, and the infection may spread into the eustachian tubes.

Bacteria reach the middle ear through the lining or the passageway of the eustachian tube and can then produce infection, which causes swelling of the lining of the middle ear, blocking of the eustachian tube, and migration of white cells from the bloodstream to help fight the infection. In this process the white cells accumulate, often

Ear, Nose, and Throat Disorders

killing bacteria and dying themselves, leading to the formation of pus, a thick yellowish-white fluid in the middle ear. As the fluid increases, the child may have trouble hearing because the eardrum and middle ear bones are unable to move as freely as they should. As the infection worsens, many children also experience severe ear pain. Too much fluid in the ear can put pressure on the eardrum and eventually tear it.

What are the effects of otitis media?

Otitis media not only causes severe pain but rarely may result in serious complications if it is not treated. An untreated infection can travel from the middle ear to the nearby parts of the head, including the brain. Although the hearing loss caused by otitis media is usually temporary, untreated otitis media may lead to permanent hearing impairment. Persistent fluid in the middle ear and chronic otitis media can reduce a child's hearing at a time that is critical for speech and language development. Children who have early hearing impairment from frequent ear infections are likely to have speech and language disabilities.

How can someone tell if a child has otitis media?

Otitis media is often difficult to detect because most children affected by this disorder do not yet have sufficient speech and language skills to tell someone what is bothering them. Common signs to look for are as follows:

- Unusual irritability
- Difficulty sleeping
- Tugging or pulling at one or both ears
- Fever
- Fluid draining from the ear
- Loss of balance
- Unresponsiveness to quiet sounds or other signs of hearing difficulty such as sitting too close to the television or being inattentive

Can anything be done to prevent otitis media?

Two vaccines approved for young children may reduce the risk of otitis media. The *Haemophilus influenzae* type B (HIB) vaccine and the pneumococcal conjugate (Prevnar®) vaccines dramatically reduce the risk of life-threatening infections from these bacteria. These same bacteria are frequent causes of otitis media, so there is reason to suspect they may be effective for prevention of this problem. However, data has been mixed regarding how large an impact they have on rates of otitis media. There is also some evidence that the influenza vaccine may reduce the risk of otitis media by up to 30 percent. It is known that children who are cared for in group settings, as well as children who live with adults who smoke cigarettes, have more ear infections. Therefore, a child who is prone to otitis media should avoid contact with sick playmates and environmental tobacco smoke. Infants who nurse from a bottle while lying down also appear to develop otitis media more frequently. Children who have been breast-fed often have fewer episodes of otitis media. Research has shown that cold and allergy medications such as antihistamines and decongestants are not helpful in preventing ear infections.

How does a child's physician diagnose otitis media?

The simplest way to detect an active infection in the middle ear is to look in the child's ear with an otoscope, a light instrument that allows the physician to examine the outer ear and the eardrum. Inflammation of the eardrum indicates an infection. There are several ways that a physician checks for middle ear fluid. The use of a special type of otoscope called a pneumatic otoscope allows the physician to blow a puff of air onto the eardrum to test eardrum movement. (An eardrum with fluid behind it does not move as well as an eardrum with air behind it.)

A useful test of middle ear function is called tympanometry. This test requires insertion of a small soft plug into the opening of the child's ear canal. The plug contains a speaker, a microphone, and a device that is able to change the air pressure in the ear canal, allowing for several measures of the middle ear. The child feels air pressure changes in the ear or hears a few brief tones. While this test provides information on the condition of the middle ear, it does not determine how well the child hears. A physician may suggest a hearing test for a child who has frequent ear infections to determine the extent of hearing loss. The hearing test is usually performed by an audiologist, a person who is specially trained to measure hearing.

How is otitis media treated?

Studies have shown that the many cases of otitis media in children will resolve spontaneously without treatment. For example, about 60 percent of children improve within twenty-four hours, and

Ear, Nose, and Throat Disorders

70 percent within seventy-two hours, without use of medications. Treatment with antibiotics only improves this slightly, and frequent use of antibiotics can lead bacteria to become resistant to the drugs. Accordingly, many experts feel that immediate treatment with antibiotics is not necessary for many children, and that the primary emphasis should be on pain relievers.

For otherwise healthy children more than two years old who are not severely ill, it may be reasonable to delay treatment for forty-eight to seventy-two hours, and only prescribe antibiotics if there is no improvement at that point. However, decisions about whether and when to treat otitis media need to be made on a case-by-case basis by the child's physician.

If an antibiotic is prescribed for otitis media, following the physician's instructions is very important. Once started, the antibiotic should be taken until it is finished. Most physicians will have the child return for a follow-up examination to see if the infection has cleared.

Unfortunately, there are many bacteria that can cause otitis media, and some have become resistant to some antibiotics. This happens when antibiotics are given for coughs, colds, flu, or viral infections where antibiotic treatment is not useful. When bacteria become resistant to antibiotics, those treatments are then less effective against infections. This means that several different antibiotics may have to be tried before an ear infection clears. Antibiotics may also produce unwanted side effects such as nausea, diarrhea, and rashes.

Once the infection clears, fluid may remain in the middle ear for several months. Middle ear fluid that is not infected often disappears after three to six weeks. Neither antihistamines nor decongestants are recommended as helpful in the treatment of otitis media at any stage in the disease process. Sometimes physicians will treat the child with an antibiotic to hasten the elimination of the fluid, but current guidelines recommend against this in most cases. If the fluid persists for more than three months and is associated with a loss of hearing, many physicians suggest the insertion of "tubes" in the affected ears. This operation, called a myringotomy, can usually be done on an outpatient basis by a surgeon, who is usually an otolaryngologist (a physician who specializes in the ears, nose, and throat). While the child is asleep under general anesthesia, the surgeon makes a small opening in the child's eardrum. A small metal or plastic tube is placed into the opening in the eardrum. The tube ventilates the middle ear and helps keep the air pressure in the middle ear equal to the air pressure in the environment. The tube normally stays in the eardrum for six to twelve months, after which time it usually comes out spontaneously. If a child has enlarged or infected adenoids, the surgeon may recommend removal of the adenoids at the same time the ear tubes are inserted. Removal of the adenoids has been shown to reduce episodes of otitis media in some children, but not those who are under four years of age. Research, however, has shown that removal of a child's tonsils does not reduce occurrences of otitis media. Tonsillotomy and adenoidectomy may be appropriate for reasons other than middle ear fluid.

Hearing should be fully restored once the fluid is removed. Some children may need to have the operation again if the otitis media returns after the tubes come out. While the tubes are in place, water should be kept out of the ears. Many physicians recommend that a child with tubes wear special ear plugs while swimming or bathing so that water does not enter the middle ear.

What research is being done on otitis media?

Several avenues of research are being explored to further improve the prevention, diagnosis, and treatment of otitis media. For example, research is better defining those children who are at high risk for developing otitis media and conditions that predispose certain individuals to middle ear infections. Emphasis is being placed on discovering the reasons why some children have more ear infections than other children. The effects of otitis media on children's speech and language development are important areas of study, as is research to develop more accurate methods to help physicians detect middle ear infections. How the defense molecules and cells involved with immunity respond to bacteria and viruses that often lead to otitis media is also under investigation. Scientists are evaluating the success of certain drugs currently being used for the treatment of otitis media and are examining new drugs that may be more effective, easier to administer, and better at preventing new infections.

Section 23.6

Perforated Eardrum

Excerpted from "Ruptured Eardrum,"
© 2008 A.D.A.M., Inc. Reprinted with permission.

A ruptured or perforated eardrum is an opening in the tympanic membrane (eardrum).

Causes

The tympanic membrane (eardrum) separates the outer ear from the middle ear. The membrane vibrates when sound waves strike it, and this starts the process that converts the sound wave into a nerve impulse that travels to the brain. When the eardrum is damaged, the hearing process is interrupted.

The eardrum also acts as a barrier to keep outside material (such as bacteria) from entering the middle ear. When the eardrum is perforated, bacteria can easily travel to the middle ear—causing an infection.

Damage to the eardrum can occur from acoustic trauma such as direct injury or barotrauma (pressure-induced damage). Inserting cotton-tipped swabs or small objects into the ear to clean them sometimes causes a perforation of the eardrum. Foreign objects in the ear are another cause of perforated eardrum.

Ear infections may cause a ruptured eardrum as the pressure of fluid in the middle ear increases. Conversely, a ruptured eardrum can cause ear infections because the eardrum is no longer intact, and bacteria can enter the middle ear.

Symptoms

- Earache or ear discomfort
- May be severe and increasing
- A sudden decrease in ear pain may occur followed by ear drainage
- Drainage from the ear (may be clear, pus, or bloody)

- Hearing loss in the affected ear (may not be complete loss of hearing)
- Ear noise/buzzing

Exams and Tests

The doctor will look in your ear with an otoscope. If the eardrum is punctured, the doctor will see an opening in it, and may even see the bones of the middle ear. Sometimes it is hard for the doctor to see the eardrum because of drainage from the ear (pus).

Audiology testing can measure the extent of hearing loss.

Treatment

A ruptured or perforated eardrum usually heals by itself within two months. The goal of treatment is to relieve pain and prevent infection.

Antibiotics may be used to prevent infection or to treat an existing infection. Analgesics, including over-the-counter medications, may be used to relieve pain.

Occasionally, the health care provider may place a patch over the eardrum while it heals. Surgical repair of the eardrum may be needed, if the eardrum does not heal on its own (tympanoplasty).

Warmth to the ear may help relieve discomfort. Keep the ear clean and dry while healing. Cotton balls should be placed in the ear while showering or shampooing to prevent water entering the ear.

Outlook (Prognosis)

A ruptured or perforated eardrum may be uncomfortable, but it usually heals by itself within two months. Any hearing loss is usually temporary.

Possible Complications

- Permanent hearing loss
- Ear infection (otitis media)

When to Contact a Medical Professional

Call your health care provider if:

- you have symptoms of a ruptured or perforated eardrum;

- you are diagnosed with a ruptured eardrum, and symptoms last longer than two months in spite of medical treatment;
- you are diagnosed with a ruptured eardrum, and you develop persistent fever, general ill feeling, or hearing loss.

Prevention

Do not insert objects into the ear canal, even to clean it. Foreign objects should only be removed by a health care provider. Have ear infections treated promptly.

Section 23.7

Sinusitis

"Sinus Infection (Sinusitis)," National Institute of Allergy and Infectious Diseases, National Institutes of Health, November 23, 2007.

Overview

You're coughing, your nose is stuffy, and you feel tired and achy. You think that you might be getting a cold. Later, when the medicines you've been taking to relieve symptoms of the common cold are not working and you've got a terrible headache, you finally drag yourself to the doctor. After listening to your history of symptoms, examining your face and forehead, and perhaps doing a sinus x-ray, the doctor says you have sinusitis.

Sinusitis means your sinuses are infected or inflamed. But this gives little indication of the misery and pain this condition can cause. Health experts usually divide sinusitis cases into the following types:

- Acute cases, which last for four weeks or less
- Subacute cases, which last four to twelve weeks
- Chronic cases, which last more than twelve weeks and can continue for months or even years
- Recurrent cases, which involve several acute attacks within a year

Health experts estimate thirty-seven million Americans are affected by sinusitis every year. Healthcare providers report nearly thirty-two million cases of chronic sinusitis to the Centers for Disease Control and Prevention annually. Americans spend $5.8 billion each year on healthcare costs related to sinusitis.

What Are Sinuses?

When people say, "I'm having a sinus attack," they usually are referring to symptoms of congestion and achiness in one or more of four pairs of cavities, or sinuses, known as paranasal sinuses. These cavities, located within the skull or bones of the head surrounding the nose, include the following:

- Frontal sinuses over the eyes in the brow area
- Maxillary sinuses inside each cheekbone
- Ethmoid sinuses just behind the bridge of the nose and between the eyes
- Sphenoid sinuses behind the ethmoids in the upper region of the nose and behind the eyes

Each sinus has an opening into the nose for the free exchange of air and mucus, and each is joined with the nasal passages by a continuous mucous membrane lining. Therefore, anything that causes a swelling in the nose—an infection, an allergic reaction, or another type of immune reaction—also can affect your sinuses.

Air trapped within a blocked sinus, along with pus or other secretions (liquid material) may cause pressure on the sinus wall. The result is the sometimes intense pain of a sinus attack. Similarly, when air is prevented from entering a paranasal sinus by a swollen membrane at the opening, a vacuum can be created that also causes pain.

Cause

Acute Sinusitis

Most cases of acute sinusitis start with a common cold, which is caused by a virus. Colds can inflame your sinuses and cause symptoms of sinusitis. Both the cold and the sinus inflammation usually go away without treatment within two weeks. If the inflammation produced by the cold leads to a bacterial infection, however, then this infection is what health experts call acute sinusitis.

Ear, Nose, and Throat Disorders

The inflammation caused by the cold results in swelling of the mucous membranes (linings) of your sinuses, and this can lead to air and mucus becoming trapped behind the narrowed openings of the sinuses. When mucus stays inside your sinuses and is unable to drain into your nose, it can become the source of nutrients (material that gives nourishment) for bacteria.

Most healthy people harbor bacteria, such as *Streptococcus pneumoniae* and *Haemophilus influenzae*, in the nose and throat, and the bacteria cause no problems. But when you have a cold, you tend to sniff or to blow your nose, and these actions cause pressure changes that can send bacteria inside the sinuses. If your sinuses then stop draining properly, bacteria that may have been living harmlessly in your nose or throat can begin to multiply in your sinuses, causing acute sinusitis.

People who suffer from allergies that affect the nose (like pollen allergy, also called hay fever), as well as people who may have chronic nasal symptoms not caused by allergy, are also prone to develop episodes of acute sinusitis. The chronic nasal problems cause the nasal membranes to swell, and the sinus passages become blocked in a manner similar to that described above for the common cold. The normally harmless bacteria in the nose and throat again lead to acute sinusitis.

Rarely, fungal infections can cause acute sinusitis. Although fungi are abundant in the environment, they usually are harmless to healthy people because the human body has a natural resistance to fungus. However, in people whose immune system is not functioning properly, fungus, such as Aspergillus, can cause acute sinusitis. (Aspergillus is commonly found growing on dead leaves, stored grain, compost piles, or in other decaying vegetation.)

In general, people who have reduced immune function (such as those with primary immune deficiency disease or human immunodeficiency virus [HIV] infection) or abnormalities in mucus secretion or mucus movement (such as those with cystic fibrosis) are more likely to suffer from sinusitis.

Chronic Sinusitis

In chronic sinusitis, the membranes of both the paranasal sinuses and the nose are thickened because they are constantly inflamed. Most experts now use the term "chronic rhinosinusitis" to describe this condition, and they also recommend that the condition be divided into rhinosinusitis with or without nasal polyps. Nasal polyps are grapelike growths of the sinus membranes that protrude into the sinuses or into the nasal passages. Polyps make it even more difficult for the sinuses to drain and for air to pass through the nose.

The causes of chronic sinusitis are largely unknown. The condition often occurs in people with asthma, the majority of whom have allergies. It is possible that constant exposure to inhaled allergens that are present year-round, such as house dust mites, pets, mold (a kind of fungus), and cockroaches cause chronic inflammation of the nose and the sinuses.

An allergic reaction to certain fungi may be responsible for at least some cases of chronic sinusitis; this condition is called "allergic fungal sinusitis." At least half of all people with chronic rhinosinusitis do not have allergies, however.

Most health experts believe that chronic rhinosinusitis is not an infectious disease (like acute sinusitis). If you suffer frequent episodes of acute sinusitis, however, you may be prone to develop chronic rhinosinusitis. Other causes of chronic rhinosinusitis may be an immune deficiency disorder (for example, primary immune deficiency disease or HIV infection) or an abnormality in the quality of mucus produced by the respiratory system (cystic fibrosis).

Another group of people who may develop chronic sinusitis are those with significant anatomic (structure) variations inside the nose, such as a deviated septum, that lead to blockage of mucus.

Symptoms

One of the most common symptoms of sinusitis is pain, and the location depends on which sinus is affected:

- If you have a pain in your forehead over the frontal sinuses when you are touched, your frontal sinuses may be inflamed.

- If your upper jaw and teeth ache, and your cheeks become tender to the touch, you may have an infection in the maxillary sinuses.

- If you have swelling of the eyelids and tissues around your eyes, and pain between your eyes, you may have inflammation of the ethmoid sinuses that are near the tear ducts in the corner of your eyes. Ethmoid inflammation also can cause a stuffy nose, a loss of smell, and tenderness when you touch the sides of your nose.

- If you have earaches, neck pain, and deep achiness at the top of your head, you may have infection in the sphenoid sinuses, although these sinuses are less frequently affected.

Most people with sinusitis have pain or tenderness in several locations, and their symptoms usually do not clearly indicate which sinuses are inflamed.

In addition to the pain, people with sinusitis frequently have thick nasal secretions that are yellow, green, or blood-tinged. Sometimes these secretions, referred to as post-nasal drip, drain in the back of the throat and are difficult to get rid of. Also, acute and chronic sinusitis are strongly associated with nasal symptoms such as a stuffy nose, as well as with a general feeling of fullness over the entire face.

Less common symptoms of sinusitis can include the following:

- Tiredness
- Decreased sense of smell
- Cough that may be more severe at night
- Sore throat
- Bad breath
- Fever

On rare occasions, acute sinusitis can result in brain infection and other serious complications.

Diagnosis

Because your nose can get stuffy when you have a condition like the common cold, you may confuse simple nasal congestion with sinusitis. A cold, however, usually lasts about seven to fourteen days and goes away without treatment. Acute sinusitis often lasts longer and typically causes more symptoms than a cold.

Your healthcare provider can usually diagnose acute sinusitis by noting your symptoms and doing a physical examination, which includes examining your nasal tissues. If your symptoms are vague or persist, your healthcare provider may order a computed tomography (CT) scan, a form of x-ray, to confirm that you have sinusitis.

Laboratory tests your healthcare provider may use to diagnose chronic sinusitis include the following:

- Blood tests to rule out conditions associated with sinusitis, like an immune deficiency disorder
- A sweat test or a blood test to rule out cystic fibrosis

- Tests on the material that is inside your sinuses to detect bacterial or fungal infection
- Biopsy of the membranes (linings) of the nose or sinuses to determine the health of the cells lining these cavities

Treatment

After diagnosing sinusitis and identifying a possible cause, your healthcare provider can suggest various treatments.

Acute Sinusitis

If you have acute sinusitis, your healthcare provider may recommend the following:

- Antibiotics to control a bacterial infection, if present
- Pain relievers to reduce any pain
- Decongestants to reduce congestion

Even if you have acute sinusitis, your provider may choose not to use an antibiotic because many cases of acute sinusitis will end on their own. But if you do not feel better after a few days you should contact your provider again.

You should use over-the-counter or prescription decongestant nose drops and sprays only for a few days. If you use these medicines for longer periods, they can lead to even more congestion and swelling of your nasal passages.

If you have an allergic disease along with sinusitis, you may also need medicine to control allergies. This may include a nasal steroid spray that reduces the swelling around the sinus passages and allows the sinuses to drain. If you already have asthma and then get sinusitis, your asthma may worsen. You should stay in close touch with your healthcare provider to modify your asthma treatment if needed.

Chronic Sinusitis

Healthcare providers often find it difficult to treat chronic sinusitis successfully. The two main forms of treatment that are used, nasal steroid sprays and long courses of oral antibiotics, alone or in combination, have not been rigorously tested in chronic sinusitis. Scientists need to do more research to determine what the best treatment is.

Ear, Nose, and Throat Disorders

Many healthcare providers also recommend using saline (saltwater) washes or sprays in the nose to help remove thick secretions and allow the sinuses to drain.

If you have severe chronic sinusitis, your healthcare provider may prescribe oral steroids, such as prednisone. Because oral steroids are powerful medicines and can have significant side effects, you should take them only when other medicines have not worked.

Surgery

When medicine fails, surgery may be the only alternative for treating chronic sinusitis. The goal of surgery is to improve sinus drainage and reduce blockage of the nasal passages. During surgery, which is usually done through the nose, the surgeon does the following:

- Enlarges the natural opening of the sinuses
- Removes any polyps
- Corrects significant anatomic deformities that contribute to the obstruction

Most people have fewer symptoms and better quality of life after surgery. In a substantial number of people, however, problems can recur after surgery, sometimes even after a short period of time.

In children, surgeons can sometimes eliminate sinus problems by removing adenoids (tissue in the back of the throat) that obstruct the nasal-sinus passages.

Prevention

There are no methods that have been scientifically tested and proven to prevent acute or chronic sinusitis. However, your healthcare provider may recommend a variety of measures that may provide you with some benefit:

- Keep your nose as moist as possible with frequent use of saline (salt) sprays.
- Avoid very dry indoor environments and use a humidifier, if necessary. But be aware that if you have allergies to molds, house dust mites, or cockroaches, a humid environment may also create problems.
- Avoid exposure to irritants, such as cigarette and cigar smoke or strong odors from chemicals.

Childhood Diseases and Disorders Sourcebook, Second Edition

- Avoid exposure to anything you're allergic to. If you have not been tested for allergies and you are getting frequent sinus infections, ask your healthcare provider to give you an allergy evaluation or to refer you to an allergy specialist.
- Avoid long periods of swimming in pools treated with chlorine, which irritates the lining of the nose and sinuses.
- Avoid water diving, which forces water into the sinuses from the nasal passages.

You may find that air travel poses a problem if you are suffering from acute or chronic sinusitis. As air pressure in a plane is reduced, pressure can build up in your head, blocking your sinuses or the eustachian tubes in your ears. As a result, you might feel discomfort in your sinuses or middle ear during the plane's ascent or descent. Some health experts recommend using decongestant nose drops or sprays before a flight to avoid this problem.

Complications

On rare occasions, acute sinusitis can result in brain infection and other serious complications.

Research

At least two-thirds of sinusitis cases are caused by two bacteria, *Streptococcus pneumoniae* and *Haemophilus influenzae*. These bacteria also can cause otitis media (middle ear infection) in children as well as pneumonia and acute worsening of chronic bronchitis in people of all ages. The National Institute of Allergy and Infectious Diseases (NIAID) is supporting many studies to better understand how these bacteria infect as well as to identify potential candidates for future vaccine strategies that could eliminate these diseases.

A project supported by NIAID is developing an advanced "sinuscope" that will permit improved airway evaluation during a medical examination, especially when a doctor is considering surgical intervention.

Scientific studies have shown a close relationship between having asthma and sinusitis. For example, the vast majority of people with moderate to severe asthma also have chronic sinusitis. Health experts have suggested that chronic sinusitis and asthma may be the same disease manifested in two parts of the respiratory system: upper and lower.

NIAID conducts and supports research on asthma that will lead to a better understanding of the causes behind chronic bronchial inflammation in asthma. This will advance our understanding of the causes of chronic sinusitis and lead to the development of more effective treatments and ways to prevent the disease.

Scientists supported by NIAID and other institutions are also investigating whether chronic sinusitis has genetic causes. They have found that certain alterations in the gene that causes cystic fibrosis may increase the likelihood of developing chronic sinusitis. This research is giving scientists new insights into the cause of the disease in some people and points to new strategies for diagnosis and treatment.

Other NIAID-supported research is examining whether chronic sinusitis can be caused by an unusual reaction to fungi normally found inside the nose and the sinuses. One study has recently shown that when blood cells from people with chronic sinusitis are exposed to fungal material, those cells make chemicals that produce inflammation. This raises the possibility that fungi may play a role in some cases of chronic sinusitis. NIAID is supporting trials of antifungal drugs to determine whether, and for whom, this new treatment strategy holds promise.

Section 23.8

Swimmer's Ear

© 2008 A.D.A.M., Inc. Excerpted with permission.

Swimmer's ear is inflammation, irritation, or infection of the outer ear and ear canal. The medical term for swimmer's ear is otitis externa.

Causes

Swimmer's ear is fairly common, especially among teenagers and young adults.

Causes of swimmer's ear include:

- swimming in polluted water;
- scratching the ear or inside the ear;
- object stuck in the ear.

Trying to clean wax from the ear canal, especially with cotton swabs or small objects, can irritate or damage the skin.

Swimmer's ear is occasionally associated with middle ear infection (otitis media) or upper respiratory infections such as colds. Moisture in the ear makes the ear more prone to infection from water-loving bacteria such as pseudomonas. Other bacteria, and rarely, fungus, can also cause infection.

Symptoms

- Ear pain—may worsen when pulling the outer ear
- Itching of the ear or ear canal
- Drainage from the ear—yellow, yellow-green, pus-like, or foul smelling

Exams and Tests

The doctor will perform a physical exam, which includes looking inside the ears. The ear, including the ear canal, appears red

Ear, Nose, and Throat Disorders

and swollen. The skin inside the ear canal may be scaly or shedding.

Touching or moving the outer ear increases the pain. The eardrum may be difficult for the doctor to see because of a swelling in the outer ear.

The doctor may take a sample of fluid from the ear and send it to a lab so any bacteria or fungus can be identified.

Treatment

The goal of treatment is to cure the infection. Medicines may include:

- ear drops containing antibiotics;
- corticosteroids to reduce itching and inflammation.

The ear canal should be cleaned of drainage. This allows the medicines to work better.

Four or five ear drops should be used at a time, so that the medicine can get into the end of the ear canal. If the ear canal is very swollen, a wick may be applied in the ear to allow the drops to travel to the end of the canal.

Analgesics may be used if pain is severe. Placing something warm against the ears may reduce pain.

Outlook (Prognosis)

Swimmer's ear responds well to treatment, but complications may occur if it is not treated. Some individuals with underlying medical problems, such as diabetes, may be more likely to get complications such as malignant otitis externa.

Possible Complications

- Chronic otitis externa
- Malignant otitis externa
- Spread of infection to other areas of the body

When to Contact a Medical Professional

Call for an appointment with your doctor if you develop any symptoms of swimmer's ear. Call your doctor if the symptoms worsen or persist despite treatment, or if new symptoms appear, including pain and redness of the skull behind the ear or persistent fever.

Prevention

Protect ears from further damage:

- Do not scratch the ears or insert cotton swabs or other objects in the ears.
- Keep ears clean and dry, and do not let water enter the ears when showering, shampooing, or bathing.
- Dry the ear thoroughly after exposure to moisture.
- Avoid swimming in polluted water.
- Use earplugs when swimming.
- Consider mixing 1 drop of alcohol with 1 drop of white vinegar and placing the mixture into the ears after they get wet. The alcohol and acid in the vinegar help prevent bacterial growth.

Section 23.9

Tonsillitis

© 2008 A.D.A.M., Inc. Reprinted with permission.

Tonsillitis is inflammation (swelling) of the tonsils.

Causes

The tonsils are lymph nodes in the back of the mouth and top of the throat. They normally help to filter out bacteria and other microorganisms to prevent infection in the body.

They may become so overwhelmed by bacterial or viral infection that they swell and become inflamed, causing tonsillitis. The infection may also be present in the throat and surrounding areas, causing pharyngitis.

Tonsillitis is extremely common, particularly in children.

Symptoms

- Difficulty swallowing
- Ear pain
- Fever, chills
- Headache
- Sore throat—lasts longer than forty-eight hours and may be severe
- Tenderness of the jaw and throat
- Voice changes, loss of voice

Exams and Tests

The health care provider will look in the mouth and throat for enlarged, visible tonsils. They are usually reddened and may have white spots on them. The lymph nodes of the jaw and neck may be enlarged and tender to the touch.

A culture of the tonsils may show bacterial infection. A culture for the streptococcus bacteria (strep) may be taken because it is the most common and most dangerous form of tonsillitis. A rapid strep test may also be performed by your physician by taking a throat swab for a quick diagnosis.

Treatment

If the cause of the tonsillitis is bacteria such as strep, antibiotics are given to cure the infection. The antibiotics may be given once as a shot, or taken for ten days by mouth.

If antibiotic pills are used, they must be taken for the full course. They must not be stopped just because the discomfort stops, or the infection will *not* be cured. Some health care providers will treat all tonsillitis with antibiotics to prevent the chance of strep-related complications. Others treat only known bacterial and strep infections.

Rest to allow the body to heal. Fluids, especially warm (not hot), bland fluids or very cold fluids may soothe the throat. Gargle with warm salt water or suck on lozenges (containing benzocaine or similar ingredients) to reduce pain.

Over-the-counter medications may be used to reduce pain and fever. Do *not* use aspirin in children if the infection could be viral, because this may be associated with Reye syndrome.

Surgery to remove the tonsils (tonsillectomy) may be necessary for some people who have repeated infections.

Outlook (Prognosis)

Tonsillitis symptoms usually lessen in two or three days after treatment starts. The infection usually is cured by then, but may require more than one course of antibiotics. Complications of untreated strep tonsillitis may be severe. A tonsillectomy may be recommended if tonsillitis is severe, comes back, or does not respond to antibiotics.

Possible Complications

- Pharyngitis—bacterial
- Pharyngitis—viral
- Dehydration from difficulty swallowing fluids
- Blocked airway from enlarged tonsils
- Peritonsillar abscess or abscess in other parts of the throat

Ear, Nose, and Throat Disorders

- Rheumatic fever and subsequent cardiovascular disorders
- Kidney failure
- Post-streptococcal glomerulonephritis

When to Contact a Medical Professional

Call your health care provider if a sore throat persists longer than forty-eight hours, is accompanied by other symptoms of tonsillitis, if symptoms worsen, or new symptoms develop.

Chapter 24

Endocrine and Growth Disorders

Chapter Contents

Section 24.1—Constitutional Growth Delay 352
Section 24.2—Growth Hormone Deficiency 354
Section 24.3—Hypothyroidism 357
Section 24.4—Idiopathic Short Stature 359
Section 24.5—Precocious Puberty 361

Section 24.1

Constitutional Growth Delay

"Constitutional Growth Delay in Children," © 2007 MAGIC Foundation (www.magicfoundation.org). Reprinted with permission.

What Is Constitutional Delay of Growth?

One of the most common diagnoses made after a growth evaluation is constitutional delay of growth. These children, often called "late bloomers," have a characteristic pattern of growth. Constitutional delay of growth (CDG) is considered more of a variant of normal growth, rather than a "disease process."

Children with constitutional delay of growth are typically born with a normal birth weight and length, but in the first two years of life, show slow growth and thus lose height percentiles. There may be delayed dental development later in childhood. A similar pattern of growth is often seen in a parent. For example, the mother might recall her first menstrual cycle occurring late, such as after age fifteen. The father might recall being short but catching up toward the end of high school.

Constitutional delay of growth is diagnosed more frequently in boys than girls but can occur in either sex. The growth rate between ages three and ten should be normal so there should not be a further loss in percentiles. If there is a concern about the growth rate, further workup is recommended. However, when peers go through pubertal growth acceleration, children with constitutional delay of growth will lose percentiles as their onset into puberty is delayed.

Bone age x-ray of the left hand and wrist is delayed in CDG, but is also delayed in many other conditions. Thus, a delayed bone age supports the diagnosis of constitutional delay of growth, but is not conclusive.

Should I Take My Child to See a Growth Specialist?

Your primary care team will help decide whether a consultation is needed. You should point out whether there was a similar pattern of growth in any of the family members.

Endocrine and Growth Disorders

Questions to Ask Your Primary Care Physician

- Is my child short but growing well, such as at least 2¼ inches per year?
- Do you think the growth pattern is consistent with constitutional delay or suggestive of another diagnosis?
- Is the bone age or skeletal age delayed?
- Does it look like my child will catch up to his or her genetic potential?

How Is Constitutional Delay of Growth Diagnosed?

Your primary care team can diagnose CDG, though sometimes a consultation with an endocrinologist is sought to confirm the diagnosis.

What Should I Expect at the Endocrinologist's Office?

The endocrinologist will take a detailed family history of heights and get an appreciation of the timing of growth of other family members. You can help out by asking grandparents about their height and timing of pubertal development.

Hand carry a copy of the growth charts. The more information you provide, the more accurate will be the assessment.

A detailed examination will be performed including a brief assessment of how far along your child is in terms of pubertal development.

There may be no laboratory tests requested, or there might be a bone age x-ray of the left hand and wrist as well as a blood test screening for other tests that can mimic constitutional delay of growth. There is no specific blood test to diagnose constitutional delay of growth.

Section 24.2

Growth Hormone Deficiency

© 2008 A.D.A.M., Inc. Reprinted with permission.

Alternative Names

Panhypopituitarism; dwarfism; pituitary dwarfism

Definition

Growth hormone deficiency involves abnormally short stature with normal body proportions. Growth hormone deficiency can be categorized as either congenital (present at birth) or acquired.

Causes

An abnormally short height in childhood may occur if the pituitary gland does not produce enough growth hormone. It can be caused by a variety of genetic mutations (such as Pit-1 gene, Prop-1 gene, growth hormone receptor gene, growth hormone gene), absence of the pituitary gland, or severe brain injury, but in most cases no underlying cause of the deficiency is found.

Growth retardation may become evident in infancy and persist throughout childhood. The child's "growth curve," which is usually plotted on a standardized growth chart by the pediatrician, may range from flat (no growth) to very shallow (minimal growth). Normal puberty may or may not occur, depending on the degree to which the pituitary can produce adequate hormone levels other than growth hormone.

Growth hormone deficiency may be associated with deficiencies of other hormones, including the following:

- Thyrotropins (control production of thyroid hormones)
- Vasopressin (controls water balance in the body)
- Gonadotropins (control production of male and female sex hormones)

Endocrine and Growth Disorders

- ACTH or adrenocorticotrophic hormone (controls the adrenal gland and its production of cortisol, dehydroepiandrosterone [DHEA], and other hormones)

Physical defects of the face and skull can also be associated with abnormalities of the pituitary or pituitary function. A small percentage of infants with cleft lip and cleft palate have decreased growth hormone levels.

Symptoms

- Slowed or absent increase in height
- Slow growth before age five
- Short stature—below fifth percentile on a standardized growth chart, an adult less than five feet tall
- Absent or delayed sexual development in an adolescent
- Headaches
- Excessive thirst with excessive urination
- Increased urine volume

Exams and Tests

A physical examination including weight, height, and body proportions will show signs of slowed growth rate and deviation from normal growth curves.

Tests may include the following:

- Hand x-ray can determine bone age.
- DEXA (dual energy x-ray absorptiometry) can also determine bone age.
- Measurement of growth hormone and associated binding protein levels (IGF-I and IGFBP-3) reveals if the growth problem is caused by dysfunction of the pituitary gland.
- Tests to measure other hormone levels (lack of growth hormone may not be an isolated problem).
- X-ray of head may show problems with the skull, such as small, enlarged, or empty sella or a space-occupying lesion.
- Magnetic resonance imaging (MRI) of the head can show the hypothalamus and pituitary glands.

Treatment

Synthetic growth hormone can be used for children with growth hormone deficiency. This treatment requires the assistance of a pediatric endocrinologist. Treatment with synthetic (recombinant) human growth hormone is generally considered to be safe, with rare side effects.

If the deficiency is an isolated growth hormone deficiency, synthetic growth hormone is given alone. If the deficiency is not isolated, other hormone replacement preparations will be required as well.

Outlook (Prognosis)

Growth rates are improved in most children treated with growth hormones, although the effectiveness may decrease with prolonged treatment.

Possible Complications

If left untreated, extremely short stature and delayed puberty will result from this condition.

In the past, some patients acquired Creutzfeldt-Jakob disease (the human form of "mad cow" disease) from human-derived growth hormone that was used to treat growth deficiencies. This medication has been removed from the market.

Synthetic growth hormone is used instead and carries no risk of infectious disease.

When to Contact a Medical Professional

Call your health care provider if your child seems abnormally short for his or her age.

Prevention

Most cases are not preventable.

Review your child's growth chart with your physician after each checkup. If your child's growth rate is dropping or your child's projected adult height is much shorter than an average height of both parents, evaluation by a specialist is recommended.

Adjusted average height of both parents is as follows:

- **For boys:** Mom's height plus 5 inches + Dad's height. Divide the end number by 2.

- **For girls:** Dad's height minus 5 inches + Mom's height. Divide the end number by 2.

Section 24.3

Hypothyroidism

"Clinical Hypothyroidism: General Information," © 2008 MAGIC Foundation (www.magicfoundation.org). Reprinted with permission.

Hypothyroidism, or a deficiency in the secretion of the thyroid hormones, thyroxine (T4) and triiodothyronine (T3), by the thyroid gland may be difficult to recognize, but usually is very easy to treat. During childhood and adolescence the hypothyroid patient presents either with an enlarged thyroid gland, also known as a goiter, or diminution in the rate of growth in height. At the time of birth the symptoms and signs of hypothyroidism are minimal or absent, and the lack of adequate thyroid hormone from birth until approximately age two years is associated with varying degrees of permanent mental retardation. For these reasons most countries in the western world and every state in the United States routinely perform screening tests within the first week of life to detect congenital hypothyroidism so that prompt treatment can be initiated to prevent mental retardation.

Causes

Hypothyroidism usually is caused by an abnormality of the immune system that results in damage and destruction of the thyroid gland. This process results either in loss of thyroid tissue or an enlargement of the thyroid. The gland has the shape of a bow tie or butterfly, and is located just below the larynx, or "Adam's apple," and in front of the trachea, or windpipe. In most instances there is no pain or tenderness associated with thyroid diseases, although patients occasionally complain of difficulty in swallowing as if there were a lump in their throat.

Signs

Often the only sign of hypothyroidism during childhood is an abnormal rate of linear growth. Actually the child may not be short compared to other children of the same age if he or she were above average in height before the disease occurred. Therefore, the most important feature of hypothyroidism is a decrease in the rate or velocity of growth in height. If the disease is recognized early and adequately treated, the child will grow at an accelerated rate until reaching the same growth percentile where the child measured prior to the onset of hypothyroidism. Hypothyroidism progresses very slowly and insidiously, making the diagnosis difficult for physicians. In the more advanced and long-standing the child may have other general symptoms of hypothyroidism, such as easy fatigability, mild weight gain in association with a reduction in appetite, constipation, an intolerance of cold weather, dry skin, and either delayed (usual) or early (rare) onset of sexual development at adolescence.

Other Possible Causes

Less often, hypothyroidism may be caused by a failure of the pituitary gland to secrete thyroid stimulating hormone, or TSH. This hormone is essential for stimulating the thyroid gland to make T4 and T3 in normal amounts. TSH may be deficient for several reasons:

- The pituitary gland is diseased, a rare cause.

- The area above the pituitary, called the hypothalamus, that is necessary to stimulate the pituitary, is diseased.

- There is a tumor, cyst, or other abnormal structure between the hypothalamus and pituitary gland that prevents the pituitary from receiving its stimulus to secrete TSH.

Usually patients with TSH deficiency also have deficient secretion of growth hormone, and may have deficient secretion of the gonadotropins, called luteinizing hormone (LH) and follicle stimulating hormone (FSH), which stimulate puberty and reproduction, and adrenocorticotropic hormone (ACTH), which is necessary for cortisol and hydrocortisone secretion by the adrenal gland.

Treatment

The treatment of hypothyroidism, regardless of the cause, is easy and inexpensive. One or two tablets of the major thyroid hormone, thyroxine (trade names in the United States are Levothroid®, Levoxyl®, and Synthroid®) once a day provides normal thyroid function and growth. The dose, depending upon the child's age, ranges between 50 ug (0.05 mg) and 200 ug (0.2 mg) although some infants require slightly lower doses. The blood levels of T4 and TSH should be monitored annually to assure that the dose remains adequate as the child grows. In most instances the treatment must be continued for life since the diseases that cause hypothyroidism are permanent rather than transient.

Every child that has a decrease in the rate of growth in height during childhood and adolescence should have blood tests to measure T4, free T4, and TSH in order to determine if the growth problem is caused by hypothyroidism.

Section 24.4

Idiopathic Short Stature

"Idiopathic Short Stature," © 2008 MAGIC Foundation (www.magicfoundation.org). Reprinted with permission.

Idiopathic short stature (also known as ISS) is a big name for children who are short with no known cause. Idiopathic short stature is a problem that can be present in both girls and boys. Many causes of short stature have been discovered over the past few years, but there are still factors that are not yet understood. ISS falls into this latter category. Although the reasons for ISS are not yet totally understood, it is known that the administration of growth-promoting treatments may help affected children.

Idiopathic short stature is defined as having a height significantly shorter than the normal population (i.e., shorter than 1.2 percent of the population of the same age and gender), a poor adult height prediction (generally defined as less than 5'4" for males and less than 4'11" for females), and no detectable cause for the short stature.

Should I Take My Child to See a Growth Specialist?

You should first take your child to visit your local pediatrician, who will refer your child to a growth specialist (pediatric endocrinologist) if necessary.

You should remember that the window of opportunity for growth ends when the growth plates fuse after puberty; therefore, the earlier you take your child for an assessment the better.

Questions to Ask Your Pediatrician

- Is my child growing at an appropriate rate for his or her age?
- Is my child within the normal range of expected position on the growth chart?
- Is my child on track to reach a normal expected height which is appropriate for our family?
- Is my child at an appropriate stage of puberty for his or her age?

How is ISS Diagnosed?

Idiopathic short stature is normally diagnosed by a pediatric endocrinologist after a full investigation of the medical history, a complete physical examination, and the exclusion of any chronic medical condition or other hormonal abnormality.

The work-up for a diagnosis of idiopathic short stature, although a simple diagnosis, may require a series of blood and/or other tests to be done to rule out various medical conditions that are known to affect height.

Do Growth-Promoting Therapies Work in Children with ISS?

Growth hormone was first approved by the Federal Drug Administration for use in patients with idiopathic short stature in 2003 based on the successful results of clinical trials conducted in the United States and in Europe.

When started at an early enough age, growth hormone can significantly increase the final height of a child with idiopathic short stature.

After completion of puberty, no further growth in height is possible. An early diagnosis is, therefore, critical to the success of the treatment.

Section 24.5

Precocious Puberty

"Precocious Puberty," © 2007 MAGIC Foundation (www.magicfoundation.org). Reprinted with permission.

Precocious puberty or central precocious puberty can be very confusing and truly unexpected. After all who knew children could go into puberty too early? There are treatments for this condition because it is not something which is healthy for children to experience for many reasons. Often children with precocious puberty look older (they are taller/more developed than other children the same age). They are expected to act as old as they look. This in combination with other factors leads to a time of great stress. We are here to help parents!

Recent news reports have stated that central precocious puberty is becoming more frequent. Many factors may contribute to children who exhibit signs of (early) precocious puberty.

The Pituitary Gland: The "Master Gland"

The pituitary gland, which is often referred to as the "master gland," regulates the release of most of the body's hormones (chemical messengers that send information to different parts of the body). It is a pea-sized gland that is located underneath the brain. The pituitary gland controls the release of thyroid, adrenal, growth, and sex hormones. The hypothalamus, located in the brain above the pituitary gland, regulates the release of hormones from the pituitary gland.

Hormones: The "Chemical Messengers"

Hormones are chemical messengers that carry information from one cell to another in the body. Hormones are carried throughout body by the blood, and are responsible for regulating many body functions. The body makes many hormones (e.g., thyroid, growth, sex, and adrenal hormones) that work together to maintain normal bodily function. Hormones involved in the control of puberty include:

- **GnRH:** Gonadotropin releasing hormone, which comes from the brain in boys and in girls. Other androgens from the adrenal glands (located near the kidneys) produce pubic and axillary hair at the time of puberty.
- **Estrogen:** A female sex hormone, which is responsible for breast development in girls. It is made mainly by the ovaries, but is also present in boys in smaller amounts.
- **Sex hormones:** Responsible for the development of pubertal signs as well as changes in behavior and the ability to have children.

Precocious puberty means having signs of puberty (e.g., pubic hair or breast development) at an earlier age than usual.

Normal Puberty

There is a wide range of ages at which individuals normally start puberty. Girls usually develop breasts and then pubic hair between the ages of eight and thirteen years. Menstrual periods typically start at twelve to thirteen years of age. Girls will often experience moodiness and become more irritable during puberty. Boys normally develop testicular enlargement and then pubic hair between the ages of nine and fourteen years. Underarm and facial hair, as well as deepening of the voice, typically occur between the ages of thirteen and sixteen years. Your child may be taller than the other children in his or her class. This is because the hormones that increase at the time of puberty also cause a spurt in growth.

Causes of Precocious Puberty

In the majority of cases of precocious puberty, the cause is unknown. In some instances, the pituitary signals the ovaries and testicles to make female and male hormones at an earlier than usual time. In other cases, signs of puberty occur prematurely because of abnormalities in the ovaries, testicles, or adrenal glands. Tests are usually necessary to determine whether the cause of precocious puberty is in the brain or in another area of the body.

Endocrine and Growth Disorders

Treatment

If your child's doctor determines that treatment is necessary, your child may receive a medication (analog or modified form of GnRH). The goals of treatment with this drug are to temporarily stop puberty and to decrease the rate of bone maturation. Rapid bone maturation will cause your child's adult height to be shorter than his or her potential height. After the first couple of months of treatment, your child's rapid growth should slow and his or her pubertal stage will remain the same or possibly regress. Many children are too young to deal with the psychological aspects of early puberty and by stopping further advances, your child may feel more like his or her friends.

GnRH analogs are given by injection daily, or at intervals of every three or four weeks. If your child receives daily medication, then a nurse will teach you how to safely give injections at home. If your child receives the medication once a month, your local physician or a visiting nurse will most likely give the injection.

Possible Treatment Side Effects

During the first six weeks of treatment your child may experience the following side-effects: Girls may have mood changes, acne, an increase in breast size, and menses. Boys may have an increase in pubic hair and testicular development as well as acne. These effects are only temporary and should be controlled by the seventh week of treatment. Other side effects your child may experience include redness and slight pain at the site of the injection. Rarely, a sterile abscess may occur. Use of a filter needle to reconstitute the depot form of the analog will help prevent this. Your child will receive medication until it is appropriate for puberty to resume. Research to date indicates that when the treatment is stopped puberty should resume and advance normally.

Follow-Up Clinic Visits

It will be important for your child to be seen every three months. This will allow the doctor to adjust the GnRH analog dose to ensure that your child is receiving the appropriate amount. Your child's height will be measured in order to determine his or her growth rate. If treatment is successful, your child's growth rate should decrease. A physical exam will be done at each visit to evaluate development, and a bone age x-ray will be done at least once a year. Hormone levels occasionally need to be checked.

Due to early puberty, your child may be taller than other children of his or her age. It is important to treat children according to their actual age rather than their size, or apparent age, since children tend to develop self-esteem and behave according to how they are treated. Parents of children with precocious puberty should remind teachers, relatives, and friends about this important relationship.

Your child may feel embarrassed by the physical effects of puberty. All children want to look and act like their friends. It is helpful to emphasize to your child that all girls and boys normally experience puberty but in his or her case it has occurred sooner than usual. It is important to tell your child that the changes in her or his body are normal. Your child should be allowed to participate in his or her usual activities, which may include spending the night with a friend, athletics, and extracurricular events. Encourage your child to discuss with you worries that he or she may be having.

Questions Many Parents Have

How should I explain this disorder to my child? Your child may have several questions regarding early puberty and its treatment. It is often helpful to reassure your child that the pubertal changes in his or her body are normal, and that most individuals will eventually have these changes but that in his or her body they happened sooner than usual.

What should we tell friends and relatives? It is not necessary to tell anyone about your child's problem; if, however, they ask about the problem and you wish to discuss this with them, explain that your child is perfectly normal but has started puberty at an earlier than normal age. If your child is receiving injections, you can explain that they are given to temporarily stop puberty, which assists these children in achieving an acceptable adult height.

What will my child's final adult height be? Final adult height depends on multiple factors. Parental heights play a significant role in the height of a child. The relationship between bone age and chronological age is also important since excessive skeletal maturation for age provides less time for growth. If puberty was detected at an early stage, then your child will have a better chance of reaching his or her expected height. If, however, puberty was detected at a later stage, then his or her bones will be more advanced and this will limit the time remaining for growth and, therefore, final adult height.

Chapter 25

Gastrointestinal Disorders

Chapter Contents

Section 25.1—Abdominal Pain 366
Section 25.2—Appendicitis 370
Section 25.3—Celiac Disease 374
Section 25.4—Cyclic Vomiting Syndrome 377
Section 25.5—Diarrhea 381
Section 25.6—Encopresis (Constipation and Soiling) 387
Section 25.7—Gastroenteritis 390
Section 25.8—Gastroesophageal Reflux 393
Section 25.9—Irritable Bowel Syndrome 397
Section 25.10—Lactose Intolerance 399

Section 25.1

Abdominal Pain

Reprinted with permission of the University of Michigan Health System, May 2008. Written by Kyla Boyse, R. N., http://www.med.umich.edu/1libr/yourchild/abpain.htm. © 2008 Regents of the University of Michigan.

What is abdominal pain?

Abdominal pain, or stomachache, affects many children. It can be a sign of infection, constipation, or a serious medical condition. The pain may also be unrelated to a medical problem, and simply be your child's way of expressing feelings of stress or anxiety (which does not mean that it doesn't truly hurt!). Abdominal pain results in many doctor and emergency room (ER) visits, as well as many missed days of school.

What is recurrent abdominal pain (RAP)?

If your health care provider has ruled out serious conditions, yet the abdominal pain is severe enough to limit your child's activity, and occurs at least once a month in a period of at least three months, your child may have recurrent abdominal pain (also called functional abdominal pain). Recurrent abdominal pain (RAP) typically affects kids ages four to twelve, and is quite common, affecting up to 15 percent of children.[1] While the exact cause is not known, the reason for your child's pain may be related to diet, anxiety, depression, increased sensitivity, or immaturity of the nervous system. RAP can be associated with anxiety, depression, headache, vomiting, pale skin, not participating in regular activities, and missing school. Kids with RAP are at greater risk of having anxiety as young adults.[2]

What is abdominal pain like for my child?

Abdominal pain has many different characteristics. The pain may be acute (starting suddenly) or chronic (present for a period of weeks or months). It may be dull, sharp, or crampy. Each type of pain and its location in the belly provides clues about the specific cause. That's why it's important to "know your child's pain" as it can help in making

Gastrointestinal Disorders

a diagnosis. Write down the things that make your child's pain worse or better, how long it lasts, other problems at the time of pain (vomiting, diarrhea). Filling out this pain diary and bringing it to your appointment will help your child's health care provider figure out what's going on.

When should I take my child to the doctor for a stomachache?

It is very important to know when to seek medical advice. Although most childhood abdominal pain has no known cause and is not dangerous, there are causes of pain that may be life threatening and require immediate medical attention. Some alarm signs and symptoms that should trigger your child's doctor to order more tests include (but are not limited to):[3]

- weight loss;
- slowed growth rate;
- lots of vomiting;
- chronic severe diarrhea;
- gastrointestinal blood loss;
- persistent pain on the right side of the abdomen;
- unexplained fever;
- a family history of inflammatory bowel disease;
- other abnormal or unexplained findings in the doctor's exam.

How can I help my child with the pain?

While your child is getting checked out, talk with your doctor about safe and effective ways to ease pain. There are times when watching for worsening pain is important and your doctor may not feel pain medication is the safest option. In this case, distraction techniques such as guided imagery may help your child cope. You could also try progressive relaxation or self-hypnosis.

What diet and medication treatments are available for the pain of RAP?

There has been limited scientific study of treatment for recurrent abdominal pain. One review of treatments[4] found the following:

- Diet changes do not result in dramatic symptom improvement. Lactose-restricting diets have not been shown to help. Increased fiber, however, is simple and inexpensive, and works for some kids.

- Peppermint oil enteric-coated capsules often decrease pain in kids who have irritable bowel (diarrhea alternating with constipation) in combination with RAP.

- Few medicines have been found to alleviate symptoms in children with RAP. A European study found famotidine (a histamine-receptor blocker) worked better than a placebo in children with dyspeptic symptoms (vomiting, burping, heartburn). This medicine is not currently available in the United States, and more research on its use is needed.

- Children diagnosed with "abdominal migraine" may benefit from the use of pizotifen (a serotonin blocker) when used to prevent an attack. More research needs to be done on this medicine, too.

How can I find out more about behavioral and alternative treatments for RAP?

One study[5] found that cognitive-behavioral therapy (CBT) helped kids with RAP to become pain-free more quickly than without CBT. There was no evidence for any negative side effects of this treatment. In the study, the CBT involved explaining RAP and how the pain would be managed, training parents, and training kids in self-management over the course of a number of training sessions.

There is good evidence to support using behavioral interventions (for example: distraction, relaxation, coping skills, and biofeedback) in reducing or eliminating RAP.[4] Treatment including biofeedback (along with adding fiber to the diet) has been shown to be more effective than adding fiber alone.[6]

While this study found that fiber and biofeedback was as effective as fiber/biofeedback/cognitive-behavioral/parental support, it may be that for some families, parental support could help.[7] Sometimes worried parents can make the situation worse (not on purpose, of course) by reinforcing their child's pain behavior. In this case, if the parents get the support they need in the stressful situation of dealing with their child's suffering with RAP, it can help the overall situation for the child.

Teaching kids self-hypnosis[8] or guided imagery shows great promise as a treatment for recurrent abdominal pain. However, both treatments need more study to prove their effectiveness as RAP treatments. Not much research has been done.

How do we choose a treatment plan?

It works best to choose treatments based on the type of RAP your child has.[4] Your doctor should also take into account any other factors that are involved. For example, if your child is anxious about school, the anxiety may be a factor—in addition to their stomachaches—in poor attendance at school. In that case, their individualized treatment plan would need to include addressing school anxiety.[6]

Your doctor can help figure out what approaches would work best for your child. You should always feel free to get a second opinion, if it would make you more comfortable.

References

1. Boyle JT. Recurrent abdominal pain: an update. *Pediatrics in Review*. 18:310–21, 1997.

2. Campo JV, Di Lorenzo C, Chiappetta L, et al. Adult outcomes of pediatric recurrent abdominal pain: do they just grow out of it? *Pediatrics* 108: e1, 2001. Available from URL: http://pediatrics.aappublications.org/cgi/content/full/108/1/e1. Accessed 10 November 2003.

3. American Academy of Pediatrics Subcommittee on Chronic Abdominal Pain. Chronic abdominal pain in children. *Pediatrics*, Mar 2005; 115: e370–e381.

4. Weydert JA. Ball TM. Davis MF. Systematic review of treatments for recurrent abdominal pain. *Pediatrics* 111:e1–e11, 2003. Available from URL: http://pediatrics.aappublications.org/cgi/content/full/111/1/e1. Accessed 23 November 2003.

5. Sanders MR, Rebgetz M, Morrison M, Bor W, Gordon A, Dadds M, Shepherd R. Cognitive-behavioral treatment of recurrent nonspecific abdominal pain in children: an analysis of generalization, maintenance, and side effects. *J Consult Clin Psychol*. 57:294–300, 1989.

6. Humphreys PA. Gevirtz RN. Treatment of recurrent abdominal pain: components analysis of four treatment protocols. *Journal of Pediatric Gastroenterology & Nutrition*. 31:47–51, 2000.

7. Banez, GA. Recurrent abdominal pain in children and adolescents: classification, epidemiology, and etiology/conceptual

models. Available from URL:http://www.med.unc.edu/wrkunits/2depts/medicine/fgidc/pediatric.htm. Accessed 10 November 2003.

8. Anbar RD. Self-hypnosis for the treatment of functional abdominal pain in childhood. *Clinical Pediatrics.* 40:447–51, 2001.

Section 25.2

Appendicitis

© 2008 A.D.A.M., Inc. Reprinted with permission.
Updated April 17, 2008.

Appendicitis is inflammation of the appendix. The appendix is a small pouch attached to your large intestine.

Causes

Appendicitis is one of the most common causes of emergency abdominal surgery in the United States. Appendicitis usually occurs when the appendix becomes blocked by feces, a foreign object, or rarely, a tumor.

Symptoms

The symptoms of appendicitis vary. It can be hard to diagnose appendicitis in young children, the elderly, and women of childbearing age.

Typically, the first symptom is pain around your belly button. The pain may be vague at first, but becomes increasingly sharp and severe. You may have reduced appetite, nausea, vomiting, and a low-grade fever.

As the inflammation in the appendix increases, the pain tends to move into your right lower abdomen and focuses directly above the appendix at a place called McBurney point.

If the appendix ruptures, the pain may lessen briefly and you may feel better. However, once the lining of the abdominal cavity becomes inflamed and infected (a condition called peritonitis), the pain worsens and you become sicker.

Gastrointestinal Disorders

Abdominal pain may be worse when walking or coughing. You may prefer to lie still because sudden movement causes pain.

Later symptoms include:

- chills;
- constipation;
- diarrhea;
- fever;
- loss of appetite;
- nausea;
- shaking;
- vomiting.

Exams and Tests

If you have appendicitis, your pain increases when the doctor suddenly releases the pressure after gently pressing on your lower right belly area. If peritonitis is present, touching the belly area may cause a spasm of the muscles.

A rectal examination may reveal abdominal or pelvic tenderness on the right side of your body.

Doctors can usually diagnose appendicitis by your description of the symptoms, the physical exam, and laboratory tests alone. In some cases, additional tests may be needed. These may include:

- abdominal computed tomography (CT) scan;
- abdominal ultrasound;
- diagnostic laparoscopy.

Note: The U.S. Food and Drug Administration recalled a drug used during some appendicitis-related imaging tests after reports of life-threatening side effects and deaths. The drug, called NeutroSpec, was used to help diagnose appendicitis in patients ages five and older who may have had the condition but did not show the usual signs and symptoms.

Treatment

If you have an uncomplicated case, a surgeon will remove your appendix soon after your doctor thinks you might have the condition.

If the operation reveals that your appendix is normal, the surgeon will remove the appendix and explore the rest of your abdomen for other causes of your pain.

If a CT scan shows that you have an abscess from a ruptured appendix, you may be treated first and have your appendix removed after the infection and inflammation have gone away.

Outlook (Prognosis)

If your appendix is removed before it ruptures, you will likely get well very soon after surgery. If your appendix ruptures before surgery, you will probably recover more slowly, and are more likely to develop an abscess or other complications.

Possible Complications

- Abnormal connections between abdominal organs or between these organs and the skin surface
- Abscess
- Infection of the surgical wound
- Peritonitis

When to Contact a Medical Professional

Call your local emergency department or emergency medical service (such as 911) if:

- your pain is severe, sudden, and sharp;
- you have a fever along with your pain;
- you are vomiting blood or have bloody diarrhea;
- you have a rigid, hard abdomen that is tender to touch;
- you are unable to pass stool, especially if you are also vomiting;
- you have chest, neck, or shoulder pain;
- you are dizzy or light-headed.

Call your health care provider if you develop abdominal pain in the lower right portion of your belly, or any other symptoms of appendicitis. Also call your doctor if:

- you have nausea and lack of appetite;

Gastrointestinal Disorders

- you are unintentionally losing weight;
- you have yellowing of your eyes or skin;
- you have bloating for more than two days;
- You have diarrhea for more than five days, or if your infant or child has had diarrhea for two days or vomiting for twelve hours (call right away if a baby under three months has diarrhea or vomiting);
- you have had abdominal discomfort for more than one week;
- you have burning with urination or you are urinating more often than usual;
- you have pain and may be pregnant;
- your pain gets worse when you take antacids or eat something.

References

Wolfe JM, Henneman PL. Acute Appendicitis. In: *Marx J. Rosen's Emergency Medicine: Concepts and Clinical Practice*. 6th ed. St. Louis, Mo: Mosby; 2006: Chap.92.

Maa J, Kirkwood JS. The Appendix. In: Townsend CM, Beauchamp RD, Evers BM, Mattox KL, eds. *Sabiston Textbook of Surgery*, 18th ed. St. Louis, Mo: WB Saunders; 2008:Chap 49.

US Food and Drug Administration. FDA Issues Public Health Advisory on use of NeutroSpec, [Technetium (99m TC) Fanolesomab], Imaging Agent for Diagnosis of Appendicitis. Rockville, MD: National Press Office; December 19, 2005. Press Release P05-104.

Lyon C, Clark DC. Diagnosis of acute abdominal pain in older patients. *Am Fam Physician*. 2006 Nov 1;74(9):1537–44. Review.

Ebell MH. Diagnosis of appendicitis: part 1. History and physical examination. *Am Fam Physician*. 2008 Mar 15;77(6):828–30. Review.

Bundy DG, Byerley JS, Liles EA, Perrin EM, Katznelson J, Rice HE. Does this child have appendicitis? *JAMA*. 2007 Jul 25;298(4):438–51. Review.

Section 25.3

Celiac Disease

"What I Need to Know about Celiac Disease," National Digestive Diseases Information Clearinghouse, National Institute of Diabetes and Digestive and Kidney Diseases, National Institutes of Health, NIH Publication No. 07-5755, August 2007.

What is celiac disease?

Having celiac disease means a person can't eat gluten, a protein found in wheat, rye, or barley. Gluten may also be found in some medicines. Celiac disease is hereditary, meaning it runs in families. The treatment for celiac disease is a gluten-free diet. Other names for celiac disease are celiac sprue and gluten intolerance.

In people with celiac disease, the body's immune system responds to gluten by damaging the lining of the small intestine. This lining has small finger-like growths called villi. The villi normally absorb nutrients from the foods we eat. When the villi are damaged, the body can't get the nutrients it needs.

People with celiac disease don't always know they have it because they don't feel sick. Or if they feel sick, they don't know celiac disease is the cause.

Is celiac disease serious?

Yes. Celiac disease can be very serious. Besides stomach pain, it can cause anemia, malnutrition, infertility, a certain skin rash, and other health problems.

What are the symptoms of celiac disease?

Symptoms of celiac disease include the following:

- Gas
- Diarrhea
- Stomach pain
- Feeling very tired

- Change in mood
- Weight loss
- A very itchy skin rash with blisters
- Slowed growth

Most people with celiac disease have one or more symptoms, but not all have digestive problems. And some people with the disease don't have any symptoms. Having one or more of these symptoms does not mean a person has celiac disease because many other disorders include these symptoms.

How is celiac disease diagnosed?

Celiac disease can be hard to discover because its symptoms are like many other digestive diseases. People with celiac disease can go untreated for many years.

If your doctor thinks you have celiac disease, you will probably need a blood test. You will need to follow your regular diet before and while being tested. If you don't, the results could be wrong.

If your test results show you might have celiac disease, the doctor will perform a biopsy to make sure celiac disease is the problem. For a biopsy, the doctor takes a small piece of tissue from your small intestine. To get to your small intestine, the doctor puts a long tube into your mouth and down into your stomach. At the end of the tube are small tools for snipping out the bit of tissue needed to view with a microscope. You will take medicine before the biopsy that makes you very sleepy. It also keeps you from feeling any pain. Many people sleep through the procedure.

How is celiac disease treated?

The only treatment for celiac disease is a gluten-free diet. A dietitian can work with you to help you learn how to select gluten-free foods. A dietitian is an expert in food and healthy eating. You will learn to check labels of foods and other items for gluten. If you eliminate gluten from your diet, your small intestine will heal. If you eat gluten, or use items that contain gluten, you will harm your small intestine.

The following list gives examples of foods you can eat and foods you should stay away from if you have celiac disease. This list is not complete. A dietitian can help you learn what other foods you can and can't eat when following a gluten-free diet.

The following foods are allowed: amaranth, arrowroot, buckwheat, cassava, corn, flax, indian rice grass, Job's tears, legumes, millet, nuts, potatoes, quinoa, rice, sago, seeds, soy, sorghum, tapioca, wild rice, and yucca.

Foods to avoid: Wheat, including einkorn, emmer, spelt, kamut, wheat starch, wheat bran, wheat germ, cracked wheat, and hydrolyzed wheat protein; barley; rye; and triticale (a cross between wheat and rye).

Other wheat products: bromated flour, durum flour, enriched flour, farina, graham flour, phosphated flour, plain flour, self-rising flour, semolina, and white flour.

Processed foods that may contain wheat, barley, or rye (most of these foods can be found gluten-free—when in doubt, check with the food manufacturer): bouillon cubes, brown rice syrup, potato chips, candy, cold cuts, hot dogs, salami, sausage, Communion wafer, French fries, gravy, imitation fish, matzo, rice mixes, sauces, seasoned tortilla chips, self-basting turkey, soups, soy sauce, and vegetables in sauce. (This list was adapted from the following resource: Thompson T. *Celiac Disease Nutrition Guide*, 2nd ed. Chicago: American Dietetic Association, 2006. © American Dietetic Association. Adapted with permission. For a complete copy of the *Celiac Disease Nutrition Guide*, please visit www.eatright.org.)

Section 25.4

Cyclic Vomiting Syndrome

Excerpted from the National Institute of Diabetes and Digestive and Kidney Diseases, National Institutes of Health, NIH Publication No. 04-4548, February 2004. Revised by David A. Cooke, M.D., July 2008.

In cyclic vomiting syndrome (CVS), people experience bouts or cycles of severe nausea and vomiting that last for hours or even days and alternate with longer periods of no symptoms. CVS occurs mostly in children, but the disorder can affect adults, too.

CVS has no known cause. Each episode is similar to the previous ones. The episodes tend to start at about the same time of day, last the same length of time, and present the same symptoms at the same level of intensity. Although CVS can begin at any age in children and adults, it usually starts between the ages of three and seven. In adults, episodes tend to occur less often than they do in children, but they last longer. Furthermore, the events or situations that trigger episodes in adults cannot always be pinpointed as easily as they can in children.

Episodes can be so severe that a person may have to stay in bed for days, unable to go to school or work. No one knows for sure how many people have CVS, but medical researchers believe that more people may have the disorder than is commonly thought (as many as one in fifty children in one study). Because other more common diseases and disorders also cause cycles of vomiting, many people with CVS are initially misdiagnosed until the other disorders can be ruled out. What is known is that CVS can be disruptive and frightening not just to people who have it, but to the entire family as well.

The Four Phases of CVS

CVS has four phases:

- Prodrome
- Episode
- Recovery
- Symptom-free interval

The prodrome phase signals that an episode of nausea and vomiting is about to begin. This phase, which is often marked by abdominal pain, can last from just a few minutes to several hours. Sometimes taking medicine early in the prodrome phase can stop an episode in progress. However, sometimes there is no warning: A person may simply wake up in the morning and begin vomiting.

The episode phase consists of nausea and vomiting; inability to eat, drink, or take medicines without vomiting; paleness; drowsiness; and exhaustion.

The recovery phase begins when the nausea and vomiting stop. Healthy color, appetite, and energy return.

The symptom-free interval phase is the period between episodes when no symptoms are present.

Triggers

Most people can identify a specific condition or event that triggered an episode. The most common trigger is an infection. Another, often found in children, is emotional stress or excitement, often from a birthday or vacation, for example. Colds, allergies, sinus problems, and the flu can also set off episodes in some people.

Other reported triggers include eating certain foods (such as chocolate or cheese), eating too much, or eating just before going to bed. Hot weather, physical exhaustion, menstruation, and motion sickness can also trigger episodes.

Symptoms

The main symptoms of CVS are severe vomiting, nausea, and retching (gagging). Episodes usually begin at night or first thing in the morning and may include vomiting or retching as often as six to twelve times an hour during the worst of the episode. Episodes usually last anywhere from one to five days, though they can last for up to ten days.

Other symptoms include pallor, exhaustion, and listlessness. Sometimes the nausea and vomiting are so severe that a person appears to be almost unconscious. Sensitivity to light, headache, fever, dizziness, diarrhea, and abdominal pain may also accompany an episode.

In addition, the vomiting may cause drooling and excessive thirst. Drinking water usually leads to more vomiting, though the water can dilute the acid in the vomit, making the episode a little less painful. Continuous vomiting can lead to dehydration, which means that the body has lost excessive water and salts.

Gastrointestinal Disorders

Diagnosis

CVS is hard to diagnose because no clear tests—such as a blood test or x-ray—exist to identify it. A doctor must diagnose CVS by looking at symptoms and medical history and by excluding more common diseases or disorders that can also cause nausea and vomiting. Also, diagnosis takes time because doctors need to identify a pattern or cycle to the vomiting.

CVS and Migraine

The relationship between migraine and CVS is still unclear, but medical researchers believe that the two are related. First, migraine headaches, which cause severe pain in the head; abdominal migraine, which causes stomach pain; and CVS are all marked by severe symptoms that start quickly and end abruptly, followed by longer periods without pain or other symptoms.

Second, many of the situations that trigger CVS also trigger migraines. Those triggers include stress and excitement.

Third, research has shown that many children with CVS either have a family history of migraine or develop migraines as they grow older.

Because of the similarities between migraine and CVS, doctors treat some people with severe CVS with drugs that are also used for migraine headaches. The drugs are designed to prevent episodes, reduce their frequency, or lessen their severity.

Treatment

CVS cannot be cured. Treatment varies, but people with CVS are generally advised to get plenty of rest; sleep; and take medications that prevent a vomiting episode, stop or alleviate one that has already started, or relieve other symptoms.

Once a vomiting episode begins, treatment is supportive. It helps to stay in bed and sleep in a dark, quiet room. Severe nausea and vomiting may require hospitalization and intravenous fluids to prevent dehydration. Sedatives may help if the nausea continues.

Sometimes, during the prodrome phase, it is possible to stop an episode from happening altogether. For example, people who feel abdominal pain before an episode can ask their doctor about taking ibuprofen (Advil®, Motrin®) to try to stop it. Other medications that may be helpful are ranitidine (Zantac®) or omeprazole (Prilosec®), which help calm the stomach by lowering the amount of acid it makes. Limited data suggests that medications used to treat migraine headaches such as sumatriptan may be effective for acute vomiting attacks. Certain potent anti-nausea drugs such as ondansetron appear to be helpful. Sedatives such as lorazepam may also have some benefit.

During the recovery phase, drinking water and replacing lost electrolytes are very important. Electrolytes are salts that the body needs to function well and stay healthy. Symptoms during the recovery phase can vary: Some people find that their appetites return to normal immediately, while others need to begin by drinking clear liquids and then move slowly to solid food.

People whose episodes are frequent and long-lasting may be treated during the symptom-free intervals in an effort to prevent or ease future episodes. Medications that help people with migraine headaches—propranolol, cyproheptadine, and amitriptyline—are sometimes used during this phase, but they do not work for everyone. Taking the medicine daily for one to two months may be necessary to see if it helps.

In addition, the symptom-free phase is a good time to eliminate anything known to trigger an episode. For example, if episodes are brought on by stress or excitement, this period is the time to find ways to reduce stress and stay calm. If sinus problems or allergies cause episodes, those conditions should be treated.

Complications

The severe vomiting that defines CVS is a risk factor for several complications:

- **Dehydration:** Vomiting causes the body to lose water quickly.

- **Electrolyte imbalance:** Vomiting also causes the body to lose the important salts it needs to keep working properly.

- **Peptic esophagitis:** The esophagus (the tube that connects the mouth to the stomach) becomes injured from the stomach acid that comes up with the vomit.

- **Hematemesis:** The esophagus becomes irritated and bleeds, so blood mixes with the vomit.

- **Mallory-Weiss tear:** The lower end of the esophagus may tear open or the stomach may bruise from vomiting or retching.

- **Tooth decay:** The acid in the vomit can hurt the teeth by corroding the tooth enamel.

Section 25.5

Diarrhea

Excerpted from "Diarrhea," National Digestive Diseases Information Clearinghouse, National Institute of Diabetes and Digestive and Kidney Diseases, National Institutes of Health, NIH Publication No. 07-2749, March 2007.

What Is Diarrhea?

Diarrhea is loose, watery stools. A person with diarrhea typically passes stool more than three times a day. People with diarrhea may pass more than a quart of stool a day. Acute diarrhea is a common problem that usually lasts one or two days and goes away on its own without special treatment. Prolonged diarrhea persisting for more than two days may be a sign of a more serious problem and poses the risk of dehydration. Chronic diarrhea may be a feature of a chronic disease.

Diarrhea can cause dehydration, which means the body lacks enough fluid to function properly. Dehydration is particularly dangerous in children and older people, and it must be treated promptly to avoid serious health problems.

People of all ages can get diarrhea and the average adult has a bout of acute diarrhea about four times a year. In the United States, each child will have had seven to fifteen episodes of diarrhea by age five.

What Causes Diarrhea?

Acute diarrhea is usually related to a bacterial, viral, or parasitic infection. Chronic diarrhea is usually related to functional disorders such as irritable bowel syndrome or inflammatory bowel disease.

A few of the more common causes of diarrhea include the following:

- **Bacterial infections:** Several types of bacteria consumed through contaminated food or water can cause diarrhea. Common culprits include *Campylobacter*, *Salmonella*, *Shigella*, and *Escherichia coli* (*E. coli*).

- **Viral infections:** Many viruses cause diarrhea, including rotavirus, Norwalk virus, Cytomegalovirus, herpes simplex virus, and viral hepatitis.

- **Food intolerances:** Some people are unable to digest food components such as artificial sweeteners and lactose—the sugar found in milk.

- **Parasites:** Parasites can enter the body through food or water and settle in the digestive system. Parasites that cause diarrhea include *Giardia lamblia*, *Entamoeba histolytica*, and *Cryptosporidium*.

- **Reaction to medicines:** Antibiotics, blood pressure medications, cancer drugs, and antacids containing magnesium can all cause diarrhea.

- **Intestinal diseases:** Inflammatory bowel disease, colitis, Crohn disease, and celiac disease often lead to diarrhea.

- **Functional bowel disorders:** Diarrhea can be a symptom of irritable bowel syndrome.

Some people develop diarrhea after stomach surgery or removal of the gallbladder. The reason may be a change in how quickly food moves through the digestive system after stomach surgery or an increase in bile in the colon after gallbladder surgery.

People who visit foreign countries are at risk for traveler's diarrhea, which is caused by eating food or drinking water contaminated with bacteria, viruses, or parasites. Traveler's diarrhea can be a problem for people visiting developing countries. Visitors to the United States, Canada, most European countries, Japan, Australia, and New Zealand do not face much risk for traveler's diarrhea.

In many cases, the cause of diarrhea cannot be found. As long as diarrhea goes away on its own, an extensive search for the cause is not usually necessary.

What Are the Symptoms of Diarrhea?

Diarrhea may be accompanied by cramping, abdominal pain, bloating, nausea, or an urgent need to use the bathroom. Depending on the cause, a person may have a fever or bloody stools.

Gastrointestinal Disorders

Diarrhea in Children

Children can have acute and chronic forms of diarrhea. Causes include bacteria, viruses, parasites, medications, functional bowel disorders, and food sensitivities. Infection with the rotavirus is the most common cause of acute childhood diarrhea. Rotavirus diarrhea usually resolves in three to nine days. Children who are six to thirty-two weeks old can be vaccinated against the virus with a vaccine called RotaTeq®.

If your child has diarrhea, do not hesitate to call the doctor for advice. Diarrhea is especially dangerous in newborns and infants, leading to dehydration in just a day or two. A child can die from dehydration within a few days. The main treatment for diarrhea in children is rehydration to replace lost fluid quickly.

Take your child to the doctor if there is no improvement after twenty-four hours or if any of the following symptoms appear:

- Stools containing blood or pus
- Black stools
- A temperature above 102 degrees
- Signs of dehydration

Medications to treat diarrhea in adults can be dangerous for children and should only be given with a doctor's guidance.

Dehydration

Diarrhea can cause dehydration, which means the body has lost too much fluid and too many electrolytes and can't function properly. Dehydration is particularly dangerous in children and in older adults and must be treated promptly to avoid serious health problems.

Signs of dehydration are as follows:

- Thirst
- Less frequent urination
- Dry skin
- Fatigue
- Light-headedness
- Dark-colored urine

Signs of dehydration in children include the following:

- Dry mouth and tongue
- No tears when crying
- No wet diapers for three hours or more
- Sunken abdomen, eyes, or cheeks
- High fever
- Listlessness or irritability
- Skin that does not flatten when pinched and released

If you suspect that you or your child is dehydrated, call the doctor immediately. Severe dehydration may require hospitalization.

Preventing Dehydration

The fluid and electrolytes lost during diarrhea need to be replaced promptly because the body cannot function without them. Electrolytes are the salts and minerals that affect the amount of water in your body, muscle activity, and other important functions.

Although water is extremely important in preventing dehydration, it does not contain electrolytes. Broth and soups that contain sodium, and fruit juices, soft fruits, or vegetables that contain potassium, help restore electrolyte levels. Over-the-counter rehydration solutions such as Pedialyte®, CeraLyte®, and Infalyte® are also good electrolyte sources and are especially recommended for use in children.

When Should a Doctor Be Consulted?

Diarrhea is not usually harmful, but it can become dangerous or signal a more serious problem. You should see the doctor if you experience any of the following:

- Diarrhea for more than three days
- Severe pain in the abdomen or rectum
- A fever of 102 degrees or higher
- Blood in your stool or black, tarry stools
- Signs of dehydration

How Is the Cause of Diarrhea Diagnosed?

Diagnostic tests to find the cause of diarrhea may include the following:

- **Medical history and physical examination:** The doctor will ask you about your eating habits and medication use and will examine you for signs of illness.
- **Stool culture:** A sample of stool is analyzed in a laboratory to check for bacteria, parasites, or other signs of disease and infection.
- **Blood tests:** Blood tests can be helpful in ruling out certain diseases.
- **Fasting tests:** To find out if a food intolerance or allergy is causing the diarrhea, the doctor may ask you to avoid lactose, carbohydrates, wheat, or other foods to see whether the diarrhea responds to a change in diet.
- **Sigmoidoscopy:** For this test, the doctor uses a special instrument to look at the inside of the rectum and lower part of the colon.
- **Colonoscopy:** This test is similar to a sigmoidoscopy, but it allows the doctor to view the entire colon.
- **Imaging tests:** These tests can rule out structural abnormalities as the cause of diarrhea.

How Is Diarrhea Treated?

In most cases of diarrhea, replacing lost fluid to prevent dehydration is the only treatment necessary. Medicines that stop diarrhea may be helpful, but they are not recommended for people whose diarrhea is caused by a bacterial infection or parasite. If you stop the diarrhea before having purged the bacteria or parasite, you will trap the organism in the intestines and prolong the problem. Rather, doctors usually prescribe antibiotics as a first-line treatment. Viral infections are either treated with medication or left to run their course, depending on the severity and type of virus.

Tips about Food

Until diarrhea subsides, try to avoid caffeine, milk products, and foods that are greasy, high in fiber, or very sweet. These foods tend to aggravate diarrhea.

As you improve, you can add soft, bland foods to your diet, including bananas, plain rice, boiled potatoes, toast, crackers, cooked carrots, and baked chicken without the skin or fat. For children, the pediatrician may also recommend a bland diet. Once the diarrhea has stopped, the pediatrician will likely encourage children to return to a normal and healthy diet if it can be tolerated.

Preventing Traveler's Diarrhea

Traveler's diarrhea happens when you consume food or water contaminated with bacteria, viruses, or parasites. You can take the following precautions to prevent traveler's diarrhea when you travel outside of the United States:

- Do not drink tap water or use it to brush your teeth.
- Do not drink unpasteurized milk or dairy products.
- Do not use ice made from tap water.
- Avoid all raw fruits and vegetables, including lettuce and fruit salads, unless they can be peeled and you peel them yourself.
- Do not eat raw or rare meat and fish.
- Do not eat meat or shellfish that is not hot when served.
- Do not eat food from street vendors.

You can safely drink bottled water—if you are the one to break the seal—along with carbonated soft drinks, and hot drinks such as coffee or tea.

Depending on where you are going and how long you will stay, your doctor may recommend that you take antibiotics before leaving to protect you from possible infection.

Hope through Research

The Division of Digestive Diseases and Nutrition at the National Institute of Diabetes and Digestive and Kidney Diseases supports basic and clinical research into gastrointestinal conditions, including diarrhea. Among other areas, researchers are studying how the processes of absorption and secretion in the digestive tract affect the content and consistency of stool, the relationship between diarrhea and *Helicobacter pylori,* motility in chronic diarrhea, and chemical compounds that may be useful in treating diarrhea.

Section 25.6

Encopresis (Constipation and Soiling)

Reprinted with permission of the University of Michigan Health System, May 2008. Written by Kyla Boyse, R.N., http://www.med.umich.edu/llibr/yourchild/encopre.htm. © 2008 Regents of the University of Michigan.

What is constipation?

When your child's bowel movements are very hard, difficult, or painful to pass, and/or occur less often than every three days, it is called constipation. This may happen if your child doesn't eat enough fiber, doesn't get enough exercise, or doesn't drink enough liquids (especially water). It can also happen if your child ignores the urge to poop because they are embarrassed to use the public bathroom, or don't want to stop playing. Constipation can make pooping painful, so that your child may hold their poop in to avoid a painful bowel movement. Functional constipation means that the constipation is not due to an underlying disease process.

What is soiling?

Soiling, overflow incontinence, or fecal incontinence, is when liquid or formed poop leaks into the child's underwear. The child has no control over this leakage. It usually happens when a big, hard blockage of poop from constipation is blocking the rectum. This is called an impaction. When a child has an impaction, poop can leak around the blockage into the underwear.

What is encopresis?

Encopresis is overflow soiling that happens because of constipation. In children with encopresis, formed, soft, or liquid poop leaks from the anus around a mass of poop that is stuck in the lower bowel. The bowel can get so stretched that your child can no longer feel the urge to poop, and the anal sphincter (the muscle around the anus that holds the poop in) can get very weak. Sometimes the poop takes up so much room that your child's bladder doesn't have enough space. This can cause bedwetting.

How common are constipation and encopresis?

About 16 to 37 percent of school-aged kids are affected by constipation. Constipation with overflow soiling affects at least 4 percent of preschool kids and 1 to 2 percent of school-aged kids. In school-aged kids, encopresis is most likely to affect boys.

How do I know when to see the doctor?

If you feel there may be a problem with your child's bowel function, don't delay. Talk to your pediatrician. Current studies show that children do better when they are diagnosed and treated earlier in the course of the problem.

You should call your child's doctor if:

- you are worried about constipation in your child;
- any constipation symptoms last longer than one week;
- you see blood on the stool (poop), or worry about small skin tears at the anus;
- your child has hemorrhoids;
- normal pushing is not enough to get the poop out;
- your child's bowel movements are painful;
- liquid or soft poop leaks out between bowel movements;
- your child is constipated and vomiting;
- your child has a swollen belly;
- you are concerned about your child's growth and weight gain.

How does the doctor tell if my child has encopresis?

The doctor will need to talk to you and your child. The doctor may need to do a finger exam of your child's rectal vault to feel whether it is full of impacted poop, and may need your child to get an abdominal x-ray and/or barium enema. Keep a "bowel movement monitoring sheet" of your child's pooping patterns, and bring it to your doctor appointment. This will help the doctor and you figure out what is going on.

Gastrointestinal Disorders

What kind of treatment will my child need?

Only a doctor should start treatment for your child. Never give laxatives, suppositories, enemas, or other bowel medication to a child without your child's doctor's instructions to do so.

Treatment may include:

- Starting with a "clean-out" to clear the impaction from the rectal vault. Your doctor may prescribe a high dose of mineral oil, enemas, or a combination of things.

- Changing your child's diet to include more fluids (especially water) and fiber-rich foods.

- Making sure your child gets lots of exercise.

- Behavioral training—which includes having your child sit on the toilet several times a day, and using rewards for sitting and for pooping. Keep the tone positive. Never try to embarrass or punish your child.

- Giving your child medicines by mouth to help soften the stools.

- Following up with your doctor on a regular schedule to make sure the impaction does not happen again.

Remember: it is very important to use both the medicines and the behavior training. You are the key to helping your child solve this problem. Consistency is important. Get your child's school to work with you on the program.

How do I work with my child's school?

Talk with your child's teacher, principal, and school nurse, to make sure they know what is going on. They will need to be involved with making sure that your child gets enough fluids during the school day, and can get to the toilet often and on time. School personnel may also need to help with your child's cleanup if they soil themselves. Teachers have an important role to play in making sure your child can take care of the problem privately, and avoid being teased by the other kids.

Section 25.7

Gastroenteritis

"Gastroenteritis," © 2008 The Cleveland Clinic Foundation, 9500 Euclid Avenue, Cleveland, OH 44195, www.clevelandclinic.org. Additional information is available from the Cleveland Clinic Health Information Center, 216-444-3771, toll-free 800-223-2273 extension 43771, or at http://www.clevelandclinic.org/health.

What is gastroenteritis?

Gastroenteritis is an inflammation of the gastrointestinal tract (the pathway responsible for digestion that includes the mouth, esophagus, stomach, and intestines). Gastroenteritis is also sometimes referred to as "stomach flu," even though it is not related to influenza.

What causes gastroenteritis?

Gastroenteritis can be caused by viral, bacterial, or parasitic infections. Viral gastroenteritis is highly contagious and is responsible for the majority of outbreaks in developed countries.

Common routes of infection include:

- food (especially seafood);
- contaminated water;
- contact with an infected person;
- unwashed hands;
- dirty utensils.

In less developed countries, gastroenteritis is more often spread through contaminated food or water.

What are the symptoms of gastroenteritis?

The main symptom of gastroenteritis is diarrhea. When the colon (large intestine) becomes infected during gastroenteritis, it loses its ability to retain fluids, which causes the person's feces to become watery. Other symptoms include:

Gastrointestinal Disorders

- abdominal pain or cramping;
- nausea;
- vomiting;
- fever;
- poor feeding (in infants);
- unintentional weight loss (may be a sign of dehydration);
- excessive sweating;
- clammy skin;
- muscle pain or joint stiffness;
- incontinence (loss of stool control).

Because of the symptoms of vomiting and diarrhea, people who have gastroenteritis can become dehydrated very quickly. It is very important to watch for signs of dehydration, which include:

- extreme thirst;
- urine that is darker in color;
- dry skin;
- dry mouth;
- sunken cheeks or eyes;
- in infants, dry diapers (for more than four to six hours).

How common is gastroenteritis?

Because gastroenteritis is so similar to diarrhea, and because so many cases do not require hospitalization, it is difficult to determine how many cases of gastroenteritis occur per year. Worldwide, it is estimated that three to five billion cases of acute diarrhea (which can be caused by many other diseases besides gastroenteritis) occur per year, with about one hundred million cases in the United States (roughly 1 to 2.5 cases of diarrhea per child). Gastroenteritis is estimated to cause about five to ten million deaths per year worldwide, and about ten thousand deaths per year in the United States.

Who is at risk for gastroenteritis?

Anyone can get the disease. People who are at a higher risk include:

- children in daycare;
- students living in dormitories;
- military personnel; and
- travelers.

People with immune systems that are weakened by disease or medications or not fully developed (i.e., infants) are usually affected most severely.

How is gastroenteritis diagnosed?

The doctor will take a medical history to make sure that nothing else is causing the symptoms. Also, the doctor might perform a rectal or abdominal examination to exclude the possibilities of inflammatory bowel disease (e.g., Crohn disease) and pelvic abscesses (pockets of pus). A stool culture (a laboratory test to identify bacteria and other organisms from a sample of feces) can be used to determine the specific virus or germ that is causing gastroenteritis.

Other diseases that could cause diarrhea and vomiting are pneumonia, septicemia (a disease caused by toxic bacteria in the bloodstream), urinary tract infection, and meningitis (an infection that causes inflammation of the membranes of the spinal cord or brain). Also, conditions that require surgery, such as appendicitis (an inflammation of the appendix), intussusception (a condition in which the intestine folds into itself, causing blockage), and Hirschsprung disease (a condition where nerve cells in the intestinal walls do not develop properly) can cause symptoms similar to gastroenteritis.

How is gastroenteritis treated?

The body can usually fight off the disease on its own. The most important factor when treating gastroenteritis is the replacement of fluids and electrolytes that are lost because of the diarrhea and vomiting. Foods that contain electrolytes and complex carbohydrates, such as potatoes, lean meats (e.g., chicken), and whole grains can help replace nutrients. You can also buy electrolyte and fluid replacement solutions at food and drug stores. Or, if hospitalization is required, the nutrients can be replaced intravenously (injected directly into the veins).

Antibiotics will not be effective if the cause of gastroenteritis is a viral infection. Doctors usually do not recommend antidiarrheal medications (e.g., loperamide) for gastroenteritis because they tend to prolong infection, especially in children.

Gastrointestinal Disorders

How can gastroenteritis be prevented?

There are several steps that you can take to reduce your risk of getting gastroenteritis, including:

- washing your hands frequently, especially after going to the bathroom and when you are working with food;
- cleaning and disinfecting kitchen surfaces, especially when working with raw meat or eggs;
- keeping raw meat, eggs, and poultry away from foods that are eaten raw;
- Drinking bottled water and avoiding ice cubes when traveling.

Section 25.8

Gastroesophageal Reflux

Excerpted from "Gastroesophageal Reflux in Children and Adolescents," National Digestive Diseases Information Clearinghouse, National Institute of Diabetes and Digestive and Kidney Diseases, National Institutes of Health, NIH Publication No. 06-5418, August 2006.

What is gastroesophageal reflux (GER)?

Gastroesophageal reflux occurs when stomach contents reflux, or back up, into the esophagus during or after a meal. The esophagus is the tube that connects the mouth to the stomach. A ring of muscle at the bottom of the esophagus opens and closes to allow food to enter the stomach. This ring of muscle is called the lower esophageal sphincter (LES). Reflux can occur when the LES opens, allowing stomach contents and acid to come back up into the esophagus.

GER often begins in infancy, but only a small number of infants continue to have GER as older children.

What are the symptoms of GER?

Almost all children and adults have a little bit of reflux, often without being aware of it. When refluxed material rapidly returns to the stomach, it does not harm the esophagus. However, in some children, the stomach contents remain in the esophagus and damage the esophageal lining. In other children, the stomach contents go up to the mouth and are swallowed again. When the refluxed material passes into the back of the mouth or enters the airways, the child may become hoarse, have a raspy voice, or a chronic cough. Other symptoms include the following:

- Recurrent pneumonia
- Wheezing
- Difficult or painful swallowing
- Vomiting
- Sore throat
- Weight loss
- Heartburn (in older children)

How is GER diagnosed?

You may want to visit an internist or a gastroenterologist. An internist specializes in internal medicine and a gastroenterologist treats diseases of the digestive system. The doctor can talk with you about your child's symptoms, examine your child, and recommend tests to determine if reflux is the cause of the symptoms. These tests check the esophagus, stomach, and small intestine for problems. Sometimes a doctor will start treatment without running tests if the symptoms strongly indicate GER.

The most common tests used to diagnose GER are the following:

- **Upper gastrointestinal (GI) series x-ray:** X-rays are taken to check for damage to the esophagus, stomach, or intestines. First, a chalky drink called barium is swallowed, which makes the images on the x-rays easier to see. A doctor cannot make a diagnosis of GER based on x-rays alone, but x-rays help rule out other problems that cause the same symptoms as GER.

- **Endoscopy:** A sedative is given before this procedure to make the child sleepy. A small, flexible tube with a very tiny camera on the end is then inserted through the mouth and esophagus and into the stomach. The camera gives the doctor a view of the lining of the esophagus, stomach, and small intestine by transmitting the images onto a television screen. During the endoscopy, the doctor can also remove a small piece of tissue in a procedure called a biopsy. Looking at the tissue with a microscope helps the doctor determine the level of acid damage and rule out problems.

- **Esophageal pH probe:** A thin, light wire with an acid sensor at its tip is inserted through the nose into the lower part of the esophagus. This probe detects and records the amount of stomach acid coming back up into the esophagus and indicates whether acid is in the esophagus when the child has symptoms such as crying, coughing, or arching her back.

Speak with your child's health care provider if any of the following occur:

- increased amounts of vomiting or persistent projectile (forceful) vomiting;
- vomiting fluid that is green or yellow or looks like coffee grounds or blood;
- difficulty breathing after vomiting or spitting up;
- pain related to eating;
- food refusal that causes weight loss or poor weight gain;
- difficult or painful swallowing.

What is the treatment for GER?

Treatment for reflux depends on the child's symptoms and age. The doctor or nurse may first suggest a trial of medication to decrease the amount of acid made in the stomach when a child or teenager is uncomfortable, has difficulty sleeping or eating, or fails to grow.

H_2-blockers, which are also called H_2- receptor agonists, are one class of medication often tried first. These drugs help keep acid from backing up into the esophagus. They are often used to treat children with GER because they come in liquid form. H_2-blockers include the following:

- Cimetidine (Tagamet®)
- Ranitidine (Zantac®)
- Famotidine (Pepcid®)
- Nizatidine (Axid®)

A second class of medications often used to reduce stomach acid is proton-pump inhibitors (PPIs), which block the production of stomach acid. PPIs have few side effects, but those that have been reported are constipation, nausea, and headaches. This class of drugs includes the following:

- Esomeprazole (Nexium®)
- Omeprazole (Prilosec®)
- Lansoprazole (Prevacid®)
- Rabeprazole (Aciphex®)
- Pantoprazole (Protonix®)

A third class of medications used to treat GER is prokinetic agents. Prokinetic agents make the LES close tighter so stomach acid cannot reflux into the esophagus. These drugs are often used in combination with acid reducers. Prokinetic agents include the following:

- Metoclopramide (Reglan®)
- Cisapride (Propulsid®)
- Erythromycin (Dispertab®, Robimycin®)
- Bethanechol (Duvoid®, Urecholine®)

Serious side effects have been reported in adults and children taking metoclopramide and cisapride, including confusion, anxiety, diarrhea, and nausea. People taking prokinetic agents should tell their doctor if they are taking other medications because there could be an adverse drug reaction.

Besides using medication, you may be able to reduce symptoms other ways:

- Have your child eat more frequent smaller meals.
- Have your child avoid eating two to three hours before bed.
- Raise the head of your child's bed six to eight inches by putting blocks of wood under the bedposts. Just using extra pillows will not help.
- Have your child avoid carbonated drinks, chocolate, caffeine, and foods that are high in fat or contain a lot of acid (citrus fruits) or spices.

If the child continues to have symptoms despite initial treatment, tests may be ordered to help find better treatments. Surgery for GER in children is rare. However, surgery may be the best option for children who have severe symptoms that do not respond to medication.

If surgery is needed, a fundoplication will be performed. During a fundoplication the upper part of the stomach is wrapped around the LES. This procedure adds pressure to the lower end of the esophagus and reduces acid reflux.

Your child's doctor can discuss the treatment options with you to help your child feel well again.

Section 25.9

Irritable Bowel Syndrome

"Irritable Bowel Syndrome in Children," National Institute of Diabetes and Digestive and Kidney Diseases, National Institutes of Health, NIH Publication No. 03-4640, May 2003. Reviewed by David A. Cooke, M.D., July 2008.

Irritable bowel syndrome (IBS) is a digestive disorder that causes abdominal pain, bloating, gas, diarrhea, and constipation—or some combination of these problems. IBS affects people of all ages, including children.

IBS is classified as a functional disorder because it is caused by a problem in how the intestines, or bowels, work. People with IBS tend to have overly sensitive intestines that have muscle spasms in response to food, gas, and sometimes stress. These spasms may cause pain, diarrhea, and constipation.

IBS may be a cause of recurring abdominal pain in children. The diagnosis of IBS is based on having abdominal pain or discomfort plus any two of the following:

- The pain is relieved by having a bowel movement.

- The onset of pain is associated with a change in the frequency of stools.

- The onset of pain is associated with a change in stool consistency.

The symptoms must be present for at least twelve weeks in the preceding twelve months, and there should be no diseases that might cause the symptoms.

In children and adolescents, IBS affects girls and boys equally and may be diarrhea-predominant, constipation-predominant, or have a variable stool pattern.

Children with IBS may also have headache, nausea, or mucus in the stool. Weight loss may occur if a child eats less to try to avoid pain. Some children first develop symptoms after a stressful event, such as teething, a bout with the flu, or problems at school or at home. Stress does not cause IBS, but it can trigger symptoms.

To diagnose IBS, the doctor will ask questions about symptoms and examine the child to rule out more serious problems or diseases. IBS is not a disease—it is a syndrome, or group of symptoms that occur together. It does not damage the intestine, so if the physical exam and other tests show no sign of disease or damage, the doctor may diagnose IBS.

In children, IBS is treated mainly through changes in diet—eating more fiber and less fat to help prevent spasms—and through bowel training to teach the child to empty the bowels at regular, specific times during the day. Medications like laxatives are rarely prescribed because children are more susceptible to addiction than adults. When laxatives are necessary, parents must follow the doctor's instructions carefully. Learning stress management techniques may also help some children.

Section 25.10

Lactose Intolerance

Excerpted from "Why Does Milk Bother Me?" National Institute of Diabetes and Digestive and Kidney Diseases, National Institutes of Health, NIH Publication No. 07-2751, February 2005.

What do I need to know about lactose intolerance?

Lactose intolerance means that you cannot digest foods with lactose in them. Lactose is the sugar found in milk and foods made with milk.

Should I worry about lactose intolerance?

No. Lactose intolerance is not serious. You should feel better soon if you eat less food with lactose or if you use products that help you digest lactose.

Why does my body have trouble digesting lactose?

You cannot digest lactose because you do not have enough lactase enzyme. The small intestine needs lactase enzyme to break down lactose. If lactose is not digested, it can cause gas and stomach cramps.

How will I feel if I have lactose intolerance?

After eating foods with lactose in them, you may feel sick to your stomach.

You may also have any of the following:

- Gas
- Diarrhea
- Swelling in your stomach

Some illnesses can cause these same problems. Your doctor can tell you if your problems are caused by lactose intolerance.

How will my doctor check for lactose intolerance?

Your doctor might use one of these tests:

- **Blood and breath tests:** You will drink a sweet drink with lactose in it. Then, your doctor will test your breath or blood for signs that you did or did not digest the lactose.
- **Stool test:** Your doctor can also find out if you digest lactose by testing your stool (bowel movement). The stool test is often used to check babies for lactose intolerance.

What can I do about lactose intolerance?

You will need to eat less of all foods with lactose. These foods include the following:

- **Foods made with milk:** Lactose is in milk and all foods made with milk, like ice cream, ice milk, sherbet, cream, butter, some cheeses, cottage cheese, and yogurt.
- **Prepared foods:** Lactose is added to some boxed, canned, frozen, and other prepared foods, like bread, cereal, lunch meats, salad dressings, mixes for cakes, cookies, pancakes, and biscuits, and frozen dinners.

How will I know if lactose is in food?

Look for certain words on food labels. These words mean the food has lactose in it:

- Butter
- Cheese
- Cream
- Dried milk
- Lactose
- Milk
- Milk solids
- Powdered milk
- Whey

Gastrointestinal Disorders

Can I eat any foods with lactose?

You may be able to eat a small amount of some foods with lactose. For example, you may be able to eat cheese or yogurt, but not drink milk. Aged cheeses, like cheddar and Swiss, have very little lactose. Or you may be able to eat some prepared foods. To find out if you can, try a small amount of the food and then see how you feel.

Some people can eat a little of certain foods that contain milk, but none of others.

Can I take anything to help me digest lactose?

You can buy pills or drops at a drug or grocery store to help you digest lactose. They are available in the following forms:

- Pills that you chew right before eating foods with lactose. These pills are called lactase enzyme caplets.

- A liquid that you add to milk before drinking. The liquid is called lactase enzyme drops.

You can also drink a special milk with less lactose in it. You can buy this milk at the grocery store. It is called lactose-reduced milk.

What else do I need to know about diet?

Drinking milk and eating foods made with milk are the most common ways to get calcium. Calcium is important for good health. If you cannot eat or drink these foods, you may need to eat other foods with calcium:

- Canned salmon with bones
- Sardines
- Collard greens
- Turnip greens
- Broccoli
- Tofu

Also, ask your doctor if you should take a calcium tablet every day.

Chapter 26

Kidney and Urologic Disorders

Chapter Contents

Section 26.1—Bedwetting and Urinary Incontinence 404
Section 26.2—Childhood Nephrotic Syndrome 409
Section 26.3—Hemolytic Uremic Syndrome 413
Section 26.4—Urinary Tract Infections 415

Section 26.1

Bedwetting and Urinary Incontinence

Excerpted from "Urinary Incontinence in Children," National Institute of Diabetes and Digestive and Kidney Diseases, National Institutes of Health, NIH Publication No. 07-4095, October 2006.

Parents or guardians of children who experience bedwetting at night or accidents during the day should treat this problem with understanding and patience. This loss of urinary control is called urinary incontinence or just incontinence. Although it affects many young people, it usually disappears naturally over time, which suggests that incontinence, for some people, may be a normal part of growing up. Incontinence at the normal age of toilet training may cause great distress. Daytime or nighttime incontinence can be embarrassing. It is important to understand that many children experience occasional incontinence and that treatment is available for most children who have difficulty controlling their bladders.

How does the urinary system work?

Urination, or voiding, is a complex activity. The bladder is a balloon-like organ that lies in the lowest part of the abdomen. The bladder stores urine, then releases it through the urethra, the canal that carries urine to the outside of the body. Controlling this activity involves nerves, muscles, the spinal cord, and the brain.

The bladder is composed of two types of muscles: the detrusor, a muscular sac that stores urine and squeezes to empty; and the sphincter, a circular group of muscles at the bottom or neck of the bladder that automatically stay contracted to hold the urine in and automatically relax when the detrusor contracts to let the urine into the urethra. A third group of muscles below the bladder (pelvic floor muscles) can contract to keep urine back.

A baby's bladder fills to a set point, then automatically contracts and empties. As the child gets older, the nervous system matures. The child's brain begins to get messages from the filling bladder and begins to send messages to the bladder to keep it from automatically emptying until the child decides it is the time and place to void.

Incontinence happens less often after age five: About 10 percent of five-year-olds, 5 percent of ten-year-olds, and 1 percent of eighteen-year-olds experience episodes of incontinence. It is twice as common in boys as in girls.

Failures in this control mechanism result in incontinence. Reasons for this failure range from simple to complex.

What causes nighttime incontinence?

After age five, wetting at night—often called bedwetting or sleepwetting—is more common than daytime wetting. Experts do not know what causes nighttime incontinence. Young people who experience nighttime wetting are usually physically and emotionally normal. Most cases probably result from a mix of factors including slower physical development, an overproduction of urine at night, a lack of ability to recognize bladder filling when asleep, and, infrequently, anxiety. For many, there is a strong family history of bedwetting, suggesting an inherited factor.

Slower physical development: Between the ages of five and ten, bedwetting may be the result of a small bladder capacity, long sleeping periods, and underdevelopment of the body's alarms that signal a full or emptying bladder. This form of incontinence will fade away as the bladder grows and the natural alarms become operational.

Excessive output of urine during sleep: Normally, the body produces a hormone that can slow the production of urine. This hormone is called antidiuretic hormone, or ADH. The body normally produces more ADH at night so that the need to urinate is lower. If the body doesn't produce enough ADH at night, the production of urine may not be slowed down, leading to bladder overfilling. If a child does not sense the bladder filling and awaken to urinate, then wetting will occur.

Anxiety: Experts suggest that anxiety-causing events occurring in the lives of children ages two to four might lead to incontinence before the child achieves total bladder control. Anxiety experienced after age four might lead to wetting after the child has been dry for a period of six months or more. Such events include angry parents, unfamiliar social situations, and overwhelming family events such as the birth of a brother or sister.

Incontinence itself is an anxiety-causing event. Strong bladder contractions leading to leakage in the daytime can cause embarrassment and anxiety that lead to wetting at night.

Genetics: Certain inherited genes appear to contribute to incontinence. In 1995, Swedish researchers announced they had found a site on human chromosome 13 that is responsible, at least in part, for nighttime wetting. If both parents were bedwetters, a child has an 80 percent chance of also being a bedwetter. Experts believe that other, undetermined genes also may be involved in incontinence.

Obstructive sleep apnea: Nighttime incontinence may be one sign of another condition called obstructive sleep apnea, in which the child's breathing is interrupted during sleep, often because of inflamed or enlarged tonsils or adenoids. Other symptoms of this condition include snoring, mouth breathing, frequent ear and sinus infections, sore throat, choking, and daytime drowsiness. In some cases, successful treatment of this breathing disorder may also resolve the associated nighttime incontinence.

Structural problems: Finally, a small number of cases of incontinence are caused by physical problems in the urinary system in children. Rarely, a blocked bladder or urethra may cause the bladder to overfill and leak. Nerve damage associated with the birth defect spina bifida can cause incontinence. In these cases, the incontinence can appear as a constant dribbling of urine.

What causes daytime incontinence?

Daytime incontinence that is not associated with urinary infection or anatomic abnormalities is less common than nighttime incontinence and tends to disappear much earlier than the nighttime versions. One possible cause of daytime incontinence is an overactive bladder. Many children with daytime incontinence have abnormal elimination habits, the most common being infrequent voiding and constipation.

An overactive bladder: Muscles surrounding the urethra—the tube that takes urine away from the bladder—have the job of keeping the passage closed, preventing urine from passing out of the body. If the bladder contracts strongly and without warning, the muscles surrounding the urethra may not be able to keep urine from passing. This often happens as a consequence of urinary tract infection (UTI) and is more common in girls.

Infrequent voiding: Infrequent voiding refers to a child's voluntarily holding urine for prolonged intervals. For example, a child may not want to use the toilets at school or may not want to interrupt enjoyable activities, so he or she ignores the body's signal of a full bladder. In these cases, the bladder can overfill and leak urine. In addition, these children often develop UTIs, leading to an irritable or overactive bladder.

Other causes: Some of the same factors that contribute to nighttime incontinence may act together with infrequent voiding to produce daytime incontinence. These factors include:

- small bladder capacity;
- structural problems;
- anxiety-causing events;
- pressure from a hard bowel movement (constipation);
- drinks or foods that contain caffeine, which increases urine output and may also cause spasms of the bladder muscle, or other ingredients to which the child may have an allergic reaction, such as chocolate or artificial coloring.

Sometimes overly strenuous toilet training may make the child unable to relax the sphincter and the pelvic floor to completely empty the bladder. Retaining urine, or incomplete emptying, sets the stage for UTIs.

What treats or cures incontinence?

Growth and development: Most urinary incontinence fades away naturally. Over time, bladder capacity increases, natural body alarms become activated, an overactive bladder settles down, production of ADH becomes normal, the child learns to respond to the body's signal that it is time to void, and stressful events or periods pass.

Many children overcome incontinence naturally—without treatment—as they grow older. The number of cases of incontinence goes down by 15 percent for each year after the age of five.

Medications: Nighttime incontinence may be treated by increasing ADH levels. The hormone can be boosted by a synthetic version known as desmopressin, or DDAVP, which is available in pill form, nasal spray, or nose drops. Desmopressin is approved for use in children.

Another medication, called imipramine, is also used to treat sleep-wetting. It acts on both the brain and the urinary bladder. Researchers estimate that these medications may help as many as 70 percent of patients achieve short-term success. Many patients, however, relapse once the medication is withdrawn.

If a young person experiences incontinence resulting from an overactive bladder, a doctor might prescribe a medicine that helps to calm the bladder muscle. This medicine controls muscle spasms and belongs to a class of medications called anticholinergics.

Bladder training and related strategies: Bladder training consists of exercises for strengthening and coordinating muscles of the bladder and urethra, and may help the control of urination. These techniques teach the child to anticipate the need to urinate and prevent urination when away from a toilet. Techniques that may help nighttime incontinence include determining bladder capacity, drinking less fluid before sleeping, and developing routines for waking up.

Unfortunately, none of these techniques guarantees success. Techniques that may help daytime incontinence include urinating on a schedule—timed voiding—such as every two hours, avoiding caffeine or other foods or drinks that you suspect may contribute to your child's incontinence, and following suggestions for healthy urination, such as relaxing muscles and taking your time.

Moisture alarms: At night, moisture alarms can awaken a person when he or she begins to urinate. These devices include a water-sensitive pad worn in pajamas, a wire connecting to a battery-driven control, and an alarm that sounds when moisture is first detected. For the alarm to be effective, the child must awaken as soon as the alarm goes off, go to the bathroom, and change the bedding. Using alarms may require having another person sleep in the same room to awaken the bedwetter.

Incontinence is also called enuresis. Primary enuresis is wetting in a person who has never been dry for at least six months. Secondary enuresis is wetting that begins after at least six months of dryness. Nocturnal enuresis is wetting that usually occurs during sleep, also called nighttime incontinence. Diurnal enuresis is wetting when awake, also called daytime incontinence.

Kidney and Urologic Disorders

Section 26.2

Childhood Nephrotic Syndrome

National Institute of Diabetes and Digestive and Kidney Diseases, National Institutes of Health, NIH Publication No. 08-4695, February 2008.

What is nephrotic syndrome?

Nephrotic syndrome is a set of signs or symptoms that may point to kidney problems. The kidneys are two bean-shaped organs found in the lower back. Each is about the size of a fist. They clean the blood by filtering out excess water and salt and waste products from food. Healthy kidneys keep protein in the blood, which helps the blood soak up water from tissues. But kidneys with damaged filters may leak protein into the urine. As a result, not enough protein is left in the blood to soak up the water. The water then moves from the blood into body tissues and causes swelling.

Both children and adults can have nephrotic syndrome. The causes of and treatments for nephrotic syndrome in children are sometimes different from the causes and treatments in adults.

Childhood nephrotic syndrome can occur at any age but is most common between the ages of eighteen months and five years. It seems to affect boys more often than girls.

A child with nephrotic syndrome has these signs:

- High levels of protein in the urine, a condition called proteinuria
- Low levels of protein in the blood
- Swelling resulting from buildup of salt and water
- Less frequent urination
- Weight gain from excess water

Nephrotic syndrome is not itself a disease. But it can be the first sign of a disease that damages the kidney's tiny blood-filtering units, called glomeruli, where urine is made.

How is childhood nephrotic syndrome diagnosed?

To diagnose childhood nephrotic syndrome, the doctor may ask for a urine sample to check for protein. The doctor will dip a strip of chemically treated paper into the urine sample. Too much protein in the urine will make the paper change color. Or the doctor may ask for a twenty-four-hour collection of urine for a more precise measurement of the protein and other substances in the urine.

The doctor may take a blood sample to see how well the kidneys are removing wastes. Healthy kidneys remove creatinine and urea nitrogen from the blood. If the blood contains high levels of these waste products, some kidney damage may have already occurred. But most children with nephrotic syndrome do not have permanent kidney damage.

In some cases, the doctor may want to examine a small piece of kidney tissue with a microscope to see if something specific is causing the syndrome. The procedure of collecting a small tissue sample from the kidney is called a biopsy, and it is usually performed with a long needle passed through the skin. The child will be awake during the procedure and receive calming drugs and a local painkiller at the site of the needle entry. A child who is prone to bleeding problems may require open surgery for the biopsy. General anesthesia will be used if surgery is required. For any biopsy procedure, the child will stay overnight in the hospital to rest and allow the health care team to address quickly any problems that might occur.

What conditions are associated with childhood nephrotic syndrome?

Minimal change disease: The condition most commonly associated with childhood nephrotic syndrome is minimal change disease. Doctors do not know what causes it. The condition is called minimal change disease because children with this form of the nephrotic syndrome have normal or nearly normal appearing kidney biopsies. If a child is diagnosed with minimal change disease, the doctor will probably prescribe prednisone, which belongs to a class of drugs called corticosteroids. Prednisone stops the movement of protein from the blood into the urine, but it does have side effects that the doctor will explain. Following the doctor's directions exactly is essential to protect the child's health. The doctor may also prescribe another type of drug called a diuretic, which reduces the swelling by helping the child urinate more frequently.

When protein is no longer present in the urine, the doctor will begin to reduce the dosage of prednisone. This process takes several weeks. Some children never get sick again, but most experience a relapse, developing swelling and protein in the urine again, usually following a viral illness. However, as long as the child continues to respond to prednisone and the urine becomes protein free, the child has an excellent long-term outlook without kidney damage.

Children who relapse frequently, or who seem to be dependent on prednisone or have side effects from it, may be given a second type of drug called a cytotoxic agent. The agents most frequently used are cyclophosphamide and chlorambucil. After reducing protein in the urine with prednisone, the doctor may prescribe the cyclophosphamide or chlorambucil for eight to twelve weeks. Alternatively, cyclosporine, a drug also used in transplant patients, may be given. Treatment with cyclosporine frequently continues over an extended period.

In recent years, doctors have explored the use of mycophenolate mofetil (MMF) instead of cytotoxic agents for children who relapse frequently. MMF is an immunosuppressant used to treat autoimmune diseases and to keep the body from rejecting a transplanted organ. MMF has not been tested for treating minimal change disease in large clinical trials, but doctors report promising results with small numbers of patients. MMF has milder side effects than cytotoxic agents, but taking immunosuppressants can raise the risk of infection and other diseases. The good news is that most children outgrow minimal change disease by their late teens with no permanent damage to their kidneys.

Focal segmental glomerulosclerosis (FSGS) and membranoproliferative glomerulonephritis (MPGN): In about 20 percent of children with nephrotic syndrome, a kidney biopsy reveals scarring or deposits in the glomeruli. The two most common diseases that damage these tiny blood-filtering units are FSGS and MPGN.

Because prednisone is less effective in treating these diseases than it is in treating minimal change disease, the doctor may use additional therapies, including cytotoxic agents. Recent experience with another class of drugs called angiotensin-converting enzyme (ACE) inhibitors, usually used to treat high blood pressure, indicates these drugs can help decrease the amount of protein leaking into the urine and keep the kidneys from being damaged in children with FSGS or MPGN.

Congenital nephropathy: Rarely, a child may be born with congenital nephropathy, a condition that causes nephrotic syndrome. The most common form of this condition is congenital nephropathy of the Finnish type (CNF), inherited as an autosomal recessive trait—meaning the gene for CNF must be inherited from both parents.

Another condition that causes nephrotic syndrome in the first months of life is diffuse mesangial sclerosis (DMS). The pattern of inheritance for DMS is not as clearly understood as the pattern for CNF, although the condition does appear to be genetic.

Since medicines have little effect on congenital nephropathy, transplantation is usually required by the second or third year of life, when the child has grown enough to receive a kidney. To keep the child healthy, the doctor may recommend infusions of the protein albumin to make up for the protein lost in urine and prescribe a diuretic to help eliminate the extra fluid that causes swelling. The child's immune system may be weakened, so antibiotics should be given at the first sign of infection.

Congenital nephropathy can disturb thyroid activity, so the child may need the substitute hormone thyroxine to promote growth and help bones mature. Some children with congenital nephropathy have excessive blood clotting, or thrombosis, which must be treated with a blood thinner like warfarin.

A child with congenital nephropathy may need tube feedings to ensure proper nutrition. In some cases, the diseased kidneys may need to be removed to eliminate proteinuria. Dialysis will then be required to replace kidney function until the child's body is big enough to receive a transplanted kidney. Peritoneal dialysis is preferable to hemodialysis for young children.

In peritoneal dialysis, a catheter is surgically placed in the abdomen and then used to introduce a solution into the abdominal cavity, or peritoneum. The solution draws wastes and extra fluid from the bloodstream. After a few hours, the solution is drained and replaced with a fresh supply. The drained solution carries the wastes and extra fluid out of the body.

Section 26.3

Hemolytic Uremic Syndrome

National Institute of Diabetes and Digestive and Kidney Diseases, National Institutes of Health, NIH Publication No. 06-4570, December 2005.

Hemolytic uremic syndrome, or HUS, is one of the most common causes of sudden, short-term kidney failure in children. In severe cases, this acute kidney failure may require several sessions of dialysis to temporarily take over the kidneys' job of filtering wastes from the blood, but most children recover without permanent damage to their health.

Course of the Disease

Most cases of HUS occur after an infection of the digestive system by *Escherichia coli* (*E. coli*) bacterium, which is found in foods like meat, dairy products, and juice when they are contaminated. Some people have contracted HUS after swimming in pools or lakes contaminated with feces. Washing and cooking foods adequately, avoiding undercooked meats, and avoiding unclean swimming areas are the best ways to protect your child from this disease.

Infection of the digestive tract is called gastroenteritis and may cause your child to vomit and have stomach cramps and bloody diarrhea. Most children who experience gastroenteritis recover fully in two or three days and do not develop HUS. In a few children, however, HUS develops when the bacteria lodged in the digestive system make toxins that enter the bloodstream and start to destroy red blood cells.

Signs and Symptoms

Symptoms of HUS may not become apparent until a week after the digestive problems. With HUS, the child remains pale, tired, and irritable. Other signs include small, unexplained bruises or bleeding from the nose or mouth that may occur because the toxins also destroy the platelets, cells that normally help the blood to clot.

You may notice that your child's urine output decreases. The urine may also appear red. Urine formation slows because the damaged red blood cells clog the tiny blood vessels in the kidneys, making them work harder to remove wastes and extra fluid from the blood. The body's inability to rid itself of excess fluid and wastes may in turn cause high blood pressure or swelling of the face, hands, feet, or entire body. This progression to acute kidney failure occurs in about half of HUS cases.

Call your child's doctor immediately if you notice unexplained bruises, unusual bleeding, swollen limbs, or generalized swelling, extreme fatigue, or decreased urine output in your child. You should call your doctor or visit an emergency room if your child goes twelve hours without urinating.

Treatment

Treatments, which consist of maintaining normal salt and water levels in the body, are aimed at easing the immediate symptoms and preventing further problems. Your child may need a transfusion of red blood cells delivered intravenously—that is, through an IV needle. Only the most severe cases require dialysis. Some children may sustain significant kidney damage that slowly develops into permanent kidney failure and will then require long-term dialysis or a kidney transplant. Some studies suggest that limiting protein in the child's diet and treating blood pressure with a medicine from a class of drugs called angiotensin-converting enzyme inhibitors, usually called ACE inhibitors, helps delay or prevent the onset of permanent kidney failure. Most children recover completely with no long-term consequences.

Some parents feel a sense of responsibility for their child's illness after a case of HUS. While the disease may have been preventable, caregivers should not feel guilty because the invisible course of the disease cannot be predicted from the initial bacterial infection, which many children experience without developing HUS. Caregivers who get their children the appropriate medical care should rest assured that they have done all that any caring parent could do.

Hope through Research

The National Institute of Diabetes and Digestive and Kidney Diseases (NIDDK) conducts and supports research to help many kinds of people with kidney disease, including children. NIDDK's Division of Kidney, Urologic, and Hematologic Diseases (DKUHD) maintains the Pediatric Nephrology Program, which supports research into the causes, treatment, and prevention of kidney diseases in children. DKUHD supports several researchers working to find ways to prevent HUS from developing after the initial infection of the digestive system.

Section 26.4

Urinary Tract Infections

> Excerpted from "Urinary Tract Infections in Children," National Institute of Diabetes and Digestive and Kidney Diseases, National Institutes of Health, NIH Publication No. 07-4246, December 2005.

Urinary tract infections (UTIs) affect about 3 percent of children in the United States every year. Throughout childhood, the risk of a UTI is 2 percent for boys and 8 percent for girls. UTIs account for more than one million visits to pediatricians' offices every year. The symptoms are not always obvious to parents, and younger children are usually unable to describe how they feel. Recognizing and treating urinary tract infections is important. Untreated UTIs can lead to serious kidney problems that could threaten the life of your child.

How does the urinary tract normally function?

The kidneys filter and remove waste and water from the blood to produce urine. They get rid of about one and a half to two quarts of urine per day in an adult and less in a child, depending on the child's age. The urine travels from the kidneys down two narrow tubes called the ureters. The urine is then stored in a balloon-like organ called the bladder (see Figure 26.1). In a child, the bladder can hold about one to one and a half ounces of urine for each year of the child's age. So, the bladder of a four-year-old child may hold about four to six ounces (less than one cup); an eight-year-old can hold eight to twelve ounces. When the bladder empties, a muscle called the sphincter relaxes and urine flows out of the body through the urethra, a tube at the bottom of the bladder. The opening of the urethra is at the end of the penis in boys (see Figure 26.2) and in front of the vagina in girls (see Figure 26.3).

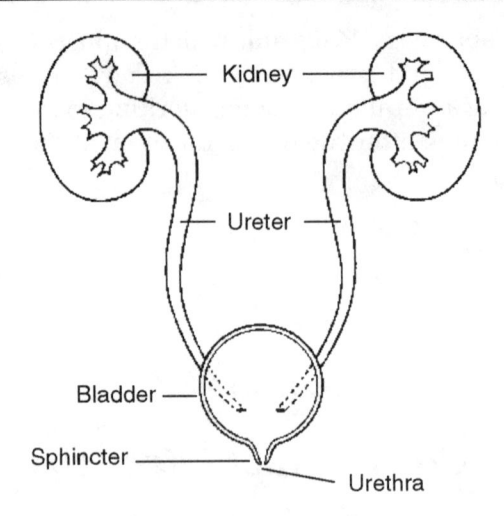

Childhood Diseases and Disorders Sourcebook, Second Edition

Figure 26.1. Front view of urinary tract

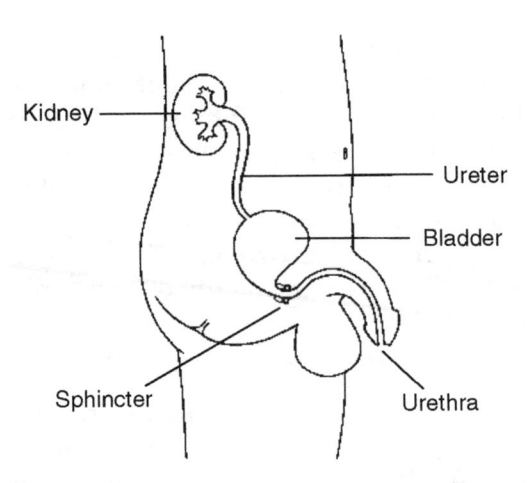

Figure 26.2. Side view of male urinary tract

How does the urinary tract become infected?

Normal urine contains no bacteria (germs). Bacteria may, at times, get into the urinary tract and the urine from the skin around the rectum and genitals by traveling up the urethra into the bladder. When this happens, the bacteria can infect and inflame the bladder and cause swelling and pain in the lower abdomen and side. This bladder infection is called cystitis.

Kidney and Urologic Disorders

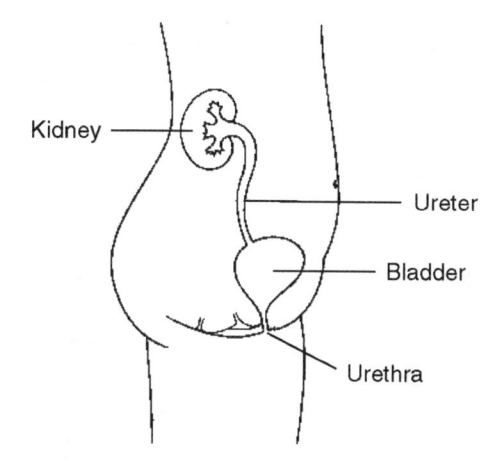

Figure 26.3. Side view of female urinary tract

If the bacteria travel up through the ureters to the kidneys, a kidney infection can develop. The infection is usually accompanied by pain and fever. Kidney infections are much more serious than bladder infections.

In some children a urinary tract infection may be a sign of an abnormal urinary tract that may be prone to repeated problems. For this reason, when a child has a urinary infection, additional tests are often recommended. In other cases, children develop urinary tract infections because they are prone to such infections, just as other children are prone to getting coughs, colds, or ear infections. Or a child may happen to be infected by a type of bacteria with a special ability to cause urinary tract infections.

Children who frequently delay a trip to the bathroom are more likely to develop UTIs. Regular urination helps keep the urinary tract sterile by flushing away bacteria. Holding in urine allows bacteria to grow. Keeping the sphincter muscle tight for a long time also makes it more difficult to relax that muscle when it is time to urinate. As a result, the child's bladder may not empty completely. This dysfunctional voiding can set the stage for a urinary infection.

What are the signs of urinary tract infection?

A urinary tract infection causes irritation of the lining of the bladder, urethra, ureters, and kidneys, just like the inside of the nose or the throat becomes irritated with a cold. If your child is an infant or only a few years old, the signs of a urinary tract infection may not be clear, since children that young cannot tell you exactly how they feel. Your child may have a high fever, be irritable, or not eat.

On the other hand, sometimes a child may have only a low-grade fever, experience nausea and vomiting, or just not seem healthy. The diaper urine may have an unusual smell. If your child has a high temperature and appears sick for more than a day without signs of a runny nose or other obvious cause for discomfort, he or she may need to be checked for a bladder infection.

An older child with bladder irritation may complain of pain in the abdomen and pelvic area. Your child may urinate often. If the kidney is infected, your child may complain of pain under the side of the rib cage, called the flank, or low back pain. Crying or complaining that it hurts to urinate and producing only a few drops of urine at a time are other signs of urinary tract infection. Your child may have difficulty controlling the urine and may leak urine into clothing or bed sheets. The urine may smell unusual or look cloudy or red.

How do you find out whether your child has a urinary tract infection?

Only by consulting a health care provider can you find out for certain whether your child has a urinary tract infection.

Some of your child's urine will be collected and examined. The way urine is collected depends on your child's age. If the child is not yet toilet trained, the health care provider may place a plastic collection bag over your child's genital area. It will be sealed to the skin with an adhesive strip. An older child may be asked to urinate into a container. The sample needs to come as directly into the container as possible to avoid picking up bacteria from the skin or rectal area. A doctor or nurse may need to pass a small tube into the urethra. Urine will drain directly from the bladder into a clean container through this tube, called a catheter. Sometimes the best way to get the urine is by placing a needle directly into the bladder through the skin of the lower abdomen. Getting urine through the tube or needle will ensure that the urine collected is pure.

Some of the urine will be examined under a microscope. If an infection is present, bacteria and sometimes pus will be found in the urine. If the bacteria from the sample are hard to see, the health care provider may place the sample in a tube or dish with a substance that encourages any bacteria present to grow. Once the germs have multiplied, they

Kidney and Urologic Disorders

can then be identified and tested to see which medications will provide the most effective treatment. The process of growing bacteria in the laboratory is known as performing a culture and often takes a day or more to complete.

The reliability of the culture depends on how long the urine stands before the culture is started. If you collect your child's urine at home, refrigerate it as soon as it is collected and carry the container to the health care provider or lab in a plastic bag filled with ice.

How are urinary tract infections treated?

Urinary tract infections are treated with bacteria-fighting drugs called antibiotics. While a urine sample is being examined, the health care provider may begin treatment with a drug that treats the bacteria most likely to be causing the infection. Once culture results are known, the health care provider may decide to switch your child to another antibiotic.

The way the antibiotic is given and the number of days that it must be taken depend in part on the type of infection and how severe it is. When a child is sick or not able to drink fluids, the antibiotic may need to be put directly into the bloodstream through a vein in the arm or hand. Otherwise, the medicine (liquid or pills) may be given by mouth or by shots. The medicine is given for at least three to five days and possibly for as long as several weeks. The daily treatment schedule recommended depends on the specific drug prescribed: The schedule may call for a single dose each day or up to four doses each day. In some cases, your child will need to take the medicine until further tests are finished.

After a few doses of the antibiotic, your child may appear much better, but often several days may pass before all symptoms are gone. In any case, your child should take the medicine for as long as the doctor recommends. Do not stop medications because the symptoms have gone away. Infections may return, and germs can resist future treatment if the drug is stopped too soon.

Children should drink fluids when they wish. Make sure your child drinks what he or she needs, but do not force your child to drink large amounts of fluid. The health care provider needs to know if the child is not interested in drinking.

What tests may be needed after the infection is gone?

Once the infection has cleared, additional tests may be recommended to check for abnormalities in the urinary tract. Repeated infections in abnormal urinary tracts may cause kidney damage. The kinds of tests ordered will depend on your child and the type of urinary infection. Because no single test can tell everything about the urinary tract that might be important, more than one of the following tests may be needed:

- **Kidney and bladder ultrasound:** An ultrasound test examines the kidney and bladder using sound waves. This test shows shadows of the kidney and bladder that may point out certain abnormalities. However, this test cannot reveal all important urinary abnormalities. It also cannot measure how well a kidney works.

- **Voiding cystourethrogram (VCUG):** This test examines the urethra and bladder while the bladder fills and empties. A liquid that can be seen on x-rays is placed into the bladder through a catheter. The bladder is filled until the child urinates. This test can reveal abnormalities of the inside of the urethra and bladder. The test can also determine whether the flow of urine is normal when the bladder empties.

- **Intravenous pyelogram:** This test examines the whole urinary tract. A liquid that can be seen on x-rays is injected into a vein. The substance travels into the kidneys and bladder, revealing possible obstructions.

- **Nuclear scans:** These tests use radioactive materials that are usually injected into a vein to show how well the kidneys work, the shape of the kidneys, and whether urine empties from the kidneys in a normal way. Each kind of nuclear scan gives different information about the kidneys and bladder. Nuclear scans expose a child to about the same amount of radiation as a conventional x-ray. At times, it can even be less.

- **Computed tomography (CT) scans and magnetic resonance imaging (MRI):** These tests provide three-dimensional images and cross-sections of the bladder and kidneys. With a typical CT scan or MRI machine, the child lies on a table that slides inside a tunnel where the images are taken. If the child's infection is complicated or difficult to see in other image tests, a CT scan or MRI can provide clearer, more detailed images to help the doctor understand the problem.

What abnormalities lead to urinary problems?

Many children who get urinary tract infections have normal kidneys and bladders. But if a child has an abnormality, it should be detected

Kidney and Urologic Disorders

as early as possible to protect the kidneys against damage. Abnormalities that could occur include the following:

- **Vesicoureteral reflux (VUR):** Urine normally flows from the kidneys down the ureters to the bladder in one direction. With VUR, when the bladder fills, the urine may also flow backward from the bladder up the ureters to the kidneys. This abnormality is common in children with urinary infections.

- **Urinary obstruction:** Blockages to urinary flow can occur in many places in the urinary tract. The ureter or urethra may be too narrow or a kidney stone at some point stops the urinary flow from leaving the body. Occasionally, the ureter may join the kidney or bladder at the wrong place and prevent urine from leaving the kidney in the normal way.

- **Dysfunctional voiding:** Some children develop a habit of delaying a trip to the bathroom because they don't want to leave their play. They may work so hard at keeping the sphincter muscle tight that they forget how to relax it at the right time. These children may be unable to empty the bladder completely. Some children may strain during urination, causing pressure in the bladder that sends urine flowing back up the ureters. Dysfunctional voiding can lead to vesicoureteral reflux, accidental leaking, and UTIs.

Do urinary tract infections have long-term effects?

Young children are at the greatest risk for kidney damage from urinary tract infections, especially if they have some unknown urinary tract abnormality. Such damage includes kidney scars, poor kidney growth, poor kidney function, high blood pressure, and other problems. For this reason it is important that children with urinary tract infections receive prompt treatment and careful evaluation.

How can urinary tract infections be prevented?

If your child has a normal urinary tract, you can help him or her avoid UTIs by encouraging regular trips to the bathroom. Make sure your child gets enough to drink if infrequent voiding is a problem. Teach your child proper cleaning techniques after using the bathroom to keep bacteria from entering the urinary tract.

Some abnormalities in the urinary tract correct themselves as the child grows, but some defects may require surgical correction. A common procedure to correct VUR is the reimplantation of the ureters.

During this surgery, the doctor repositions the connection between the ureter and the bladder so that urine will not back up into the ureters and kidneys. In recent years, doctors have treated some cases of VUR by injecting collagen, or a similar substance, into the bladder wall, just below the opening where the ureter joins the bladder. This injection creates a kind of valve that keeps urine from flowing back into the ureter. The injection is delivered to the inside of the bladder through a catheter passed through the urethra, so there is no need for a surgical incision.

Chapter 27

Liver Disorders

Chapter Contents

Section 27.1—Alpha-1 Antitrypsin Deficiency 424
Section 27.2—Autoimmune Hepatitis 428

Section 27.1

Alpha-1 Antitrypsin Deficiency

"Alpha-1 Antitrypsin Deficiency (AATD)," is reprinted with permission from the Cincinnati Children's Hospital Medical Center website, http://www.cincinnatichildrens.org. © 2006 Cincinnati Children's Hospital Medical Center. All rights reserved.

What is alpha-1 antitrypsin deficiency (AATD)?

Alpha-1 antitrypsin deficiency (AATD) is a common, serious disease that is passed down from parents to children. It can cause liver and lung disease. The liver makes a protein called alpha-1 antitrypsin that goes into the bloodstream. This protein protects the lungs and allows them to work normally. If there is not enough alpha-1 antitrypsin, it is called alpha-1 antitrypsin deficiency (AATD).

Alpha-1 antitrypsin deficiency is the most common genetic cause of liver disease in children and is the most common genetic disease for which liver transplantation is done.

Some studies suggest one in three thousand Americans have AATD, and that 95 percent of these individuals have not been diagnosed.

What causes alpha-1 antitrypsin deficiency?

Alpha-1 antitrypsin is a protein that is made in the liver and then released into the bloodstream. Sometimes a gene mutation produces an abnormal form of this protein which cannot be released from the liver, which means it cannot enter the bloodstream.

Alpha-1 antitrypsin's job is to protect tissues in the body from being digested by enzymes released from inflammatory cells. Enzymes may then attack the lung and/or liver tissue.

In very young children, alpha-1 antitrypsin then accumulates in the liver, causing damage to the liver. Approximately 10 percent of infants born with the severe deficiency have liver disease that is fatal without a liver transplant.

Alpha-1-antitrypsin deficiency is an inherited condition and does not appear unless a person receives the same defective gene from both parents. If both parents carry an abnormal gene for alpha-1 antitrypsin deficiency disease there is:

- a 25 percent chance their child will develop the disorder;
- a 50 percent chance their child will receive one defective gene from one of the parents, which means the child will not show symptoms of the disorder but is a "carrier";
- a 25 percent chance their child will receive both normal genes, one from each parent, and will be unaffected.

What are the signs and symptoms?

Jaundice that doesn't clear up may be the first sign of an alpha-1 antitrypsin deficiency in an infant. Other symptoms in infancy may include:

- elevated liver enzyme levels;
- dark urine, pale stools;
- itching;
- enlarged liver;
- bleeding;
- ascites (the accumulation of a watery fluid that is produced by membranes when they are inflamed in the tissue that lines the belly);
- feeding difficulties;
- poor growth or failure to thrive.

Other children may not show signs of this condition until early childhood. First signs may include:

- elevated liver enzyme levels;
- easily tired;
- loss of appetite;
- swelling of the legs or belly;
- enlargement or inflammation of the liver;
- jaundice, fever;
- enlarged spleen;

- ascites (the accumulation of a watery fluid that is produced by membranes when they are inflamed in the tissue that lines the belly);
- pruritus (severe itching of the skin);
- panniculitis (rare form of skin disease that is an inflammation of fat just beneath the skin, causing the skin to harden and form lumps).

How is it diagnosed?

Alpha-1 antitrypsin deficiency uses a simple blood test that measures the type of alpha-1 antitrypsin circulating in the blood. This test can tell whether a person is deficient or is a carrier. The blood test can be done soon after a baby is born if it is known that members of the baby's family carry the alpha-1 antitrypsin deficiency gene. A test also is available to check if a baby in the womb has the condition.

Liver disease resulting from alpha-1 antitrypsin deficiency can be determined by abnormal changes found in blood, urine, and liver function tests. A doctor can tell by feel during a physical exam if something is not normal. A computed tomography (CT) scan, and ultrasound and radioisotope scans of the liver and spleen also can detect damage. A liver biopsy can confirm the diagnosis.

If bilirubin (a liquid produced in the liver that removes toxins from the body and helps break down fat in food) levels are higher than normal, it may be a sign of alpha-1 antitrypsin deficiency. Increased levels of certain enzymes and abnormal ratios of certain proteins may also indicate liver disease.

What is the treatment?

Alpha-1 antitrypsin deficiency affects children differently. One child may not show any signs of liver disease and another child may be seriously affected. Only a small percentage of children develop liver disease because of the deficiency.

There is no cure for alpha-1 antitrypsin deficiency. If liver disease has developed, a liver transplant is currently the only option available for survival. The goal of treatment is to relieve the symptoms:

- Medicine may be given for severe itching or jaundice.
- Diuretics may be used to help reduce body fluid buildup.
- A healthy diet and vitamin supplements can provide essential nutrients and may increase overall quality of daily living. Eating

a number of smaller meals during the day keeps the digestive process from interfering with breathing.
- Vitamin/nutrition supplements may increase the effectiveness of the digestive process and increase energy levels.
- Shunts (a kind of bypass) may be surgically inserted to lower the pressure within the blood vessels in the liver for people with liver disease caused by alpha-1 antitrypsin deficiency.

Transplantation can result in a cure of alpha-1 antitrypsin deficiency. If a transplant is the best treatment option, the doctor and the other members of the patient care team focus on preventing complications. They will treat symptoms while your child waits for a donated liver. A liver transplant totally replaces the abnormal liver cells that produce the abnormal alpha-1 antitrypsin deficiency and corrects the protein abnormality.

It is critical for a child with AATD to avoid smoking or being exposed to second-hand smoke.

What is the long-term prognosis?

There is good chance of avoiding liver disease since only about 10 percent of children with alpha-1 antitrypsin deficiency develop significant liver disease. Liver transplants have been effective in reversing the symptoms of liver failure due to alpha-1 antitrypsin deficiency.

Section 27.2

Autoimmune Hepatitis

"Autoimmune Hepatitis," is reprinted with permission from the Cincinnati Children's Hospital Medical Center website, http://www.cincinnatichildrens.org. © 2006 Cincinnati Children's Hospital Medical Center. All rights reserved.

What is autoimmune hepatitis?

Autoimmune hepatitis is a condition in which a person's own immune system attacks the liver, causing inflammation and liver cell death. The inflammation continues and gets worse over time. If not treated, this can lead to irreversible cirrhosis (a disease of the liver caused by liver cells that do not work properly), and eventually liver failure.

Autoimmune hepatitis is classified as either type I or II.

Type I is the most common form in North America. It occurs at any age and is more common in females than males. About half of those with type I have other autoimmune disorders such as thyroiditis, Graves disease, Sjögren syndrome, autoimmune anemia, and ulcerative colitis.

Type II is less common, and often affects girls ages two to fourteen.

What are the causes of autoimmune hepatitis?

When the immune system is working correctly, it protects the body from infections caused by bacteria and viruses. In the case of an autoimmune disease, the body does not recognize certain cells and body parts as part of itself. The body then goes to war against itself, damaging the body part it thinks is foreign.

When the immune system attacks the liver in this way, it is called autoimmune hepatitis. Autoimmune hepatitis is not caused by a virus or bacteria, so it is not a contagious disease. In fact, it is not known what triggers the immune system to react against the liver.

What are signs and symptoms of autoimmune hepatitis?

Fatigue (when you feel tired all the time) is one of the most common symptoms of autoimmune hepatitis. Often when patients experience fatigue along with some of the disease's other symptoms—including abdominal pain and aching joints—the cause is mistaken for a mild case of the flu.

Other symptoms may include:

- enlarged liver;
- itching;
- skin rashes;
- dark urine;
- nausea;
- vomiting;
- pale or gray-colored stools;
- loss of appetite.

When autoimmune hepatitis progresses to severe cirrhosis, there may be jaundice (yellow coloring to the skin and eyes), swelling of the belly caused by fluid, bleeding in the intestines, or mental confusion. Also, females may stop having their menstrual periods.

How is it autoimmune hepatitis diagnosed?

Your child's doctor will make a diagnosis based on their symptoms, blood tests, and liver biopsy.

A routine blood test for liver enzymes can reveal a pattern typical of hepatitis, but further tests, especially for autoantibodies, are needed to diagnose autoimmune hepatitis.

Antibodies are proteins made by the immune system to fight off bacteria and viruses. In autoimmune hepatitis, two antibodies that may develop in the blood are the ANA (antinuclear antibody) and the SMA (smooth muscle antibodies). Also, gamma globulin, a certain type of blood protein, will be elevated when autoimmune hepatitis is present.

A liver biopsy is needed to determine how much inflammation and scarring has developed.

How is it autoimmune hepatitis treated?

With the right treatment, autoimmune hepatitis usually can be controlled. In fact, recent studies show that continued treatment not only stops the disease from getting worse, but it may actually reverse some of the damage.

Medicine: The primary treatment is medicine to suppress (or slow down) an overactive immune system. Both types of autoimmune hepatitis are treated with daily doses of a steroid called prednisone.

Your child's doctor may start your child on a high dose and lower the dose as the disease is controlled. The goal is to find the lowest possible dose that will control your child's disease.

Another medication, azathioprine, is also used to treat this disease. Like prednisone, azathioprine slows down the immune system, but in a different way.

Treatment with azathioprine helps lower the dose of prednisone needed, thereby reducing steroid side effects. Your doctor may prescribe azathioprine in addition to prednisone once the disease is under control.

Most people with autoimmune hepatitis will need to take prednisone, with or without azathioprine, for years. Some people take it for life. These steroids may slow down the disease, but everyone is different.

In about one out of every four people, treatment eventually can be stopped. However, it is important to carefully monitor your child's condition and report any new symptoms to the doctor because the disease may return and be even more severe, especially during the first few months after stopping treatment.

Side effects: Both prednisone and azathioprine have side effects. Prednisone can cause fluid retention, weight gain, and the face to swell. Azathioprine can lower your child's white blood count and sometimes cause nausea and poor appetite.

Liver transplantation: People who progress to end-stage liver disease (liver failure) may need a liver transplant. The outcome for patients with autoimmune hepatitis is excellent. Survival rates at transplant centers for this condition are well over 90 percent, with a good quality of life after recovery.

What is the long-term prognosis?

The outlook for children with autoimmune hepatitis is generally favorable. In about seven out of ten people the disease goes into remission, with symptoms becoming less severe within two years of starting treatment.

However, some people whose disease goes into remission will see it return within three years, so treatment may be necessary on and off for years, if not for life.

Chapter 28

Musculoskeletal Disorders

Chapter Contents

Section 28.1—Bowlegs and Knock-Knee 432
Section 28.2—Flat Feet 435
Section 28.3—Growing Pains 438
Section 28.4—Intoeing 440
Section 28.5—Juvenile Rheumatoid Arthritis 442
Section 28.6—Juvenile Dermatomyositis 446
Section 28.7—Marfan Syndrome 452
Section 28.8—Muscular Dystrophy 455
Section 28.9—Osgood-Schlatter Disease 460
Section 28.10—Scoliosis 462

Section 28.1

Bowlegs and Knock-Knee

Reprinted from "Bowlegs" and "Knock Knee," © 2005 Dartmouth-Hitchcock Medical Center (www.dhmc.org). Reprinted with permission.

Bowlegs

Alternative name: Genu Varum

What are bowlegs?

Bowlegs is a term used to describe a condition in which, when a person stands with their feet and ankles together, their knees remain far apart.

What are the signs of bowlegs?

- Knees remain far apart when both feet and ankles are touching.
- Patient is over three years old and still has bowlegs.

How are bowlegs caused?

Babies and small children are bowlegged due to their position in the womb. Usually when an infant starts walking, the legs will straighten out and correct the problem. Other causes of bowlegs include:

- Blount disease, a growth-related condition, in which the inner part of the bone just below the knee develops a curvature due to the weight placed on the knee;
- bone dysplasia (abnormal bone growth or development);
- rickets (rachitis).

How does a doctor tell if a patient has bowlegs?

The doctor will take some of the following steps to see if a patient has bowlegs:

- Make a visual exam of the legs, after which a doctor can often confirm that a patient has the condition.
- Order an x-ray to help in diagnosis.

How are bowlegs treated?

Usually, there is no treatment recommended for bowlegs, especially in young children. Braces may be used in Blount disease. Surgery is rarely needed to correct the problem. In rickets, supplements of vitamin D and calcium are prescribed.

Knock-Knee

Alternate name: Genu Valgum

What is knock-knee?

Knock-knee is a term used to describe an unusually large distance between the ankles when the knees are touching. It happens mainly in children and is not normally anything to worry about. Up to three-quarters of children between the age of three and five have the condition and it usually corrects itself by the age of about seven. Treatment may be needed if the knock-knee does not correct itself or if it is caused by an underlying medical problem.

What are the signs of knock-knee?

- When the knees are touching, the feet and ankles are far apart.
- Walking difficulties.
- An awkward way of walking (gait).

What causes knock-knee?

Most children develop some degree of knock-knee when they are starting school. It happens when the child's weight falls to the outside of the knee joint. This is usually part of normal development.

Sometimes, knock-knee can be a result of a disease or a symptom of another condition. Some childhood diseases that could cause knock-knee are:

- rickets, caused by lack of vitamin D.

How does a doctor tell if a patient has knock-knee?

The doctor will take some of the following steps to see if a patient has knock-knee:

- Look at the legs, hips, and feet.
- Watch how the patient walks.
- Measure the distance between the ankles when the knees are lightly touching.
- Order an x-ray to see if there is an underlying problem with the bones.

How is knock-knee treated?

Usually, there is no treatment recommended for knock-knee, especially in children under the age of eight. In severe cases of knock-knee that continue past the age of ten and into adolescence, surgery may be considered to correct the problem.

Some of the following treatments can be recommended:

- The inside edge of the heel of the shoes may be raised a little to try to correct the line of the leg.

Section 28.2

Flat Feet

"Pes Planus," © 2008 A.D.A.M., Inc.
Reprinted with permission. Updated May 12, 2008.

Alternative Names

Pes planovalgus; flat feet; fallen arches; pronation of feet

Definition

Pes planus is a condition where the arch or instep of the foot collapses and comes in contact with the ground. In some individuals, this arch never develops.

Causes

Flat feet are a common condition. In infants and toddlers, the longitudinal arch is not developed and flat feet are normal. The arch develops in childhood, and by adulthood, most people have developed normal arches.

When flat feet persist, most are considered variations of normal. Most feet are flexible and an arch appears when the person stands on his or her toes. Stiff, inflexible, or painful flat feet may be associated with other conditions and require attention.

Painful flat feet in children may be caused by a condition called tarsal coalition. In tarsal coalition, two or more of the bones in the foot fuse together, limiting motion and often leading to a flat foot.

Most flat feet do not cause pain or other problems. Flat feet may be associated with pronation, a leaning inward of the ankle bones toward the center line. Shoes of children who pronate, when placed side by side, will lean toward each other (after they have been worn long enough for the foot position to remodel their shape).

Foot pain, ankle pain, or lower leg pain (especially in children) may be a result of flat feet and should be evaluated by a health care provider.

Symptoms

- Absence of longitudinal arch of foot when standing
- Foot pain
- Heel tilts away from the midline of the body more than usual

Exams and Tests

Examination of the foot is sufficient for the health care provider to make the diagnosis of flat foot. However, the underlying cause must be determined. If an arch develops when the patient stands on their toes, then the flat foot is called flexible and no treatment or further work-up is necessary.

If there is pain associated with the foot or if the arch does not develop with toe-standing, x-rays are necessary. If a tarsal coalition is suspected, a computed tomography (CT) scan is often ordered. If a posterior tibial tendon injury is suspected, your health care provider may recommend magnetic resonance imaging (MRI).

Treatment

Flexible flat feet that are painless do not require treatment. If pain due to flexible flat feet occurs, an orthotic (arch supporting insert in the shoe) can bring relief. With the increased interest in running, many shoe stores carry shoes for normal feet and pronated feet. The shoes designed for pronated feet make long-distance running easier and less tiring as they correct for the positional abnormality.

Rigid or painful flat feet require the evaluation of a health care provider. The exact treatment depends on the cause of the flat feet. For tarsal coalition, treatment starts with rest and possibly casting.

If this fails to improve the pain, surgery may be necessary to either resect the fused bone or actually completely fuse several bones in a corrected position. For problems with the posterior tibial tendon, treatment may start with rest, anti-inflammatory medications, and shoe inserts or ankle braces.

In more advanced cases, surgery may be necessary to clean the tendon, repair the tendon, or actually fuse some of the joints of the foot in a corrected position in very advanced cases.

Outlook (Prognosis)

Most cases of flat feet are painless and no problems are to be expected. The prognosis of painful flat feet again depends on the cause of the condition. Usually treatment is successful, regardless of the cause.

If a fusion is required then there is some loss of ankle motion, especially turning the foot inward and outward, but otherwise patients with fusions report tremendous improvement in pain and function.

Possible Complications

Flat feet are not really associated with any complications except pain. Some causes of flat feet can be successfully treated without surgery if caught early, but occasionally, surgery is the last option to relieve pain.

While usually successful, surgery sometimes does not result in satisfactory results for all patients. Some have persistent pain and other possible surgical complications include infection and failure of fused bones to heal.

When to Contact a Medical Professional

Call your health care provider if you experience persistent pain in your feet or your child complains of foot pain or lower leg pain.

Prevention

Most cases are not preventable.

References

Hosalkar HS, Spiegel DA, Davidson RS. The Foot and Toes. In: Kliegman RM, Behrman RE, Jenson HB, Stanton BF, eds. *Nelson Textbook of Pediatrics*. 18th ed. Philadelphia, Pa: Saunders Elsevier; 2007; Chap. 673.

Section 28.3

Growing Pains

"Growing Pains," November 2007, reprinted with permission from www.KidsHealth.org. Copyright © 2007 The Nemours Foundation. This information was provided by KidsHealth, one of the largest resources online for medically reviewed health information written for parents, kids, and teens. For more articles like this one, visit www.KidsHealth.org, or www.TeensHealth.org.

Your eight-year-old son wakes up crying in the night complaining that his legs are throbbing. You rub them and soothe him as much as you can, but you're uncertain about whether to give him any medication or take him to the doctor.

Sound familiar? Your child is probably experiencing growing pains, a normal occurrence in about 25 to 40 percent of children. They generally strike during two periods: in early childhood, among three- to five-year-olds, and later on, in eight- to twelve-year-olds.

What causes them?

No firm evidence exists to show that the growth of bones causes pain. The most likely causes are the aches and discomforts resulting from the jumping, climbing, and running that active children do during the day. The pains can occur after a child has had a particularly athletic day.

What are the signs and symptoms?

Growing pains always concentrate in the muscles, rather than the joints. Most children report pains in the front of their thighs, in the calves, or behind the knees. Whereas joints affected by more serious diseases are swollen, red, tender, or warm, the joints of children experiencing growing pains appear normal.

Although growing pains often strike in late afternoon or early evening before bed, there are occasions when pain can wake a slumbering child. The intensity of the pain varies from child to child, and most kids don't experience the pains every day.

How are growing pains diagnosed?

One symptom that doctors find most helpful in making a diagnosis of growing pains is how the child responds to touch while in pain. Children who have pain for a serious medical disease don't like to be handled because movement tends to increase the pain. But children with growing pains respond differently—they feel better when they're held, massaged, and cuddled.

Growing pains are what doctors call a diagnosis of exclusion. This means that other conditions should be ruled out before a diagnosis of growing pains is made. A thorough history and physical examination by your child's doctor can usually accomplish this. In rare instances, blood and x-ray studies may be required before a final diagnosis of growing pains is made.

How can you help your child?

Some things that may help alleviate the pain include:

- massaging the area;
- stretching;
- placing a heating pad on the area;
- giving ibuprofen or acetaminophen (never give aspirin to a child under twelve due to its association with Reye syndrome, a rare but potentially fatal disease).

When should I call my child's doctor?

Alert your child's doctor if any of the following symptoms occur with your child's pain:

- Persistent pain, pain in the morning, or swelling or redness in one particular area or joint
- Pain associated with a particular injury
- Fever
- Limping
- Unusual rashes
- Loss of appetite
- Weakness
- Tiredness
- Uncharacteristic behavior

These signs are not due to growing pains and should be evaluated by a child's doctor.

Although growing pains often point to no serious illness, they can be upsetting to a child—or a parent. Because a child seems completely cured of the aches in the morning, parents sometimes suspect that the child faked the pains. However, this usually is not the case. Support and reassurance that growing pains will pass as children grow up can help them relax.

Section 28.4

Intoeing

"Intoeing," © 2005 Dartmouth-Hitchcock Medical Center (www.dhmc.org). Reprinted with permission.

Alternative name: pigeon toe

What is intoeing?

Intoeing is when the tips of your feet are turned inward instead of pointing straight forward when walking. It is usually found in children at different ages. In many cases of intoeing in children under the age of eight, the condition corrects itself. There are three different types of intoeing:

- Curved foot (metatarsus adductus), in which the feet point inward from the middle of foot to the toes—sometimes looks like clubfoot
- Twisted shin bone (tibial torsion), in which the leg bone is twisted and causes the feet to turn inward
- Twisted thigh bone (persistent femoral anteversion), in which the hip joint is turned more inward and causes legs and feet to turn inward

What are the signs of intoeing?

- Stumbling

Musculoskeletal Disorders

- Noticeable turning in of feet
- Walking difficulties
- An awkward way of walking (gait)

What causes intoeing?

There is no known cause of intoeing but it can sometimes run in families.

How does a doctor tell if a patient has intoe?

The doctor will take some of the following steps to see if a patient has intoe:

- Look at the legs and feet.
- Watch the walking pattern of the patient.
- Order an x-ray to get a clear view of the bones.

How is intoeing treated?

In children under the age of eight, there is no treatment recommended for intoeing. After a time, the intoeing corrects itself.

Notes below on the three types of intoeing include the recommended treatment when the problem does not correct itself:

- **Curved foot (metatarsus adductus):** Usually this problem corrects itself within the first four to six months of life. If the intoeing is severe, putting on a cast or special shoes might be used to help in realigning the foot and correcting the problem. Surgery is very rarely used for this type of intoeing.

- **Twisted shin bone (tibial torsion):** Usually this problem corrects itself before the child is five years old. In severe cases, surgery is done to reset the bone. Special shoes, exercise programs, and splints have not proved effective.

- **Twisted thigh bone (persistent femoral anteversion):** Usually this problem corrects itself before the child is five years old. In severe cases, surgery is done to reset the bone. Special shoes, exercise programs, and splints have not proved effective.

Section 28.5

Juvenile Rheumatoid Arthritis

"Juvenile Rheumatoid Arthritis," June 2008, reprinted with permission from www.KidsHealth.org. Copyright © 2008 The Nemours Foundation. This information was provided by KidsHealth, one of the largest resources online for medically reviewed health information written for parents, kids, and teens. For more articles like this one, visit www.KidsHealth.org, or www.TeensHealth.org.

It may begin with a swollen knuckle, a spiking fever, or an unexplainable rash. But no matter what symptoms appear, hearing the word "arthritis" in a diagnosis for your child can be unexpected and confusing.

Arthritis is an inflammation of the joints that is characterized by swelling, heat, and pain. Nearly three hundred thousand children in the United States have some sort of arthritis. Arthritis can be short-term—lasting for just a few weeks or months, then going away forever—or it can be chronic and last for months or years. In rare cases, it can last a lifetime.

The most prevalent form of juvenile arthritis is juvenile rheumatoid arthritis, or JRA. It affects approximately fifty thousand children in the United States. JRA also called juvenile idiopathic arthritis (JIA) because it is very different from adult rheumatoid arthritis.

What Causes JRA?

It's not known exactly what causes JRA in kids. Research indicates that it is an autoimmune disease. In autoimmune diseases, white blood cells lose the ability to tell the difference between the body's own healthy cells and harmful invaders like bacteria and viruses. The immune system, which is supposed to protect the body from these harmful invaders, instead releases chemicals that can damage healthy tissues and cause inflammation and pain.

To effectively manage and minimize the effects of arthritis, an early and accurate diagnosis is essential. By understanding the symptoms and characteristics of each type of JRA, you can help your child maintain an active, productive lifestyle.

Types of Juvenile Rheumatoid Arthritis

Typically, juvenile rheumatoid arthritis appears between the ages of six months and sixteen years. The first signs often are joint pain or swelling and reddened or warm joints. Many rheumatologists (doctors specializing in joint disorders) find that the greater the number of joints affected, the more severe the disease and the less likely that the symptoms will eventually go into total remission.

The three major types of juvenile rheumatoid arthritis are:

- Oligoarticular JRA, which affects four or fewer joints. Symptoms include pain, stiffness, or swelling in the joints. The knee and wrist joints are the most commonly affected. An inflammation of the iris (the colored area of the eye) may occur with or without active joint symptoms. This inflammation, called iridocyclitis, iritis, or uveitis, can be detected early by an ophthalmologist.

- Polyarticular arthritis, which affects more girls than boys. Symptoms include swelling or pain in five or more joints. The small joints of the hands are affected as well as the weight-bearing joints such as the knees, hips, ankles, feet, and neck. In addition, a low-grade fever may appear, as well as bumps or nodules on the body on areas subjected to pressure from sitting or leaning.

- Systemic JRA, which affects the whole body. Symptoms include high fevers that often increase in the evenings and then may suddenly drop to normal. During the onset of fever, the child may feel very ill, appear pale, or develop a rash. The rash may suddenly disappear and then quickly appear again. The spleen and lymph nodes may also become enlarged. Eventually many of the body's joints are affected by swelling, pain, and stiffness.

Signs and Symptoms

The first signs of arthritis can be subtle or obvious. Signs may include limping or a sore wrist, finger, or knee. Joints may suddenly swell and remain enlarged. Stiffness in the neck, hips, or other joints can also occur. Rashes may suddenly appear and disappear, developing in one area and then another. High fevers that tend to spike in the evenings and suddenly disappear are characteristic of systemic juvenile rheumatoid arthritis.

Diagnosis

To diagnose JRA, the doctor will take a detailed medical history and conduct a thorough physical examination. The doctor may order x-rays or blood tests to exclude other conditions that can produce similar symptoms.

Other tests that may be done include:

- CBC (complete blood count), a common blood test used to evaluate all the basic cellular components of blood, including red blood cells, white blood cells, and platelets. Abnormalities in the numbers and appearances of these cells can be useful in the diagnosis of many medical conditions.
- Blood culture, a test to detect bacteria that cause infections in the bloodstream. This may be done to rule out infections.
- Bone marrow examination, a test that allows doctors to look at blood where it's formed (in the bone marrow) to rule out conditions such as leukemia.
- Erythrocyte sedimentation rate, which checks how rapidly red blood cells settle to the bottom of a test tube. This rate often increases in people when inflammation is occurring in the body.
- A test for rheumatoid factor, an antibody produced in the blood of children with some forms of JRA. But it's much more commonly found in adults with rheumatoid arthritis.
- ANA (antinuclear antibody), a blood test to detect autoimmunity. It's also useful in predicting which children are likely to have eye disease with JRA.
- A bone scan, to detect changes in bone and joints to evaluate the causes of unexplained bone and joint pain.

In some cases, the doctor may want an orthopedic surgeon to examine your child's joints and take samples of joint fluid or synovium (the lining of the joints) for examination and testing.

Doctors also may test for certain infections such as Lyme disease that may cause similar symptoms or occur along with the arthritis.

Treatments

In many cases, JRA may be treated with a combination of medication, physical therapy, and exercise. In specific situations, your child may require injection of corticosteroids into the joint or surgery. Your child's health care providers, including the primary care physician, rheumatologist, and physical therapist, will work together to develop the best method of treatment.

The goals of treatment are to relieve pain and inflammation, slow down or prevent the destruction of joints, and restore use and function of the joints to promote optimal growth, physical activity, and social and emotional development in your child.

Medications: For inflammation and pain, the doctor or pediatric rheumatologist may prescribe nonsteroidal anti-inflammatory drugs (NSAIDs), like ibuprofen (such as Advil® or Motrin®). These drugs may help reduce inflammation and pain by limiting the release of harmful chemicals from white blood cells.

Higher or lower dosages may be needed, depending upon your child's response to the medication. The doctor or rheumatologist should explain what the medication is meant to do and what side effects, if any, your child may experience. It's important for your child to continue taking the medication until the doctor says to stop.

If NSAIDs do not control inflammation of the joints, your doctor may prescribe other medications such as methotrexate. You can also ask for information about newer treatments that might be available.

Physical therapy: An appropriate physical therapy program is essential in the management of any type of arthritis. A physical therapist will explain the importance of certain activities and recommend exercises suited to your child's specific condition. The therapist may recommend range-of-motion exercises to restore flexibility in stiff, sore joints and other exercises to help build strength and endurance.

Regular exercise: When pain strikes, it's natural for your child to want to sit still. But it's important to maintain a regular exercise program. Muscles must be kept strong and healthy so they can help support and protect joints. Regular exercise also helps to maintain range of motion.

At home and at school, your child should maintain regular exercise and physical fitness programs. Safe activities include walking, swimming, and bicycling (especially on indoor stationary bikes). Always be certain your child warms up the muscles through stretching before exercising. Making exercise a family activity can increase the level of fun and enthusiasm.

Consult the doctor and physical therapist about sports restrictions. Some, especially impact sports, can be hazardous to weakened joints and bones. In addition, make sure your child eats a balanced diet that includes plenty of calcium to promote bone health.

Section 28.6

Juvenile Dermatomyositis

"Juvenile Dermatomyositis (JDM)," is reprinted with permission from the Cincinnati Children's Hospital Medical Center website, http://www.cincinnatichildrens.org. © 2007 Cincinnati Children's Hospital Medical Center. All rights reserved.

What is juvenile dermatomyositis?

Juvenile dermatomyositis (JDM) is a disease in children that causes skin rash (dermato) and muscle inflammation (myositis) resulting in weak muscles.

JDM is a type of autoimmune disease. The immune system is a group of cells that functions to protect the body from infections. In autoimmune diseases like JDM, these cells fight the body's own tissues and cells, resulting in inflammation and tissue damage.

JDM is different from adult dermatomyositis. In JDM, there is no increased risk of cancer. However, blood vessel involvement is frequent and often severe. Also, calcium deposition (calcinosis) is common, especially in the recovery phase.

Who gets JDM?

JDM occurs in children under the age of sixteen and affects three thousand to five thousand children in the United States. Each year there are about three new cases of JDM per million people. JDM occurs twice as often in girls as in boys. The average age of onset is seven years and rarely occurs under the age of two. JDM is encountered worldwide, but is more frequently reported in North America and may be more common in the African-American population. There appears to be a clustering of new cases in the spring and summer.

What causes JDM?

We do not know what causes JDM. Although a number of factors have been investigated, no single factor has been identified as the cause. One view commonly held by researchers in this area (but not scientifically proven) is that myositis requires the combination of two factors—infection and genetics. In this theory, the body has an abnormal response to a virus infection. The immune system attacks and clears the virus, but does not stop this process and begins attacking the body's own tissue(s). There is some evidence to show that some individuals are more likely to have this type of abnormal immune response and that this tendency for the immune system to react in this way is at least partially inherited.

This is not a simple genetic inheritance as seen in other forms of muscle disease such as muscular dystrophy, as it is very, very rare for other family members to develop JDM. In some individuals there appear to be genes or groups of genes which either allow for the immune system to cause the illness to occur or fail to protect the person from developing it.

We do know that JDM is not contagious. Furthermore, there is nothing you could have done more or less of that would have prevented your child from developing this disease.

What are the symptoms of JDM?

In most children, the onset of JDM is characterized by fever in the range of 101 to 104 degrees Fahrenheit and easy fatigue. Almost all children with JDM have less energy and do fewer activities or just refuse to do certain tasks because they know they cannot do them successfully. Weight loss and poor appetite may occur.

The two most characteristic findings in JDM at the time of diagnosis are skin rash and muscle weakness. Muscle weakness and pain often begin gradually. The skin rash generally starts in the first few weeks after the onset of muscle symptoms. However, the skin rash may be absent and many physicians may fail to recognize this disease during its early stages. JDM often goes unrecognized for several months after the onset of symptoms.

The skin rash and muscle weakness are caused by involvement of the blood vessels in the skin and muscles. Blood vessels in the digestive tract can sometimes also become involved resulting in gastrointestinal symptoms. Symptoms can range from mild to rarely life-threatening. Children with JDM can demonstrate periods where symptoms are not present, called remission. The following is a list of the most common findings seen in JDM patients.

Skin rash: The first sign of JDM is often slow development of a skin rash. You may notice your child's eyelids and cheeks become red or purplish and the eyelids may become puffy. This may be misdiagnosed as allergies. Red patches that look like dry skin appear over the knuckles, elbows, and knees. This may be misdiagnosed as eczema. The rash is made worse by sunlight.

Muscle weakness: The muscles closer to the trunk (neck, shoulders, hips) will slowly become very weak. Common movements like climbing stairs and getting up from the floor or chair may become difficult. Your child may complain that their muscles are sore and that they have less energy. In very severe cases of JDM, the muscles used for swallowing can be affected. This can result in choking on food. Your child's voice may also sound faint. If you notice these symptoms occurring, contact the doctor immediately.

Stiff and swollen joints: Your child may complain of stiff and sore joints. The joints or the muscles around them may become inflamed. The inflammation doesn't usually last long or cause joint damage.

Contractures: A contracture is a shortened muscle that causes a joint to remain in a bent position. This can result through the healing process (as the muscle heals, it may scar) or through lack of exercise. Contractures can be avoided by daily exercises and physical therapy.

Ulcers: The ulcers in JDM are caused by breakdown of the tissue surrounding an involved blood vessel that is not providing enough circulation to the tissue. These ulcers most commonly occur in the skin and gastrointestinal tract. When they occur in the skin, they are sores that have a crater-like appearance with an obvious border to the ulcer. These ulcers are very slow to heal and do not scab easily. They vary in severity of the pain from painless to very painful. If a child with JDM develops an ulcer, even a very small one, you need to inform your child's doctors quickly so that treatment can be started. The JDM-related ulcers can occur in any part of the gastrointestinal tract (from the esophagus to the rectum). Your child may complain of pain with swallowing, severe abdominal pain, or bloody stools. In some instances there is very little pain but just dark or bloody stools. If any of these occur in your child you need to contact your doctor immediately.

Calcium deposits: Some children with JDM develop calcium deposit under the skin or in the muscle. The calcium deposits vary in size but are always firm feeling—like little rocks under the skin. Deposits in the muscle can impair muscle movement. In some cases these calcium deposits will break through the skin and drain. These draining areas may become infected. Contact your doctor if this happens.

How is JDM diagnosed?

There is no specific blood test for JDM. To make the diagnosis of JDM requires a combination of information from different sources. The doctor will ask many questions about your child's symptoms (for example, when did the symptoms start?) and perform a detailed physical examination paying special attention to skin and muscles. The doctor will check for rash involving the eyelids, face, knuckles, knees, and elbows. The doctor will also perform a muscle strength exam. Lab tests (blood and urine) will be performed. The most characteristic finding in the lab tests is increased level of one or more muscle-related enzymes (for example creatine phosphokinase [CPK], aldolase, serum glutamic oxaloacetic transaminase [SGOT]). Magnetic resonance imaging (MRI) is a way to view the muscles. MRI does not involve s-ray exposure. MRI can be used to either help make the diagnosis of JDM or to find inflamed muscles most suitable for muscle biopsy. Muscle biopsy provides the most specific information about your child's inflamed muscles and blood vessels. If your child needs a biopsy, the surgeon will remove a small piece of muscle and the pathologist will look at it under the microscope to see if there is any inflammation. Doctors sometimes do not perform muscle biopsies if the child has a typical rash and demonstrates muscle weakness and muscle enzyme elevation in the blood tests.

What is the treatment for JDM?

There is no cure for JDM. However, there are effective treatments that can reduce or eliminate the symptoms and allow people with JDM to lead active, healthy lives. The goals of any treatment program for JDM are to control muscle inflammation and damage, maintain and improve muscle strength and function, relieve pain, control or prevent other symptoms, and help the child and the family to learn to live with the illness. To reach these goals, doctors work with families to find a treatment plan that works best for them. Treatment usually includes medication, physical therapy, and education. As your child's symptoms change, the treatment plan may also be changed. Some common drug therapies are listed below.

Prednisone: Prednisone is the most commonly used drug in the group of medications called steroids, corticosteroids, or glucocorticoids. Other drugs in this group are Solu-Medrol® or prednisolone. Prednisone (or one of the other steroids) is the initial treatment for children with JDM in most instances. Prednisone works quickly to suppress the immune system and help control inflammation in the muscles, joints, and skin. This drug is similar to cortisone, a hormone produced naturally in the body. At first, high doses of this drug are given until your child's muscle enzyme tests and strength improve. As your child gets better, the dose will be gradually reduced. In many instances children will remain on prednisone for at least two years. Side effects depend on both the dose used and the duration of therapy. Common side effects include weight gain, increased appetite, increased risk for infections, and facial swelling. Over a long period of time, the drug can also cause decreased calcium content in the bones, cataracts, high blood pressure, and slowed growth rate. The doctor will try to lower the dose as soon as possible to lessen the side effects, while keeping the disease under control.

Methotrexate: For patients with more severe symptoms that are not controlled by prednisone or as a treatment to allow for fewer steroids to be used, methotrexate is often used. Methotrexate also suppresses the immune system. Methotrexate is also used to treat cancer but in much higher doses. The effect in the body (both in the way that it affects the immune system as well as side effects) of methotrexate in the doses used for treatment of children with JDM are much milder that that seen in treatment of cancer. The doctor will use as low a dose as possible and will usually use it in combination with prednisone. Methotrexate can be given as a pill or by injection. It is given once per week. Common side effects include mouth sores and stomach upset, which can be controlled by taking a vitamin called folic acid. Less common side effects include increased liver enzymes and an increased risk of getting infections.

Hydroxychloroquine (brand name of drug is Plaquenil®): Hydroxychloroquine is a drug that is sometimes used to treat the rash in children with JDM. The drug is given as a pill, usually once daily, and is given in combination with other drugs that control the other symptoms in children with JDM. Hydroxychloroquine is generally tolerated very well. Some will develop stomach upset. Approximately one in every three thousand to five thousand people who take hydroxychloroquine will accumulate pigment in the retina of the eye.

If this is allowed to progress then it could interfere with a person's vision. For this reason, an ophthalmologist (eye doctor) needs to check your child's eyes every six months while your child is taking hydroxychloroquine. If the eye doctor detects any pigment accumulation, the hydroxychloroquine will be stopped before any visual problems develop.

Cyclosporine (brand names Neoral® or Sandimmune®): If prednisone and methotrexate don't fully control your child's JDM your doctor may use cyclosporine. This is another type of immune suppressive drug that was originally developed for organ transplantation. Cyclosporine in combination with methotrexate can help lower the prednisone dose without causing repeat episodes of disease. Side effects that may occur include extra hair growth on the face and arms, swelling of gums, and high blood pressure.

Intravenous immunoglobulin (IVIG): IVIG is a blood-derived product that has been used in the treatment of children with JDM. IVIG consists of purified antibodies which are proteins that the body's immune system uses to fight infection. The mechanism of action is unclear, but IVIG has been shown to slow down the inflammatory process. IVIG is given through a needle into a vein (intravenous or IV) in the hospital, usually once a month. Side effects like headache, fever, and vomiting can occur, but they are usually prevented by pretreating with Tylenol, Benadryl, and sometimes the addition of a steroid.

What is the outcome of JDM?

JDM is a treatable disease. Most children go into remission within two years and may have their medications eliminated. However, some children may have active disease longer than two years, and some may have more severe symptoms than others. Some children with JDM can have repeat episodes of the disease or may have the type of disease that does not easily respond to medications. It is impossible at this time to predict how your child will respond. The most important thing is to take all the medicine your doctor prescribes and perform physical therapy. Despite the challenges children with JDM and their families face, the majority of children grow up to lead an active, productive life.

Section 28.7

Marfan Syndrome

"Learning about Marfan Syndrome," National Human Genome Research Institute, National Institutes of Health, November 27, 2007.

What is Marfan syndrome?

Marfan syndrome is one of the most common inherited disorders of connective tissue. It is an autosomal dominant condition occurring once in every ten thousand to twenty thousand individuals. There is a wide variability in clinical symptoms in Marfan syndrome with the most notable occurring in eye, skeleton, connective tissue, and cardiovascular systems.

Marfan syndrome is caused by mutations in the FBN1 gene. FBN1 mutations are associated with a broad continuum of physical features ranging from isolated features of Marfan syndrome to a severe and rapidly progressive form in newborns.

What are the symptoms of Marfan syndrome?

The most common symptom of Marfan syndrome is myopia (nearsightedness from the increased curve of the retina due to connective tissue changes in the globe of the eye). About 60 percent of individuals who have Marfan syndrome have lens displacement from the center of the pupil (ectopia lentis). Individuals who have Marfan syndrome also have an increased risk for retinal detachment, glaucoma, and early cataract formation.

Other common symptoms of Marfan syndrome involve the skeleton and connective tissue systems. These include bone overgrowth and loose joints (joint laxity). Individuals who have Marfan syndrome have long, thin arms and legs (dolichostenomelia). Overgrowth of the ribs can cause the chest bone (sternum) to bend inward (pectus excavatum or funnel chest) or push outward (pectus carinatum or pigeon breast). Curvature of the spine (scoliosis) is another common skeletal symptom that can be mild or severe and progressively worsen with age. Scoliosis shortens the trunk and also contributes to the arms and legs appearing too long.

Musculoskeletal Disorders

Cardiovascular malformations are the most life threatening symptom of Marfan syndrome. They include dilated aorta just as it leaves the heart (at the level of the sinuses of Valsalva), mitral valve prolapse, tricuspid valve prolapse, enlargement of the proximal pulmonary artery, and a high risk for aortic tear and rupture(aortic dissection).

How is Marfan syndrome diagnosed?

The diagnosis of Marfan syndrome is a clinical diagnosis that is based on family history and the presence of characteristic clinical findings in ocular, skeletal, and cardiovascular systems. There are four major clinical diagnostic features:

- Dilatation or dissection of the aorta at the level of the sinuses of Valsalva
- Ectopia lentis (dislocated lens of the eye)
- Lumbosacral dural ectasia determined by computed tomography (CT) scan or magnetic resonance imaging (MRI)
- Four of the eight typical skeletal features

Major criteria for establishing the diagnosis in a family member also include having a parent, child, or sibling who meets major criteria independently, the presence of an FBN-1 mutation known to cause the syndrome, or a haplotype around FBN-1 inherited by descent and identified in a familial Marfan patient (also known as genetic linkage to the gene).

The FBN1 gene is the gene associated with the true Marfan syndrome. Genetic testing of the FBN1 gene identifies 70 to 93 percent of the mutations and is available in clinical laboratories. However patients negative for the test for gene mutation should be considered for evaluation for other conditions that have similar features of Marfan syndrome such as Dietz syndrome, Ehlers-Danlos syndrome, and homocystinuria. To unequivocally establish the diagnosis in the absence of a family history requires a major manifestation from two systems and involvement of a third system. If a mutation known to cause Marfan syndrome is identified, the diagnosis requires one major criterion and involvement of a second organ system.

To establish the diagnosis in a relative of a patient known to have Marfan Syndrome (index case) requires the presence of a major criterion in the family history and one major criterion in an organ system with involvement of a second organ system.

What is the treatment for Marfan syndrome?

Individuals who have Marfan syndrome are treated by a multidisciplinary medical team that includes a geneticist, cardiologist, ophthalmologist, orthopedist, and cardiothoracic surgeon.

Eye problems are generally treated with eyeglasses. When lens dislocation interferes with vision or causes glaucoma, surgery can be performed and an artificial lens implanted.

Skeletal problems such as scoliosis and pectus excavatum may require surgery. For those individuals who have pes planus (flat feet) arch supports and orthotics can be used to decrease leg fatigue and muscle cramps.

Medication, such as beta blockers, is used to decrease the stress on the aorta at the time of diagnosis or when there is progressive aortic dilatation. Surgery to repair the aorta is done when the aortic diameter is greater than 5 mm in adults and older children, when the aortic diameter increases by 1.0 mm per year, or when there is progressive aortic regurgitation.

Cardiovascular surveillance includes yearly echocardiograms to monitor the status of the aorta. Currently the use of beta blocker medications has delayed but not prevented the need to eventually perform aortic surgery.

Recent work on angiotensin II receptor blockers, another blood pressure medication like beta blockers, has shown additional promise to protect the aorta from dilatation. Clinical trials will be starting soon to see if this drug can prevent the need for surgery better than beta blockers have.

Individuals who have Marfan syndrome are advised to avoid contact and competitive sports and isometric exercise like weight lifting and other static forms of exercise. They can participate in aerobic exercises like swimming. They are also advised to avoid medications such as decongestants and foods that contain caffeine which can lead to chronic increases in blood pressure and stretch the connective tissue in the cardiovascular system.

Is Marfan syndrome inherited?

Marfan syndrome is inherited in families in an autosomal dominant manner. Approximately 75 percent of individuals who have Marfan syndrome have a parent who also has the condition (inherited). Approximately 25 percent of individuals who have Marfan syndrome have the condition as a result of a new (de novo) mutation. When a parent has Marfan syndrome, each of his or her children has a 50 percent chance (one chance in two) to inherit the FBN1 gene. While Marfan syndrome is not always inherited, it is always heritable.

When a child with Marfan syndrome is born to parents who do not show features of the Marfan syndrome, it is likely the child has a new mutation. In this family situation, the chance for future siblings (brothers and sisters of the child with Marfan syndrome) to be born with Marfan syndrome is less than 50 percent. But the risk is still greater than the general population risk of one in ten thousand. The risk is higher for siblings because there are rare families where a Marfan gene mutation is in some percentage of the germline cells of one of the parents (testes or ovaries).

Prenatal testing for Marfan syndrome is available when the gene mutation is known, and also using a technique called linkage analysis (tracking the gene for Marfan syndrome in a family using genetic markers).

Section 28.8

Muscular Dystrophy

"Muscular Dystrophy," reproduced with permission from Moseley C.: Your Orthopaedic Connection. Rosemont, IL, American Academy of Orthopaedic Surgeons, © 2007.

Muscular dystrophy (MD) is a group of rare diseases that cause muscle fibers to weaken and break down. MD affects the skeletal or voluntary muscles that control movement in the arms, legs, and trunk. It also can affect the heart and other involuntary muscles, such as those in the gut. MD passes from parent to child (genetic) and worsens over time (progressive).

There are nine major types of MD affecting people of all ages, from infancy to middle age or later. The two most common types of MD that affect children are Duchenne muscular dystrophy (DMD) and Becker muscular dystrophy (BMD).

Both DMD and BMD affect boys almost exclusively; girls are rarely affected.

MD is a sex-linked recessive disease. It typically passes from a mother (who has no symptoms) to her son.

Symptoms

Both Duchenne MD and Becker MD cause weak muscles, lack of coordination, and progressive disability.

Duchenne Muscular Dystrophy

Duchenne MD begins with muscle loss in the pelvis, upper arms, and legs. The first signs and symptoms of DMD develop between ages two to five years. Symptoms include:

- difficulty walking, such as lateness in learning how to walk (older than eighteen months), having a waddling gait, or walking on the toes or balls of the feet;
- difficulty running or jumping because of weakness in leg muscles;
- frequent falls, stumbling, and difficulty climbing stairs;
- difficulty standing from a lying or sitting position;
- reduced endurance;
- enlarged calf muscles;
- mild mental retardation (in some patients).

Many children with DMD lose their ability to walk by late childhood and require wheelchairs. As muscles continue to weaken in the back and chest, most children develop curvature of the spine (scoliosis). By adolescence, DMD usually progresses to weaken the heart and respiratory muscles.

Becker Muscular Dystrophy

Becker MD begins with muscle loss in the hips, pelvis, thighs, and shoulders. BMD is basically a milder form of Duchenne MD. Symptoms include:

- physical difficulties similar to Duchenne muscular dystrophy;
- waddling gait, perhaps walking on toes or sticking out the abdomen to balance weak muscles.

BMD progresses more slowly over the course of decades, and is a milder and less predictable disease. Some men with BMD need wheelchairs by age thirty years or later; others manage for many years with minor aids, such as a walking cane.

If you think your child may have MD, see your doctor as soon as possible for diagnosis and comprehensive care.

Diagnosis

To diagnose MD, the doctor will take a complete medical history of your child and the family. The doctor will also perform a thorough physical examination of your child and may use laboratory tests to confirm the diagnosis of MD.

Patient History

Tell the doctor if other family members have any signs or symptoms of MD. Be sure to mention if your child has any other health problems. Also, tell the doctor at what age your child achieved growth milestones, such as learning how to walk.

Physical Examination

The doctor will want to see how your child stands up from a sitting position on the floor. Children with DMD use the Gower maneuver to stand up. They start out on their hands and feet, planting their feet widely apart and pushing up their bottom first. Then they use their hands to push up on their knees and thighs. The doctor will also want to watch your child walk. He or she may carefully test the child's muscles and nervous system.

Laboratory Tests

The doctor may use certain laboratory tests to confirm that your child has MD.

Blood tests: The doctor checks a blood sample for high levels of the enzyme creatine kinase, which can indicate muscle damage.

Electromyography: The doctor puts small electrodes into muscle to measure electrical activity. Changes in the pattern of activity can show disease.

Muscle biopsy: The doctor removes a small piece of muscle to study in the laboratory. This can distinguish various forms of MD from other muscle diseases.

Genetic testing: Sometimes, the doctor can study a blood sample to identify an abnormal gene and diagnose MD.

Treatment

Duchenne MD has a more certain and severe disease process than Becker MD. Doctors do not yet have a cure for any type of MD. Fortunately, timely interventions can help slow progression of complications and maximize your child's quality of life.

Nonsurgical Treatment

The goals of nonsurgical treatment of MD include keeping the child's body flexible, upright, and mobile, and helping the child function independently for as long as possible.

The doctor may recommend various nonsurgical treatments:

- **Physical therapy and bracing to prevent contractures:** The doctor may prescribe daily stretching exercises to improve the child's ability to walk. Regular, moderate physical therapy may help maintain range of motion in stiff or "frozen" joints. Walking braces for the ankle-foot or the knee-ankle-foot can help support weak muscles and keep the body flexible, slowing progression of contractures.

- **Medications:** Sometimes a doctor may prescribe anti-inflammatory corticosteroid medications to improve muscle strength and delay progression of DMD. These medications can cause serious side effects.

- **Assistive devices:** Rehabilitative devices such as canes, walkers, wheelchairs, strollers, and electric wheelchairs can help maintain the child's mobility and independence. Sometimes it helps to make modifications to your home, such as widening doorways and installing wheelchair ramps. Eventually, as respiratory muscles weaken, the child may also need the assistance of a breathing device, or ventilator.

Surgical Treatment

- **Surgical release of contractures:** A surgeon may cut through tendons to relieve contractures (tendon release surgery). Some surgeries can help the child continue to walk.

Musculoskeletal Disorders

- **Spinal fusion for scoliosis:** Scoliosis in a wheelchair-dependent child with MD can become so severe that it aggravates breathing problems. Having spine surgery before this happens can help with breathing function, lessen back pain, and improve sitting balance. All of these factors improve the child's quality of life. The doctor may recommend surgery when the spinal curve reaches a certain size (greater than 20 degrees). A surgeon will perform a spinal fusion using metal rods to hold the back in a straighter position.

Coping with Muscular Dystrophy

Like all children, those with MD need to feel loved, valued, and safe. They need to develop strong self-esteem. Parents, siblings, other family members, and friends can help by seeing the child first, not the disease.

Keep a positive attitude, communicate openly and honestly, and be patient and optimistic. By giving your love, support, and encouragement, you can help your child have a happy and rewarding life, despite the challenges of MD. Some tips for coping:

- Encourage your child to stay independent for as long as possible.

- Answer your child's questions about MD. Give an older child more information about the disease, and allow him or her to take part in medical decision making.

- Ask for and accept help from other people. Family members of people with MD face significant physical, emotional, and financial commitments.

- Don't blame yourself for your child's MD. At various times, everyone in the family may experience all the stages of grief—denial, anger, bargaining, depression, and acceptance. As MD progresses, crisis points can trigger powerful emotions. Consider joining a support group to learn coping strategies and to know that you are not alone.

Section 28.9

Osgood-Schlatter Disease

"Osgood-Schlatter Disease," © 2008 Children's Healthcare of Atlanta (www.choa.org). Reprinted with permission.

Osgood-Schlatter disease is an overuse condition of the knee, frequently diagnosed in growing and active athletes. The condition results in pain and swelling in the area below the knee, on the upper part of the tibia (shin bone). It is commonly seen in preteen and teenage boys and girls when they are at the peak of their growth potential.

Osgood-Schlatter disease involves a bump or knot that arises from the upper end of the shin bone, just below the knee. It causes pain with a lot of rigorous activities, particularly running or jumping.

Osgood-Schlatter disease occurs at the insertion of the quadriceps mechanism (thigh muscle and tendon) into the tibia (shin bone). The muscle inserts into the patella (knee cap) and from there, the patellar tendon runs down to one of the apophyses (growth centers) called the tibial tubercle. The knee is a hinge joint.

The quadriceps pull the tibia forward (extension) while the hamstrings pull the tibia backward (flexion). This produces the rhythmic and often rigorous back and forth motion of walking or running. In the case of Osgood-Schlatter disease, the pull of the patellar tendon overworks the apophysis of the tibial tubercle. This produces an inflammation which is uncomfortable. In addition, the body begins to lay down more bone to reinforce the area and the prominence (that all of us have) begins to enlarge.

Are X-rays Necessary?

X-rays may be ordered by a doctor to confirm the diagnosis or to exclude other problems. Often, the diagnosis is made based upon the clinical information and the doctor's experience. X-rays are more likely to be ordered if the condition affects only one side, or if there are other factors raising the doctor's concern to other possible diagnoses.

What Can Be Done?

Treatment is focused on decreasing the symptoms in the athlete. The majority of cases respond quickly by applying ice to the knee, modifying activity and taking anti-inflammatory medicine for ten to fourteen days at a time.

In some instances, a knee pad or sleeve may be used to apply pressure, provide support, and protect the tender area from being bumped.

There are rarely long lasting side effects of Osgood-Schlatter disease. In a very small percentage of cases, a tiny piece of bone forms in the end of the patellar tendon. This bone fragment can be painful and may require removal through a minor outpatient surgical procedure.

While the symptoms can be very frustrating to the active, competitive athlete, keep in mind that reassurance and symptomatic treatment are usually adequate in managing the condition.

Relief Treatments

Physical therapy: Physical therapy may be ordered by the primary care doctor to instruct the athlete in proper quadriceps and hamstring stretching, and strengthening exercises.

Ice: Icing can be a very effective anti-inflammatory treatment. The best time to apply ice is immediately after the workout, such as the car ride home from the game or practice field. One effective way to ice is to apply an ice cup massage. Fill several Styrofoam cups with water and freeze them. When frozen, tear off one inch around the cup's rim to create a frozen snow cone. The ice should be applied directly to the sore area in a circular massaging motion until the area becomes numb, usually about ten to fifteen minutes. This can be repeated every sixty to ninety minutes, several times a day.

Medicine: Anti-inflammatory medicine or nonsteroidal anti-inflammatory drugs (NSAIDs) can be another effective treatment. A doctor may suggest an over-the-counter medicine, such as ibuprofen (Motrin® or Advil®) or naproxen (Aleve®), or prescribe a medicine. For those young athletes who can swallow pills, Aleve works well because it needs to be taken only twice a day (morning and night).

It does not need to be taken during school or right before workouts. Ibuprofen should be taken three times a day. Anti-inflammatory medicine should be taken for ten to fourteen days to allow the medicine to build up to therapeutic levels in the body. Taking medicine every now and then allows the levels to drop; this decreases the effectiveness of the medication.

Activity modification: Because Osgood-Schlatter disease is rarely a serious problem and does not involve the joint, activities do not often need to be stopped completely. Minimizing certain activities such as sprinting, jumping, or squatting during a workout may lessen the discomfort. For sports where a direct blow to the knee is possible, such as football, basketball, soccer, and lacrosse, a knee pad may offer protection.

Section 28.10

Scoliosis

Excerpted from "Questions and Answers about Scoliosis in Children and Adolescents," National Institute of Arthritis and Musculoskeletal and Skin Diseases, July 2001. Reviewed by David A. Cooke, M.D., July 2008.

What is scoliosis?

Scoliosis is a musculoskeletal disorder in which there is a sideways curvature of the spine, or backbone. The bones that make up the spine are called vertebrae. Some people who have scoliosis require treatment. Other people, who have milder curves, may only need to visit their doctor for periodic observation.

Who gets scoliosis?

People of all ages can have scoliosis, but this section focuses on children and adolescents. Of every one thousand children, three to five develop spinal curves that are considered large enough to need treatment. Adolescent idiopathic scoliosis (scoliosis of unknown cause) is the most common type and occurs after the age of ten. Girls are more likely than boys to have this type of scoliosis. Since scoliosis can run in families, a child who has a parent, brother, or sister with idiopathic scoliosis should be checked regularly for scoliosis by the family physician.

Idiopathic scoliosis can also occur in children younger than ten years of age, but is very rare. Early onset or infantile idiopathic scoliosis occurs in children less than three years old. It is more common in Europe than in the United States. Juvenile idiopathic scoliosis occurs in children between the ages of three and ten.

What causes scoliosis?

In 80 to 85 percent of people, the cause of scoliosis is unknown; this is called idiopathic scoliosis. Before concluding that a person has idiopathic scoliosis, the doctor looks for other possible causes, such as injury or infection. Causes of curves are classified as either nonstructural or structural.

Nonstructural (functional) scoliosis: A structurally normal spine that appears curved. This is a temporary, changing curve. It is caused by an underlying condition such as a difference in leg length, muscle spasms, or inflammatory conditions such as appendicitis. Doctors treat this type of scoliosis by correcting the underlying problem.

Structural scoliosis: A fixed curve that doctors treat case by case. Sometimes structural scoliosis is one part of a syndrome or disease, such as Marfan syndrome, an inherited connective tissue disorder. In other cases, it occurs by itself. Structural scoliosis can be caused by neuromuscular diseases (such as cerebral palsy, poliomyelitis, or muscular dystrophy), birth defects (such as hemivertebra, in which one side of a vertebra fails to form normally before birth), injury, certain infections, tumors (such as those caused by neurofibromatosis, a birth defect sometimes associated with benign tumors on the spinal column), metabolic diseases, connective tissue disorders, rheumatic diseases, or unknown factors (idiopathic scoliosis).

How does the doctor diagnose scoliosis?

The doctor takes the following steps to evaluate a patient for scoliosis:

- **Medical history:** The doctor talks to the patient and the patient's parent or parents and reviews the patient's records to look for medical problems that might be causing the spine to curve, for example, birth defects, trauma, or other disorders that can be associated with scoliosis.

- **Physical examination:** The doctor looks at the patient's back, chest, pelvis, legs, feet, and skin. The doctor checks if the patient's shoulders are level, whether the head is centered, and whether opposite sides of the body look level. The doctor also examines the back muscles while the patient is bending forward to see if one side of the rib cage is higher than the other. If there is a significant asymmetry (difference between opposite sides of the body), the doctor will refer the patient to an orthopedic spine specialist (a doctor who has experience treating people with scoliosis). Certain changes in the skin, such as so-called café au lait (coffee-with-milk-colored) spots, can suggest that the scoliosis is caused by a birth defect.

- **X-ray evaluation:** Patients with significant spinal curves, unusual back pain, or signs of involvement of the central nervous system (brain and spinal cord) such as bowel and bladder control problems need to have an x-ray. The x-ray should be done with the patient standing with his or her back to the x-ray machine. The view is of the entire spine on one long (36-inch) film. Occasionally, doctors ask for more tests to see if there are other problems.

- **Curve measurement:** The doctor measures the curve on the x-ray image. He or she finds the vertebrae at the beginning and end of the curve and measures the angle of the curve Curves that are greater than 20 degrees require treatment.

Doctors group curves of the spine by their location, shape, pattern, and cause. They use this information to decide how best to treat the scoliosis.

Location: To identify a curve's location, doctors find the apex of the curve (the vertebra within the curve that is the most off-center); the location of the apex is the "location" of the curve. A thoracic curve has its apex in the thoracic area (the part of the spine to which the ribs attach). A lumbar curve has its apex in the lower back. A thoracolumbar curve has its apex where the thoracic and lumbar vertebrae join.

Shape: The curve usually is S- or C-shaped.

Pattern: Curves frequently follow patterns that have been studied in previous patients. The larger the curve is, the more likely it will progress (depending on the amount of growth remaining).

Does scoliosis have to be treated? What are the treatments?

Many children who are sent to the doctor by a school scoliosis screening program have very mild spinal curves that do not need treatment. When a child does need treatment, the doctor may send him or her to an orthopedic spine specialist.

The doctor will suggest the best treatment for each patient based on the patient's age, how much more he or she is likely to grow, the degree and pattern of the curve, and the type of scoliosis. The doctor may recommend observation, bracing, or surgery.

Observation: Doctors follow patients without treatment and re-examine them every four to six months when the patient is still growing (is skeletally immature) and has an idiopathic curve of less than 25 degrees.

Bracing: Doctors advise patients to wear a brace to stop a curve from getting any worse when the patient is still growing and has an idiopathic curve that is more than 25 to 30 degrees; has at least two years of growth remaining, has an idiopathic curve that is between 20 and 29 degrees, and, if a girl, has not had her first menstrual period; or is still growing and has an idiopathic curve between 20 and 29 degrees that is getting worse.

As a child nears the end of growth, the indications for bracing will depend on how the curve affects the child's appearance, whether the curve is getting worse, and the size of the curve.

Surgery: Doctors advise patients to have surgery to correct a curve or stop it from worsening when the patient is still growing, has a curve that is more than 45 degrees, and has a curve that is getting worse.

Are there other ways to treat scoliosis?

Some people have tried other ways to treat scoliosis, including manipulation by a chiropractor, electrical stimulation, dietary supplements, and corrective exercises. So far, studies of the following treatments have not been shown to prevent curve progression, or worsening:

- Chiropractic manipulation
- Electrical stimulation
- Nutritional supplementation
- Exercise

Studies have shown that exercise alone will not stop progressive curves. However, patients may wish to exercise for the effects on their general health and well-being.

Which brace is best?

The decision about which brace to wear depends on the type of curve and whether the patient will follow the doctor's directions about how many hours a day to wear the brace.

There are two main types of braces. Braces can be custom-made or can be made from a prefabricated mold. All must be selected for the specific curve problem and fitted to each patient. To have their intended effect (to keep a curve from getting worse), braces must be worn every day for the full number of hours prescribed by the doctor until the child stops growing.

Milwaukee brace: Patients can wear this brace to correct any curve in the spine. This brace has a neck ring.

Thoracolumbosacral orthosis (TLSO): Patients can wear this brace to correct curves whose apex is at or below the eighth thoracic vertebra. The TLSO is an underarm brace, which means that it fits under the arm and around the rib cage, lower back, and hips.

If the doctor recommends surgery, which procedure is best?

Many surgical techniques can be used to correct the curves of scoliosis. The main surgical procedure is correction, stabilization, and fusion of the curve. Fusion is the joining of two or more vertebrae. Surgeons can choose different ways to straighten the spine and also different implants to keep the spine stable after surgery. (Implants are devices that remain in the patient after surgery to keep the spine aligned.) The decision about the type of implant will depend on the cost; the size of the implant, which depends on the size of the patient; the shape of the implant; its safety; and the experience of the surgeon. Each patient should discuss his or her options with at least two experienced surgeons.

Patients and parents who are thinking about surgery may want to ask the following questions:

- What are the benefits of surgery for scoliosis?
- What are the risks of surgery for scoliosis?

- What techniques will be used for the surgery?
- What devices will be used to keep the spine stable after surgery?
- Where will the incisions be made?
- How straight will the patient's spine be after surgery?
- How long will the hospital stay be?
- How long will it take to recover from surgery?
- Is there chronic back pain after surgery for scoliosis?
- Will the patient's growth be limited?
- How flexible will the spine remain?
- Can the curve worsen or progress after surgery?
- Will additional surgery be likely?
- Will the patient be able to do all the things he or she wants to do following surgery?

Can people with scoliosis exercise?

Although exercise programs have not been shown to affect the natural history of scoliosis, exercise is encouraged in patients with scoliosis to minimize any potential decrease in functional ability over time. It is very important for all people, including those with scoliosis, to exercise and remain physically fit. Girls have a higher risk than boys of developing osteoporosis (a disorder that results in weak bones that can break easily) later in life. The risk of osteoporosis is reduced in women who exercise regularly all their lives; and weight-bearing exercise, such as walking, running, soccer, and gymnastics, increases bone density and helps prevent osteoporosis. For both boys and girls, exercising and participating in sports also improves their general sense of well-being.

What are researchers trying to find out about scoliosis?

Researchers are looking for the cause of idiopathic scoliosis. They have studied genetics, growth, structural and biochemical alterations in the discs and muscles, and central nervous system changes. The changes in the discs and muscles seem to be a result of scoliosis and not the cause. Scientists are still hopeful that studying changes in the central nervous system in people with idiopathic scoliosis may reveal a cause of this disorder.

Childhood Diseases and Disorders Sourcebook, Second Edition

Researchers continue to examine how a variety of braces, surgical procedures, and surgical instruments can be used to straighten the spine or to prevent further curvature. They are also studying the long-term effects of a scoliosis fusion and the long-term effects of untreated scoliosis.

Chapter 29

Neurological Disorders

Chapter Contents

Section 29.1—Brain Tumors 470
Section 29.2—Cerebral Palsy 485
Section 29.3—Epilepsy 492
Section 29.4—Febrile Seizures 499
Section 29.5—Headache 503
Section 29.6—Neurofibromatosis 508
Section 29.7—Tourette Syndrome 515

Section 29.1

Brain Tumors

"Pediatric FAQ," © 2008 National Brain Tumor Foundation (www.braintumor.org). Reprinted with permission.

What is a brain tumor?

A brain tumor is an abnormal mass of tissue in which some cells grow and multiply uncontrollably, apparently unregulated by the mechanisms that control normal cells. The growth of a tumor takes up space within the skull and interferes with normal brain activity. A tumor can cause damage by increasing pressure in the brain, by shifting the brain or pushing against the skull, and by invading and damaging nerves and healthy brain tissue. The location of a brain tumor influences the type of symptoms that occur. This is because different functions are controlled by different parts of the brain.

Brain tumors rarely metastasize (spread) to other parts of the body outside of the central nervous system (CNS). The CNS includes the brain and spinal cord.

Some tumor types are more common in children than in adults. When childhood brain tumors occur in adults, they often occur in a different part of the brain than in children. Brain tumors in children are often located in the brain stem and cerebellum, while in adults they often occur in the cerebral hemispheres. Although most primary tumors attack members of both sexes with equal frequency, some, such as meningiomas, occur more frequently in women, while others, such as medulloblastomas, more commonly afflict boys and young men.

The prognosis for brain tumor patients is as individual as the patients themselves. Your child's doctors will help you understand the possible consequences of your child's specific tumor.

What are the common symptoms of brain tumors in children?

Some of the general symptoms of brain tumors in children are headaches; vomiting (usually in the morning and without nausea);

unsteadiness or loss of balance; seizures; double vision or vision problems; decreased coordination; fatigue or sleepiness; weakness on one side of the body; increased size of the head; uncontrolled eye movements; irritability; and behavioral changes.

Symptoms are often vague in children, especially in very young children who are not able to fully describe their symptoms. Some of these symptoms can occur in a variety of more common childhood illnesses. The difference with brain tumors is that these symptoms persist and get worse over time. If your child is experiencing any of the above-mentioned symptoms, it is important to see a doctor and get a definitive diagnosis.

Pediatric brain tumors are not contagious. Their causes are unknown.

What is the difference between a benign brain tumor and a malignant (cancerous) brain tumor?

Benign brain tumors are slow-growing tumors that can be removed or destroyed if in an accessible location. Malignant tumors (brain cancer) are rapidly growing tumors that invade or infiltrate and destroy normal brain tissue. No one is certain why, but some benign brain tumors may change over time to become malignant.

Tumors are graded to indicate how quickly they are growing. Most medical institutions use the World Health Organization (WHO) classification system to identify brain tumors. The WHO classifies brain tumors by cell origin and how the cells behave, from the least aggressive (benign) to the most aggressive (malignant). Some tumor types are assigned a grade, which signifies the rate of growth. There are variations in grading systems, depending on the tumor type. The classification and grade of an individual tumor help predict its likely behavior.

The distinction between benign and malignant can be ambiguous. Some benign tumors can be as dangerous as malignant ones if in a dangerous or inaccessible location, such as the brain stem. Conversely, some malignant tumors can be cured.

Although they may fall into a specific classification or category, brain tumors are specific to each individual. Brain tumors have vastly different characteristics and patterns of growth due to the molecular makeup of the individual tumor.

How are pediatric brain tumors diagnosed?

A brain tumor diagnosis usually involves several steps, which can include a neurological examination, brain scan(s), and/or a biopsy.

Should a child's symptoms lead the doctor to suspect a tumor, a neurological examination will be given. This is a series of tests to measure the function of the child's nervous system and physical and mental alertness. If responses to the neurological exam are not normal, the doctor may order a scan.

A brain scan is a picture of the internal structures in the brain. A specialized machine takes a scan in much the same way a digital camera takes a photograph. Using computer technology, a scan compiles an image of the brain by photographing it from various angles. Magnetic resonance imaging (MRI) and computerized tomography (CT) scans may confirm the presence and location of a tumor. Other studies, such as an electroencephalogram (EEG) or examination of cerebrospinal fluid (CSF) may also be done.

MRI (magnetic resonance imaging) is a scanning device that uses magnetic fields and computers to capture images of the brain on film. It does not use x-rays. It provides pictures from various planes, which permit doctors to create a three-dimensional image of the tumor. The MRI detects signals emitted from normal and abnormal tissue, providing clear images of most tumors.

CT or CAT scan (computed tomography) combines sophisticated x-ray and computer technology. CT can show a combination of soft tissue, bone, and blood vessels. CT images can determine some types of tumors, as well as help detect swelling, bleeding, and bone and tissue calcification.

CT is a valuable diagnostic tool and its use has been increasing rapidly. However, CT scans involve exposure to ionizing radiation, which is known to cause cancer. This is a concern for children, because they are more sensitive to radiation than adults. It is wise for parents of children who have brain tumors to keep a record of their x-ray history. This information can help doctors make informed decisions and minimize radiation overexposure.

Some types of scans use a contrast agent, which helps the doctor to see the difference between normal and abnormal brain tissue. The contrast agent is injected into a vein and flows into brain tissue. Abnormal brain tissue absorbs more dye than normal tissue. Contrast agents may cause allergic reactions in some patients. Gadolinium, the contrast agent used with an MRI, may cause temporary headaches but has no other known side effects. Usually, iodine is the contrast agent used during a CT scan. If your child is allergic to iodine, tell your doctor beforehand.

The most accurate diagnosis of a brain tumor is made with surgery, which permits the neurosurgeon to see the tumor and obtain a specimen for a pathological examination.

Neurological Disorders

A biopsy is a surgical procedure in which a sample of tissue is taken from the tumor site and examined under a microscope. The biopsy will provide information on types of abnormal cells present in the tumor. The purpose of a biopsy is to discover the type and grade of a tumor. An open biopsy is done during a craniotomy. A craniotomy involves removing a piece of the skull in order to get access to the brain. After the tumor is resected (completely removed) or debulked (partially removed), the bone is usually put back into place. A closed biopsy (also called stereotactic or needle biopsy) may be performed when the tumor is in an area of the brain that is difficult to reach. In a closed biopsy, the neurosurgeon drills a small hole into the skull and passes a narrow, hollow needle into the tumor to remove a sample of tissue.

Once a sample is obtained, a pathologist examines the tissue under a microscope and writes a pathology report containing an analysis of the brain tissue. Sometimes the pathologist may not be able to make an exact diagnosis. This may be because more than one grade of tumor cells exists within the same tumor. In some cases, the tissue may be sent to another institution for additional analysis.

How are pediatric brain tumors treated?

The standard treatments for brain tumors are surgery, radiation therapy, and chemotherapy. In some cases when the tumor is slow growing, the treatment team may delay surgery and use frequent scans to monitor the tumor's growth.

Sometimes surgery alone will cure a brain tumor. In general, radiation and chemotherapy treatments are used as secondary or adjuvant treatments for tumors that cannot be managed using only surgery. However, radiation and chemotherapy may be used without surgery if the tumor is inoperable. Use of radiation therapy is avoided in children below the age of three because it causes significant long-term damage to the developing brain.

In many cases, at the time of diagnosis, treatment decisions must be made quickly, especially with regard to surgery. When possible, the doctor and family will discuss a treatment plan based on the type and location of the tumor. In treating brain tumors, a multidisciplinary treatment team, made up of various specialists, is generally considered the preferred approach. Neurosurgeons, neurologists, radiation oncologists, pathologists, and other medical professionals may be part of the treatment team.

The goal of brain surgery, or resection, is to remove as much of a tumor as possible without causing damage to critical neurological functions.

When only part of a tumor can be resected, it is possible that the tumor will recur (grow back). However, a partial resection can sometimes relieve symptoms and improve the effectiveness of other therapies.

Some childhood brain tumors block the flow of cerebrospinal fluid (CSF) in the ventricles (spaces within the brain), leading to hydrocephalus (water on the brain). This condition causes increased intracranial pressure, leading to neurological problems. In such cases, the neurosurgeon will implant a ventriculoperitoneal (VP) shunt to drain the excess fluid from the ventricles into the abdominal cavity and relieve the pressure in the brain. This type of surgery is performed under general anesthesia. A small hole is drilled into the skull and a small catheter (tube) is passed into a ventricle of the brain. A valve which controls the flow of fluid is attached to the catheter to keep the fluid away from the brain. Another catheter is attached to the valve and tunneled under the skin, behind the ear, down the neck and chest, and into the peritoneal (abdominal) cavity. The excess fluid is reabsorbed by the body. Ask your neurosurgeon about the type of shunt, potential problems and what symptoms to look out for that might indicate a problem, and the expected duration of shunt placement.

Radiation therapy uses high-energy x-rays or other types of ionizing radiation to stop cancer cells from dividing. Radiation therapy may be used when surgery is not advised, for tumors that cannot be completely resected, or after surgery to prevent or delay tumor recurrence. Radiation therapy can stop or slow the growth of inoperable tumors.

Conventional radiation therapy delivers radiation to an entire region of the brain. The radiation is fractionated into many small doses and given over a period of time (usually five to seven weeks, excluding weekends). Depending on the location, type, and size of the tumor(s), the treatment may be either focused or whole brain radiation therapy (WBRT). Focused radiation therapy aims x-rays at the tumor and area surrounding it. WBRT aims radiation at the entire brain.

Stereotactic radiosurgery (SRS) delivers a single, high dose of radiation in a one-day session. A head frame or mask is used to hold the head in position, then CT or MRI scans are taken. With the aid of computer imaging, the location of the tumor is accurately calculated. The radiation is delivered directly to the tumor, often from several different directions. Size and location of the tumor are important eligibility criteria for SRS.

The goal of radiation therapy is to give the maximum amount of radiation to tumor cells while sparing healthy brain tissue.

Chemotherapy uses chemicals (drugs) that have a toxic effect on tumor cells as they divide. Chemotherapy is usually taken orally or by injection, and may be given alone or in combination with other treatments. Chemotherapy is given in cycles, which consist of "on" and "off" phases—days of treatment followed by periods of time between treatments. Cycles vary depending on the drug or drugs used. Chemotherapy is usually a secondary therapy. It is also used to delay or replace radiation treatment in young children.

Most chemotherapy drugs enter and affect the entire body, causing a range of side effects. Side effects are caused when the drugs damage normal cells that are dividing. Reactions can range from mild to severe. All side effects should be reported to the doctor. There are treatments available to alleviate many of these problems. Antiemetics (antinausea drugs) have greatly reduced the nausea chemotherapy patients have experienced in the past. Your child's doctors will work with you to minimize or prevent anticipated side effects. In some cases, the type of chemotherapy drug may be changed.

How do I choose my child's treatment team?

There are many medical centers with teams that specialize in treating pediatric brain tumor patients. There is no one "best" doctor, but there are issues to consider that can help guide you in choosing the doctor that is best for your child. Good communication is key to a good relationship with your doctors. If you ask your questions and get them answered, the experience will be easier for you and your family. If you are not comfortable with your doctor, consider changing doctors.

Getting a second opinion is important if your child's doctor does not have experience with brain tumors or if you want to confirm your primary physician's recommendation. Ask your doctor for a referral to a specialist. You can also research different treatment centers, or call the National Brain Tumor Foundation. They can provide you with phone numbers of comprehensive cancer centers and medical centers of excellence specific to pediatric brain tumors.

There are many important questions to ask when choosing a treatment center. Does the center have specialists in neurosurgery, neurology, neuro-oncology and radiation oncology? What types of imaging technology are available? How many patients does the medical center diagnose and treat per year?

Where can I go for social and emotional support?

Many people rely on family and friends or their spiritual community for support. Medical social workers can connect you with local resources. Support groups, including internet-based groups, can often provide contact with other people in a similar situation. A good support system is important to help families cope with the crisis brought on by a child's brain tumor diagnosis.

There are organizations with resources available to help patients and their families cope with the disease. Some hold summer camps for children with cancer and their siblings. Wish-fulfillment agencies grant wishes for children with life-threatening illnesses.

What about returning to school?

Frequent or prolonged absence from the classroom may disrupt the learning process. A child with a brain tumor may face the additional challenge of physical changes in the structure of the brain, which affect the thought and learning processes. It is important to identify these changes and to adopt teaching and learning strategies that capitalize on the child's strengths and compensate for the child's weaknesses. These changes can best be identified by neuropsychological testing.

Neuropsychological testing measures cognitive skills (memory, learning, language), motor skills, and social skills. It is used to help schools plan for optimal educational interventions. Child development centers associated with major medical centers generally have neuropsychologists who are skilled not only in administering testing but also in making recommendations for optimal functioning of the child. Many insurance companies require a letter of necessity from your child's doctor to cover this service. Once a child's educational needs have been identified, those involved in meeting these needs must decide upon a plan of action (called an individualized educational plan or IEP) to ensure that these needs are met.

Prior to a full return to school, the social worker or school liaison on your child's treatment team can help your child to participate in school activities to the best of his or her current ability and energy. This can be done through partial attendance, hospital-based schooling, or "home-bound" tutoring. When your child is able to return to school more fully, there are several steps you can take to ease that transition.

How a child is feeling on any given day will also affect his or her academic performance. The attitude of the child's teacher and peers toward the child who is ill may also affect his or her behavior and performance in school.

Some children can continue to attend school while in treatment. Many are at risk of problems with their self-image and relationships

Neurological Disorders

with peers, especially if educators and classmates misunderstand the side effects of the child's illness and treatments. To make the transition back to school easier, the teacher and school nurse should be encouraged to prepare classmates by supplying them with information and answering their questions. Some medical centers provide a child life worker and health care practitioner who can help prepare the class for your child's return. Ask your child's healthcare team about how they can help.

Which Brain Tumors Are Most Common in Children?

Some tumor types are more common in children than in adults. The most common types of childhood tumors are brain stem gliomas, craniopharyngiomas, ependymomas, juvenile pilocytic astrocytomas, medulloblastomas, optic nerve gliomas, pineal tumors, primitive neuroectodermal tumors (PNET), and rhabdoid tumors.

Brain Stem Glioma

Characteristics

- Named for its location at the base of the brain.
- Can range from low grade to high grade.
- Occurs most often in children between three and ten years of age, but can occur in adults.

Symptoms

- Headaches
- Nausea
- Speech or balance abnormalities
- Difficulty swallowing
- Weakness or numbness of the arms and/or legs
- Facial weakness
- Double vision

Symptoms can develop slowly and subtly and may go unnoticed for months. In other cases, the symptoms may arise abruptly. A sudden onset of symptoms tends to occur with rapidly growing, high-grade tumors.

Treatment

Surgery may not be an option because the brain stem controls vital life functions and can easily be damaged. Radiation therapy can reduce symptoms and help slow the tumor's growth. Low-grade brain stem gliomas can have very long periods of remission.

Craniopharyngioma

Characteristics

- Most common in the parasellar region, an area at the base of the brain and near the optic nerves.
- Also grows in the regions of the optic nerves and the hypothalamus, near the pituitary gland.
- Tends to be low grade.
- Often accompanied by a cyst.
- Originates in cells left over from early fetal development.
- Occurs in children and men and women in their fifties and sixties.

Symptoms

- Headaches
- Visual changes
- Weight gain
- Delayed development in children

Treatment

Surgery is the most common treatment. Radiation therapy may be used.

Ependymoma

Ependymal tumors begin in the ependyma, cells that line the passageways in the brain where cerebral spinal fluid (CSF) is produced and stored. Ependymomas are classified as either supratentorial (in the cerebral hemispheres) or infratentorial (in the back of the brain). Variations of this tumor type include subependymoma, subependymal giant-cell astrocytoma, and malignant ependymoma. Ependymoblastoma, which occurs in infants and children under three years, is no longer considered a subtype of ependymoma. For ependymoblastoma, see primitive neuroectodermal tumor (PNET) below.

Characteristics

- Usually localized to one area of the brain.
- Develops from cells that line the hollow cavities at the bottom of the brain and the canal containing the spinal cord.
- Can be slow growing or fast growing.
- May be located in the ventricles.
- May block the ventricles, causing hydrocephalus (water on the brain).
- Sometimes extends to the spinal cord.
- Common in children, and among men and women in their forties and fifties.
- Occurrence peaks at age five and again at age thirty-four.
- Accounts for 2 percent of all brain tumors.

Symptoms

- Severe headaches
- Nausea and vomiting
- Difficulty walking
- Fatigue and sleepiness
- Problems with coordination
- Neck pain or stiffness
- Visual problems

Treatment

The doctor will perform tests to determine if it has spread to the spinal cord. Surgery followed by radiation therapy is the usual course of treatment. A shunt may be needed to treat hydrocephalus caused by blockage of the ventricles.

Juvenile Pilocytic Astrocytoma (JPA)

This tumor is also known as a pilocytic astrocytoma, or by the initials JPA. Astrocytoma tumors develop from star-shaped glial cells (astrocytes) that support nerve cells. Astrocytomas are the most common primary CNS tumor. Astrocytomas are generally classified as low or high grade. Low-grade astrocytomas are slow growing. High-grade astrocytomas (grades three and four) grow more quickly. Juvenile pilocytic astrocytoma is a low-grade (grade one) tumor. Symptoms tend to be subtle and may take one to two years to diagnose. This is because the brain can often adapt to a slow-growing tumor for a period of time. High-grade tumors may present with changes that are sudden and dramatic.

Characteristics

- Slow growing, with relatively well-defined borders.
- Grows in the cerebrum, optic nerve pathways, brain stem, and cerebellum.
- Occurs most often in children and teens.
- Accounts for 2 percent of all brain tumors.

Symptoms

- Headaches
- Seizures or convulsions
- Difficulty thinking or speaking
- Behavioral or cognitive changes (related to thinking, reasoning, and memory)
- Weakness or paralysis in one part or one side of the body
- Loss of balance
- Vision changes
- Nausea or vomiting

Treatment

Surgery is the standard treatment. If the tumor cannot be completely resected, radiation or chemotherapy may be given. Chemotherapy may be given to very young children instead of radiation therapy to avoid damage to the developing brain. Some of these tumors can progress to a higher grade, so it is important to be diligent about following up with the medical team after treatment.

Medulloblastoma

Characteristics

- A type of primitive neuroectodermal tumor (PNET) (see following).
- Often located in the cerebellum or near the brain stem.
- Can spread to the spinal cord through the CSF.
- May obstruct the fourth ventricle, causing hydrocephalus.
- Occurs most often in children under the age of ten, but may occur in adults.
- Slightly more common in males than females.

Symptoms

- Headaches
- Early morning vomiting
- Lethargy or sleepiness
- Lack of coordination
- Double vision
- Behavioral or personality changes
- Signs of pressure seen behind the eye when examined with an ophthalmoscope

Treatment

Surgery is the standard treatment when possible. Chemotherapy is usually part of the treatment plan. Radiation of the brain and spine is often recommended in adults and children over three years of age. A shunt may be needed to treat hydrocephalus. This tumor may recur years later if not totally resected.

Optic Nerve Glioma

Characteristics

- Named for its location on or near the nerve pathways between the eyes and the brain.
- Can range from low grade to high grade.
- Occurs most often in infants and children, but can occur in adults.

Symptoms

- Headaches
- Progressive loss of vision
- Double vision

Treatment

Surgery is standard treatment, usually followed by radiation therapy or chemotherapy. Chemotherapy may be given to very young children instead of radiation therapy to avoid damage to the developing brain.

Pineal Tumor

A malignant form of pineal tumor is called pineoblastoma.

Characteristics

- Named for its location in or around the pineal gland (near the center of the brain).
- Can range from low grade to high grade.
- Can produce an excess of melatonin, a hormone that controls the sleep/wake cycle.
- Can block the ventricles, causing hydrocephalus.
- High-grade pineal tumors can spread to the spinal cord through the CSF.
- Common types include germ cell tumors, pineal parenchymal tumors, and gliomas.
- Occurs most often in children and young adults.

Symptoms

- Headaches
- Nausea and vomiting
- Fatigue
- Double vision
- Memory problems

Neurological Disorders

Treatment

Surgery is standard treatment when possible. Radiation therapy may be used as primary treatment in adults and children over three. Chemotherapy may be given to delay the use of radiation therapy in very young patients. Clinical trials using chemotherapy drugs are available for pineal tumors. A shunt may be needed to treat hydrocephalus caused by blockage of the ventricles. Treatment for high-grade (malignant) pineal tumors such as a pineoblastoma may involve radiation to the brain and spine to control spread through the CSF. Clinical trials using chemotherapy or biological therapy following radiation therapy are being investigated.

Primitive Neuroectodermal Tumors (PNET)

There are several tumor types in this category. Names of specific PNETs may be based on the tumor location. Examples include pineoblastoma (located in the pineal region), medulloblastoma (located in the cerebellum), and cerebral cortex PNET (located in the cerebral cortex).

Characteristics

- Highly aggressive and tend to spread throughout the CNS.
- Grow from undeveloped brain cells.
- Commonly include cysts and calcification (calcium deposits).
- Tend to be large.
- Occur most often in young children.

Symptoms

- Can vary depending on location of tumor
- Weakness or change in sensation on one side of the body
- Morning headache or headache that goes away after vomiting
- Nausea and vomiting
- Seizures
- Unusual sleepiness or lethargy
- Behavioral or personality changes
- Unexplained weight loss or weight gain

Treatment

Surgery is the standard treatment when possible. In adults and children over three years of age, surgery may be followed by radiation therapy to the whole brain and spinal cord, and chemotherapy. In children under three years of age, surgery may be followed by chemotherapy or a clinical trial of chemotherapy to delay or reduce the need for radiation therapy.

Rhabdoid Tumor

Characteristics

- Rare.
- Highly aggressive and tends to spread throughout the CNS.
- Often appears in multiple sites in the body, especially the kidneys.
- Difficult to classify; may be confused with medulloblastoma or PNETs.
- Occurs most often in young children but can also occur in adults.

Symptoms

- Vary depending on location of tumor in the brain or body.
- An orbital tumor may cause the eye to protrude.
- Balance problems may occur.
- External tumors cause noticeable lumps; internal tumor symptoms vary based on location.

Treatment

Whenever possible, surgery is performed to remove as much of the tumor as possible. This is usually followed by chemotherapy and radiation therapy. In children under three years of age, surgery may be followed by chemotherapy alone. Clinical trials are being studied using autologous bone marrow transplantation after high-dose chemotherapy for recurrent or multiple rhabdoid tumors.

Section 29.2

Cerebral Palsy

"Cerebral Palsy," © 2007 March of Dimes Birth Defects Foundation. All rights reserved. For additional information, contact the March of Dimes at their website www.marchofdimes.com.

Cerebral palsy refers to a group of conditions that affect movement, balance, and posture. Affected children have abnormalities in one or more parts of the brain that affect the ability to control muscles. Symptoms range from mild to severe but do not get worse as the child gets older. With treatment, most children can significantly improve their abilities.

Many children with cerebral palsy have other conditions that require treatment. These include mental retardation, learning disabilities, seizures, abnormal physical sensations (difficulties with sense of touch), and problems with vision, hearing, and speech.

How common is cerebral palsy?

Cerebral palsy usually is diagnosed by three years of age. About 2 to 3 children in 1,000 are affected.[1] About 800,000 children and adults of all ages in the United States have cerebral palsy.[2]

What are the different types of cerebral palsy?

There are three major types of cerebral palsy. Some individuals may have symptoms of more than one type.

Spastic cerebral palsy: About 70 to 80 percent of affected individuals have the spastic type, in which muscles are stiff, making movement difficult.[1] Spastic diplegia is a form of spastic cerebral palsy in which both legs are affected. Affected children may have difficulty walking because tight muscles in the hips and legs cause legs to turn inward and cross at the knees (called scissoring). In spastic hemiplegia, only one side of the body is affected, often with the arm more severely affected than the leg. Most severe is spastic quadriplegia, in which all four limbs, the trunk and face are affected. Children with spastic quadriplegia usually cannot walk. They often have mental retardation, difficulty speaking, and seizures.

Athetoid or dyskinetic cerebral palsy: About 10 to 20 percent of affected individuals have the athetoid form, which affects the entire body.[1] It is characterized by fluctuations in muscle tone (varying from too tight to too loose) and sometimes is associated with uncontrolled movements (which can be slow and writhing or rapid and jerky). Affected children often have trouble learning to control their bodies well enough to sit and walk. Because muscles of the face and tongue can be affected, there also can be difficulties with sucking, swallowing and speech.

Ataxic cerebral palsy: About 5 to 10 percent of affected individuals have the ataxic form, which affects balance and coordination. They may walk with an unsteady gait with feet far apart. They have difficulty with motions that require precise coordination, such as writing.

What are the causes of cerebral palsy?

Cerebral palsy usually is caused by factors that disrupt normal development of the brain before birth. In some cases, genetic defects may contribute to brain malformations and "miswiring" of nerve cell connections in the brain, resulting in cerebral palsy.[2] Other cases are caused by injuries to the developing brain, such as a fetal stroke. Contrary to common belief, few cases of cerebral palsy are caused by a lack of oxygen reaching the fetus during labor and delivery.[2]

A small number of babies develop brain injuries in the first months or years of life that can result in cerebral palsy.[2] These injuries may be caused by brain infection (such as meningitis) and head injuries. In many cases, the cause of cerebral palsy in a child is not known.

Certain risk factors make it more likely that a baby will develop cerebral palsy. However, most babies with one of these risk factors do not develop cerebral palsy. Risk factors for cerebral palsy include:

- **Prematurity:** Premature babies (those born before thirty-seven completed weeks of pregnancy) who weigh less than 3 1/3 pounds are between twenty and eighty times more likely to develop cerebral palsy than full-term babies.[3] Many of these tiny babies suffer from bleeding in the brain, which can damage delicate brain tissue, or develop periventricular leukomalacia, destruction of nerves around the fluid-filled cavities (ventricles) in the brain.

- **Infections during pregnancy:** Certain infections in the mother can cause brain damage and result in cerebral palsy. Examples of these infections include rubella, cytomegalovirus (usually mild viral infection), herpes (viral infections that can cause genital sores), and toxoplasmosis (a usually mild parasitic infection). Maternal infections involving the placental membranes (chorioamnionitis) may contribute to cerebral palsy in full-term as well as premature babies.[2] A 2003 study at the University of California at San Francisco found that full-term babies were four times more likely to develop cerebral palsy if they were exposed to chorioamnionitis in the womb.[4]

- **Insufficient oxygen reaching the fetus:** This may occur when the placenta is not functioning properly or it tears away from the wall of the uterus before delivery.

- **Asphyxia during labor and delivery:** Until recently, it was widely believed that asphyxia (lack of oxygen) during a difficult delivery was the cause of most cases of cerebral palsy. Studies now show that birth complications, including asphyxia, contribute to only 5 to 10 percent of cases of cerebral palsy.[2]

- **Severe jaundice:** Jaundice, a yellowing of the skin and whites of the eyes, is caused by the buildup of a pigment called bilirubin in the blood. Mild cases of jaundice usually clear up without treatment and do not harm the baby. However, jaundice can occasionally become severe. Affected babies have high levels of bilirubin in the blood. Without treatment, high bilirubin levels can pose a risk of permanent brain damage, resulting in athetoid cerebral palsy. Certain blood diseases, such as Rh disease, can cause severe jaundice and brain damage, resulting in cerebral palsy. Rh disease is an incompatibility between the blood of the mother and her fetus. It usually can be prevented by giving an Rh-negative woman an injection of a blood product called Rh immune globulin around the twenty-eighth week of pregnancy and again after the birth of an Rh-positive baby.

- **Blood clotting disorders (thrombophilias):** These disorders in either mother or baby may increase the risk of cerebral palsy.

What are some early signs of cerebral palsy?

Some children with cerebral palsy may have delays in learning to roll over, sit, crawl, or walk. The Centers for Disease Control and

Prevention (CDC) recommends that parents contact their child's provider if they see any of the following signs:[5]

- A child more than two months old who:
  - has difficulty controlling her head when picked up;
  - has stiff legs that cross or "scissor" when picked up.
- A child more than six months old who:
  - reaches with only one hand while keeping the other in a fist.
- A child more than ten months old who:
  - crawls by pushing off with one hand and leg while dragging the opposite hand and leg.
- A child more than twelve months old who:
  - cannot crawl;
  - cannot stand with support.

How is cerebral palsy diagnosed?

Cerebral palsy is diagnosed mainly by evaluating how a baby or young child moves. The provider evaluates the child's muscle tone; children with cerebral palsy may appear floppy or stiff. Some may have variable muscle tone (too loose at times and too tight at other times).

The provider checks the child's reflexes and looks to see if the baby has developed a preference for using his right or left hand. While most babies do not develop a hand preference (become right- or left-handed) until at least twelve months of age, some babies with cerebral palsy do so before six months of age.

Another important sign of cerebral palsy is the persistence of certain reflexes, called primitive reflexes. These reflexes are normal in younger infants but generally disappear by six to twelve months of age. The provider also takes a careful medical history and attempts to rule out any other disorders that could be causing the symptoms.

The provider may suggest brain imaging tests, such as magnetic resonance imaging (MRI), computed tomography (CT scan), or ultrasound. These tests sometimes can help identify the cause of cerebral palsy. Ultrasound often is recommended in premature babies who are considered at risk for cerebral palsy to help diagnose brain abnormalities that are frequently associated with cerebral palsy. In some children with cerebral palsy, especially those who are mildly affected, brain

Neurological Disorders

imaging tests show no abnormalities, suggesting that microscopically small areas of brain damage can cause symptoms.

About half of babies who are suspected to be at higher risk for cerebral palsy at twelve months of age appear to outgrow their symptoms by age two.[6]

How is cerebral palsy treated?

A team of health care professionals works with the child and family to identify the child's needs and create an individualized treatment plan to help the child reach his or her maximum potential. The team is generally coordinated by one health care professional and may include pediatricians, physical medicine and rehabilitation physicians, orthopedic surgeons, physical and occupational therapists, ophthalmologists (eye doctors), speech/language pathologists, social workers, and psychologists.

The child usually begins physical therapy soon after diagnosis. Therapy improves motor skills (such as sitting and walking) and muscle strength and helps prevent contractures (shortening of muscles that limits joint movement). Sometimes braces, splints, or casts are used along with physical therapy to help prevent contractures and to improve function of the hands or legs. If contractures are severe, surgery may be recommended to lengthen affected muscles.

Drugs sometimes are recommended to ease spasticity or to reduce abnormal movement. Unfortunately, oral drug treatment often is not very helpful. Sometimes injection of drugs, such as Botox (botulinum toxin), directly into spastic muscles is helpful. The effects may last several months.

A new type of drug treatment is showing promise in children with moderate to severe spasticity. During a surgical procedure, a pump is implanted under the skin that continuously delivers the anti-spasmodic drug baclofen.

For some children with spastic cerebral palsy, a surgical technique called selective dorsal rhizotomy may permanently reduce spasticity and improve the ability to sit, stand, and walk. In this procedure, doctors identify and cut some of the nerve fibers at the base of the spine that are contributing most to spasticity. This procedure usually is recommended only for children with severe spasticity who have not responded well to other treatments.[2]

Occupational therapists work with the child on skills required for daily living, including feeding and dressing. Children with speech problems work with a speech therapist or, in more severe cases, learn to use a computerized voice synthesizer that can speak for them. Computers have become an important tool for children and adults with cerebral palsy in terms of therapy, education, recreation, and employment.

Some children with cerebral palsy may benefit from the many mechanical aids available today, including walkers, positioning devices (to allow a child with abnormal posture to stand correctly), customized wheelchairs, and specially adapted scooters and tricycles.

Can cerebral palsy be prevented?

In many cases, the cause of cerebral palsy is not known, so there is nothing that can be done to prevent it. However, some causes of cerebral palsy can be prevented by eliminating or managing certain risk factors.

Rh disease and congenital rubella syndrome used to be common causes of cerebral palsy. Now Rh disease usually can be prevented when an Rh-negative pregnant woman receives appropriate care. Women can be tested for immunity to rubella before pregnancy and vaccinated if they are not immune. A woman can help reduce her risk of preterm delivery when she seeks early (ideally starting with a preconception visit) and regular prenatal care and avoids cigarettes, alcohol, and illicit drugs.

Babies with severe jaundice can be treated with special lights (phototherapy) and blood transfusions (exchange transfusions), when indicated. Head injuries in babies and young children often can be prevented when babies ride in car seats properly positioned in the back seat of the car and when children wear helmets when riding bicycles. Routine vaccination of babies (with the Hib vaccine) prevents many cases of meningitis, another cause of brain damage in the early months.

Is the March of Dimes conducting research on cerebral palsy?

The March of Dimes supports a number of grants on prenatal brain development and factors that may disrupt it.

One grantee is studying how developing nerve cells in the fetal brain respond to prolonged oxygen deprivation. This can improve understanding of how lack of oxygen before or around the time of birth can injure the developing brain and how such brain injuries can be prevented or treated.

Another grantee is investigating how intrauterine infections may contribute to brain injuries that result in cerebral palsy, with the goal of developing drug treatments to help prevent these injuries.

A grantee also is studying specific learning disabilities in young children with cerebral palsy in order to develop improved interventions.

Many other March of Dimes grantees are seeking improved ways of preventing preterm delivery, an important risk factor for cerebral palsy.

References

1. Centers for Disease Control and Prevention (CDC). Cerebral Palsy. October 4, 2004, accessed September 14, 2007.

2. National Institute of Neurological Disorders and Stroke. Cerebral Palsy: Hope Through Research. NIH Publication Number 06-159, updated 7/13/07.

3. Platt, M., et al. Trends in Cerebral Palsy Among Infants of Very Low Birthweight (<1500 g) or Born Prematurely (<32 Weeks) in 16 European Centres: A Database Study. *Lancet*, volume 369, January 6, 2006, pages 43–50.

4. Wu, Y.W., et al. Chorioamnionitis and Cerebral Palsy in Term and Near-Term Infants. *Journal of the American Medical Association*, volume 290, number 20, November 26, 2003, pages 2677–84.

5. Centers for Disease Control and Prevention (CDC). Learn the Signs, Act Early: Cerebral Palsy Fact Sheet. December 7, 2006.

6. Pellegrino, Louis. Cerebral palsy, in Batshaw, M.L. (ed.), *Children With Disabilities*, Fifth Edition, Baltimore, MD, Paul H. Brooks Publishing Company, 2002, pages 433–66.

Section 29.3

Epilepsy

© 2008 A.D.A.M., Inc. Reprinted with permission.

Alternative Names

Seizure disorder

Definition

Epilepsy is a brain disorder involving repeated seizures of any type.

Causes

Seizures ("fits") are episodes of disturbed brain function that cause changes in attention or behavior. They are caused by abnormal excited electrical signals in the brain.

Sometimes seizures are related to a temporary condition, such as exposure to drugs, withdrawal from certain drugs, or abnormal levels of sodium or glucose in the blood. In such cases, repeated seizures may not recur once the underlying problem is corrected.

In other cases, injury to the brain (for example, stroke or head injury) causes brain tissue to be abnormally excitable. In some people, an inherited abnormality affects nerve cells in the brain, which leads to seizures.

Some seizures are idiopathic, which means the cause can not be identified. Such seizures usually being between age five and twenty, but can occur at any age. People with this condition have no other neurological problems, but often have a family history of seizures or epilepsy.

Disorders affecting the blood vessels, such as stroke and transient ischemic attack (TIA), are the most common cause of seizures after age sixty. Degenerative disorders such as senile dementia Alzheimer type can also lead to seizures.

Some of the more common causes of seizures include:

Neurological Disorders

- Developmental problems, genetic conditions present at birth, or injuries near birth (seizures usually begin in infancy or early childhood);
- Metabolic abnormalities may affect people of any age and may be a result of diabetes complications:
  - electrolyte imbalances;
  - kidney failure, uremia (toxic accumulation of wastes);
  - nutritional deficiencies;
  - phenylketonuria (PKU)—can cause seizures in infants;
  - other metabolic diseases, such as inborn error of metabolism;
  - use of cocaine, amphetamines, alcohol, or certain other recreational drugs;
  - withdrawal from alcohol;
  - withdrawal from drugs, particularly barbiturates and benzodiazepines;
- Brain injury:
  - most common in young adults;
  - seizures usually begin within two years after the injury;
  - early seizures (within two weeks of injury) do not necessarily mean that chronic (ongoing) seizures (epilepsy) will develop;
- Tumors and brain lesions (such as hematomas):
  - may affect any age but are more common after age thirty;
  - partial (focal) seizures most common to start with;
  - may lead to generalized tonic-clonic seizures;
- Infections:
  - may affect people of all ages;
  - may be a reversible cause of seizures;
  - brain infections like meningitis and encephalitis can produce seizures;
  - brain abscess;
  - acute severe infections of any part of the body;

- chronic infections (such as neurosyphilis);
- complications of acquired immunodeficiency syndrome (AIDS) or other immune disorders.

Seizure disorders affect about 0.5 percent of the population. Approximately 1.5 to 5.0 percent of the population may have a seizure in their lifetime. Epilepsy can affect people of any age.

Risk factors include a family history of epilepsy, head injury, or other condition that causes damage to the brain.

The following factors may present a risk for worsening of seizures in a person with a previously well-controlled seizure disorder:

- Pregnancy
- Lack of sleep
- Skipping doses of epilepsy medications
- Use of alcohol or other recreational drugs
- Certain prescribed medications
- Illness

Symptoms

The severity of symptoms can vary greatly, from simple staring spells to loss of consciousness and violent convulsions. For many patients, the event is the same thing over and over, while some people have many different types of seizures that cause different symptoms each time. The type of seizure a person has depends on a variety of many things, such as the part of the brain affected and the underlying cause of the seizure.

An aura consisting of a strange sensation (such as tingling, smell, or emotional changes) occurs in some people prior to each seizure. Seizures may occur repeatedly without explanation.

Note: Disorders that may cause symptoms resembling seizures include transient ischemic attacks (TIAs), rage or panic attacks, and other disorders that cause loss of consciousness.

Symptoms of Generalized Seizures

Generalized seizures affect all or most of the brain. They include petit mal and grand mal seizures.

Petit mal seizures:

Neurological Disorders

- minimal or no movements (usually, except for "eye blinking")—may appear like a blank stare;
- brief sudden loss of awareness or conscious activity—may only last seconds;
- recurs many times;
- occurs most often during childhood;
- decreased learning (child often thought to be daydreaming).

Tonic-clonic (grand mal) seizures:

- whole body, violent muscle contractions;
- rigid and stiff;
- affects a major part of the body;
- loss of consciousness;
- breathing stops temporarily, followed by sighing;
- incontinence of urine;
- tongue or cheek biting;
- confusion following the seizure;
- weakness following the seizure (Todd paralysis).

Symptoms of Partial Seizures (Simple and Complex)

Partial seizures may be complex or simple. Partial seizures affect only a portion of the brain.

Symptoms of simple partial (focal) seizures may include:

- muscle contractions of a specific body part;
- abnormal sensations;
- nausea;
- sweating;
- skin flushing;
- dilated pupils.

Symptoms of partial complex seizures may include:

- automatism (automatic performance of complex behaviors without conscious awareness);

- abnormal sensations;
- nausea;
- sweating;
- skin flushing;
- dilated pupils;
- recalled or inappropriate emotions;
- changes in personality or alertness;
- may or may not lose consciousness;
- problems with smell or taste—if the epilepsy is focused in the temporal lobe of the brain.

Exams and Tests

The diagnosis of epilepsy and seizure disorders requires a history of recurrent seizures of any type. A physical examination (including a detailed neuromuscular examination) may be normal, or it may show abnormal brain function related to specific areas of the brain.

An electroencephalograph (EEG), a reading of the electrical activity in the brain, may confirm the presence of various types of seizures. It may, in some cases, indicate the location of the lesion causing the seizure. EEGs can often be normal in between seizures, so it may be necessary to do prolonged EEG monitoring.

Tests may include various blood tests to rule out other temporary and reversible causes of seizures, including:

- complete blood count (CBC);
- blood chemistry;
- blood glucose;
- liver function tests;
- kidney function tests;
- tests for infectious diseases;
- CSF (cerebrospinal fluid) analysis.

Tests for the cause and location of the problem may include:

- head computed tomography (CT) or magnetic resonance imaging (MRI) scan;
- lumbar puncture (spinal tap).

Treatment

If an underlying cause for recurrent seizures (such as infection) has been identified and treated, seizures may stop. Treatment may include surgery to repair tumors or brain lesions.

Anticonvulsants taken by mouth may reduce the number of future seizures. How well medicine works depends on each individual's response to the drug. The type of medicine used depends on seizure type, and dosage may need to be adjusted from time to time. Some seizure types respond well to one medication and may respond poorly (or even be made worse) by others. Some medications need to be monitored for side effects and blood levels.

Epilepsy that does not respond to the use of several medications is called refractory epilepsy. Certain people with this type of epilepsy may benefit from brain surgery to remove the abnormal brain cells that are causing the seizures. Others may be helped with a vagal nerve stimulator, which is implanted in the chest. This stimulator can help reduce the number of seizures.

Sometimes, children are placed on a special diet to help prevent seizures. One is the ketogenic diet.

Patients should wear medical alert jewelry so that prompt medical treatment can be obtained if a seizure occurs.

Support Groups

The stress caused by having seizures (or being a caretaker of someone with seizures) can often be helped by joining a support group. In these groups, members share common experiences and problems.

Outlook (Prognosis)

Epilepsy may be a chronic, lifelong condition. In some cases, the need for medications may be reduced or eliminated over time. Certain types of childhood epilepsy resolve or improve with age. A seizure-free period of four years may indicate that reduction or elimination of medications is possible.

Death or permanent brain damage from seizures is rare, but can occur if the seizure is prolonged or two or more seizures occur close together (status epilepticus). Death or brain damage are most often caused by prolonged lack of breathing and resultant death of brain tissue from lack of oxygen. There are some cases of sudden, unexplained death in patients with epilepsy.

Serious injury can occur if a seizure occurs during driving or when operating dangerous equipment, so these activities may be restricted for people with poorly controlled seizure disorders.

Infrequent seizures may not severely restrict the person's lifestyle. Work, school, and recreation do not necessarily need to be restricted.

Possible Complications

- Prolonged seizures or numerous seizures without complete recovery between them (status epilepticus).
- Injury from falls, bumps, or self-inflicted bites.
- Injury from having a seizure while driving or operating machinery.
- Inhaling fluid into the lungs and subsequent aspiration pneumonia.
- Permanent brain damage (stroke or other damage).
- Difficulty with learning.
- Side effects of medications.
- Many anti-epileptic medications cause birth defects—women wishing to become pregnant should alert their doctor in advance in order to adjust medications.

When to Contact a Medical Professional

Call your local emergency number (911) if this the first time a person has had a seizure or a seizure is occurring in someone without a medical identification (ID) bracelet (instructions explaining what to do). In the case of someone who has had seizures before, call the ambulance for any of these emergency situations:

- This is a longer seizure than the person normally has, or an unusual number of seizures for the person.
- Repeated seizures over a few minutes.
- Repeated seizures where consciousness or normal behavior is not regained between them (status epilepticus).

Call your health care provider if any new symptoms occur, including possible side effects of medications (drowsiness, restlessness, confusion, sedation, or others), nausea/vomiting, rash, loss of hair, tremors or abnormal movements, or problems with coordination.

Prevention

Generally, there is no known way to prevent epilepsy. However, adequate diet and sleep, and abstinence from drugs and alcohol, may decrease the likelihood of precipitating a seizure in people with epilepsy.

Reduce the risk of head injury by wearing helmets during risky activities; this can help lessen the chance of developing epilepsy.

Section 29.4

Febrile Seizures

Excerpted from "Febrile Seizures Fact Sheet," National Institute of Neurological Disorders and Stroke, National Institutes of Health, NIH Publication No. 06-3930, December 27, 2007.

What are febrile seizures?

Febrile seizures are convulsions brought on by a fever in infants or small children. During a febrile seizure, a child often loses consciousness and shakes, moving limbs on both sides of the body. Less commonly, the child becomes rigid or has twitches in only a portion of the body, such as an arm or a leg, or on the right or the left side only. Most febrile seizures last a minute or two, although some can be as brief as a few seconds while others last for more than fifteen minutes.

The majority of children with febrile seizures have rectal temperatures greater than 102 degrees F. Most febrile seizures occur during the first day of a child's fever. Children prone to febrile seizures are not considered to have epilepsy, since epilepsy is characterized by recurrent seizures that are not triggered by fever.

How common are febrile seizures?

Approximately one in every twenty-five children will have at least one febrile seizure, and more than one-third of these children will have additional febrile seizures before they outgrow the tendency to have them. Febrile seizures usually occur in children between the ages of six months and five years and are particularly common in toddlers. Children rarely develop their first febrile seizure before the age of six months or after three years of age. The older a child is when the first febrile seizure occurs, the less likely that child is to have more.

What makes a child prone to recurrent febrile seizures?

A few factors appear to boost a child's risk of having recurrent febrile seizures, including young age (less than fifteen months) during the first seizure, frequent fevers, and having immediate family members with a history of febrile seizures. If the seizure occurs soon after a fever has begun or when the temperature is relatively low, the risk of recurrence is higher. A long initial febrile seizure does not substantially boost the risk of recurrent febrile seizures, either brief or long.

Are febrile seizures harmful?

Although they can be frightening to parents, the vast majority of febrile seizures are harmless. During a seizure, there is a small chance that the child may be injured by falling or may choke from food or saliva in the mouth. Using proper first aid for seizures can help avoid these hazards.

There is no evidence that febrile seizures cause brain damage. Large studies have found that children with febrile seizures have normal school achievement and perform as well on intellectual tests as their siblings who don't have seizures. Even in the rare instances of very prolonged seizures (more than one hour), most children recover completely.

Between 95 and 98 percent of children who have experienced febrile seizures do not go on to develop epilepsy. However, although the absolute risk remains very small, certain children who have febrile seizures face an increased risk of developing epilepsy. These children include those who have febrile seizures that are lengthy, that affect only part of the body, or that recur within twenty-four hours, and children with cerebral palsy, delayed development, or other neurological abnormalities. Among children who don't have any of these risk factors, only one in one hundred develops epilepsy after a febrile seizure.

What should be done for a child having a febrile seizure?

Parents and caregivers should stay calm and carefully observe the child. To prevent accidental injury, the child should be placed on a protected surface such as the floor or ground. The child should not be held or restrained during a convulsion. To prevent choking, the child should be placed on his or her side or stomach. When possible, the parent should gently remove all objects in the child's mouth. The parent should never place anything in the child's mouth during a convulsion. Objects placed in the mouth can be broken and obstruct the child's airway. If the seizure lasts longer than ten minutes, the child should be taken immediately to the nearest medical facility. Once the seizure has ended, the child should be taken to his or her doctor to check for the source of the fever. This is especially urgent if the child shows symptoms of stiff neck, extreme lethargy, or abundant vomiting.

How are febrile seizures diagnosed and treated?

Before diagnosing febrile seizures in infants and children, doctors sometimes perform tests to be sure that seizures are not caused by something other than simply the fever itself. For example, if a doctor suspects the child has meningitis (an infection of the membranes surrounding the brain), a spinal tap may be needed to check for signs of the infection in the cerebrospinal fluid (fluid that bathes the brain and spinal cord). If there has been severe diarrhea or vomiting, dehydration could be responsible for seizures. Also, doctors often perform other tests such as examining the blood and urine to pinpoint the cause of the child's fever.

A child who has a febrile seizure usually doesn't need to be hospitalized. If the seizure is prolonged or is accompanied by a serious infection, or if the source of the infection cannot be determined, a doctor may recommend that the child be hospitalized for observation.

How are febrile seizures prevented?

If a child has a fever most parents will use fever-lowering drugs such as acetaminophen or ibuprofen to make the child more comfortable, although there are no studies that prove that this will reduce the risk of a seizure. One preventive measure would be to try to reduce the number of febrile illnesses, although this is often not a practical possibility.

Prolonged daily use of oral anticonvulsants, such as phenobarbital or valproate, to prevent febrile seizures is usually not recommended because of their potential for side effects and questionable effectiveness for preventing such seizures.

Children especially prone to febrile seizures may be treated with the drug diazepam orally or rectally, whenever they have a fever. The majority of children with febrile seizures do not need to be treated with medication, but in some cases a doctor may decide that medicine given only while the child has a fever may be the best alternative. This medication may lower the risk of having another febrile seizure. It is usually well tolerated, although it occasionally can cause drowsiness, a lack of coordination, or hyperactivity. Children vary widely in their susceptibility to such side effects.

What research is being done on febrile seizures?

Some studies suggest that women who smoke or drink alcohol during their pregnancies are more likely to have children with febrile seizures, but more research needs to be done before this link can be clearly established. Scientists are also working to pinpoint factors that can help predict which children are likely to have recurrent or long-lasting febrile seizures.

Investigators continue to monitor the long-term impact that febrile seizures might have on intelligence, behavior, school achievement, and the development of epilepsy. For example, scientists conducting studies in animals are assessing the effects of seizures and anticonvulsant drugs on brain development.

Investigators also continue to explore which drugs can effectively treat or prevent febrile seizures and to check for side effects of these medicines.

Section 29.5

Headache

"Headaches in Children," © 2007 American Headache Society (www.achenet.org). Reprinted with permission.

Did you know?

- Headaches can be a common problem in children.
- Somewhere between 4 and 10 percent of children have migraine headaches.
- Many adults with headaches started having their headaches as children, with 20 percent reporting the onset before age ten.
- Most headaches in children are benign—meaning they are not symptoms of some serious disorder or disease.
- Migraine headaches often run in families, so information on other family member's headaches are important.
- Headache may interfere with participation in activities and school and can be a significant health problem.

What is a primary headache?

Headaches can be divided into two categories, primary or secondary.

Primary refers to headaches that occur on their own and not as the result of some other health problem. Primary headaches include migraine, migraine with aura, tension-type headache, and cluster headache.

Secondary refers to headaches that result from some cause or condition, such as a head injury or concussion, blood vessel problems, medication side effects, infections in the head or elsewhere in the body, sinus disease, or tumors. There are many different causes for secondary headaches, ranging from rare, serious diseases to easily treated conditions.

When to call the doctor about your child's headache?

You should consult your family doctor if headaches are frequent or severe or include unusual symptoms. Your physician may ask you to describe features of your headache (for example, the location of the pain, pain severity, and any other symptoms associated with the headache attack). To rule out possibility of secondary headache, the physician may decide to order special tests, including a computed tomography (CT) scan or magnetic resonance imaging (MRI). Worrisome symptoms that should be brought to your doctor's attention include:

- headaches that wake a child from sleep;
- early morning vomiting without nausea (upset stomach);
- worsening or more frequent headaches;
- personality changes;
- complaints that "this is the worst headache I've ever had!";
- the headache is different than previous headaches;
- headaches with fever or a stiff neck;
- headaches that follow an injury.

Why do you need to know what kind of headache your child is having?

As you may be aware, children suffer from a number of different types of headaches. It is important to rule out any dangerous cause for their headache that may classify it as a "secondary headache." It also is important to understand what type of headache your child has because it will impact treatment, level of disability, and lifestyle factors that will impact how to take care of a child with headaches. For example, a child with migraine may have a common factor that precedes their attack, such as fasting or low blood sugar. Therefore, it is important to know how to avoid conditions that may increase the risk of an attack and have medications that are specific for the headache being treated.

What is a tension-type headache (episodic)?

This type of headache has also been called a tension headache, muscle contraction headache, stress-related headache, and "ordinary headache." These headaches can be either episodic or chronic and may include tightness in the muscles of the head or neck. A tension-type headache can last from thirty minutes to several days. Chronic tension headaches may persist for many months. The pain usually occurs on both sides of the head, is steady and nonthrobbing. Some people say "it feels like a band tightening around my head." The pain is usually mild to moderate in severity. Most of the time the headache does not affect the person's activity level.

Tension-type headaches are usually not associated with other symptoms, such as nausea or vomiting. Some people may experience sensitivity to light or sound with the headache, but not both. Muscle tightness may be noticed by some patients but doesn't always have to occur.

What is a migraine headache (episodic)?

Migraine headaches are recurrent headaches that occur at intervals of days, weeks, or months. There may or may not be a pattern to the attacks—for example, teenage girls may tend to have attacks associated with their menstrual cycle. Migraines generally have some of the following symptoms and characteristics:

- Untreated, they can last from one to seventy-two hours in children. Sleep or medical treatment can reduce this time period.
- Headache starts on one side of the head. This may vary from headache to headache and in children, they may start in the front or in both temples.
- Throbbing or pounding pain during the headache.
- Pain is rated as moderate to severe.
- Pain gets worse with exertion. The pain may be so severe that it is difficult or almost impossible to continue with normal daily activities.
- Nausea, vomiting, and/or stomach pain commonly occur with the attacks.
- Light and/or sound sensitivity is also common.
- Pain may be relieved with rest or sleep.
- Other members of the family have had migraines or "sick headaches."
- Auras, or a visual disturbance, may occur in some children between five and sixty minutes prior to the headache. These auras

are recognized as blurry vision, flashing lights, colored spots, or even dizziness.

What can we do to prevent my child's headaches?

Taking good care of your child can decrease the frequency and severity of his or her headaches:

- Drink plenty of fluid (four to eight glasses per day).:
  - Caffeine should be avoided.
  - Sports drinks may help during a headache as well as during exercise by keeping sugar and sodium levels normal.
- Regular and sufficient sleep:
  - Fatigue and overexertion can trigger headaches.
  - Most children and adolescents need to sleep eight to ten hours each night and keep a regular sleep schedule to help prevent headaches.
- Eat balanced meals at regular times:
  - Skipping meals can cause low blood sugar, hypoglycemia, which can trigger a headache.
  - Avoid foods that trigger headaches in your child.
  - Minimize stress and overcommitments.
  - Avoid overcrowded schedules or stressful and potentially upsetting situations.
- Follow prescribed treatment plan:
  - Also, if your child's doctor prescribed daily medication to reduce headache frequency (called preventive or prophylactic medication), remember to have him or her take it every day, whether he or she is having headaches or not.

What should I do if my child gets a headache?

Have your child take pain medication for his or her headache as soon as they feel pain. He or she may be taking over-the-counter medication or prescription medication when they get a headache. Follow the doctor's instructions in using the medication and treatment plan.

Neurological Disorders

Keep a record of your child's headaches. Write down everything that might relate to your child's headache (foods, odors, situations), how long it lasted, and how much pain the headache caused.

Learn the sings and symptoms that might be associated with a headache so you can recognize an oncoming episode.

Help teach your child on what to do when a headache starts. Your child needs to be able to treat his or her headaches at school and at home.

Your child should not be afraid to tell you about their headache.

Your child will need to know what to do at school, so you may need to work with the nurse to establish the treatment plan that the physician has established for your child. This may require that both you and the physician get involved in working with the school to implement a successful treatment plan.

How do you know your child "really" does have a headache?

Recognizing the signs and symptoms of a headache will help you and your child take control of them. For example, we can see a child may be getting a headache or has a headache because:

- they sit quietly in a chair, bed, or sofa and do not watch TV;
- they do not want to exert themselves;
- they may fall asleep at an unusual time;
- they may have nausea, vomiting, or other stomach-related symptoms;
- light and noise may bother them;
- they may seem lethargic or fatigued.

Looking for signs of headache will help you and your child realize that the disability associated with headache is real and should not be dismissed.

Section 29.6

Neurofibromatosis

Excerpted from "Neurofibromatosis Fact Sheet," National Institute of Neurological Disorders and Stroke, National Institutes of Health, NIH Publication No. 06-2126, updated December 13, 2007.

What are the neurofibromatoses?

The neurofibromatoses are a group of three genetically distinct but related disorders of the nervous system that cause tumors to grow around the nerves. Tumors begin in the cells that make up the myelin sheath, a thin membrane that envelops and protects nerve fibers, and often spread into adjacent areas. The type of tumor that develops depends on its location in the body and the kind of cells involved. The most common tumors are neurofibromas, which develop in the tissue surrounding peripheral nerves. Most tumors are noncancerous, although occasionally they become cancerous over time.

Why these tumors occur still isn't completely known, but it appears to be mainly related to mutations in genes that play key roles in suppressing tumor growth in the nervous system. These mutations keep the genes—identified as NF1 and NF2—from making specific proteins that control cell production. Without these proteins, cells multiply out of control and form tumors.

An estimated 100,000 Americans have a neurofibromatosis (the singular form of neurofibromatoses) disorder, which occurs in both sexes and in all races and ethnic groups. Scientists have classified the disorders as neurofibromatosis type 1 (NF1), neurofibromatosis type 2 (NF2), and a type that was once considered to be a variation of NF2 but is now called schwannomatosis.

What is NF1?

NF1 is the most common neurofibromatosis, occurring in 1 in 3,000 to 4,000 individuals in the United States. Although many affected people inherit the disorder, between 30 and 50 percent of new cases occur because of a spontaneous genetic mutation from unknown causes. Once this mutation has taken place, the mutant gene can be passed on to succeeding generations.

What are the signs and symptoms of NF1?

To diagnose NF1, a doctor looks for two or more of the following:

- Six or more light brown spots on the skin (often called "cafe-au-lait" spots), measuring more than 5 millimeters in diameter in children, or more than 15 millimeters across in adolescents and adults
- Two or more neurofibromas, or one plexiform neurofibroma (a neurofibroma that involves many nerves)
- Freckling in the area of the armpit or the groin
- Two or more growths on the iris of the eye (known as Lisch nodules or iris hamartomas)
- A tumor on the optic nerve (optic glioma)
- Abnormal development of the spine (scoliosis), the temple (sphenoid) bone of the skull, or the tibia (one of the long bones of the shin)
- A first-degree relative (parent, sibling, or child) with NF1

What other symptoms or conditions are associated with NF1?

Many children with NF1 have larger than normal head circumference and are shorter than average. Hydrocephalus, the abnormal buildup of fluid in the brain, is a possible complication of the disorder. Headache and epilepsy are also more likely in individuals with NF1 than in the normal population. Cardiovascular complications are associated with NF1, including congenital heart defects, high blood pressure (hypertension), and constricted, blocked, or damaged blood vessels (vasculopathy). Children with NF1 may have poor linguistic and visual-spatial skills, and perform less well on academic achievement tests, including those that measure reading, spelling, and math skills. Learning disabilities, such as attention deficit hyperactivity disorder (ADHD), are common in children with NF1.

When do symptoms appear?

Symptoms, particularly the most common skin abnormalities—café-au-lait spots, neurofibromas, Lisch nodules, and freckling in the armpit and groin—are often evident at birth or shortly afterwards, and almost always by the time a child is ten years old.

Because many features of these disorders are age dependent, a definitive diagnosis may take several years.

What is the prognosis for someone with NF1?

NF1 is a progressive disorder, which means most symptoms will worsen over time, although a small number of people may have symptoms that stay the same and never get any worse. It isn't possible to predict the course of any individual's disorder. In general, most people with NF1 will develop mild to moderate symptoms, and if complications arise they will not be life threatening. Most people with NF1 have a normal life expectancy.

How is NF1 treated?

Since doctors don't know how to prevent or stop neurofibromas from growing, surgery is often recommended to remove them. Several surgical options exist, but there is no general agreement among doctors about when surgery should be performed or which surgical option is best. Individuals considering surgery should carefully weigh the risks and benefits of all their options to determine which surgical treatment is right for them. There are also surgical and chemical techniques that can reduce the size of eye tumors (optic gliomas) when vision is threatened. In addition, some bone malformations, such as scoliosis, can be surgically corrected. In the rare instances when tumors become malignant (3 to 5 percent of all cases), treatment may include surgery, radiation, or chemotherapy.

Treatments for other conditions associated with NF1 are aimed at controlling or relieving symptoms. Headache and epileptic seizures are treated with medications. Since there is a higher than average risk for learning disabilities, children with NF1 should undergo a detailed neurological exam before they enter school. Once these children enter school, if teachers or parents suspect there is evidence of a learning disability (or disabilities), they should request an evaluation that includes an IQ test and the standard range of tests to evaluate verbal and spatial skills. Children with learning disabilities are eligible for special education services under the provisions of the Individuals with Disabilities Education Act (IDEA).

Neurological Disorders

What is NF2?

This rare disorder affects about 1 in 40,000 people. NF2 is characterized by slow-growing tumors on the eighth cranial nerve. This nerve has two branches: the acoustic branch helps people hear by transmitting sound sensations to the brain; the vestibular branch helps people maintain their balance. The tumors of NF2, called vestibular schwannomas because of their location and the types of cells that compose them (Schwann cells, which form the myelin sheath around nerves), press against and sometimes even damage the nerves they surround. In some cases they will also damage nearby vital structures such as other cranial nerves and the brainstem, leading to a potentially life-threatening situation.

Individuals with NF2 are at risk for developing other types of nervous system tumors such as spinal schwannomas, which grow within the spinal cord and between the vertebrae, and meningiomas, which are tumors that grow along the membranes covering the brain and spinal cord.

What are the signs and symptoms of NF2?

To diagnose NF2, a doctor looks for the following:

- Bilateral vestibular schwannomas
- A family history of NF2 (parent, sibling, or child) plus a unilateral vestibular schwannoma before age thirty

Or any two of the following:

- Glioma
- Meningioma
- Schwannoma
- Juvenile posterior subcapsular lenticular opacity (juvenile cortical cataract)

When do symptoms appear?

Signs of NF2 may be present in childhood but are so subtle that they can be overlooked, especially in children who don't have a family history of the disorder. Typically, symptoms of NF2 are noticed between eighteen and twenty-two years of age. The most frequent first symptom is hearing loss or ringing in the ears (tinnitus). Less often, the first visit to a doctor will be because of disturbances in balance, vision impairment (such as vision loss from cataracts), weakness in an arm or leg, seizures, or skin tumors.

What is the prognosis for someone with NF2?

Because NF2 is so rare, few studies have been done to look at the natural progression of the disorder. The course of NF2 varies greatly among individuals, although inherited NF2 appears to run a similar course among affected family members. Generally, vestibular schwannomas grow slowly, and balance and hearing deteriorate over a period of years. A recent study suggests that an earlier age of onset is associated with faster tumor growth and a greater mortality risk.

How is NF2 treated?

NF2 is best managed at a specialty clinic with an initial screening and annual follow-up evaluations. Improved diagnostic technologies, such as MRI (magnetic resonance imaging), can reveal tumors as small as a few millimeters in diameter, which allows for early treatment. Vestibular schwannomas grow slowly, but they can grow large enough to completely engulf the eighth cranial nerve. Early surgery, to completely remove the tumor while it's still small, might be advisable to preserve hearing and balance. There are several surgical options, depending on tumor size and the extent of hearing loss. Some techniques preserve the auditory nerve and enable individuals to retain some hearing; other techniques may involve removing the nerve and replacing it with an electronic auditory implant in the brainstem to restore hearing.

Surgery is available to correct cataracts and retinal abnormalities. A strategy of watchful waiting might be more appropriate for slowly growing brain and spinal tumors, which have higher risks of surgical complications.

What is schwannomatosis?

Schwannomatosis is a newly recognized neurofibromatosis that is genetically and clinically distinct from NF1 and NF2. Like NF2 it occurs rarely. Inherited forms of the disorder account for only 15 percent of all cases. Researchers still don't fully understand what causes the tumors and the intense pain that are characteristics of the disorder.

What are the signs and symptoms of schwannomatosis?

The distinguishing feature of schwannomatosis is the development of multiple schwannomas everywhere in the body except on the vestibular nerve. The dominant symptom is excruciatingly intense pain, which develops when a schwannoma enlarges, compresses nerves, or presses on adjacent tissue. Some people experience additional neurological symptoms, such as numbness, tingling, or weakness in the fingers and toes. Patients with schwannomatosis never have neurofibromas.

About one-third of those with schwannomatosis have tumors limited to a single part of the body, such as an arm, a leg, or a segment of the spine. Some people develop many schwannomas; others develop only a few.

What is the prognosis for someone with schwannomatosis?

Anyone with schwannomatosis experiences some degree of pain, but the intensity varies. A small number of people have such mild pain that they are never diagnosed with the disorder. Most people have significant pain, which can be managed with medications or surgery. In some extreme cases, pain will be so severe and disabling it will keep people from working or leaving the house.

How is schwannomatosis treated?

There is no currently accepted medical treatment or drug for schwannomatosis, but surgical management is often effective. When tumors are completely removed pain usually subsides, although it may recur if new tumors form. When surgery isn't possible, ongoing monitoring and management of pain in a multidisciplinary pain clinic is advisable.

Are there prenatal tests for the neurofibromatoses?

Clinical genetic testing can confirm the presence of a mutation in the NF1 gene with an accuracy of 95 percent. Some families and doctors may choose to use a genetic test to confirm an uncertain diagnosis when there is no family history of the disorder and when waiting for additional symptoms to appear would put an unnecessary emotional burden on the family. Prenatal testing for the NF1 mutation is also possible using amniocentesis or chorionic villus sampling procedures. Genetic testing for the NF2 mutation is sometimes available but is accurate in only 65 percent of those tested. Genetic counselors can provide information about these procedures and help families cope with the results.

What research is being done on the neurofibromatoses?

In the mid-1990s, research teams supported by the National Institute of Neurological Disorders and Stroke (NINDS) located the exact position of the NF1 gene on chromosome 17. The gene has been cloned and its structure continues to be analyzed. The NF1 gene makes a large and complex protein called neurofibromin, which is primarily active in nervous system cells as a regulator of cell division, functioning as a kind of molecular brake to keep cells from overmultiplying. In addition to work on NF1, intensive efforts have led to the identification of the NF2 gene on chromosome 22. As in NF1, the NF2 gene product is a tumor-suppressor protein (termed merlin or schwannomin).

Ongoing NINDS-sponsored research continues to discover additional genes that appear to play a role in tumor suppression or growth. Continuing research on these genes and their proteins is beginning to reveal how this novel family of growth regulators controls how and where tumors form and grow. Understanding the molecular pathways and mechanisms that govern these key proteins and their activities will offer scientists exciting opportunities to design drugs that could replace the missing proteins in people who have the neurofibromatoses and return their cell production to normal.

The NINDS currently supports basic and clinical research to understand how the genetic mutations that cause the benign tumors of NF1 can also cause abnormal development of neurons and neural networks during fetal development. This abnormal development can lead to the learning disabilities and cognitive deficits of children with the disorder.

The NINDS also encourages research aimed at developing improved methods of diagnosing the neurofibromatoses and at identifying factors that contribute to the wide variations of symptoms and severity of the disorders.

Just as important, the NINDS is supporting ongoing research with a large group of children with NF1 to help doctors answer the question that most parents ask when their child is diagnosed with the disorder: "What can we expect when our child goes to school?" Using magnetic resonance imaging (MRI), which shows brain structure, functional MRI, which shows areas of the brain at work, and neuropsychological tests that measure specific cognitive skills, researchers are looking for associations between brain abnormalities and specific cognitive disabilities. Finding these links would give doctors an indication of the kinds of learning disabilities parents and their children could anticipate in the future and help them develop early intervention programs.

Section 29.7

Tourette Syndrome

Excerpted from "Tourette Syndrome Fact Sheet," National Institute of Neurological Disorders and Stroke, National Institutes of Health, NIH Publication No. 05-2163, updated December 11, 2007.

What is Tourette syndrome?

Tourette syndrome (TS) is a neurological disorder characterized by repetitive, stereotyped, involuntary movements and vocalizations called tics. The disorder is named for Dr. Georges Gilles de la Tourette, the pioneering French neurologist who in 1885 first described the condition in an eighty-six-year-old French noblewoman.

The early symptoms of TS are almost always noticed first in childhood, with the average onset between the ages of seven and ten years. TS occurs in people from all ethnic groups; males are affected about three to four times more often than females. It is estimated that two hundred thousand Americans have the most severe form of TS, and as many as one in one hundred exhibit milder and less complex symptoms such as chronic motor or vocal tics or transient tics of childhood. Although TS can be a chronic condition with symptoms lasting a lifetime, most people with the condition experience their worst symptoms in their early teens, with improvement occurring in the late teens and continuing into adulthood.

What are the symptoms?

Tics are classified as either simple or complex. Simple motor tics are sudden, brief, repetitive movements that involve a limited number of muscle groups. Some of the more common simple tics include eye blinking and other vision irregularities, facial grimacing, shoulder shrugging, and head or shoulder jerking. Simple vocalizations might include repetitive throat clearing, sniffing, or grunting sounds. Complex tics are distinct, coordinated patterns of movements involving several muscle groups. Complex motor tics might include facial grimacing combined with a head twist and a shoulder shrug. Other complex motor tics may actually appear purposeful, including sniffing or touching objects, hopping, jumping, bending, or twisting. Simple vocal tics may include throat clearing, sniffing/snorting, grunting, or barking. More complex vocal tics include words or phrases. Perhaps the most dramatic and disabling tics include motor movements that result in self-harm such as punching oneself in the face or vocal tics including coprolalia (uttering swear words) or echolalia (repeating the words or phrases of others). Some tics are preceded by an urge or sensation in the affected muscle group, commonly called a premonitory urge. Some with TS will describe a need to complete a tic in a certain way or a certain number of times in order to relieve the urge or decrease the sensation.

Tics are often worse with excitement or anxiety and better during calm, focused activities. Certain physical experiences can trigger or worsen tics, for example tight collars may trigger neck tics, or hearing another person sniff or throat-clear may trigger similar sounds. Tics do not go away during sleep but are often significantly diminished.

What is the course of TS?

Tics come and go over time, varying in type, frequency, location, and severity. The first symptoms usually occur in the head and neck area and may progress to include muscles of the trunk and extremities. Motor tics generally precede the development of vocal tics and simple tics often precede complex tics. Most patients experience peak tic severity before the mid-teen years with improvement for the majority of patients in the late teen years and early adulthood. Approximately 10 percent of those affected have a progressive or disabling course that lasts into adulthood.

Can people with TS control their tics?

Although the symptoms of TS are involuntary, some people can sometimes suppress, camouflage, or otherwise manage their tics in an effort to minimize their impact on functioning. However, people with TS often report a substantial buildup in tension when suppressing their tics to the point where they feel that the tic must be expressed. Tics in response to an environmental trigger can appear to be voluntary or purposeful but are not.

What causes TS?

Although the cause of TS is unknown, current research points to abnormalities in certain brain regions (including the basal ganglia, frontal lobes, and cortex), the circuits that interconnect these regions, and the neurotransmitters (dopamine, serotonin, and norepinephrine) responsible for communication among nerve cells. Given the often complex presentation of TS, the cause of the disorder is likely to be equally complex.

What disorders are associated with TS?

Many with TS experience additional neurobehavioral problems including inattention; hyperactivity and impulsivity (attention deficit hyperactivity disorder—ADHD) and related problems with reading, writing, and arithmetic; and obsessive-compulsive symptoms such as intrusive thoughts/worries and repetitive behaviors. For example, worries about dirt and germs may be associated with repetitive hand washing, and concerns about bad things happening may be associated with ritualistic behaviors such as counting, repeating, or ordering and arranging. People with TS have also reported problems with depression or anxiety disorders, as well as other difficulties with living, that may or may not be directly related to TS. Given the range of potential complications, people with TS are best served by receiving medical care that provides a comprehensive treatment plan.

How is TS diagnosed?

TS is a diagnosis that doctors make after verifying that the patient has had both motor and vocal tics for at least one year. The existence of other neurological or psychiatric conditions, including childhood-onset involuntary movement disorders such as dystonia, or psychiatric disorders characterized by repetitive behaviors/movements (for example, stereotypic behaviors in autism and compulsive behaviors in obsessive-compulsive disorder [OCD]) can also help doctors arrive at a diagnosis. Common tics are not often misdiagnosed by knowledgeable clinicians. But atypical symptoms or atypical presentation (for example, onset of symptoms in adulthood) may require specific specialty expertise for diagnosis. There are no blood or laboratory tests needed for diagnosis, but neuroimaging studies, such as magnetic resonance imaging (MRI), computerized tomography (CT), and electroencephalogram (EEG) scans, or certain blood tests may be used to rule out other conditions that might be confused with TS.

It is not uncommon for patients to obtain a formal diagnosis of TS only after symptoms have been present for some time. The reasons for this are many. For families and physicians unfamiliar with TS, mild and even moderate tic symptoms may be considered inconsequential, part of a developmental phase, or the result of another condition. For example, parents may think that eye blinking is related to vision problems or that sniffing is related to seasonal allergies. Many patients are self-diagnosed after they, their parents, other relatives, or friends read or hear about TS from others.

How is TS treated?

Because tic symptoms do not often cause impairment, the majority of people with TS require no medication for tic suppression. However, effective medications are available for those whose symptoms interfere with functioning. Neuroleptics are the most consistently useful medications for tic suppression; a number are available but some are more effective than others (for example, haloperidol and pimozide). Unfortunately, there is no one medication that is helpful to all people with TS, nor does any medication completely eliminate symptoms. In addition, all medications have side effects. Most neuroleptic side effects can be managed by initiating treatment slowly and reducing the dose when side effects occur. The most common side effects of neuroleptics include sedation, weight gain, and cognitive dulling. Neurological side effects such as tremor, dystonic reactions (twisting movements or postures), parkinsonian-like symptoms, and other dyskinetic (involuntary) movements are less common and are readily managed with dose reduction. Discontinuing neuroleptics after long-term use must be done slowly to avoid rebound increases in tics and withdrawal dyskinesias. One form of withdrawal dyskinesia called tardive dyskinesia is a movement disorder distinct from TS that may result from the chronic use of neuroleptics. The risk of this side effect can be reduced by using lower doses of neuroleptics for shorter periods of time.

Other medications may also be useful for reducing tic severity, but most have not been as extensively studied or shown to be as consistently useful as neuroleptics. Additional medications with demonstrated efficacy include alpha-adrenergic agonists such as clonidine and guanfacine. These medications are used primarily for hypertension but are also used in the treatment of tics. The most common side effect from these medications that precludes their use is sedation.

Effective medications are also available to treat some of the associated neurobehavioral disorders that can occur in patients with TS.

Neurological Disorders

Recent research shows that stimulant medications such as methylphenidate and dextroamphetamine can lessen ADHD symptoms in people with TS without causing tics to become more severe. However, the product labeling for stimulants currently contraindicates the use of these drugs in children with tics/TS and those with a family history of tics. Scientists hope that future studies will include a thorough discussion of the risks and benefits of stimulants in those with TS or a family history of TS and will clarify this issue. For obsessive-compulsive symptoms that significantly disrupt daily functioning, the serotonin reuptake inhibitors (clomipramine, fluoxetine, fluvoxamine, paroxetine, and sertraline) have been proven effective in some patients.

Psychotherapy may also be helpful. Although psychological problems do not cause TS, such problems may result from TS. Psychotherapy can help the person with TS better cope with the disorder and deal with the secondary social and emotional problems that sometimes occur. More recently, specific behavioral treatments that include awareness training and competing response training, such as voluntarily moving in response to a premonitory urge, have shown effectiveness in small controlled trials. Larger and more definitive NIH-funded studies are underway.

Is TS inherited?

Evidence from twin and family studies suggests that TS is an inherited disorder. Although early family studies suggested an autosomal dominant mode of inheritance (an autosomal dominant disorder is one in which only one copy of the defective gene, inherited from one parent, is necessary to produce the disorder), more recent studies suggest that the pattern of inheritance is much more complex. Although there may be a few genes with substantial effects, it is also possible that many genes with smaller effects and environmental factors may play a role in the development of TS. Genetic studies also suggest that some forms of ADHD and OCD are genetically related to TS, but there is less evidence for a genetic relationship between TS and other neurobehavioral problems that commonly co-occur with TS. It is important for families to understand that genetic predisposition may not necessarily result in full-blown TS; instead, it may express itself as a milder tic disorder or as obsessive-compulsive behaviors. It is also possible that the gene-carrying offspring will not develop any TS symptoms.

The sex of the person also plays an important role in TS gene expression. At-risk males are more likely to have tics and at-risk females are more likely to have obsessive-compulsive symptoms.

People with TS may have genetic risks for other neurobehavioral disorders such as depression or substance abuse. Genetic counseling of individuals with TS should include a full review of all potentially hereditary conditions in the family.

What is the prognosis?

Although there is no cure for TS, the condition in many individuals improves in the late teens and early twenties. As a result, some may actually become symptom-free or no longer need medication for tic suppression. Although the disorder is generally lifelong and chronic, it is not a degenerative condition. Individuals with TS have a normal life expectancy. TS does not impair intelligence. Although tic symptoms tend to decrease with age, it is possible that neurobehavioral disorders such as depression, panic attacks, mood swings, and antisocial behaviors can persist and cause impairment in adult life.

What is the best educational setting for children with TS?

Although students with TS often function well in the regular classroom, ADHD, learning disabilities, obsessive-compulsive symptoms, and frequent tics can greatly interfere with academic performance or social adjustment. After a comprehensive assessment, students should be placed in an educational setting that meets their individual needs. Students may require tutoring, smaller or special classes, and in some cases special schools.

All students with TS need a tolerant and compassionate setting that both encourages them to work to their full potential and is flexible enough to accommodate their special needs. This setting may include a private study area, exams outside the regular classroom, or even oral exams when the child's symptoms interfere with his or her ability to write. Untimed testing reduces stress for students with TS.

What research is being done?

Knowledge about TS comes from studies across a number of medical and scientific disciplines, including genetics, neuroimaging, neuropathology, clinical trials (medication and non-medication), epidemiology, neurophysiology, neuroimmunology, and descriptive/diagnostic clinical science.

Genetic studies: Currently, investigators funded by the National Institutes of Health (NIH) are conducting a variety of large-scale genetic studies. Rapid advances in the technology of gene finding will allow for genome-wide screening approaches in TS, and finding a gene or genes for TS would be a major step toward understanding genetic risk factors. In addition, understanding the genetics of TS genes will strengthen clinical diagnosis, improve genetic counseling, lead to the clarification of pathophysiology, and provide clues for more effective therapies.

Neuroimaging studies: Within the past five years, advances in imaging technology and an increase in trained investigators have led to an increasing use of novel and powerful techniques to identify brain regions, circuitry, and neurochemical factors important in TS and related conditions.

Neuropathology: Within the past five years, there has been an increase in the number and quality of donated postmortem brains from TS patients available for research purposes. This increase, coupled with advances in neuropathological techniques, has led to initial findings with implications for neuroimaging studies and animal models of TS.

Clinical trials: A number of clinical trials in TS have recently been completed or are currently underway. These include studies of stimulant treatment of ADHD in TS and behavioral treatments for reducing tic severity in children and adults. Smaller trials of novel approaches to treatment such as dopamine agonist and GABAergic medications also show promise.

Epidemiology and clinical science: Careful epidemiological studies now estimate the prevalence of TS to be substantially higher than previously thought, with a wider range of clinical severity. Furthermore, clinical studies are providing new findings regarding TS and coexisting conditions. These include subtyping studies of TS and OCD, an examination of the link between ADHD and learning problems in children with TS, a new appreciation of sensory tics, and the role of coexisting disorders in rage attacks. One of the most important and controversial areas of TS science involves the relationship between TS and autoimmune brain injury associated with group A beta-hemolytic streptococcal infections or other infectious processes. There are a number of epidemiological and clinical investigations currently underway in this intriguing area.

Chapter 30

Respiratory and Lung Conditions

Chapter Contents

Section 30.1—Asthma 524
Section 30.2—Bronchitis 528
Section 30.3—Cystic Fibrosis 531

Section 30.1

Asthma

"You Can Control Your Asthma,"
Centers for Disease Control and Prevention, 2006.

What Is Asthma?

Asthma is a disease that affects your lungs. It is the most common long-term disease of children, but adults have asthma, too. Asthma causes repeated episodes of wheezing, breathlessness, chest tightness, and nighttime or early morning coughing. If you have asthma, you have it all the time, but you will have asthma attacks only when something bothers your lungs.

We know that if someone in your family has asthma, you are also more likely to have it. In most cases, we don't know what causes asthma, and we don't know how to cure it. You can control your asthma by knowing the warning signs of an attack, staying away from things that trigger an attack, and following the advice of your health care provider. When you control your asthma, you won't have symptoms like wheezing or coughing, you'll sleep better, you won't miss work or school, you can take part in all physical activities, and you won't have to go to the hospital.

How Is Asthma Diagnosed?

Asthma can be hard to diagnose, especially in children under five years of age. Regular physical checkups that include checking your lung function and checking for allergies can help your health care provider make the right diagnosis.

During a checkup, the health care provider will ask you questions about whether you cough a lot, especially at night, and whether your breathing problems are worse after physical activity or during a particular time of year. Health care providers will also ask about other symptoms such as chest tightness, wheezing, and colds that last more than ten days. They will ask you whether your family members have or have had asthma, allergies, or other breathing problems, and they

Respiratory and Lung Conditions

will ask you questions about your home. The health care provider will also ask you about missing school or work and about any trouble you may have doing certain activities.

A lung function test, called spirometry, is another way to diagnose asthma. A spirometer measures the largest amount of air you can exhale, or breathe out, after taking a very deep breath. The spirometer can measure airflow before and after you use asthma medicine.

What Is an Asthma Attack?

An asthma attack happens in your body's airways, which are the paths that carry air to your lungs. As the air moves through your lungs, the airways become smaller, like the branches of a tree are smaller than the tree trunk. During an asthma attack, the sides of the airways in your lungs swell, and the airways shrink. Less air gets in and out of your lungs, and mucus that your body produces clogs up the airways even more. The attack may include coughing, chest tightness, wheezing, and trouble breathing. Some people call an asthma attack an "episode."

What Causes an Asthma Attack?

An asthma attack can occur when you are exposed to things in the environment such as house dust mites and tobacco smoke. These are called asthma triggers. Some of the most important triggers are listed below.

How Is Asthma Treated?

You can control your asthma and avoid an attack by taking your medicine exactly as your health care provider tells you to do and by avoiding things that can cause an attack.

Everyone with asthma does not take the same medicine. Some medicines can be inhaled, or breathed in, and some can be taken as a pill. Asthma medicines come in two types—quick-relief and long-term control. Quick-relief medicines control the symptoms of an asthma attack. If you need to use your quick-relief medicines more and more, you should visit your health care provider to see if you need a different medicine. Long-term control medicines help you have fewer and milder attacks, but they don't help you if you're having an asthma attack.

Asthma medicines can have side effects, but most side effects are mild and soon go away. Ask your health care provider about the side effects of your medicines.

The important thing to remember is that you can control your asthma. With your health care provider's help, make your own asthma management plan so that you know what to do based on your own symptoms. Decide who should have a copy of your plan and where he or she should keep it. Take your long-term control medicine even when you don't have symptoms.

Important Asthma Triggers

Environmental tobacco smoke (secondhand smoke): Environmental tobacco smoke is often called "secondhand smoke" because it is smoke that is breathed in not by a smoker but by a second person nearby. Parents, friends, and relatives of children with asthma should try to stop smoking and should never smoke around a person with asthma. They should only smoke outdoors and not in the family home or car. They should not allow others to smoke in the home, and they should make sure their child's school is smoke-free.

Dust mites: Dust mites are in almost everybody's home, but they don't cause everybody to have asthma attacks. If you have asthma, dust mites may be a trigger for an attack. To help prevent asthma attacks, use mattress covers and pillow case covers to make a barrier between dust mites and yourself. Don't use down-filled pillows, quilts, or comforters. Remove stuffed animals and clutter from your bedroom.

Outdoor air pollution: Pollution caused by industrial emissions and automobile exhaust can cause an asthma attack. Pay attention to air quality forecasts on radio and television and plan your activities for when air pollution levels will be low if air pollution aggravates your asthma.

Cockroach allergen: Cockroaches and their droppings may trigger an asthma attack. Get rid of cockroaches in your home and keep them from coming back by taking away their food and water. Cockroaches are usually found where food is eaten and crumbs are left behind. Remove as many water and food sources as you can because cockroaches need food and water to survive. Vacuum or sweep areas that might attract cockroaches at least every two or three days. You can also use roach traps or gels to decrease the number of cockroaches in your home.

Pets: Furry pets may trigger an asthma attack. When a furry pet is suspected of causing asthma attacks, the simplest solution is to find the pet another home. If pet owners are too attached to their pets or are unable to locate a safe, new home for the pet, they should keep the pet out of the bedroom of the person with asthma.

Pets should be bathed weekly and kept outside as much as possible. People with asthma are not allergic to their pet's fur, so trimming your pet's fur will not help your asthma. If you have a furry pet, vacuum often to clean up anything that could cause an asthma attack. If your floors have a hard surface, such as wood or tile, and are not carpeted, damp mop them every week.

Mold: When mold is inhaled or breathed in, it can cause an asthma attack. Get rid of mold in all parts of your home to help control your asthma attacks. Keep the humidity level in your home between 35 and 50 percent. In hot, humid climates, you may need to use an air conditioner or a dehumidifier or both. Fix water leaks, which allow mold to grow behind walls and under floors.

Other triggers: Strenuous physical exercise; some medicines; bad weather such as thunderstorms, high humidity, or freezing temperatures; and some foods and food additives can trigger an asthma attack.

Strong emotional states can also lead to hyperventilation and an asthma attack.

Learn what triggers your attacks so that you can avoid the triggers whenever possible and be alert for a possible attack when the triggers cannot be avoided.

Remember, you can control your asthma!

Section 30.2

Bronchitis

"Bronchitis," © Cedars-Sinai Medical Center. All rights reserved. Reprinted with permission. The text of this document is available online at http://www.csmc.edu/6941.html. Accessed February 27, 2008.

The bronchi are the two main airways that branch down from the trachea (the airway that starts in the back of the throat and goes into the chest). When the parts of the walls of the bronchi become swollen and tender (inflamed), the condition is called bronchitis. The inflammation causes more mucus to be produced, which narrows the airway and makes breathing more difficult.

There are several types of bronchitis:

- Acute bronchitis can last for up to ninety days.

- Chronic bronchitis can last for months or sometimes years. If chronic bronchitis decreases the amount of air flowing to the lungs, it is considered to be a sign of chronic obstructive pulmonary disease.

- Infectious bronchitis usually occurs in the winter due to viruses, including the influenza virus. Even after a viral infection has passed, the irritation of the bronchi can continue to cause symptoms. Infectious bronchitis can also be due to bacteria, especially if it follows an upper respiratory viral infection. It is possible to have viral and bacterial bronchitis at the same time.

- Irritative bronchitis (or industrial or environmental bronchitis) is caused by exposure to mineral or vegetable dusts or fumes from strong acids, ammonia, some organic solvents, chlorine, hydrogen sulfide, sulfur dioxide, and bromine.

Symptoms

Symptoms will vary somewhat depending on the underlying cause of the bronchitis. When the bronchitis is due to an infection the symptoms may include the following:

Respiratory and Lung Conditions

- A slight fever of 100 to 101°F with severe bronchitis. The fever may rise to 101 to 102°F and last three to five days even after antibiotics are started.
- A runny nose.
- Aches in the back and muscles.
- Chills.
- Coughing that starts out dry is often the first sign of acute bronchitis. Small amounts of white mucus may be coughed up if the bronchitis is viral. If the color of the mucus changes to green or yellow, it may be a sign that a bacterial infection has also set in. The cough is usually the last symptom to clear up and may last for weeks.
- Feeling tired.
- Shortness of breath that can be triggered by inhaling cold, outdoor air or smelling strong odors. This happens because the inflamed bronchi may narrow for short periods of time, cutting down the amount of air that enters the lungs. Wheezing, especially after coughing, is common.
- Sore throat.

Bronchitis does not usually lead to serious complications (e.g., acute respiratory failure or pneumonia) unless the patient has a chronic lung disease, such as chronic obstructive pulmonary disease or asthma.

Causes and Risk Factors

An infection or irritating substances, gases, or particles in the air can cause acute bronchitis. Smokers and people with chronic lung disease are more prone to repeated attacks of acute bronchitis. This is because the mucus in their airways doesn't drain well. Others at risk of getting acute bronchitis repeatedly are people with chronic sinus infections or allergies; children with enlarged tonsils and adenoids; and people who don't eat properly.

Diagnosis

To diagnose bronchitis, a physician performs a physical examination, listens for wheezing with a stethoscope, and evaluates symptoms, making sure they are not due to pneumonia. A sample of sputum from a cough may be examined because its color—clear or white versus yellow or green—may suggest whether the bronchitis is due to a viral infection or a bacterial infection, respectively. A chest x-ray may be needed to rule out pneumonia, and if the cough lasts more than two months, a chest x-ray may be done to rule out another lung disease, such as lung cancer.

Treatment

Depending on the symptoms and cause of the bronchitis, treatment options include the following:

- Antibiotics may be ordered to treat acute bronchitis that appears to be caused by a bacterial infection or for people who have other lung diseases that put them at a greater risk of lung infections.

- Bronchodilators, which open up the bronchi, may be used on a short-term basis to open airways and reduce wheezing.

- Cool-mist humidifiers or steam vaporizers can be helpful for wheezing or shortness of breath. Leaning over a bathroom sink full of hot water with a towel loosely draped over the head can also be help open the airways.

- Corticosteroids given in an inhaler are sometimes prescribed to help the cough go away, reduce inflammation, and make the airways less reactive. They are most often given when the cough remains after the infection is no longer present.

- Cough medicines should be used carefully. While they can be helpful to suppress a dry, bothersome cough, they should not be used to suppress a cough that produces a lot of sputum. When the cough is wet, expectorants can help thin the secretions and make them easier to cough up. When a lot of mucus is present, coughing is important to clear the lungs of fluid.

- For viral bronchitis, antibiotics will not be effective. If influenza causes the bronchitis, treatment with antiviral drugs may be helpful.

- Over-the-counter pain relievers, such as aspirin, acetaminophen, or ibuprofen, can be used for pain relief and fever reduction. Children with bronchitis should not be given aspirin; instead they should take acetaminophen or ibuprofen.

- Plenty of fluids—enough to keep the urine pale (except for the first urination of the day, when it is usually darker).
- Rest, especially if a fever is present.

Section 30.3

Cystic Fibrosis

"Frequently Asked Questions," © 2007 Cystic Fibrosis Foundation (www.cff.org). Reprinted with permission.

What is cystic fibrosis?

Cystic fibrosis (CF) is a life-threatening disease that causes mucus to build up and clog some of the organs in the body, particularly in the lungs and pancreas. When mucus clogs the lungs, it can make breathing very difficult. The thick mucus also causes bacteria (or germs) to get stuck in the airways, which causes inflammation (or swelling) and infections that leads to lung damage.

Mucus also can block the digestive tract and pancreas. The mucus stops digestive enzymes from getting to the intestines. The body needs these enzymes to break down food, which provides important nutrients to help us grow and stay healthy. People with cystic fibrosis often need to replace these enzymes with capsules they take with their meals and snacks to help digest the food and get the proper nutrition.

How do people get cystic fibrosis?

Cystic fibrosis is a genetic disease. That means people inherit it from their parents through genes (or deoxyribonucleic acid [DNA]), which also determine a lot of other characteristics including height, hair color, and eye color. Genes, found in the nucleus of all the body's cells, control cell function by serving as the blueprint for the production of proteins.

The defective gene that is responsible for causing cystic fibrosis is on chromosome 7. To have cystic fibrosis, a person must inherit two copies of the defective CF gene—one copy from each parent. If both parents are carriers of the CF gene (i.e., they each have one copy of the defective gene), their child will have a 25 percent chance of inheriting both defective copies and having cystic fibrosis, a 50 percent chance of inheriting one defective copy and being a carrier, and a 25 percent chance of not having CF or carrying the gene.

Who gets cystic fibrosis?

Approximately thirty thousand people in the United States have cystic fibrosis. An additional ten million more—or about one in every thirty-one Americans—are carriers of the defective CF gene, but do not have the disease. The disease is most common in Caucasians, but it can affect all races.

The severity of cystic fibrosis symptoms is different from person to person. The most common symptoms are:

- very salty-tasting skin;
- persistent coughing, at times with phlegm;
- Frequent lung infections, like pneumonia or bronchitis;
- wheezing or shortness of breath;
- poor growth/weight gain in spite of a good appetite;
- frequent greasy, bulky stools or difficulty in bowel movements;
- small, fleshy growths in the nose called nasal polyps.

Sometimes people are told that they have asthma or chronic bronchitis when they really have cystic fibrosis. New research shows that the severity of CF symptoms is partly based on the types of CF gene mutations (defects). Scientists have found more than 1,500 different mutations of the CF gene.

How is CF diagnosed?

Most people are diagnosed with CF at birth or before the age of two. A doctor who sees the symptoms will order either a sweat test or a genetic test to confirm the diagnosis.

A sweat test is the most common test used to diagnose cystic fibrosis. A small electrode is placed on the skin (usually on the arm) to stimulate the sweat glands. Sweat is then collected and the amount of chloride, a component of salt in the sweat, is measured. A high level of chloride—a score of more than 60 mmol/L (a measure of concen-

Respiratory and Lung Conditions

tration)—means that the person has cystic fibrosis. Scores between 40 mmol/L and 60 mmol/L are considered to be on the borderline and need to be looked at on a case-by-case basis. Scores of less than 40 mmol/L are considered negative for CF. The best place to receive a reliable sweat test is at a Cystic Fibrosis Foundation–accredited care center.

In a genetic test, a blood sample or cells from the inside of the cheek is taken and sent to a laboratory to see if any of the various mutations of the CF gene are found. A genetic test is often used if the results from a sweat test are unclear.

How does CF affect the lungs?

Scientists have many different ideas about what goes wrong in the lungs of a person with cystic fibrosis, but it all begins with defective CF genes. Normally, the healthy CF gene makes a protein—known as CFTR (cystic fibrosis conductance transmembrane regulator)—that is found in the cells that line various organs, like the lungs and the pancreas. This protein controls the movement of electrically charged particles, like chloride and sodium (components of salt) in and out of these cells. When the protein is defective, as in cystic fibrosis, the salt balance in the body is disturbed. Because there is too little salt and water on the outside of the cells, the thin layer of mucus that helps keep the lungs free of germs becomes very thick and difficult to move. And because it is so hard to cough out, this mucus will clog the airways and lead to infections that damage lungs.

Is cystic fibrosis fatal?

Currently, there is no cure for cystic fibrosis. However, specialized medical care, aggressive drug treatments, and therapies, along with proper CF nutrition, can lengthen and improve the quality of life for those with CF.

The best way for people with cystic fibrosis to fight their disease is to work with their medical caregivers at a CF Foundation–accredited care center. The care center partners with people who have CF to help keep them in the best health possible.

What is a typical day for someone with CF?

Because the severity of CF differs widely from person to person, and CF lung infections flare up from time to time, there may not be a "typical" day. However, each day most people with CF:

- take pancreatic enzyme supplement capsules with every meal and most snacks (even babies who are breastfeeding may need to take enzymes);

- take multivitamins;

- do some form of airway clearance at least once and sometimes up to four or more times a day;

- take aerosolized medicines—these are liquid medications that are made into a mist or aerosol and then inhaled through a nebulizer.

What is the life expectancy for people who have CF (in the United States)?

There is no way to accurately predict how long people with cystic fibrosis will live, as many different factors may affect a person's health. Severity of disease and time of diagnosis are two such factors. Many people have a mild case of CF, while others can have moderate or severe cases. In addition, some adults with cystic fibrosis have only recently begun to use new treatments, while an infant diagnosed at birth will have the advantages of starting specialized treatments that were not available even a decade ago.

Using data from the CF Foundation Patient Registry, which is gathered from patients treated at CF Foundation–accredited care centers, we do know that more than 40 percent of all people with CF in this country are eighteen years or older. In addition, we have calculated the predicted median age of survival. This number is based on a statistical method of using life table analyses developed by insurance companies to calculate trends in survival.

In 2005, the predicted median age of survival rose to 36.5 years, up from 32 in 2000. The predicted median age of survival is the age to which half of the current CF Patient Registry population would be expected to survive, given the ages of the patients in the registry and the distribution of deaths in 2005.

The steady rise of the median predicted age of survival suggests how improvements in treatment are advancing the lives for those with CF. In 1955, children with CF were not expected to live even to first grade. Today, thanks to continued Foundation-supported research and specialized care, an increasing number of people with cystic fibrosis are living into adulthood and leading healthier lives that include careers, marriage, and families of their own.

Respiratory and Lung Conditions

What treatments or therapies are available?

The best treatments and therapies for cystic fibrosis vary from person to person. CF medical caregivers at a CF Foundation–accredited care center will work closely with the person with CF to create an individualized plan as to what drugs and therapies are needed.

Since cystic fibrosis affects the lungs of most patients, a large part of the medical treatment is to clear mucus from the airways by using different airway clearance techniques. These techniques use vibrations to help loosen the mucus in the lungs so it can be coughed out.

There are several medications that treat lung infections and can help people with cystic fibrosis breathe better. They are:

- **Mucus thinners:** Medicine that thins mucus, making it easier to cough out.
- **Antibiotics:** Drugs that can kill or slow the growth of germs called bacteria. One commonly used CF drug is TOBI®, or "tobramycin for inhalation."
- **Anti-inflammatories:** Drugs, like ibuprofen, that help to reduce inflammation or swelling of the body tissues. People with CF have inflammation in their lungs. This is one cause of the lung damage.
- **Bronchodilators:** Medicine that opens the airways for easier breathing.

Where can people with CF get the best care?

Because CF is a complex disease that affects so many parts of the body, proper care requires specialized knowledge. The best place to get that care is at one of the more than 115 nationwide CF Foundation–accredited care center.

Each center must meet strict guidelines to get the foundation's "stamp of approval" every year. Care center staff includes a whole group of specialists, including doctors, nurses, respiratory or physical therapists, dietitians, and social workers. This talented group works with each individual who has CF to meet that person's specific needs and to keep them as healthy as possible.

The latest potential treatments for CF are being tested in clinical trials at many CF Foundation–accredited care centers. Patients can help by volunteering to participate in a clinical trial that will help to advance research for a cure.

Does a lung transplant cure CF?

No. A lung transplant will not cure CF because the defective genes that cause the disease are in all of the cells in the body, not just in the lungs. At this time, scientists are not sure how to "fix" genes permanently. While a transplant does give a person with CF a new set of lungs, the rest of the cells in the body still have CF and may already be damaged by the disease. Further, organ rejection drugs can cause other health problems.

What about gene therapy? Is it a treatment for people with CF?

When scientists found the most common gene that causes CF in 1989, there was much excitement about the possibility of developing gene therapy. Gene therapy is the process by which healthy genes are delivered into cells and tissues of the body using such "vehicles" as a specially engineered virus. Researchers need to add enough healthy genes to override the effects of the defective ones. If it is successfully done, gene therapy has the potential of curing cystic fibrosis as it addresses the root cause of the disease (the faulty CF gene) and not merely the symptoms.

Scientists are currently exploring the use of gene therapy for many diseases but have had little success. That is because it has been very hard to find a safe and reliable way to deliver healthy genes into the cells and tissues of the body. For this reason, we cannot predict when and if gene therapy will become available as a treatment. Gene therapy, like any other medical research, must be safe and effective before it can be used as a treatment. Research is ongoing in both the clinic and the laboratory.

What is a clinical trial?

Once researchers have shown that a new drug is safe and potentially effective in the laboratory, a study is designed to evaluate it in people. This study is known as a clinical trial. If the Food and Drug Administration approves the clinical trial, the study can begin in people.

Researchers find volunteers with CF who fit the criteria for the specific clinical trial. Some trials, for instance, may be targeted only at children or only at people with digestive problems. Other trials may only be for people with CF whose lung function is within a certain range. Some clinical trials actually begin with volunteers who are healthy and do not have CF at all. Researchers observe how the drug behaves in the body under highly controlled and monitored circumstances, and whether the treatment is helpful to people with CF.

With more than twenty-five drugs in clinical trials and several in the laboratory, researchers will need more people than ever to volunteer for clinical trials. The best way to make sure that this important research continues for people with CF is to contact a care center near you to get involved.

Is there any help available to pay for CF care?

Many people with CF use Cystic Fibrosis Services, Inc., a mail-order specialty pharmacy that is a subsidiary of the Cystic Fibrosis Foundation. It provides access to CF medications and offers patient assistance programs, as well as helps resolve complex insurance issues. CF Services is a participating provider with more than five thousand insurance plans and nearly forty state and federally funded programs. Visit www.cfservicespharmacy.com or call 800-541-4959.

Pharmaceutical companies often offer a range of patient assistance programs—from giving out samples of new CF products, to providing free nutritional supplements, to accepting voucher payments for medications.

When will there be a cure?

The Cystic Fibrosis Foundation works as fast as possible and funds some of the best and brightest minds in science to find a cure. Because CF researchers are blazing new trails in drug development and gene therapy, experts have no way of saying for sure when a cure will be available. Certainly many children today have the chance to live long and full lives. In fact, for the first time in the history of the disease, many people with CF are now living into adulthood—more than 40 percent of people with CF in the United States are age eighteen or older.

The "aging" of the cystic fibrosis community is largely due to the increase in innovative new treatments and specialized medical care. But a better quality of life and partially increased length of life are simply not enough. That is why the Cystic Fibrosis Foundation is working tirelessly to expand and strengthen the drug development pipeline of potentially life-saving new therapies while, at the same time, supporting a vital care center network.

Our challenge is finding enough patients to join clinical trials to keep the research moving forward. Without patient volunteers, research and progress are not possible.

How can people help to advance science/research/support?

Cystic fibrosis research is definitely a team effort. Scientists across the world are working to understand and better combat this complex disease, with the hope that one or more of the many approaches to therapies will lead to a cure.

People can help advance the research in several ways:

- By volunteering for clinical trials in their area.
- By raising money and getting involved, that will fund these cutting-edge research avenues.
- By contacting a CF Foundation chapter office to ask about fund-raising events to participate in and help raise the money that drives the science ahead!

Chapter 31

Skin Conditions

Chapter Contents

Section 31.1—Eczema/Atopic Dermatitis 540
Section 31.2—Psoriasis 543

Section 31.1

Eczema/Atopic Dermatitis

This information is reprinted with the permission of DermNet, the website of the New Zealand Dermatological Society. Visit www.dermnet.org.nz for patient information on numerous skin conditions and their treatment. © 2008 New Zealand Dermatological Society.

What Is Atopic Dermatitis?

Atopic dermatitis is a chronic, itchy skin condition that is very common in children but may occur at any age. It is also known as eczema and atopic eczema. It is the most common form of dermatitis.

Atopic dermatitis usually occurs in people who have an "atopic tendency." This means they may develop any or all of three closely linked conditions: atopic dermatitis, asthma, and hay fever (allergic rhinitis). Often these conditions run within families with a parent, child, or sibling also affected. A family history of asthma, eczema, or hay fever is particularly useful in diagnosing atopic dermatitis in infants.

Atopic dermatitis is not contagious! It arises because of a complex interaction of genetic and environmental factors. These include skin irritants, the weather, temperature, and nonspecific triggers.

What Does Atopic Dermatitis Look Like?

There is quite a variation in the appearance of atopic dermatitis between individuals. From time to time, most people have acute flares with inflamed, red, sometimes blistered and weepy patches. In between flares, the skin may appear normal or suffer from chronic eczema with dry, thickened and itchy areas.

The presence of infection or an additional skin condition, the creams applied, the age of the person, their ethnic origin, and other factors can alter the way eczema looks and feels.

There are however some general patterns to where the eczema is found on the body according to the age of the affected person.

Skin Conditions

Infants

Infants less than one year old often have widely distributed eczema. The skin is often dry, scaly, and red with small scratch marks made by sharp baby nails.

The cheeks of infants are often the first place to be affected by eczema.

The diaper area is frequently spared due to the moisture retention of diapers. Just like other babies, they can develop irritant diaper dermatitis, if wet or soiled diapers are left on too long.

Toddlers and Preschoolers

As children begin to move around, the eczema becomes more localized and thickened. Toddlers scratch vigorously and the eczema may look very raw and uncomfortable.

Eczema in this age group often affects the extensor (outer) aspects of joints, particularly the wrists, elbows, ankles, and knees. It may also affect the genitals.

As the child becomes older the pattern frequently changes to involve the flexor surfaces of the same joints (the creases) with less extensor involvement. The affected skin often becomes lichenified (i.e., dry and thickened from constant scratching and rubbing).

In some children the extensor pattern of eczema persists into later childhood.

School-Age Children

Older children tend to have the flexural pattern of eczema and it most often affects the elbow and knee creases. Other susceptible areas include the eyelids, earlobes, neck, and scalp.

They can develop recurrent acute itchy blisters on the palms, fingers, and sometimes on the feet, known as pompholyx or vesicular hand/foot dermatitis.

Many children develop a "nummular" pattern of atopic dermatitis. This refers to small coin-like areas of eczema scattered over the body. These round patches of eczema are dry, red, and itchy and may be mistaken for ringworm (a fungal infection).

Mostly the eczema improves during school years and it may completely clear up by the teens, although the barrier function of the skin is never entirely normal.

Adults

Adults who have atopic dermatitis may present in various different ways.

They may continue to have a diffuse pattern of eczema but the skin is often more dry and lichenified than in children.

Commonly adults have persistent localized eczema, possibly confined to the hands, eyelids, flexures, nipples, or all of these areas.

Recurrent staphylococcal infections may be prominent.

Atopic dermatitis is a major contributing factor to occupational irritant contact dermatitis. This most often affects hands that are frequently exposed to water, detergents, and/or solvents.

Hand dermatitis in adult atopics tends to be dry and thickened but may also be blistered.

Does Atopic Dermatitis Persist Forever?

Atopic dermatitis affects 15 to 20 percent of children but only 1 to 2 percent of adults. It is impossible to predict whether eczema will improve by itself or not in an individual.

It is unusual for an infant to be affected with atopic dermatitis before the age of four months but they may suffer from infantile seborrhoic dermatitis or other rashes prior to this. The onset of atopic dermatitis is usually before two years of age although it can manifest itself in older people for the first time.

Atopic dermatitis is often worst between the ages of two and four but it generally improves after this and may clear altogether by the teens.

Certain occupations such as farming, hairdressing, domestic and industrial cleaning, domestic duties, and care giving expose the skin to various irritants and sometimes allergens. This aggravates atopic dermatitis. It is wise to bear this in mind when considering career options—it is usually easier to choose a more suitable occupation from the outset than to change it later.

Treatment

Treatment of atopic dermatitis may be required for many months and possibly years.

It nearly always requires:

- reduction of exposure to trigger factors (where possible);
- regular emollients (moisturizers);
- intermittent topical steroids.

In some cases management may also include one of more of the following:

Skin Conditions

- topical calcineurin inhibitors such as pimecrolimus cream or tacrolimus ointment;
- antibiotics;
- antihistamines;
- phototherapy;
- oral corticosteroids;
- ciclosporin;
- azathioprine.

Section 31.2

Psoriasis

"Medical Facts about Psoriasis in Children," © 2007 National Psoriasis Foundation (www.psoriasis.org). Reprinted with permission.

No one knows exactly what causes psoriasis, though scientists believe it is an immune-mediated disease. With psoriasis, skin cells reproduce in three to four days instead of twenty-eight to thirty days, as is normal. While normal skin cells are shed unnoticed, psoriasis skin cells build up and form raised, scaly lesions. It affects people differently, and its course is not easy to predict.

Skin involved with psoriasis becomes red from the increased blood supply to the rapidly dividing cells. The white scale, called plaque, is composed of dead skin cells that build up on the skin's surface. Psoriasis goes through an unpredictable cycle: flares, improvement, remission, and reappearance.

The severity of each case is categorized by the percent of the body involved with psoriasis:

- Mild cases involve only a few lesions.
- Moderate cases cover 3 to 10 percent of the body. (The palm of your hand represents 1 percent of the body's skin surface.)
- Severe cases involve more than 10 percent of the skin surface, and, in rare cases, may include all of a person's skin.

It is not contagious. People do not "catch" psoriasis from other people, nor can they transmit the disease to others. Psoriasis does not spread on an individual's skin because of self-contagion.

The more you understand about psoriasis, the more you'll be able to help the children who have psoriasis manage the disease. Here are answers to the most common medical questions about psoriasis.

What is psoriasis?

Psoriasis is a noncontagious, chronic (lifelong) skin disease. The condition is caused by skin cells maturing in three to four days, instead of the usual twenty-eight to thirty days. It is characterized by reddening of the skin, lesions, and white plaques. A person with psoriasis may have only a few lesions, or may have widespread lesions across most of the body.

What causes psoriasis?

Researchers are not certain what causes the disease. It is believed to be an immune-mediated disease. Genetics seems to play a part, as do environmental factors. Scientists believe that a biochemical stimulus triggers the abnormally high skin cell growth.

Who gets psoriasis?

While all races have the disease, Caucasians tend to have a slightly higher incidence. It appears most often between the ages of fifteen and thirty-five, though it can strike in infancy or old age. Psoriasis in infants may be difficult to diagnose and can sometimes be mistaken for eczema. About a third of all patients will present in childhood with psoriasis. Experts say that about 10 percent of all patients with psoriasis get it before the age of ten; this group seems to be more genetically predisposed to psoriasis.

How is psoriasis diagnosed?

There is no specific medical test for psoriasis. A physician usually makes the diagnosis after examining the skin, scalp, nails, and, sometimes a biopsy under a microscope.

Is all psoriasis alike?

There are several forms of psoriasis:

Skin Conditions

- **Plaque:** most common type, characterized by inflamed skin lesions topped with white scales
- **Guttate:** small dot-like lesions
- **Pustular:** blister-like lesions of noninfectious fluid (pustules)
- **Inverse:** appears in skin folds
- **Erythrodermic:** redness and swelling, exfoliation of dead skin and pain

About 10 to 30 percent of people with psoriasis also have psoriatic arthritis, which usually affects the feet and hands. It can affect a few joints, or it can be severe or disabling.

Is there a cure for psoriasis?

There is no cure at present. However, many different treatments—topical and systemic—can clear psoriasis for periods of time. Experimentation is often required to find a treatment that works for an individual.

Infants: Treatment is very conservative. Vaseline petroleum jelly and moisturizers can be a good first step. An Aveeno oatmeal bath and Benadryl cream can help relieve the itching, but a physician must be consulted before starting any treatment with an infant.

Children: For mild psoriasis, sunlight may be helpful. For moderate cases, regular ultraviolet light or narrow band ultraviolet light therapy can help clear the lesions. Many cases have been triggered by strep infection, so antibiotics may help clear the bacteria that could have triggered the psoriasis.

Teens: Ultraviolet light therapy can help clear the psoriasis. Oral medications may have different side effects for teens, and potent topical steroids need to be applied with caution because they can be absorbed too quickly.

Chapter 32

Vision Problems

Chapter Contents

Section 32.1—Amblyopia 548
Section 32.2—Conjunctivitis (Pinkeye) 550
Section 32.3—Far- and Nearsightedness 553
Section 32.4—Retinitis Pigmentosa 555
Section 32.5—Strabismus 557

Section 32.1

Amblyopia

Excerpted from "Amblyopia," National Eye Institute, January 2008.

What Is Amblyopia?

The brain and the eye work together to produce vision. Light enters the eye and is changed into nerve signals that travel along the optic nerve to the brain. Amblyopia is the medical term used when the vision in one of the eyes is reduced because the eye and the brain are not working together properly. The eye itself looks normal, but it is not being used normally because the brain is favoring the other eye. This condition is also sometimes called lazy eye.

How Common Is Amblyopia?

Amblyopia is the most common cause of visual impairment in childhood. The condition affects approximately two to three out of every one hundred children. Unless it is successfully treated in early childhood, amblyopia usually persists into adulthood, and is the most common cause of monocular (one eye) visual impairment among children and young and middle-aged adults.

What Causes Amblyopia?

Amblyopia may be caused by any condition that affects normal visual development or use of the eyes. Amblyopia can be caused by strabismus, an imbalance in the positioning of the two eyes. Strabismus can cause the eyes to cross in (esotropia) or turn out (exotropia). Sometimes amblyopia is caused when one eye is more nearsighted, farsighted, or astigmatic than the other eye. Occasionally, amblyopia is caused by other eye conditions such as cataract.

How Is Amblyopia Treated in Children?

Treating amblyopia involves making the child use the eye with the reduced vision (weaker eye). Currently, there are two ways used to do this:

Vision Problems

Atropine: A drop of a drug called atropine is placed in the stronger eye once a day to temporarily blur the vision so that the child will prefer to use the eye with amblyopia. Treatment with atropine also stimulates vision in the weaker eye and helps the part of the brain that manages vision develop more completely.

Patching: An opaque, adhesive patch is worn over the stronger eye for weeks to months. This therapy forces the child to use the eye with amblyopia. Patching stimulates vision in the weaker eye and helps the part of the brain that manages vision develop more completely.

Previously, eye care professionals often thought that treating amblyopia in older children would be of little benefit. However, surprising results from a nationwide clinical trial show that many children age seven through seventeen with amblyopia may benefit from treatments that are more commonly used on younger children. This study shows that age alone should not be used as a factor to decide whether or not to treat a child for amblyopia.

National Eye Institute–Supported Research

Findings from the clinical study, An Evaluation of Treatment of Amblyopia in Children 7 To <18 Years Old (ATS3), show that many children age seven through seventeen with amblyopia (lazy eye) may benefit from treatments that are more commonly used on younger children. Previously, eye care professionals often thought that treating amblyopia in older children would be of little benefit.

The National Eye Institute is currently supporting the Amblyopia Treatment Study: Occlusion Versus Pharmacologic Therapy for Moderate Amblyopia (ATS) to determine whether patching or eye drops is a better treatment for amblyopia. Recent results for the ATS found that the atropine eye drops, when placed in the unaffected eye once a day, work as well as eye patching and may encourage better compliance.

In addition, A Randomized Trial Comparing Part-time Versus Minimal-time Patching for Moderate Amblyopia (Two v. Six) is being conducted to determine whether the visual acuity improvement obtained with part-time (six hours) patching is equivalent to the visual acuity improvement obtained with minimal patching (two hours) for moderate amblyopia. Recent findings show that patching the unaffected eye of children with moderate amblyopia for two hours daily works as well as patching the eye for six hours. Shorter patching time should lead to better compliance with treatment and improved quality of life for children with amblyopia.

Section 32.2

Conjunctivitis (Pinkeye)

"Conjunctivitis," © 2007 Illinois Department of Public Health (www.idph.state.il.us). Reprinted with permission.

What is conjunctivitis?

Conjunctivitis is an inflammation of the thin, clear membrane (conjunctiva) that covers the white of the eye and the inside surface of the eyelids. Conjunctivitis, commonly known as "pink eye," is most often caused by a virus but also can be caused by bacterial infection, allergies (e.g., cosmetics, pollen), and chemical irritation.

How is it spread?

Anyone can get conjunctivitis. It can spread fairly easily from person to person, especially in dormitories, schools, or other places where large numbers of persons congregate. People commonly get conjunctivitis by coming into contact with the tears or other eye discharges of an infected person, and then touching their own eyes. Hands, towels, and washcloths can spread conjunctivitis. Symptoms normally appear a few days after contact with an infected person or an object contaminated with the virus (such as a towel).

Individuals with conjunctivitis may be contagious as long as symptoms persist or the eye appears abnormal. Risk of conjunctivitis increases with use of contact lenses, and touching/rubbing the eyes without hand washing first.

What are the symptoms of conjunctivitis?

Symptoms of conjunctivitis may include the following:

- Eye redness and irritation
- Sensitivity to bright light
- Itchiness or a gritty sensation in the eye
- Swollen eyelids

Vision Problems

- Tearing and discharge (Discharge may make the eyelids and eyelashes stick together or have crusty debris, especially in the morning.)

Viral conjunctivitis often begins with fairly sudden onset of pain or the feeling of dust in the eye. Infection may begin in only one eye but often spreads to involve both.

Should I contact a doctor if I develop symptoms of conjunctivitis?

You should contact your health care provider:

- if you have symptoms of conjunctivitis and they do not improve in twenty-four to forty-eight hours;
- if you have conjunctivitis and wear contact lenses;
- if you have vision problems or significant eye pain; or
- if you develop fever.

Other concerns, including the duration of your conjunctivitis symptoms, whether or not your symptoms are improving as expected, etc., should also be shared with your health care provider.

How is conjunctivitis treated?

Treatment varies with the cause. There is no curative treatment for common viral conjunctivitis; it usually will go away by itself in one to six weeks. Lubricating eye drops sometimes help to ease symptoms. (Do not share these eye drops with other persons.) If symptoms last for more than twenty-four to forty-eight hours, or vision is affected, it is important to be seen by a health care practitioner. Other kinds of conjunctivitis often have specific treatments that may be prescribed.

A person with conjunctivitis should follow these general guidelines:

- If medication has been prescribed, use exactly as directed for the full course of treatment. (All treatments used for conjunctivitis should be thrown away when no longer needed.)
- Be sure to wash hands with soap and water before and after using eye medication.
- Wash hands frequently during waking hours with soap and water (fifteen seconds), and use paper towels or blow dry.

- Avoid touching your eyes. Gently wipe discharge from the eye using disposable tissues.
- Use warm or cool water compresses to reduce discomfort.
- Do not use eye makeup. Discard eye makeup if used when conjunctivitis was present because organisms may remain in makeup and cause a reoccurrence.

Should contact lens wearers take special precautions?

- Disinfect lenses, also clean and disinfect storage case.
- Do not use eye drops or ointment with the lens in place.
- Do not wear contact lenses until eyes are entirely clear of conjunctivitis.
- If using disposable lenses, discard; after infection clears, use new lenses.

Can conjunctivitis be prevented?

Conjunctivitis can be prevented by practicing good hygiene:

- Wash hands frequently with soap and water.
- Use clean paper towels to dry hands.
- Avoid touching the hands of others or rubbing the eyes.
- Avoid exposure to eye irritants such as perfumes and smoke.
- Throw away or machine wash towels, tissues, and other items that touch the eyes after each use.
- Avoid sharing towels and washcloths.
- Avoid sharing eye drops, eye makeup, contact lens solution, tissues, and other items used on the face.

Section 32.3

Far- and Nearsightedness

"Farsightedness (Hyperopia)" and "Nearsightedness (Myopia)," © St. Luke's Cataract & Laser Institute. Reprinted with permission. The text of these documents is available online at http://www.stlukeseye.com/Conditions/Hyperopia.asp and http://www.stlukeseye.com/Conditions/Myopia.asp; accessed January 29, 2008.

Farsightedness (Hyperopia)

Overview

Farsightedness, or hyperopia, occurs when light entering the eye focuses behind the retina, instead of directly on it. This is caused by a cornea that is flatter, or an eye that is shorter, than a normal eye. Farsighted people usually have trouble seeing up close, but may also have difficulty seeing far away as well.

Young people with mild to moderate hyperopia are often able to see clearly because their natural lens can adjust or accommodate to increase the eye's focusing ability. However, as the eye gradually loses the ability to accommodate (beginning at about forty years of age), blurred vision from hyperopia often becomes more apparent.

Signs and Symptoms

- Difficulty seeing up close
- Blurred distance vision (occurs with higher amounts of hyperopia)
- Eye fatigue when reading
- Eye strain (headaches, pulling sensation, burning)
- Crossed eyes in children

Detection and Diagnosis

Hyperopia is detected with a vision test called a refraction. Young patients' eyes are dilated for this test so they are unable to mask their farsightedness with accommodation. This is called a wet refraction.

Treatment

The treatment for hyperopia depends on several factors such as the patient's age, activities, and occupation. Young patients may or may not require glasses or contact lenses, depending on their ability to compensate for their farsightedness with accommodation. Glasses or contact lenses are required for older patients.

Refractive surgery is an option for adults who wish to see clearly without glasses. Laser assisted in-situ keratomileusis (LASIK), clear lens extraction and replacement, laser thermal keratoplasty (LTK), and intraocular contact lenses are all procedures that can be performed to correct hyperopia.

Nearsightedness (Myopia)

Overview

Nearsightedness, or myopia, occurs when light entering the eye focuses in front of the retina instead of directly on it. This is caused by a cornea that is steeper, or an eye that is longer, than a normal eye. Nearsighted people typically see well up close, but have difficulty seeing far away.

This problem is often discovered in school-age children who report having trouble seeing the chalkboard. Nearsightedness usually becomes progressively worse through adolescence and stabilizes in early adulthood. It is an inherited problem.

Signs and Symptoms

- Blurry distance vision
- Vision seems clearer when squinting

Detection and Diagnosis

Nearsightedness is detected with a vision test and refraction.

Treatment

The treatment for nearsightedness depends on several factors such as the patient's age, activities, and occupation. Vision can corrected with glasses, contacts, or surgery. Refractive procedures such as LASIK can be considered for adults when the prescription has remained stable for at least one year.

Section 32.4

Retinitis Pigmentosa

Excerpted from "Learning about Retinitis Pigmentosa,"
National Human Genome Research Institute, National Institutes
of Health, November 27, 2007.

What is retinitis pigmentosa?

Retinitis pigmentosa (RP) is the name given to a group of inherited eye diseases that affect the retina (the light-sensitive part of the eye). RP causes the breakdown of photoreceptor cells (cells in the retina that detect light). Photoreceptor cells capture and process light, helping us to see. As these cells break down and die, patients experience progressive vision loss.

The most common feature of all forms of RP is a gradual breakdown of rods (retinal cells that detect dim light) and cones (retinal cells that detect light and color). Most forms of RP first cause the breakdown of rod cells. These forms of RP, sometimes called rod-cone dystrophy, usually begin with night blindness. Night blindness is somewhat like the experience normally sighted individuals encounter when entering a dark movie theatre on a bright, sunny day. However, patients with RP cannot adjust well to dark and dimly lit environments.

What are the symptoms of retinitis pigmentosa?

As the disease progresses and more rod cells break down, patients lose their peripheral vision (tunnel vision). Individuals with RP often experience a ring of vision loss in their periphery, but retain clear central vision. Others report the sensation of tunnel vision, as though they see the world through a straw. Many patients with retinitis pigmentosa retain a small degree of central vision throughout their life.

Other forms of RP, sometimes called cone-rod dystrophy, first affect central vision. Patients first experience a loss of central vision that cannot be corrected with glasses or contact lenses. With the loss of cone cells also come disturbances in color perception. As the disease progresses, rod cells degenerate, causing night blindness and peripheral vision.

Childhood Diseases and Disorders Sourcebook, Second Edition

Symptoms of RP are most often recognized in children, adolescents, and young adults, with progression of the disease continuing throughout the individual's life. The pattern and degree of visual loss are variable.

What causes retinitis pigmentosa?

Retinitis pigmentosa is an inherited disorder, and therefore not caused by injury, infection, or any other external or environmental factors. People suffering from RP are born with the disorder already programmed into their cells. Doctors can see the first signs of retinitis pigmentosa in affected children as early as age ten. Research suggests that several different types of gene mutations (changes in genes) can send faulty messages to the retinal cells, which leads to their progressive degeneration. In most cases, the disorder is linked to a recessive gene, a gene that must be inherited from both parents in order to cause the disease. But dominant genes and genes on the X chromosome also have been linked to retinitis pigmentosa. In these cases, only one parent has passed the disease gene. In some cases, a new mutation causes the disease to occur in a person who does not have a family history of the disease. The disorder also can show up as part of other syndromes, such as Bassen-Kornzweig disease or Kearns-Sayre syndrome.

How is retinitis pigmentosa treated?

There is no known cure for retinitis pigmentosa. However, there are a few treatment options, such as light avoidance and/or the use of low-vision aids to slow down the progression of RP. Some practitioners also consider vitamin A as a possible treatment option to slow down the progression of RP. Research suggests taking high doses of vitamin A (15,000 IU/day) may slow progression a little in some people, but the results are not strong. Taking too much vitamin A can be toxic and the effects of vitamin A on the disease is relatively weak. More research must be conducted before this is a widely accepted form of therapy.

Research is also being conducted in areas such as gene therapy research, transplant research, and retinal prosthesis. Since RP is usually the result of a defective gene, gene therapy has become a widely explored area for future research. The goal of such research would be to discover ways healthy genes can be inserted into the retina. Attempts at transplanting healthy retinal cells into sick retinas are being made experimentally and have not yet been considered as clinically safe and successful. Retinal prosthesis is also an important area of exploration because the prosthesis, a man-made device intended to replace

Vision Problems

a damaged body part, can be designed to take over the function of the lost photoreceptors by electrically stimulating the remaining healthy cells of the retina. Through electrical stimulation, the activated ganglion cells can provide a visual signal to the brain. The visual scene captured by a camera is transmitted via electromagnetic radiation to a small decoder chip located on the retinal surface. Data and power are then sent to a set of electrodes connected to the decoder. Electrical current passing from individual electrodes stimulate cells in the appropriate areas of the retina corresponding to the features in the visual scene.

Section 32.5

Strabismus

"Strabismus (Crossed or Turned Eye)," © St. Luke's Cataract & Laser Institute. Reprinted with permission. The text of this document is available online at http://www.stlukeseye.com/Conditions/Strabismus.asp; accessed January 29, 2008.

Overview

Strabismus is a problem caused by one or more improperly functioning eye muscles, resulting in a misalignment of the eyes. Normally, each eye focuses on the same spot but sends a slightly different message to the brain. The brain superimposes the two images, giving vision depth and dimension. Here's an easy way to see how the eyes work together: hold your finger at arm's length. While looking at your finger, close one eye, then the other. Notice how your finger changes position. Even though the images are slightly different, the brain interprets them as one.

Each eye has six muscles that work in unison to control movements. The brain controls the eye muscles, which keep the eyes properly aligned. It is critical that the muscles function together for the brain to interpret the image from each eye as a single one.

Strabismus must be detected early in children because they are so adaptable. If a child sees double, his or her brain quickly learns to suppress or block out one of the images to maintain single vision. In a very short time, the brain permanently suppresses vision from the turned eye, causing a weak or amblyopic eye. Children may also develop a head tilt or turn to compensate for the problem and eliminate the double image. Unlike children, adults with a newly acquired strabismus problem typically see double.

There are many causes of strabismus. It can be inherited, or it may be caused by trauma, certain diseases, and sometimes eye surgery.

Signs and Symptoms

Adults are much more likely to be bothered by symptoms from strabismus than young children. It is unusual for a child to complain of double vision. Children should undergo vision screening exams to detect problems early. The younger the child is when strabismus is detected and treated, the better the chance of normal vision. The following are common signs and symptoms:

- Turned or crossed eye
- Head tilt or turn
- Squinting
- Double vision (in some cases)

Detection and Diagnosis

Strabismus is detected with a comprehensive eye exam and special tests used to evaluate the alignment of the eyes such as the Krimsky test and prism testing.

Treatment

The appropriate treatment for strabismus is dependent on several factors including the patient's age, the cause of the problem, and the type and degree of the eye turn. Treatment may include patching, corrective glasses, prisms, or surgery.

With patching, the better eye is covered, forcing the child to use the weaker eye. Over time, the brain adjusts to using the weaker eye and vision gradually improves. For this treatment to be effective, it must be done at a young age before the child can develop amblyopia.

Surgery is sometimes performed for both adults and children to straighten a crossed eye. The procedure may be done with local or general anesthesia. There are several different surgical techniques used to correct strabismus. The appropriate one is dependent on the muscle involved and the degree of the eye turn.

Part Four

Developmental and Pediatric Mental Health Concerns

Chapter 33

Autism Spectrum Disorders

Even though autism was first described in the 1940s, little was really known about the disorder until the 1990s. Even today, there is a great deal that researchers, scientists, and health care providers don't know about autism.

But there are things that we do know about autism. This chapter offers broad information about autism and answers some of the more common questions that parents and families often have about the disorder.

What is autism?

Autism is a complex neurobiological disorder of development that lasts throughout a person's life. It is sometimes called a developmental disability because it usually starts before age three, in the developmental period, and because it causes delays or problems in many different skills that arise from infancy to adulthood.

The main signs and symptoms of autism involve[1] language, social behavior, and behaviors concerning objects and routines:

- **Communication:** Both verbal (spoken) and nonverbal (unspoken, such as pointing, eye contact, or smiling)

- **Social interactions:** Such as sharing emotions, understanding how others think and feel (sometimes called empathy), and

---

Reprinted from "Autism Overview: What We Know," National Institute of Child Health and Human Development, National Institutes of Health, NIH Publication No. 05-5592, updated January 2007.

holding a conversation, as well as the amount of time a person spends interacting with others

- **Routines or repetitive behaviors:** Often called stereotyped behaviors, such as repeating words or actions, obsessively following routines or schedules, playing with toys or objects in repetitive and sometimes inappropriate ways, or having very specific and inflexible ways of arranging items

People with autism might have problems talking with you, or they might not look you in the eye when you talk to them. They may have to line up their pencils before they can pay attention, or they may say the same sentence again and again to calm themselves down. They may flap their arms to tell you they are happy, or they might hurt themselves to tell you they are not. Some people with autism never learn how to talk. These behaviors not only make life challenging for people who have autism, but also take a toll on their families, their health care providers, their teachers, and anyone who comes in contact with them.

Because different people with autism can have very different features or symptoms, health care providers think of autism as a "spectrum" disorder—a group of disorders with a range of similar features. Based on their specific strengths and weaknesses, people with autism spectrum disorders (ASDs) may have mild symptoms or more serious symptoms, but they all have an ASD. This chapter uses the terms "ASD" and "autism" to mean the same thing.

What conditions are in the ASD category?

Currently, the ASD category includes the following:

- Autistic disorder (also called "classic" autism)
- Asperger syndrome
- Pervasive developmental disorder not otherwise specified (or atypical autism)[2]

In some cases, health care providers use a broader term—pervasive developmental disorders (PDD)—to describe autism. The PDD category includes the ASDs mentioned above, plus childhood disintegrative disorder and Rett syndrome.

Depending on specific symptoms, a person with autism may fall into the ASD or the PDD category. Sometimes, the terms "ASD" and "PDD" are used to mean the same thing because autism is in both categories.

What causes autism?

Scientists don't know exactly what causes autism at this time.

Much evidence supports the idea that genetic factors—that is, genes, their function, and their interactions—are one of the main underlying causes of ASDs. But, researchers aren't looking for just one gene. Current evidence suggests that as many as ten or more genes on different chromosomes may be involved in autism, to different degrees.

Some genes may place a person at greater risk for autism, called susceptibility. Other genes may cause specific symptoms or determine how severe those symptoms are. Or, genes with changes or mutations might add to the symptoms of autism because the genes or gene products aren't working properly.

Research has also shown that environmental factors, such as viruses, may also play a role in causing autism.

While some researchers are examining genes and environmental factors, other researchers are looking at possible neurological, infectious, metabolic, and immunologic factors that may be involved in autism.

Because the disorder is so complex, and because no two people with autism are exactly alike, autism is probably the result of many causes.

Is there a link between autism and vaccines?

To date, there is no conclusive scientific evidence that any part of a vaccine or any combination of vaccines causes autism, even though researchers have carried out many studies to answer this important question. There is also no proof that any material used to make or preserve vaccines plays a role in causing autism.

Although there have been reports of studies that relate vaccines to autism, the findings have not held up under further investigation. Researchers have been unable to replicate the studies that reportedly found a link between autism and vaccines.

There is a great deal of research and discussion on the topic of vaccines and autism—too much to cover here. The U.S. Centers for Disease Control and Prevention (CDC) conducts and supports most of the federal epidemiological studies that seek to answer questions about vaccines and autism.

Currently, the CDC provides the most accurate and up-to-date information about research on autism and vaccine research, both supported by the federal government and funded independently.

How many people have autism?

Currently, researchers don't know the exact number of people with an ASD in the United States.

Researchers use different ways to determine prevalence that often give different results.

Some estimates of prevalence rely on previously published studies. Researchers review all the published data on a topic and take the averages of these calculations to determine prevalence. Independent researchers[3] recently conducted two such reviews. Based on these studies, the best conservative estimate[4] of the prevalence of ASDs in the United States is that one child in one thousand children has an ASD.

Is autism more common now than it was in the past?

Researchers are not certain whether autism is more prevalent now than in the past for a number of reasons. Although more cases of autism are being identified, it is not clear why. Some of the increase may result from better education about the symptoms of autism or from more accurate diagnoses of autism.

The new definition of autism as a spectrum disorder means that even people with mild symptoms can be classified as having an ASD, which could also account for the increase in identified cases. As research moves forward using the current definition of ASDs, more definite numbers may be available to answer this question.

Is autism more common in certain groups of people?

Current figures show that autism occurs in all racial, ethnic, and social groups equally, with individuals in one group no more or less likely to have ASDs than those in other groups. Three groups are at higher-than-normal risk for ASDs:

- **Boys:** Statistics show that boys are three to four times more likely[5] to be affected by autism than are girls.

- **Siblings of those with ASDs:** Among families that have one child with an ASD, recurrence of ASD in another sibling is between[6] 2 percent and 8 percent, a figure much higher than in the general population.

- **People with certain other developmental disorders:** For certain disorders, including Fragile X syndrome, mental retardation, and tuberous sclerosis, autism is common in addition to the primary symptoms of the disorder.

Autism Spectrum Disorders

When do people usually show signs of autism?

A number of the behavioral symptoms[7] of autism are observable by eighteen months of age, including: problems with eye contact, not responding to one's name, joint attention problems, underdeveloped skills in pretend play and imitation, and problems with nonverbal communication and language.

Some studies also note that, although more subtle, some signs of autism are detectable at eight months[8] of age.

In general, the average age of autism diagnosis is currently three years old. In many cases, a delay in the child's starting to speak around age two brings problems to parents' attention, even though other, less noticeable signs may be present at an earlier age.[9]

Studies[10] also show that a subgroup of children with ASDs experiences a "regression," meaning they stop using the language, play, or social skills they had already learned. This regression usually happens between the first and second birthdays.

Researchers are still learning about the features of regression in ASDs, and whether the features differ from those shown by individuals who show signs of autism in early life.

What are some of the possible signs of autism?

Parents, caregivers, family members, teachers, and others who spend a lot of time with children can look for "red flags." Some may mean a delay in one or more areas of development, while others are more typical of ASDs. Possible red flags for autism are as follows:

- The child does not respond to his or her name.
- The child cannot explain what he or she wants.
- The child's language skills are slow to develop or speech is delayed.
- The child doesn't follow directions.
- At times, the child seems to be deaf.
- The child seems to hear sometimes, but not other times.
- The child doesn't point or wave "bye-bye."
- The child used to say a few words or babble, but now he or she doesn't.
- The child throws intense or violent tantrums.
- The child has odd movement patterns.
- The child is overly active, uncooperative, or resistant.

- The child doesn't know how to play with toys.
- The child doesn't smile when smiled at.
- The child has poor eye contact.
- The child gets "stuck" doing the same things over and over and can't move on to other things.
- The child seems to prefer to play alone.
- The child gets things for him- or herself only.
- The child is very independent for his or her age.
- The child does things "early" compared to other children.
- The child seems to be in his or her "own world."
- The child seems to tune people out.
- The child is not interested in other children.
- The child walks on his or her toes.
- The child shows unusual attachments to toys, objects, or schedules (i.e., always holding a string or having to put socks on before pants).
- The child spends a lot of time lining things up or putting things in a certain order.

In addition, your child's health care provider will send your child for an evaluation if you report any of the following behaviors; such an evaluation would consider ASDs, among other possible causes.[12]

Your child may need further evaluation if he or she:

- does not babble or coo by twelve months of age;
- does not gesture (point, wave, grasp, etc.) by twelve months of age;
- does not say single words by sixteen months of age;
- does not say two-word phrases on his or her own (rather than just repeating what someone says to him or her) by twenty-four months of age;
- has *any* loss of *any* language or social skill at *any* age.

Autism Spectrum Disorders

What should I do if I think my child has a developmental problem or autism?

Tell your child's health care provider immediately if you think something is wrong. According to the American Academy of Pediatrics (AAP)[13], "Pediatricians should listen carefully to parents discussing their child's development. [Parents] are reliable sources of information and their concerns should be valued and addressed immediately."

Your child's health care provider will note your comments and concerns, will ask some other questions, and will determine the best plan of action. In some cases, the health care provider will ask you to complete a questionnaire about your child to get more specific information about symptoms. To rule out certain conditions, the health care provider will also test your child's hearing and check your child's lead level before deciding on a course of action.

If red flags are present, and if the lead and hearing tests show no problems, your child's health care provider may refer you to a specialist in child development or another specialized health care professional. The specialist will conduct a number of tests to determine whether or not your child has autism or an ASD.

What if I don't notice any symptoms?

If you don't report any of these signs, your child's health care provider will continue to check for problems at every well-baby and well-child visit.[14] If your child's health care provider does not routinely check your child with such tests, you should ask that he or she do so.

In this developmental screening, the provider asks questions related to normal development that can help measure your child's specific progress. Typically, these questions are similar to the red flags listed earlier. Based on your answers, the health care provider may send your child for further evaluation.

The AAP recommends[15] that health care providers ask questions about different aspects of development. These questions include (but are not limited to) those listed here.

Does your child:

- Not speak as well as other children his or her age?
- Have poor eye contact?
- Act as if he or she is in his or her own world?
- Seem to "tune out" others?
- Not smile when smiled at?

- Seem unable to tell you what he or she wants, and so takes your hand and leads you to what he or she wants, or gets it him- or herself?
- Have trouble following simple directions?
- Not play with toys in a usual way?
- Not bring things to you to "show" you something?
- Not point to interesting things or direct your attention to items of interest?
- Have unusually long or severe temper tantrums?
- Show an unusual attachment to objects, especially "hard" ones, such as a flashlight or key chain, instead of "soft" ones, such as a blanket or stuffed animal?
- Prefer to play alone?
- Not pretend or play "make believe" (if the child is older than age two)?

Is there a cure for autism?

To date, there is no cure for autism, but sometimes, children with ASDs make so much progress that they no longer show the full syndrome of autism when they are older.

Research[16] shows that early diagnosis and interventions delivered early in life, such as in the preschool period, are more likely to result in major positive effects on later skills and symptoms. The sooner a child begins to get help, the more opportunity for learning. Because a young child's brain is still forming, early intervention gives children the best start possible and the best chance of developing their full potential. Even so, no matter when a person is diagnosed with autism, it's never too late to benefit from treatment. People of all ages with ASDs at all levels of ability generally respond positively to well-designed interventions.

Public Law 108-77: Individuals with Disabilities Education Improvement Act (2004) and Public Law 105-17: *Individuals with Disabilities Act, or IDEA*[17] (1997) require your child's primary care provider to refer you and your family to an early intervention service. Every state operates an early intervention program for children from birth to age three; children with autism should qualify for these services. Early intervention programs typically include behavioral methods, early developmental education, communication skills, occupational and physical therapy, and structured social play.

Autism Spectrum Disorders

What are the treatments for autism?

Currently there is no definitive, single treatment for ASDs. However, there are a variety of ways to help minimize the symptoms and maximize learning. Persons with an ASD have the best chance of using all of their individual capabilities and skills if they receive appropriate behavioral and other therapies, education, and medication. In some cases, these treatments can help people with autism function at near-normal levels.

Some possible treatments for autism are explained in the following. If you have a question about treatment, you should talk to a health care provider who specializes in caring for people with autism.

Behavioral Therapy and Other Therapeutic Options

In general, behavior management therapy works to reinforce wanted behaviors and reduce unwanted behaviors. At the same time, these methods also suggest what caregivers should do before or between episodes of problem behaviors, and what to do during or after these episodes. Behavioral therapy is often based on applied behavior analysis (ABA). Different applications of ABA commonly used for people with autism include: positive behavioral interventions and support (PBS), pivotal response training (PRT), incidental teaching, milieu therapy, verbal behavior, and discrete trial teaching (DTT), among others.

Keep in mind that other therapies, beyond ABA, may also be effective for persons with autism. Talk to your health care provider about the best options for your child.

A variety of health care providers can also help individuals with ASDs and their families to work through different situations:

- Speech-language therapists can help people with autism improve their general ability to communicate and interact with others effectively, as well as develop their speech and language skills. These therapists may teach nonverbal ways of communicating and may improve social skills that involve communicating with others. They may also help people to better use words and sentences, and to improve rate and rhythm of speech and conversation.

- Occupational therapists can help people with autism find ways to adjust tasks and conditions that match their needs and abilities. Such help may include finding a specially designed computer mouse and keyboard to ease communication, or identifying skills that build on a person's interests and individual capabilities.

Occupational therapists may also do many of the same types of activities as physical therapists do (see following).

- Physical therapists design activities and exercises to build motor control and to improve posture and balance. For example, they can help a child who avoids body contact to participate in activities and games with other children.

Special services are often available to preschool and school-aged children, as well as to teens, through the local public school system. In many cases, services provided by specialists in the school setting are free. More intense and individualized help is available through private clinics, but the family usually has to pay for private services, although some health insurance plans may help cover the cost.

Educational and School-Based Options

Children with ASDs are guaranteed free, appropriate public education under federal laws. *Public Law 108-77: Individuals with Disabilities Education Improvement Act*[17] (2004) and *Public Law 105-17: The Individuals with Disabilities Education Act—IDEA*[18] (1997) make it possible for children with disabilities to get free educational services and educational devices to help them learn as much as they can. Each child is entitled to these services from age three through high school, or until age twenty-one, whichever comes first.

The laws state that children must be taught in the least restrictive environment appropriate for that individual child. This statement does not mean that each child must be placed in a regular classroom. Instead, the laws mean that the teaching environment should be designed to meet a child's learning needs, while minimizing restrictions on the child's access to typical learning experiences and interactions. Educating persons with ASDs often includes a combination of one-to-one, small group, and regular classroom instruction.

To qualify for special education services, the child must meet specific criteria as outlined by federal and state guidelines. You can contact a local school principal or special education coordinator to learn how to have your child assessed to see if he or she qualifies for services under these laws.

If your child qualifies for special services, a team of people, including you and your family, caregivers, teachers, school psychologists, and other child development specialists, will work together to design an Individualized Educational Plan (IEP)[19] for your child. An IEP includes specific academic, communication, motor, learning, functional, and socialization goals for a child based on his or her educational needs. The team also decides how best to carry out the IEP, such as determining any devices or special assistance the child needs, and identifying the developmental specialists who will work with the child.

The special services team should evaluate and re-evaluate your child on a regular basis to see how your child is doing and whether any changes are needed in his or her plan.

A number of parents' organizations, both national and local, provide information on therapeutic and educational services and how to get these services for a child. Check the local phone book for more information.

Medication Options

Currently, there is no medication that can cure ASDs or all of the associated symptoms. Further, the Food and Drug Administration (FDA) has not approved any drugs specifically for the treatment of autism or its causes. But, in many cases, medication can treat some of the symptoms associated with ASDs. (Please note that the National Institute of Child Health and Human Development [NICHD] does not endorse or support the use of any of these medications for treating symptoms of ASDs, or for other conditions for which the medications are not FDA approved.)

Medication can improve the behavior of a person with autism. Health care providers often use medications to deal with a specific behavior, such as reducing self-injurious behavior. With the symptom minimized, the person with autism can focus on other things, including learning and communication. Some of these medications have serious risks involved with their use; others may make symptoms worse at first or may take several weeks to become effective.

Not every medication helps every person with symptoms of autism. Health care providers usually prescribe medication on a trial basis, to see if it helps. Your child's health care provider may have to try different dosages or different combinations of medications to find the most effective plan. Families, caregivers, and health care providers need to work together to make sure that medications are working and that the overall medication plan is safe.

Medications used to treat the symptoms of autism[20] may include (but are not limited to) the following:

- **Selective serotonin re-uptake inhibitors (SSRIs):** These are a group of antidepressants that treat problems resulting from an imbalance in one of the body's chemical systems, that are sometimes present in autism. These medications may reduce the frequency and intensity of repetitive behaviors; decrease irritability, tantrums, and aggressive behavior; and improve eye contact.

- **Tricyclics:** These are another type of antidepressant used to treat depression and obsessive compulsive behaviors. Although these drugs tend to cause more side effects than the SSRIs, sometimes they are more effective for certain people.

- **Psychoactive or anti-psychotic medications:** These affect the brain of the person taking them. Use of this group of drugs is the most widely studied treatment for autism. In some people with ASDs, these drugs may decrease hyperactivity, reduce stereotyped behaviors, and minimize withdrawal and aggression.

- **Stimulants:** These may be useful in increasing focus and decreasing hyperactivity in people with autism, particularly in higher-functioning individuals. Because of the risk of side effects, health care providers should monitor those using these drugs carefully and often.

- **Anti-anxiety drugs:** These can help relieve anxiousness and panic disorders associated with autism.

What is secretin and is it an effective treatment for autism?

Secretin is a hormone produced by the small intestine that helps in digestion. Currently, the FDA approves a single dose of secretin only for use in diagnosing digestive problems.

In the 1990s, news reports described a few persons with autism whose behavior improved after getting secretin during a diagnostic test.

However, a series[21] of clinical trials funded by the NICHD and conducted through the Network on the Neurobiology and Genetics of Autism: Collaborative Programs of Excellence in Autism (CPEAs) found no difference in improvement between those taking secretin and those taking placebo. In fact, of the five case-controlled clinical trials published on secretin, not one showed secretin as any better than placebo, no matter what the dosage or frequency. For this reason, secretin is not recommended as a treatment for ASDs.

Are there other disorders associated with ASDs?

In about 5 percent[22] of autism cases, another disorder is also present. Studying this kind of co-occurrence helps researchers who are trying to pinpoint the genes involved in autism. Similar disorders or disorders with similar symptoms may have similar genetic origins. In cases of one disorder commonly occurring with another, it could be that one is actually a risk factor for the other. This kind of information can provide clues to what actually happens in autism.

Some of these co-occurring disorders include the following:

- **Epilepsy or seizure disorder:** Nearly one-third[23] of those with autism also show signs of epilepsy by adulthood. In most cases, medication can control and treat epilepsy effectively.

- **Tuberous sclerosis:** About 6 percent[24] of those with autism also have tuberous sclerosis, a disorder that shares many symptoms with autism, including seizures that result from lesions (cuts) on the brain.

- **Fragile X syndrome:** Nearly 2.1 percent[25] of those with autism also have Fragile X, the most common inherited form of mental retardation.

- **Mental retardation:** About 25 percent[26] of persons with autism also have some degree of mental retardation.

Many people have treatable conditions in addition to their autism. Sleep disorders, allergies, and digestive problems are commonly seen in those with ASDs, and many of these can be treated with environmental interventions or medication. Treatment for these conditions may not cure autism, but it can improve the quality of life for people who have autism and their families.

References

1. Filipek, et al. (2000). Practice Parameter: Screening and Diagnosis of Autism—Report of the Quality Standards Subcommittee of the American Academy of Neurology and the Child Neurology Society. *Neurology*, 55:468–79.

2. *Diagnostic and Statistics Manual, fourth edition.* (1994). American Psychiatric Association: Washington, DC.

3. Fombonne, 2002; and Gilberg and Wing, 1999. As cited in: Immunization Safety Review Committee, Institute of Medicine, National Academy of Sciences. (2004). *Immunization Safety Review: Vaccines and Autism*. National Academy Press: Washington, DC.

4. Immunization Safety Review Committee, Institute of Medicine, National Academy of Sciences. (2004). *Immunization Safety Review: Vaccines and Autism*. National Academy Press: Washington, DC.

5. Volkmar, 1993; and McLennen, 1993. As cited in: Ashley-Koch, et al. (1999). Genetic Studies of Autistic Disorder and Chromosome 7. *Genomics*, 61:227–36.

6. Gillberg, 2000; Chakrabarti, 2001; and Chudley, 1998. As cited in: Muhle, et al. (2004). The genetics of autism. *Pediatrics*, 113(5):e472–e486.

7. Lord, 1995; Stone, 1999; and Charman, 1997. As cited in: Filipek et al. (2000). Practice Parameter: Screening and Diagnosis of Autism—Report of the Quality Standards Subcommittee of the American Academy of Neurology and the Child Neurology Society. *Neurology*, 55:468–79.

8. Cox, 1999; Mars, 1998; Werner, 2000; and Baranek, 1999. As cited in: Filipek, et al. (2000). Practice Parameter: Screening and Diagnosis of Autism—Report of the Quality Standards Subcommittee of the American Academy of Neurology and the Child Neurology Society. *Neurology*, 55:468–79.

9. Johnson, CP. (2004). New tool helps primary care physicians diagnose autism early. *AAP News*, 24(2):74.

10. Goldberg, 2003; and Rodier, 1998. As cited in: Lord, et al. (2004). Regression and word loss in autistic spectrum disorders. *Journal of Child Psychology and Psychiatry*, 45(5):936–55.

11. Filipek et al. (1999). Screening and diagnosis of autistic spectrum disorders. *Journal of Autism and Developmental Disorders*, 29(6):439–84.

12. Filipek et al. (2000). Practice Parameter: Screening and Diagnosis of Autism—Report of the Quality Standards Subcommittee of the American Academy of Neurology and the Child Neurology Society. *Neurology*, 55:468–79.

13. Media Resource Team, American Academy of Pediatrics (AAP). (2001). Guidelines on Diagnosis and Management of Autism. E-News, May 2001 [Electronic Version]. Retrieved

November 5, 2004, from http://aappolicy.aappublications.org/cgi/content/full/pediatrics;107/5/1221 (Registration Required).

14. Committee on Children with Disabilities, AAP. (2001). The pediatrician's role in the diagnosis and management of autistic spectrum disorder in children. *Pediatrics*, 107:1221–26.

15. Committee on Children with Disabilities, AAP. (2001). Technical report: The pediatrician's role in the diagnosis and management of autistic spectrum disorder in children. Pediatrics, 107:e85. Retrieved November 4, 2004, from http://www.pediatrics.org/cgi/content/full/107/5/385.

16. Dawson, 1997; Hurth, 1999; Rogers, 1989; Hoyson, 1984; Lovaas, 1987; Harris, 1991; McEachin, 1993; Greenspan, 1997; Smith, 1997; and Smith, 1998. As cited in Committee on Children with Disabilities, AAP. (2001). The pediatrician's role in the diagnosis and management of autistic spectrum disorder in children. *Pediatrics*, 107:1221–26.

17. For complete information about IDEA, visit http://www.ed.gov/offices/OSERS/Policy/IDEA/regs.html.

18. For complete information about IDEA, visit http://www.ed.gov/offices/OSERS/Policy/IDEA/regs.html.

19. Adapted from NICHD, NIH, DHHS. (2003). Are there treatments for Fragile X syndrome? Families and Fragile X Syndrome (NIH Pub. No. 03-3402). U.S. Government Printing Office: Washington, DC; pages 24–31.

20. Adapted from: Potenza and McDougle. (2001). New Findings on the Causes and Treatment of Autism. CNS Spectrums, Medical Broadcast Limited. Retrieved November 8, 2004, from http://www.patientcenters.com/autism/news/med_referencehtml.

21. Study confirms secretin no more effective than placebo in treating autistic symptoms, NICHD, November 2001. Retrieved November 08, 2004, from http://www.nichd.nih.gov/new/releases/newskey.cfm?from=autism.

22. Gillberg. (1998). Chromosomal disorders and autism. *Journal of autism and developmental disorders*, 28:415–25.

23. Tuchman, et al. (2002). Epilepsy in autism. *Lancet Neurology*, 1:352–58.

24. Fombonne, et al. (1997). Autism and associated medical disorders in a French epidemiological survey. *Child and Adolescent Psychiatry*, 36:1561–69.

25. Kielinen, et al. (2004). Associated medical disorders and disabilities in children with autistic disorder. *Autism*, 8(1):49–60.

26. Sigman M, Dissanayake C, Arbelle S, and Ruskin E. (1997). Cognition and emotion in children with autism. In Cohen and Volkmar (Eds.) *Handbook of Autism and Pervasive Developmental Disorders*, second edition (pp. 248–65). Wiley and Sons: NY.

Chapter 34

Attention Deficit Hyperactivity Disorder

Attention deficit hyperactivity disorder, sometimes called ADHD, is a chronic condition and the most commonly diagnosed behavioral disorder among children and adolescents. It affects between 3 and 5 percent of school-aged children in a six-month period.

Children and adolescents with attention deficit hyperactivity disorder have difficulty controlling their behavior in school and social settings. They also tend to be accident-prone. Although some of these young people may not earn high grades in school, most have normal or above-normal intelligence.

What are the signs of attention deficit hyperactivity disorder?

There are three different types of attention deficit hyperactivity disorder, and each has different symptoms. The types are inattentive, hyperactive-impulsive, and combined attention deficit hyperactivity disorder.

Children with the inattentive type may:

- have short attention spans;
- be distracted easily;

Excerpted from "Children and Adolescents with Attention-Deficit/Hyperactivity Disorder," United States Department of Health and Human Services, Substance Abuse and Mental Health Services Administration, April 2003. Revised by David A Cooke, M.D., July 2008.

- not pay attention to details;
- make many mistakes;
- fail to finish things;
- have trouble remembering things;
- not seem to listen;
- not be able to stay organized.

Children with the hyperactive-impulsive type may:

- fidget and squirm;
- be unable to stay seated or play quietly;
- run or climb too much or when they should not;
- talk too much or when they should not;
- blurt out answers before questions are completed;
- have trouble taking turns;
- Interrupt others.

The most common type is combined attention deficit hyperactivity disorder, which, as the name implies, is a combination of the inattentive and the hyperactive-impulsive types.

A diagnosis of one of the attention deficit hyperactivity disorders is usually made when children have several of the above symptoms that begin before age seven and last at least six months. Generally, symptoms have to be observed in at least two different settings, such as home and school, before a diagnosis is made.

How common is attention deficit hyperactivity disorder?

Attention deficit hyperactivity disorder is found in as many as one in every twenty children. Boys are four times more likely than girls to have the disorder.

What causes attention deficit hyperactivity disorder?

Many causes of attention deficit hyperactivity disorder have been studied, but no one cause seems to apply to all young people with the disorder. Viruses, harmful chemicals in the environment, genetics, problems during pregnancy or delivery, or anything that impairs brain development can play a role in causing the disorder.

Attention Deficit Hyperactivity Disorder

What help is available for families?

Many treatments, some with scientific basis and some without, have been recommended for children and adolescents with attention deficit hyperactivity disorder. Traditional approaches to treatment involve medications and/or behavior therapy.

Many types of medications have been used to treat attention deficit hyperactivity disorder. The most widely used drugs are stimulants. Stimulants increase activity in parts of the brain that appear to be underactive in children and adolescents with attention deficit hyperactivity disorder. Experts believe that this is why stimulants improve attention and reduce impulsive, hyperactive, or aggressive behavior. A newer nonstimulant medication, amoxetine, is helpful in some children. For some children and adolescents, certain antidepressants may also help alleviate symptoms of the disorder. Tranquilizers also have been effective for some individuals. Care must be taken when prescribing and monitoring all medications, and it is important to note that these are not the only medications that may be prescribed for this disorder.

Like most medications, those used to treat attention deficit hyperactivity disorder have side effects. These medications may cause some children to lose weight, have reduced appetites, and temporarily grow more slowly. Others may have trouble falling asleep. However, many doctors believe the benefits of these medications outweigh the possible side effects. Often, health care providers can alleviate side effects by adjusting the dosage.

Another treatment approach, called behavior therapy, involves using techniques and strategies to modify the behavior of children with the disorder. Behavior therapy may include:

- instruction for parents and teachers on how to manage and modify children's or adolescents' behavior, such as rewarding good behaviors;
- daily report cards to link efforts between home and school, where parents reward children or adolescents for good school performance and behavior;
- summer and Saturday programs;
- special classrooms that use intensive behavior modification;
- specially trained classroom aides.

While a combination of stimulants and behavior therapy is believed to be helpful, it is not clear how long the benefits from this approach last. The federal government's National Institute of Mental Health is supporting research on the long-term benefits of various treatments, as well as research to determine if medication and behavior treatment are more effective when combined. Ongoing research efforts also are aimed at identifying new medicines and treatments.

Can attention deficit hyperactivity disorder be prevented?

Given that there are many suspected causes of attention deficit hyperactivity disorder, prevention may be difficult. However, as a precaution, it is always wise for expectant mothers to receive prenatal care and stay away from alcohol, tobacco, and other harmful chemicals during pregnancy. It also makes good sense for mothers to obtain good health care for their children. These recommendations may be particularly important when attention deficit hyperactivity disorder is suspected in other family members.

What else can parents do?

When it comes to attention deficit hyperactivity disorder, parents and other caregivers should be careful not to jump to conclusions. A high energy level alone in a child or adolescent does not mean that he or she has attention deficit hyperactivity disorder. The diagnosis depends on whether the child or adolescent can focus well enough to complete tasks that suit his or her age and intelligence. This ability is most likely to be noticed by a teacher. Since some children with attention deficit hyperactivity disorder have many different types of needs and often require special accommodations to help them function, input from teachers should be taken seriously.

If parents or caregivers suspect attention deficit hyperactivity disorder, they should take the following steps:

- Make an appointment with a psychiatrist, psychologist, child neurologist, or behavioral pediatrician for an evaluation. (Ask the child's doctor for a referral.)

- Be patient if the young person is diagnosed with attention deficit hyperactivity disorder, and recognize that progress takes time.

- Instill a sense of competence in the child or adolescent. Promote his or her strengths, talents, and feelings of self-worth.

- Remember that, in many instances, failure, frustration, discouragement, low self-esteem, and depression cause more problems than the disorder itself.

Attention Deficit Hyperactivity Disorder

- Get accurate information from libraries, hotlines, or other sources.
- Ask questions about treatments and services.
- Talk with other families in their communities.
- Find family network organizations.

Children with attention deficit hyperactivity disorder may qualify for free services within public schools. Most children with attention deficit hyperactivity disorder or other disabilities are eligible to receive special education services under the Individuals with Disabilities Education Act (IDEA). This act guarantees appropriate services and a public education to children ages three to twenty-one with disabilities.

Chapter 35

Auditory Processing Disorder

What is auditory processing?

Auditory processing is a term used to describe what happens when your brain recognizes and interprets the sounds around you. Humans hear when energy that we recognize as sound travels through the ear and is changed into electrical information that can be interpreted by the brain. The "disorder" part of auditory processing disorder (APD) means that something is adversely affecting the processing or interpretation of the information.

Children with APD often do not recognize subtle differences between sounds in words, even though the sounds themselves are loud and clear. For example, the request "Tell me how a chair and a couch are alike" may sound to a child with APD like "Tell me how a couch and a chair are alike." It can even be understood by the child as "Tell me how a cow and a hair are alike." These kinds of problems are more likely to occur when a person with APD is in a noisy environment or when he or she is listening to complex information.

APD goes by many other names. Sometimes it is referred to as central auditory processing disorder (CAPD). Other common names are auditory perception problem, auditory comprehension deficit, central auditory dysfunction, central deafness, and so-called word deafness.

Excerpted from "Auditory Processing Disorder in Children," National Institute on Deafness and Other Communication Disorders, February 2004. Reviewed by David A. Cooke, M.D., July 2008.

What causes auditory processing difficulty?

We are not sure. Human communication relies on taking in complicated perceptual information from the outside world through the senses, such as hearing, and interpreting that information in a meaningful way. Human communication also requires certain mental abilities, such as attention and memory. Scientists still do not understand exactly how all of these processes work and interact or how they malfunction in cases of communication disorders. Even though your child seems to "hear normally," he or she may have difficulty using those sounds for speech and language.

The cause of APD is often unknown. In children, auditory processing difficulty may be associated with conditions such as dyslexia, attention deficit disorder, autism, autism spectrum disorder, specific language impairment, pervasive developmental disorder, or developmental delay. Sometimes this term has been misapplied to children who have no hearing or language disorder but have challenges in learning.

What are the symptoms of possible auditory processing difficulty?

Children with auditory processing difficulty typically have normal hearing and intelligence. However, they have also been observed to:

- have trouble paying attention to and remembering information presented orally;
- have problems carrying out multistep directions;
- have poor listening skills;
- need more time to process information;
- have low academic performance;
- have behavior problems;
- have language difficulty (e.g., they confuse syllable sequences and have problems developing vocabulary and understanding language);
- have difficulty with reading, comprehension, spelling, and vocabulary.

How is suspected auditory processing difficulty diagnosed in children?

You, a teacher, or a daycare provider may be the first person to notice symptoms of auditory processing difficulty in your child. So talking to your child's teacher about school or preschool performance is a good idea. Many health professionals can also diagnose APD in your child. There may need to be ongoing observation with the professionals involved.

Much of what will be done by these professionals will be to rule out other problems. A pediatrician or a family doctor can help rule out possible diseases that can cause some of these same symptoms. He or she will also measure growth and development. If there is a disease or disorder related to hearing, you may be referred to an otolaryngologist—a physician who specializes in diseases and disorders of the head and neck.

To determine whether your child has a hearing function problem, an audiologic evaluation is necessary. An audiologist will give tests that can determine the softest sounds and words a person can hear and other tests to see how well people can recognize sounds in words and sentences. For example, for one task, the audiologist might have your child listen to different numbers or words in the right and the left ear at the same time. Another common audiologic task involves giving the child two sentences, one louder than the other, at the same time. The audiologist is trying to identify the processing problem.

A speech-language pathologist can find out how well a person understands and uses language. A mental health professional can give you information about cognitive and behavioral challenges that may contribute to problems in some cases, or he or she may have suggestions that will be helpful. Because the audiologist can help with the functional problems of hearing and processing, and the speech-language pathologist is focused on language, they may work as a team with your child. All of these professionals seek to provide the best outcome for each child.

What current research is being conducted?

In recent years, scientists have developed new ways to study the human brain through imaging. Imaging is a powerful tool that allows the monitoring of brain activity without any surgery. Imaging studies are already giving scientists new insights into auditory processing. Some of these studies are directed at understanding auditory processing disorders. One of the values of imaging is that it provides an objective, measurable view of a process. Many of the symptoms described as related to APD are described differently by different people.

Imaging will help identify the source of these symptoms. Other scientists are studying the central auditory nervous system. Cognitive neuroscientists are helping to describe how the processes that mediate sound recognition and comprehension work in both normal and disordered systems.

What treatments are available for auditory processing difficulty?

Much research is still needed to understand APD problems, related disorders, and the best intervention for each child or adult. Several strategies are available to help children with auditory processing difficulties. Some of these are commercially available, but have not been fully studied. Any strategy selected should be used under the guidance of a team of professionals, and the effectiveness of the strategy needs to be evaluated. Researchers are currently studying a variety of approaches to treatment. Several strategies you may hear about include the following:

- Auditory trainers are electronic devices that allow a person to focus attention on a speaker and reduce the interference of background noise. They are often used in classrooms, where the teacher wears a microphone to transmit sound and the child wears a headset to receive the sound. Children who wear hearing aids can use them in addition to the auditory trainer.

- Environmental modifications such as classroom acoustics, placement, and seating may help. An audiologist may suggest ways to improve the listening environment, and he or she will be able to monitor any changes in hearing status.

- Exercises to improve language-building skills can increase the ability to learn new words and increase a child's language base.

- Auditory memory enhancement, a procedure that reduces detailed information to a more basic representation, may help. Also, informal auditory training techniques can be used by teachers and therapists to address specific difficulties.

- Auditory integration training may be promoted by practitioners as a way to retrain the auditory system and decrease hearing distortion. However, current research has not proven the benefits of this treatment.

Chapter 36

Developmental Delay

What is developmental delay?

Developmental delay is when your child does not reach their developmental milestones at the expected times. It is an ongoing, major delay in the process of development. If your child is slightly or only temporarily lagging behind, that is not called developmental delay. Delay can occur in one or many areas—for example, motor, language, social, or thinking skills.

Developmental delay is usually a diagnosis made by a doctor based on strict guidelines. Usually, though, the parent is the first to notice that their child is not progressing at the same rate as other children the same age. If you think your child may be "slow," or "seems behind," talk with their doctor about it. In some cases, your general pediatrician might pick up a delay during a well child visit or other meetings. It will probably take several visits and possibly a referral to a developmental specialist to be sure that the delay is not just a temporary lag. Special testing can also help gauge your child's developmental level.

The first three years of a child's life are an amazing time of development . . . and what happens during those years stays with a child for a lifetime. That's why it's so important to watch for signs of delays in development, and to get help from professionals if you suspect

---

Reprinted with permission of the University of Michigan Health System, May 2008. Written by Kyla Boyse, R.N., http://www.med.umich.edu/llibr/yourchild/devdel.htm.© 2008 Regents of the University of Michigan.

problems. The sooner a developmentally delayed child gets early intervention, the better their progress will be.

What causes developmental delay?

Developmental delay can have many different causes, such as genetic causes (like Down syndrome), or complications of pregnancy and birth (like prematurity or infections). Often, however, the specific cause is unknown. Some causes can be easily reversed if caught early enough, such as hearing loss from chronic ear infections, or lead poisoning.

What should I do if I suspect my child has developmental delay?

If you think your child may be delayed, you should take them to their primary care provider, or to a developmental and behavioral pediatrician or pediatric neurologist. An alternative to seeing a specialist is to work through your local school system (see below). If your child seems to be losing ground—in other words, starts to not be able to do things they could do in the past—you should have them seen right away. If your child is developmentally delayed, the sooner you get a diagnosis, the sooner you can begin appropriate treatment and the better the progress your child can make.

What can the school system do for my child?

Ask your school system in writing for an evaluation of your child, even if your child is a baby, toddler, or preschooler. They are required to provide it, at no cost to you. The purpose of an evaluation is to find out why your child is not meeting their developmental milestones or not doing well in school. A team of professionals will work with you to evaluate your child. If they do not find a problem, you can ask the school system to pay for an independent educational evaluation (IEE). There are strict rules about this, so you may not get it. You can also have your child tested again privately, and pay for it yourself. But check with your school district first to make sure they will accept the private test results. By law, the school system must consider the results of the second evaluation when deciding if your child can get special services.

What is early intervention?

Every state has an early intervention program that you will want to get your child into right away. If you live in Michigan, your doctor may refer you to the Early On Program in your local school district. (Outside Michigan, you can find your state's early intervention services through the National Dissemination Center for Children with Disabilities [NICHCY] website.) Early On (and all states' early intervention programs) offer many different services and will help set up an individualized program for your family. It is called an individual family service plan (IFSB).

It is most important to start treatment as early as possible, and make sure it involves lots of one-on-one interaction with your child.

What is special education?

Special education means "educational programming designed specifically for the individual." It can really help your child do better in school. If your school-aged child qualifies for special education, they will have an individualized education program (IEP) designed just for them.

What happens as my child grows up and eventually becomes an adult?

Transition planning is planning to get your child ready to lead a rewarding life as an adult. As your child gets closer to adulthood, they will need an IEP transition plan. Transition planning begins at age fourteen. It is part of the IEP every year after that. At age sixteen, planning will begin for how your child will transition from school into the community. The goal is for your child to become as independent as possible. Your child should take part in the planning, because their input will help make the plan more successful.

Chapter 37

Dyslexia

What Is Dyslexia?

When a person has difficulties with reading, writing, spelling, and maybe even speaking, no matter how hard he or she tries, the problem could be a learning disability known as dyslexia.

Dyslexia is a lifelong language processing disorder that hinders the development of oral and written language skills. Children and adults with dyslexia can be highly intelligent, however they have a neurological disorder that causes the brain to process and interpret information differently.

Since so much of what happens in a classroom is based on reading and writing, it's important to identify dyslexia as early as possible and devise strategies to help a child succeed academically.

What Are the Effects of Dyslexia?

Dyslexia can have different effects on different people, depending on the severity of the learning disability and the success of efforts to develop alternate learning methods. Traditionally dyslexia causes problems with reading, writing, and spelling and those problems manifest themselves differently in each person. In fact, some children with dyslexia show few signs of difficulty with early reading and writing, but have more trouble with later complex language

---

© 2008 by National Center for Learning Disabilities, Inc. All rights reserved. Modified with permission.

skills, such as grammar, reading comprehension, and more in-depth writing.

Dyslexia can also make it difficult for people to express themselves clearly. It can be challenging for them to use vocabulary and to structure their thoughts during conversation. Others struggle to understand when people speak to them, not because they don't hear, but because of their difficulty processing verbal information. This is particularly true with abstract thoughts and nonliteral language, such as idiomatic expressions, jokes, and proverbs.

Perhaps most importantly, all of these effects can have a disastrous impact on a person's self-image. Without help, children often get frustrated with learning. The stress of dealing with schoolwork often makes children with dyslexia lose the motivation to continue on and overcome the hurdles they face.

Is Dyslexia Common?

According to the National Institute of Health, up to 15 percent of the U.S. population has significant difficulty learning to read. Dyslexia occurs among people of all economic and ethnic backgrounds. People are born with dyslexia. Often other members of the family also have dyslexia.

What Are the Warning Signs?

The following are common signs of dyslexia in people of all ages, but that does not mean that a person displaying these signs necessarily has a learning disability. If a person continues to display difficulty over time in the areas outlined below, testing for dyslexia should be considered:

- Understanding that words are made up of sounds (known as phonological awareness)

- Assigning correct sounds to letters—alone and when combined to form words

- Pronouncing words properly—blending sounds into speech

- Spelling words

- Learning the alphabet, numbers, days of the week—basic sequential information

- Reading with age-appropriate speed and accuracy

- Reading comprehension
- Learning numbers facts
- Answering open-ended questions, such as math or word problems
- Organizing thoughts, time, or a sequence of tasks
- Learning a foreign language

How Is Dyslexia Identified?

Identifying dyslexia must be done through a formal evaluation by trained professionals. The evaluation investigates a person's ability to understand and use spoken and written language and looks at specific areas of strength and weakness in the skills that are needed for reading. Family history, intellectual ability, educational background, social environment, and other factors that can affect learning are also taken into account.

Treating Dyslexia

Recognizing dyslexia early in life is a key factor in how much the learning disability will affect a person's development. Unfortunately, adults with unidentified dyslexia often work in jobs below their intellectual capacity. But with help from a tutor, teacher, or other trained professionals, almost all people with dyslexia can become good readers and writers. Incorporating the following strategies into the learning process can help overcome the difficulties of dyslexia:

- Early exposure to oral reading, writing, drawing, and practice to encourage development of print knowledge, basic letter formation and recognition skills, and linguistic awareness (the relationship between sound and meaning)
- Practice reading different kinds of texts (i.e., books, magazines, advertisements, comics)
- Multi-sensory, structured language instruction and practice using sight, sound, and touch when introducing new ideas
- Modifying classroom procedures to allow for extra time to complete assignments, help with note-taking, oral testing and other means of assessment
- Using books-on-tape and assistive technology such as screen readers and voice recognition computer software

- Help with the emotional issues that arise from struggling to overcome academic difficulties

Reading and writing are fundamental skills for daily living, however it is important to emphasize other aspects of learning and expression. Like all people, those with dyslexia enjoy activities that tap into their strengths and interests. As multidimensional thinkers, visual fields such as design, art, architecture, engineering and surgery, which do not emphasize language skills, may appeal to them.

Chapter 38

Fragile X Syndrome

What is fragile X syndrome?

Fragile X syndrome (FXS) is the most common known cause of intellectual disability, also known as mental retardation, and developmental disability that can be inherited (passed from one generation to the next). The exact number of people who have FXS is unknown, but it is estimated that about one in four thousand males and one in six thousand to eight thousand females have the disorder. Although FXS occurs in both males and females, females generally have milder symptoms. Signs that a child has FXS include not sitting, walking, or talking as early as other children. This is known as having developmental delays. Often, there are other physical and behavioral signs, but features of FXS vary and signs can be subtle and easy to miss. Children often have a typical facial appearance that gets more noticeable with age. These features include a large head, long face, and prominent ears, chin, and forehead. Children who have FXS might also have learning disabilities, speech and language delays, and behavioral problems such as attention deficit hyperactivity disorder (ADHD). Males who have FXS usually have some degree of intellectual disability that can range from mild to severe. Females with FXS can have normal intelligence or some degree of intellectual disability with or without learning disabilities. Autism spectrum disorders (ASDs) also occur more frequently in children with FXS.

Centers for Disease Control and Prevention, 2006.

What causes fragile X syndrome?

Fragile X syndrome (FXS) is caused by a change (mutation) in a gene on the X chromosome. Genes contain codes, or recipes, for proteins. Proteins are very important biological components (parts) in all forms of life. The gene on the X chromosome that causes FXS is called the Fragile X Mental Retardation 1 (FMR1) gene. The FMR1 gene makes a protein that is needed for normal brain development. In FXS, the protein is not made.

How is FXS different from other genetic disorders?

Most genetic disorders are caused by changes (mutations) in a gene that causes a change in the recipe for its protein. This causes the protein to be made incorrectly so that it does not work normally. Some genetic disorders are caused by making too much or too little of a protein due to a single change in the part of the gene that controls how much protein is made. FXS is one of a small class of genetic disorders, called trinucleotide repeat disorders, which is caused by a more complicated change in the gene. In the case of FXS, this complex change turns off the gene so no protein product is made.

Deoxyribonucleic acid (DNA) is made up of four chemical building blocks called nucleotides: A, C, T, and G. Trinucleotide repeat disorders have a chain of three of these nucleotides that are repeated over and over again. In most people, the number of repeats is small. If the number of repeats is large, the gene does not work properly. In FXS, the pattern of CGG is repeated over and over again in the FMR1 gene, and when it reaches a certain number of repeats, the gene is turned off. A normal FMR1 gene has between about six and forty-five CGG repeats. People with FXS have over two hundred CGG repeats. When there are over two hundred CGG repeats, this is referred to as a full mutation. The gene turns off because of a process called methylation. When the gene is turned off, no protein is made. Without the protein, the person develops FXS.

When the number of CGG repeats falls between the normal range and the full mutation, then a person is said to have a premutation (about fifty-five to two hundred repeats). People who have a premutation do not have FXS because the FMR1 gene still works even with so many repeats. Until recently, people who carried the premutation were not thought to have any health problems related to FXS. However, in the past ten years, researchers have discovered that both men and women who have a premutation may have specific health problems including nervous system disorders, infertility, and problems with learning and behavior.

Fragile X Syndrome

When there are about forty-five to fifty-five CGG repeats in the FMR1 gene, it is in the intermediate or gray zone range. People with intermediate or gray zone changes have a slightly higher chance of having learning disabilities.

Are full mutations the only cause of FXS?

Over 95 percent of people with FXS have a full mutation. However, a small number of people with FXS have a normal number of repeats. Instead, they have a small change (mutation) somewhere else in the FMR1 gene that causes a faulty protein to be made. Because the protein does not work, the symptoms are the same as in FXS due to full mutations, but it will run in families in a slightly different way. In these families, FXS will be inherited like other X-linked disorders.

There is also another gene that is very similar to FMR1. It is called FMR2 and it also makes a protein that is needed for brain development. Changes in the FMR2 gene are much less common, but they cause FXS-like intellectual disability, also known as mental retardation. FMR2 is also on the X chromosome, so FMR2 intellectual disability is inherited in families like other X-linked disorders. This means that intellectual disability caused by FMR2 changes run in the family in patterns similar to FXS. Therefore, families with FMR2 intellectual disability are sometimes mistakenly believed to have FXS. Genetic testing can distinguish between the two conditions.

How does fragile X run in families?

The FMR1 gene is on the X chromosome. Like all chromosomes, the X chromosome is passed from parent to child. Females have two X chromosomes, and males have one X chromosome and one Y chromosome.

People with a normal number of repeats: In addition to being X-linked, the inheritance pattern of FXS in families is affected by the number of CGG repeats in the gene. Most people have about six to forty-five repeats in their FMR1 genes. Repeats of this size are stable in families. That is, the number of repeats does not change when passed from parent to child.

People with an intermediate number of repeats: People who have an intermediate repeat size (about forty-five to fifty-five) are not at risk for having children with FXS. However, when the gene is passed on to their children, the number of repeats can grow to a premutation size. Children who have a premutation are then at risk for having children with FXS. Therefore, a person with an intermediate-size repeat is at risk for having grandchildren with FXS.

People with a premutation: A premutation repeat (about fifty-five to two hundred repeats) can grow to a full mutation when the gene is passed from a mother to a child. Therefore, a woman with a premutation is at risk for having a child with FXS. The more repeats she has, the more likely it is to grow to a full mutation when passed to her children. On the other hand, in men, the premutation does not grow, so men with premutations do not pass on a full mutation. A man with a premutation will pass the premutation to his daughters, because he passes on his X chromosome to all his daughters. Sons of men with premutations will not be affected, because boys get a Y chromosome from their fathers instead of an X chromosome.

People with a full mutation: If men with FXS (over two hundred repeats) have children, they do not pass on the full mutation. Rather, the full mutation shrinks back to a premutation size and their daughters will have premutations. The sons of males with FXS will not be affected, because boys get a Y chromosome from their fathers instead of an X chromosome.

Females who have a full mutation have a 50 percent chance with each pregnancy of passing on the full mutation to her children.

What health problems can affect people who have a fragile X premutation?

People with premutation FMR1 genes do not have FXS. However, sometimes they have other symptoms, such as the following nervous system disorders, infertility, and problems with learning and behavior:

- **Fragile X-associated tremor/ataxia syndrome (FXTAS):** FXTAS is a disorder of the nervous system that leads to tremors, problems with walking and balance (called ataxia), memory loss, and mood disorders. Studies have shown that at least 30 percent of men with the premutation who are older than fifty years of age develop FXTAS. Women who have a premutation are less likely to be affected by FXTAS, but if they develop FXTAS, it happens at a later age than in men.

Fragile X Syndrome

- **Premature ovarian failure (POF):** Normally, women will stop having menstrual cycles and experience menopause around fifty-one years of age. Women with premature ovarian failure (POF) stop having menstrual cycles and have symptoms of menopause before forty years of age. POF occurs in about 1 to 4 percent of women in the general population; however, it occurs in about 22 percent of women who have a premutation for FXS. Therefore, women who carry a premutation are at risk for fertility problems in addition to the risk of having children who have FXS. Women who have a full mutation for FXS have the same risk for POF as women in the general population.

- **Problems with learning and behavior:** The effects on learning and behavior in men and women with the FMR1 premutation are unclear. Women with the premutation might be more likely to have mood disorders and learning disabilities. Behavioral issues such as attention deficit hyperactivity disorder (ADHD) and autism spectrum disorders (ASDs) might also be more common than in the general population. However, more studies need to be done to look at the relationship between the premutation and learning and behavioral effects.

Why do people with premutations have symptoms that are different than those in FXS?

In people who have FXS, the FMR1 gene has a very large number of CGG repeats, which causes the gene to be turned off. As a result, there is no protein made. FXS is the result of the lack of a specific protein.

People with premutations do not have FXS because they still make some of the protein from the FMR1 gene. However, the premutation can affect how the gene works. Genes contain the recipes for proteins. Before the protein is made, a temporary copy of the gene is created. This temporary copy is made of ribonucleic acid (RNA), a chemical very similar to DNA. In FMR1 genes with a premutation repeat, the gene makes extra RNA. The extra RNA affects how some cells work, which causes the symptoms described previously. Scientists do not yet understand exactly how the extra RNA causes these health problems.

How is fragile X syndrome diagnosed?

FXS can be diagnosed by testing a person's DNA from a blood sample. A physician or genetic counselor must order the test. The DNA is tested to see how many repeats are present in the FMR1 gene. If a full mutation is not detected, the physician or genetic counselor can order other tests to look for other changes in the FMR1 or the FMR2 gene. However, because these types of changes are so much less common, the other tests are not always ordered. The results of DNA tests can affect other family members and raise many issues. Therefore, anyone who is thinking about FXS testing should consider having genetic counseling prior to getting tested.

Chapter 39

Learning Disabilities

Sara's Story

When Sara was in the first grade, her teacher started teaching the students how to read. Sara's parents were really surprised when Sara had a lot of trouble. She was bright and eager, so they thought that reading would come easily to her. It didn't. She couldn't match the letters to their sounds or combine the letters to create words.

Sara's problems continued into second grade. She still wasn't reading, and she was having trouble with writing, too. The school asked Sara's mom for permission to evaluate Sara to find out what was causing her problems. Sara's mom gave permission for the evaluation.

The school conducted an evaluation and learned that Sara has a learning disability. She started getting special help in school right away.

Sara's still getting that special help. She works with a reading specialist and a resource room teacher every day. She's in the fourth grade now, and she's made real progress! She is working hard to bring her reading and writing up to grade level. With help from the school, she'll keep learning and doing well.

What Are Learning Disabilities?

Learning disability is a general term that describes specific kinds of learning problems. A learning disability can cause a person to have

---

National Dissemination Center for Children with Disabilities, January 2004. Reviewed by David A. Cooke, M.D., July 2008.

trouble learning and using certain skills. The skills most often affected are: reading, writing, listening, speaking, reasoning, and doing math.

Learning disabilities (LD) vary from person to person. One person with LD may not have the same kind of learning problems as another person with LD. Sara, in our example above, has trouble with reading and writing. Another person with LD may have problems with understanding math. Still another person may have trouble in each of these areas, as well as with understanding what people are saying.

Researchers think that learning disabilities are caused by differences in how a person's brain works and how it processes information. Children with learning disabilities are not "dumb" or "lazy." In fact, they usually have average or above average intelligence. Their brains just process information differently.

The definition of "learning disability" just below comes from the Individuals with Disabilities Education Act (IDEA). The IDEA is the federal law that guides how schools provide special education and related services to children with disabilities. The special help that Sara is receiving is an example of special education.

There is no "cure" for learning disabilities. They are lifelong. However, children with LD can be high achievers and can be taught ways to get around the learning disability. With the right help, children with LD can and do learn successfully.

IDEA's Definition of "Learning Disability"

Our nation's special education law, the Individuals with Disabilities Education Act (IDEA), defines a specific learning disability as "a disorder in one or more of the basic psychological processes involved in understanding or in using language, spoken or written, that may manifest itself in an imperfect ability to listen, think, speak, read, write, spell, or do mathematical calculations, including conditions such as perceptual disabilities, brain injury, minimal brain dysfunction, dyslexia, and developmental aphasia."

However, learning disabilities do not include "learning problems that are primarily the result of visual, hearing, or motor disabilities, of mental retardation, of emotional disturbance, or of environmental, cultural, or economic disadvantage."

How Common Are Learning Disabilities?

Very common! As many as one out of every five people in the United States has a learning disability. Almost three million children (ages

Learning Disabilities

six through twenty-one) have some form of a learning disability and receive special education in school. In fact, over half of all children who receive special education have a learning disability (Twenty-fourth Annual Report to Congress, U.S. Department of Education, 2002).

What Are the Signs of a Learning Disability?

There is no one sign that shows a person has a learning disability. Experts look for a noticeable difference between how well a child does in school and how well he or she could do, given his or her intelligence or ability. There are also certain clues that may mean a child has a learning disability. We've listed a few below. Most relate to elementary school tasks, because learning disabilities tend to be identified in elementary school. A child probably won't show all of these signs, or even most of them. However, if a child shows a number of these problems, then parents and the teacher should consider the possibility that the child has a learning disability.

When a child has a learning disability, he or she:

- may have trouble learning the alphabet, rhyming words, or connecting letters to their sounds;
- may make many mistakes when reading aloud, and repeat and pause often;
- may not understand what he or she reads;
- may have real trouble with spelling;
- may have very messy handwriting or hold a pencil awkwardly;
- may struggle to express ideas in writing;
- may learn language late and have a limited vocabulary;
- may have trouble remembering the sounds that letters make or hearing slight differences between words;
- may have trouble understanding jokes, comic strips, and sarcasm;
- may have trouble following directions;
- may mispronounce words or use a wrong word that sounds similar;
- may have trouble organizing what he or she wants to say or not be able to think of the word he or she needs for writing or conversation;

- may not follow the social rules of conversation, such as taking turns, and may stand too close to the listener;
- may confuse math symbols and misread numbers;
- may not be able to retell a story in order (what happened first, second, third); or
- may not know where to begin a task or how to go on from there.

If a child has unexpected problems learning to read, write, listen, speak, or do math, then teachers and parents may want to investigate more. The same is true if the child is struggling to do any one of these skills. The child may need to be evaluated to see if he or she has a learning disability.

What About School?

Learning disabilities tend to be diagnosed when children reach school age. This is because school focuses on the very things that may be difficult for the child—reading, writing, math, listening, speaking, reasoning. Teachers and parents notice that the child is not learning as expected. The school may ask to evaluate the child to see what is causing the problem. Parents can also ask for their child to be evaluated.

With hard work and the proper help, children with LD can learn more easily and successfully. For school-aged children (including preschoolers), special education and related services are important sources of help. School staff work with the child's parents to develop an individualized education program, or IEP. This document describes the child's unique needs. It also describes the special education services that will be provided to meet those needs. These services are provided at no cost to the child or family.

Supports or changes in the classroom (sometimes called accommodations) help most students with LD. Some common accommodations are listed below in "Tips for Teachers." Assistive technology can also help many students work around their learning disabilities. Assistive technology can range from "low-tech" equipment such as tape recorders to "high-tech" tools such as reading machines (which read books aloud) and voice recognition systems (which allow the student to "write" by talking to the computer).

It's important to remember that a child may need help at home as well as in school. The resources listed below will help families and teachers learn more about the many ways to help children with learning disabilities.

Learning Disabilities

Tips for Parents

Learn about LD. The more you know, the more you can help yourself and your child.

Praise your child when he or she does well. Children with LD are often very good at a variety of things. Find out what your child really enjoys doing, such as dancing, playing soccer, or working with computers. Give your child plenty of opportunities to pursue his or her strengths and talents.

Find out the ways your child learns best. Does he or she learn by hands-on practice, looking, or listening? Help your child learn through his or her areas of strength.

Let your child help with household chores. These can build self-confidence and concrete skills. Keep instructions simple, break down tasks into smaller steps, and reward your child's efforts with praise.

Make homework a priority. Read more about how to help your child be a success at homework.

Pay attention to your child's mental health (and your own!). Be open to counseling, which can help your child deal with frustration, feel better about himself or herself, and learn more about social skills.

Talk to other parents whose children have learning disabilities. Parents can share practical advice and emotional support.

Meet with school personnel and help develop an educational plan to address your child's needs. Plan what accommodations your child needs, and don't forget to talk about assistive technology!

Establish a positive working relationship with your child's teacher. Through regular communication, exchange information about your child's progress at home and at school.

Tips for Teachers

Learn as much as you can about the different types of LD.

Seize the opportunity to make an enormous difference in this student's life! Find out and emphasize what the student's strengths and interests are. Give the student positive feedback and lots of opportunities for practice.

Review the student's evaluation records to identify where specifically the student has trouble. Talk to specialists in your school (e.g., special education teacher) about methods for teaching this student. Provide instruction and accommodations to address the student's special needs. Examples include:

- breaking tasks into smaller steps, and giving directions verbally and in writing;
- giving the student more time to finish schoolwork or take tests;
- letting the student with reading problems use textbooks-on-tape;
- letting the student with listening difficulties borrow notes from a classmate or use a tape recorder; and
- letting the student with writing difficulties use a computer with specialized software that spell checks, grammar checks, or recognizes speech.

Learn about the different testing modifications that can really help a student with LD show what he or she has learned.

Teach organizational skills, study skills, and learning strategies. These help all students but are particularly helpful to those with LD.

Work with the student's parents to create an educational plan tailored to meet the student's needs.

Establish a positive working relationship with the student's parents. Through regular communication, exchange information about the student's progress at school.

Chapter 40

Stuttering

Stuttering is a speech disorder in which the normal flow of speech is disrupted by frequent repetitions or prolongations of speech sounds, syllables, or words or by an individual's inability to start a word. The speech disruptions may be accompanied by rapid eye blinks, tremors of the lips and/or jaw, or other struggle behaviors of the face or upper body that a person who stutters may use in an attempt to speak. Certain situations, such as speaking before a group of people or talking on the telephone, tend to make stuttering more severe, whereas other situations, such as singing or speaking alone, often improve fluency.

Who stutters?

It is estimated that over three million Americans stutter. Stuttering affects individuals of all ages but occurs most frequently in young children between the ages of two and six who are developing language. Boys are three times more likely to stutter than girls. Most children, however, outgrow their stuttering, and it is estimated that less than 1 percent of adults stutter.

Many individuals who stutter have become successful in careers that require public speaking. The list of individuals includes Winston Churchill, actress Marilyn Monroe, actors James Earl Jones, Bruce Willis, and Jimmy Stewart, and singers Carly Simon and Mel Tillis, to name only a few.

Excerpted from National Institute on Deafness and Other Communication Disorders, May 2002. Reviewed by David A. Cooke, M.D., July 2008.

What causes stuttering?

Scientists suspect a variety of causes. There is reason to believe that many forms of stuttering are genetically determined. The precise mechanisms causing stuttering are not understood.

The most common form of stuttering is thought to be developmental, that is, it is occurring in children who are in the process of developing speech and language. This relaxed type of stuttering is felt to occur when a child's speech and language abilities are unable to meet his or her verbal demands. Stuttering happens when the child searches for the correct word. Developmental stuttering is usually outgrown.

Another common form of stuttering is neurogenic. Neurogenic disorders arise from signal problems between the brain and nerves or muscles. In neurogenic stuttering, the brain is unable to coordinate adequately the different components of the speech mechanism. Neurogenic stuttering may also occur following a stroke or other type of brain injury.

Other forms of stuttering are classified as psychogenic or originating in the mind or mental activity of the brain such as thought and reasoning. Whereas at one time the major cause of stuttering was thought to be psychogenic, this type of stuttering is now known to account for only a minority of the individuals who stutter. Although individuals who stutter may develop emotional problems such as fear of meeting new people or speaking on the telephone, these problems often result from stuttering rather than causing the stuttering. Psychogenic stuttering occasionally occurs in individuals who have some types of mental illness or individuals who have experienced severe mental stress or anguish.

Scientists and clinicians have long known that stuttering may run in families and that there is a strong possibility that some forms of stuttering are, in fact, hereditary. No gene or genes for stuttering, however, have yet been found.

How is stuttering diagnosed?

Stuttering is generally diagnosed by a speech-language pathologist, a professional who is specially trained to test and treat individuals with voice, speech, and language disorders. The diagnosis is usually based on the history of the disorder, such as when it was first noticed and under what circumstances, as well as a complete evaluation of speech and language abilities.

Stuttering

How is stuttering treated?

There are a variety of treatments available for stuttering. Any of the methods may improve stuttering to some degree, but there is at present no cure for stuttering. Stuttering therapy, however, may help prevent developmental stuttering from becoming a lifelong problem. Therefore a speech evaluation is recommended for children who stutter for longer than six months or for those whose stuttering is accompanied by struggle behaviors.

Developmental stuttering is often treated by educating parents about restructuring the child's speaking environment to reduce the episodes of stuttering. Parents are often urged to do the following:

- Provide a relaxed home environment that provides ample opportunities for the child to speak. Setting aside specific times when the child and parent can speak free of distractions is often helpful.

- Refrain from criticizing the child's speech or reacting negatively to the child's disfluencies. Parents should avoid punishing the child for any disfluencies or asking the child to repeat stuttered words until they are spoken fluently.

- Resist encouraging the child to perform verbally for people.

- Listen attentively to the child when he or she speaks.

- Speak slowly and in a relaxed manner. If a parent speaks this way, the child will often speak in the same slow, relaxed manner.

- Wait for the child to say the intended word. Don't try to complete the child's thoughts.

- Talk openly to the child about stuttering if he or she brings up the subject.

Many of the currently popular therapy programs for persistent stuttering focus on relearning how to speak or unlearning faulty ways of speaking. The psychological side effects of stuttering that often occur, such as fear of speaking to strangers or in public, are also addressed in most of these programs.

Other forms of therapy utilize interventions such as medications or electronic devices. Medications or drugs which affect brain function often have side effects that make them difficult to use for long-term treatment. Electronic devices which help an individual control fluency may be more of a bother than a help in most speaking situations and are often abandoned by individuals who stutter.

Unconventional methods of stuttering therapy also exist. It is always a good policy to check the credentials, experience, and goals of the person offering treatment. Avoid working with anyone who promises a "cure" for stuttering.

What research is being done about stuttering?

Stuttering research is exploring ways to improve the diagnosis and treatment of stuttering as well as to identify its causes. Emphasis is being placed on improving the ability to determine which children will outgrow their stuttering and which children will stutter the rest of their lives. Stuttering characteristics are being examined to help identify groups of individuals who have similar types of stuttering and therefore may have a common cause. Research is also being conducted that will help locate the possible genes for the types of stuttering that tend to run in families. Modern medical tools such as PET (positron emission tomography) scans and functional MRI (magnetic resonance imaging) scans are offering insight into the brain organization of individuals who stutter. The effectiveness of different types of treatment is also being examined, and new treatments are being developed.

Chapter 41

Anxiety Disorders

What are anxiety disorders?

Children and adolescents with anxiety disorders typically experience intense fear, worry, or uneasiness that can last for long periods of time and significantly affect their lives. If not treated early, anxiety disorders can lead to the following:

- Repeated school absences or an inability to finish school
- Impaired relations with peers
- Low self-esteem
- Alcohol or other drug use
- Problems adjusting to work situations
- Anxiety disorder in adulthood

What are the types and signs of anxiety disorders?

Many different anxiety disorders affect children and adolescents. Several disorders and their signs are described below.

Generalized anxiety disorder: Children and adolescents with generalized anxiety disorder engage in extreme, unrealistic worry

---

"Children and Adolescents with Anxiety Disorders," United States Department of Health and Human Services, Substance Abuse and Mental Health Services Administration, April 2003. Reviewed by David A. Cooke, M.D.

about everyday life activities. They worry unduly about their academic performance, sporting activities, or even about being on time. Typically, these young people are very self-conscious, feel tense, and have a strong need for reassurance. They may complain about stomachaches or other discomforts that do not appear to have any physical cause.

Separation anxiety disorder: Children with separation anxiety disorder often have difficulty leaving their parents to attend school or camp, stay at a friend's house, or be alone. Often, they "cling" to parents and have trouble falling asleep. Separation anxiety disorder may be accompanied by depression, sadness, withdrawal, or fear that a family member might die. About one in every twenty-five children experiences separation anxiety disorder.

Phobias: Children and adolescents with phobias have unrealistic and excessive fears of certain situations or objects. Many phobias have specific names, and the disorder usually centers on animals, storms, water, heights, or situations, such as being in an enclosed space. Children and adolescents with social phobias are terrified of being criticized or judged harshly by others. Young people with phobias will try to avoid the objects and situations they fear, so the disorder can greatly restrict their lives.

Panic disorder: Repeated "panic attacks" in children and adolescents without an apparent cause are signs of a panic disorder. Panic attacks are periods of intense fear accompanied by a pounding heartbeat, sweating, dizziness, nausea, or a feeling of imminent death. The experience is so scary that young people live in dread of another attack. Children and adolescents with the disorder may go to great lengths to avoid situations that may bring on a panic attack. They also may not want to go to school or to be separated from their parents.

Obsessive-compulsive disorder: Children and adolescents with obsessive-compulsive disorder, sometimes called OCD, become trapped in a pattern of repetitive thoughts and behaviors. Even though they may recognize that the thoughts or behaviors appear senseless and distressing, the pattern is very hard to stop. Compulsive behaviors may include repeated hand washing, counting, or arranging and rearranging objects. About two in every one hundred adolescents experience obsessive-compulsive disorder.

Post-traumatic stress disorder: Children and adolescents can develop post-traumatic stress disorder after they experience a very stressful event. Such events may include experiencing physical or

Anxiety Disorders

sexual abuse; being a victim of or witnessing violence; or living through a disaster, such as a bombing or hurricane. Young people with post-traumatic stress disorder experience the event over and over through strong memories, flashbacks, or other kinds of troublesome thoughts. As a result, they may try to avoid anything associated with the trauma. They also may overreact when startled or have difficulty sleeping.

How common are anxiety disorders?

Anxiety disorders are among the most common mental, emotional, and behavioral problems to occur during childhood and adolescence. About thirteen of every one hundred children and adolescents ages nine to seventeen experience some kind of anxiety disorder; girls are affected more than boys. About half of children and adolescents with anxiety disorders have a second anxiety disorder or other mental or behavioral disorder, such as depression. In addition, anxiety disorders may coexist with physical health conditions requiring treatment.

Who is at risk?

Researchers have found that the basic temperament of young people may play a role in some childhood and adolescent anxiety disorders. For example, some children tend to be very shy and restrained in unfamiliar situations, a possible sign that they are at risk for developing an anxiety disorder. Research in this area is very complex, because children's fears often change as they age.

Researchers also suggest watching for signs of anxiety disorders when children are between the ages of six and eight. During this time, children generally grow less afraid of the dark and imaginary creatures and become more anxious about school performance and social relationships. An excessive amount of anxiety in children this age may be a warning sign for the development of anxiety disorders later in life.

Studies suggest that children or adolescents are more likely to have an anxiety disorder if they have a parent with anxiety disorders. However, the studies do not prove whether the disorders are caused by biology, environment, or both. More data are needed to clarify whether anxiety disorders can be inherited.

What help is available for young people with anxiety disorders?

Children and adolescents with anxiety disorders can benefit from a variety of treatments and services. Following an accurate diagnosis, possible treatments include the following:

- Cognitive-behavioral treatment, in which young people learn to deal with fears by modifying the ways they think and behave
- Relaxation techniques
- Biofeedback (to control stress and muscle tension)
- Family therapy
- Parent training
- Medication

While cognitive-behavioral approaches are effective in treating some anxiety disorders, medications work well with others. Some people with anxiety disorders benefit from a combination of these treatments. More research is needed to determine what treatments work best for the various types of anxiety disorders.

What can parents do?

If parents or other caregivers notice repeated symptoms of an anxiety disorder in their child or adolescent, they should take the following steps:

- Talk with the child's health care provider. He or she can help to determine whether the symptoms are caused by an anxiety disorder or by some other condition and can also provide a referral to a mental health professional.
- Look for a mental health professional trained in working with children and adolescents, who has used cognitive-behavioral or behavior therapy and has prescribed medications for this disorder, or has cooperated with a physician who does.
- Get accurate information from libraries, hotlines, or other sources.
- Ask questions about treatments and services.
- Talk with other families in their communities.
- Find family network organizations.

People who are not satisfied with the mental health care they receive should discuss their concerns with the provider, ask for information, and/or seek help from other sources.

Chapter 42

Bipolar Disorder

What is bipolar disorder?

Bipolar disorder is a mental illness that causes extreme mood swings. This condition is also called manic-depressive illness. It may be caused by a chemical imbalance in the brain.

Bipolar disorder sometimes runs in families. If you have a parent who has bipolar disorder, you have a greater chance of having it. Both men and women can have bipolar disorder. People of all ages can have it.

What are some of the signs of bipolar disorder?

At times, a person who has bipolar disorder may feel very happy, full of energy, and able to do anything. The person might not even want to rest when he or she feels this way. This feeling is called mania (say: "may-nee-ah"). At other times, a person who has bipolar disorder may feel very sad and depressed. The person may not want to do anything when he or she feels this way. This is called depression. People with bipolar disorder can quickly go from mania to depression and back again.

Other signs of mania may include the following:

- Feeling very irritable or angry

Reprinted with permission from "Bipolar Disorder," November 2006, http://familydoctor.org/online/famdocen/home/common/mentalhealth/depression/625.html. Copyright ©2006 American Academy of Family Physicians. All rights reserved.

- Thinking and talking so fast that other people can't follow your thoughts
- Not sleeping at all
- Feeling very powerful and important
- Having trouble concentrating
- Spending too much money
- Abusing alcohol and drugs
- Having sex without being careful to prevent pregnancy or disease

Other signs of depression may include the following:

- No interest or pleasure in things you used to enjoy, including sex
- Feeling sad or numb
- Crying easily or for no reason
- Feeling slowed down, or feeling restless and irritable
- Feeling worthless or guilty
- Change in appetite; unintended change in weight
- Trouble recalling things, concentrating, or making decisions
- Headaches, backaches, or digestive problems
- Problems sleeping, or wanting to sleep all of the time
- Feeling tired all of the time
- Thoughts about death and suicide

How is bipolar disorder treated?

Bipolar disorder can be treated by your family doctor. Your family doctor may want you to see a psychiatrist too. You and your doctors will work together to control your mood swings and make sure you stay well.

Bipolar disorder is treated with medicines to stop the mood swings. Mood stabilizers are used to even out highs and lows in your mood. Antidepressant medicine can help reduce the symptoms of depression. Your doctor may add other medicines as you need them. These medicines don't start to work right away, but you will start to notice a difference in your moods after a few weeks. Be sure to take your medicines just as your doctor tells you.

Bipolar Disorder

Counseling can help you with stress, family concerns, and relationship problems. It's important to get counseling if you have bipolar disorder.

What can I do to help myself get better?

Read about bipolar disorder and tell your family what you learn. Your doctor can suggest resources to help you learn more.

Have a regular routine. Go to bed and wake up at about the same time every day. Eat your meals and exercise at regular times.

Take your medicine every day, and don't stop taking it even if you start feeling better. Avoid caffeine and over-the-counter medicines for colds, allergies, and pain. Ask your doctor before you drink alcohol or use any other medicines.

Try to avoid stress.

Learn the early warning signs of your illness. Tell your doctor when you notice changes in your mood or behavior.

Join a local support group. You and your family can share information and experiences with the support group.

Chapter 43

Conduct Disorder

What is conduct disorder?

Children with conduct disorder repeatedly violate the personal or property rights of others and the basic expectations of society. A diagnosis of conduct disorder is likely when symptoms continue for six months or longer. Conduct disorder is known as a "disruptive behavior disorder" because of its impact on children and their families, neighbors, and schools.

Another disruptive behavior disorder, called oppositional defiant disorder, may be a precursor of conduct disorder. A child is diagnosed with oppositional defiant disorder when he or she shows signs of being hostile and defiant for at least six months. Oppositional defiant disorder may start as early as the preschool years, while conduct disorder generally appears when children are older. Oppositional defiant disorder and conduct disorder are not co-occurring conditions.

What are the signs of conduct disorder?

Symptoms of conduct disorder include the following:

- Aggressive behavior that harms or threatens other people or animals

---

"Children and Adolescents with Conduct Disorder," United States Department of Health and Human Services, Substance Abuse and Mental Health Services Administration, April 2003. Reviewed by David A. Cooke, M.D., July 2008.

- Destructive behavior that damages or destroys property
- Lying or theft
- Truancy or other serious violations of rules
- Early tobacco, alcohol, and substance use and abuse
- Precocious sexual activity

Children with conduct disorder or oppositional defiant disorder also may experience the following:

- Higher rates of depression, suicidal thoughts, suicide attempts, and suicide
- Academic difficulties
- Poor relationships with peers or adults
- Sexually transmitted diseases
- Difficulty staying in adoptive, foster, or group homes
- Higher rates of injuries, school expulsions, and problems with the law

How common is conduct disorder?

Conduct disorder affects 1 to 4 percent of nine- to seventeen-year-olds, depending on exactly how the disorder is defined. The disorder appears to be more common in boys than in girls and more common in cities than in rural areas.

Who is at risk for conduct disorder?

Research shows that some cases of conduct disorder begin in early childhood, often by the preschool years. In fact, some infants who are especially "fussy" appear to be at risk for developing conduct disorder. Other factors that may make a child more likely to develop conduct disorder include the following:

- Early maternal rejection
- Separation from parents, without an adequate alternative caregiver
- Early institutionalization
- Family neglect
- Abuse or violence

Conduct Disorder

- Parental mental illness
- Parental marital discord
- Large family size
- Crowding
- Poverty

What help is available for families?

Although conduct disorder is one of the most difficult behavior disorders to treat, young people often benefit from a range of services that include the following:

- Training for parents on how to handle child or adolescent behavior
- Family therapy
- Training in problem-solving skills for children or adolescents
- Community-based services that focus on the young person within the context of family and community influences

What can parents do?

Some child and adolescent behaviors are hard to change after they have become ingrained. Therefore, the earlier the conduct disorder is identified and treated, the better the chance for success. Most children or adolescents with conduct disorder are probably reacting to events and situations in their lives. Some recent studies have focused on promising ways to prevent conduct disorder among at-risk children and adolescents. In addition, more research is needed to determine if biology is a factor in conduct disorder.

Parents or other caregivers who notice signs of conduct disorder or oppositional defiant disorder in a child or adolescent should take the following steps:

- Pay careful attention to the signs, try to understand the underlying reasons, and then try to improve the situation.
- If necessary, talk with a mental health or social services professional, such as a teacher, counselor, psychiatrist, or psychologist specializing in childhood and adolescent disorders.
- Get accurate information from libraries, hotlines, or other sources.

- Talk to other families in their communities.
- Find family network organizations.

People who are not satisfied with the mental health services they receive should discuss their concerns with their provider, ask for more information, or seek help from other sources.

Chapter 44

Depression

What is depression?

Depression is a disorder characterized by persistent depressed (sad) mood which may last months or even years. It can occur at any age through the lifespan.

We do not yet completely understand the processes in the brain and the mind that lead to or sustain a depression. Some people seem to be at greater genetic risk for depression than others, just like some people are at greater genetic risk for hypertension, obesity, adult-onset diabetes, and other "complex" genetic disorders (disorders where the risk is associated with a number of genes, each of which somewhat increase the risk, rather than diseases associated with a single gene which "causes" the disease). Environmental factors on average have about as much influence on who gets a depression as do genetic factors. Again, this makes depression almost exactly like other similar "complex" genetic disorders with strong environmental contributions (e.g., hypertension, obesity, adult-onset diabetes). Adverse life stresses, perhaps particularly interpersonal "loss" events (e.g., death of a parent) increase the hazard for a depression.

Reprinted from "Depression in Children and Adolescents," reviewed by Neal Ryan, M.D., September 2003. Copyright NAMI: The Nation's Voice on Mental Illness. Reprinted with permission. Editor's note added by David A. Cooke, M.D., Health Reference Series Medical Advisor, November 2007.

What are the different kinds of depression?

Many classification systems have been proposed for depression. However, there is overwhelming evidence for at least two distinct type of depression:

- Unipolar depression
- Bipolar disorder or manic depressive disorder

Unipolar depression consists of one or more episodes of moderate to severe depression with persistent depressed mood and other symptoms of depression including suicidal ideation, suicide attempts, inability to experience pleasure when doing normally pleasurable activities, impaired concentration, change in appetite, change in weight, difficulty sleeping, and/or increased sleep. The disorder is usually recurrent—if you get it once you are likely to get it again in the future.

Bipolar disorder is characterized by periods of depression essentially identical to that seen in unipolar depression and periods of euphoric (too happy) or extremely irritable mood at the same time as the person has other symptoms of mania including much less need for sleep, very rapid speech, dramatic increase in activities, hypersexuality, and/or "racing" (very rapid and confused) thoughts.

How often do children get depression?

About 2 percent of school-age children (i.e., children six to twelve years of age) appear to have a major depression at any one time. With puberty, the rate of depression increases to about 4 percent major depression overall. With adolescence, girls, for the first time, have a higher rate of depression than boys. This greater risk for depression in women persists for the rest of life. Depression is diagnosable before school age (e.g., ages two to five), where it is somewhat more rare but definitely occurs. Overall, approximately 20 percent of youth will have one or more episodes of major depression by the time they become adults.

Do children with depression need treatment? Will they just "grow out of it"?

Episodes of depression in children appear to last six to nine months on average but in some children they last for years at a time. When children are in an episode they do less well at school, have impaired relationships with their friends and family, suffer inside, and have an increased risk for attempted and completed suicide. Because there are effective treatments, to ignore it and hope for the best while the child suffers is not a reasonable approach.

How can you tell if your child is depressed?

Signs that frequently help parents or others know that a child should be evaluated for depression include: the child talking about feeling persistently sad or blue; the child who talks about suicide or being better off dead; the child who is suddenly much more irritable, has a marked deterioration in school or home functioning, or no longer engages in previously pleasurable social interactions with friends.

Because the depressed child may not show significant behavioral disturbance, sometimes parents "hope for the best" or fail to get a child evaluated who shows signs of suffering internally but not disrupting the family.

What are the treatments for depressed children and adolescents?

There are two main groups of treatments for the depressed child with demonstrated evidence of efficacy:

- Psychotherapy
- Pharmacotherapy

Because the course of major depression is fluctuating and because there is a general positive effect on the child (or adult) with depression just from the process of seeing and talking with another caring individual about their depression, to say that a treatment is effective we require that it work better than nonspecific psychotherapy (e.g., talking to a nice and empathic person) in the case of psychotherapies or placebo medication pills given by a warm and friendly person in the case of pharmacotherapies. Thus, the treatments described below have an additional specific effect as well as all the benefit of the human contact and nonspecific discussion of the depression. These are the best we know how to do at present.

The two different specific psychotherapies which show efficacy in children and/or adolescents are cognitive behavioral therapy (CBT) and interpersonal therapy (IPT). CBT concentrates on changing the negative attributional bias (seeing every cup as half-empty) associated with major depression.

Despite a number of studies, there is essentially no evidence to suggest that older-generation tricyclic antidepressants (e.g., Tofranil®,

Elavil®) work for depression in children or adolescents. There are published studies finding efficacy for two selective serotonin reuptake inhibitors (SSRIs), fluoxetine (Prozac®) and sertraline (Zoloft®), in child and adolescent depression. There are ongoing studies and studies which are completed and have been presented at national meetings but not yet published for other antidepressants in child and adolescent major depression. Some of these studies are positive and others have failed to show efficacy (though individual studies frequently fail to find evidence of efficacy even for known effective treatments because of simple bad luck—studies are mathematically much more informative if positive than if negative).

In the middle of 2003 there were Federal Drug Administration (for paroxetine) and pharmaceutical company (for venlafaxine) reports of low but increased rates of impulsive/suicidal behaviors in depressed youth randomized to those active compounds when compared to depressed youth randomized to placebo in the same studies. While there were no completed suicides in these studies in any group, these findings are worrisome and demand increased attention to the question of whether or not some antidepressants may increase the hazard of suicide. At present, the data necessary to understand these studies has not been published or released to the field. [See chapter 40 of this volume for more information.]

OK, what is the right treatment for my depressed child?

Given that both psychotherapeutic and pharmacological approaches have demonstrated efficacy, what is the right treatment for a particular child? Ultimately, we don't have the answer to that question yet though there are two large ongoing multi-site studies which will help us. When considering monotherapy with either talking or pharmacological approaches we do know that all of these approaches have something like a 60 percent good to excellent clinical response rate, which means that many youth do not respond or do not respond adequately to the first treatment and will require augmentation or change of treatment.

Therefore, the youth, family, and clinician should together choose a first treatment that seems best for that individual and give that treatment an adequate trial (e.g., eight to twelve weeks). At the end of that time if the treatment isn't working, it should be changed—try the treatment for at least two to three months but no longer before evaluating it and modifying or completely scrapping as indicated by the progress.

Depression

How long should my child stay on treatment?

Medications are typically continued at least six months after response before tapering off. Many therapists will decrease the frequency of session but continue some maintenance therapy longer than the initial eight to twelve weeks of treatment. Treatment for a first episode of depression is likely to last at least six to twelve months with either treatment.

For recurring depression, many clinicians will maintain prophylactic treatment for considerably longer periods (e.g., years).

Editor's Note

In March 2004, a warning regarding possible increased suicide risk in adolescents was added to newer-generation antidepressants, and in February 2005, this was extended to all antidepressants. In spite of a great deal of data analysis, it remains unclear whether antidepressant therapy increases risk of suicide in children and adolescents. The fact that this group of patients is at high risk for suicide even in the absence of treatment makes it difficult to tease out small differences. There is conflicting data from different studies, and sharp differences in opinion among experts in the area. At this point, the Food and Drug Administration has not recommended against use of these medications, but does recommend close monitoring after treatment is started.

Chapter 45

Obsessive-Compulsive Disorder

What Is Obsessive-Compulsive Disorder?

Obsessive-compulsive disorder, or OCD, is a medical disorder that causes repetitive, unpleasant thoughts (obsessions) or behaviors (compulsions) that are difficult to control. Unlike ordinary worries or habits, these obsessions and compulsions may consume significant amounts of time (more than an hour per day), may interfere with a person's daily schedule, and may cause significant distress. OCD affects approximately 1 percent of children and adolescents. The tendency to develop this disorder involves complex genetic and environmental factors.

Examples of obsessions include recurrent concern about germ contamination, persistent worry that a family member may become sick, or excessive preoccupation with perfection or tidiness. Compulsions, also known as rituals, include repetitive behaviors (such as washing hands, checking locks) and repetitive thoughts (such as silently counting, praying, or repeating words) that the person feels must be completed. A person who has compulsions believes that performing these rituals will prevent a frightening event (for example, "If I count to three every time I talk to my mother, then she won't die").

People with obsessive-compulsive disorder may try to ignore these thoughts or avoid the behaviors but are generally unable able to do

---

The following material is reprinted with permission from www.schoolpsychiatry.org, a website for parents, educators, and clinicians that addresses the needs of children and teens who have mental health conditions. Copyright © 2006 by the Massachusetts General Hospital Department of Psychiatry.

so. Whereas adults with OCD may recognize that their obsessions or compulsions are not rational, a child or adolescent may not have that awareness.

What Does Obsessive-Compulsive Disorder Look Like in Children and Adolescents?

The thoughts and behaviors associated with obsessive-compulsive disorder are often perplexing to parents, teachers, and peers. Recognizing the symptoms of obsessive-compulsive disorder may be challenging, as the symptoms can easily be misinterpreted as willful disregard, oppositionality, or meaningless worry. In addition, children and adolescents may try to hide their symptoms or may not know how to express their underlying worries. Often, a parent or teacher sees only the end result of the symptom (hours in the bathroom, extended time alone in the bedroom, or tantrums when the child cannot do something his or her way).

Symptoms may vary over time and may change in the way they appear, which can further complicate diagnosis. Children may be able to resist the obsessions and compulsions at school but not at home. The symptoms may fluctuate, with more symptoms at stressful periods and fewer symptoms at other times. Other medical conditions can mimic the disorder, and other conditions may co-occur with the disorder.

If left untreated, the condition may lead to considerable worry or limitations in other areas of the child's life. Peer relationships, school functioning, and family functioning all may suffer. Depression may develop. In some situations, in response to the extreme anxiety, social isolation, and limited activities, a child may develop thoughts of self-harm or not wanting to be alive. A trained clinician (such as a child psychiatrist, child psychologist, or pediatric neurologist) should integrate information from home, school, and the clinical visit to make a diagnosis.

At Home

Symptoms of obsessive-compulsive disorder at home are often more intrusive than at school. Life for the child and the family can become very stressful, and all family members, including the child, may feel powerless to change rigid patterns of behavior.

At home, children with OCD may have a combination of the symptoms listed below:

- **Repeated obsessional thoughts that they find unpleasant:** Unlike ordinary worries, these obsessions (such as fear of

Obsessive-Compulsive Disorder

becoming fatally ill) are not generally realistic. Often the child may deny these thoughts or behaviors, or be embarrassed by them.

- **Repeated actions to prevent a feared consequence:** Examples include hand washing to avoid germ contamination and excessive tidying to prevent extreme discomfort or fatal consequence).

- **Consuming obsessions and compulsions:** The child or adolescent is continually preoccupied with these worries (for example, a child avoids nearly all contact with objects due to fear of contamination, or an adolescent bathes and washes hands for hours each day).

- **Extreme distress if others interrupt a ritual:** Children may have extended tantrums if a parent insists that the child move on to the next task.

- **Difficulty explaining unusual behavior:** Children with OCD may not be able to explain what their worries are or why they feel compelled to repeat their behaviors.

- **Attempts to hide obsessions or compulsions:** Children and adolescents are often ashamed of their worries or habits and will make great efforts to keep their thoughts or rituals a secret.

- **Resistance to stopping the obsessions or compulsions:** For example, parental reassurance that the child will not become ill from touching an item does not reassure the child. Frequently, children cannot ignore their symptoms and, instead, feel they must continue their rituals.

- **Concern that they are "crazy" because of their thoughts:** Children with OCD may recognize that they think differently than others their age. Consequently, these children often have low self-esteem.

At School

The differences in behaviors seen at home and at school can be significant. At school, students may be successful in suppressing symptoms, while they may be unable to do so at home. Families often seek treatment once symptoms affect school performance.

At school, a child with OCD may have a combination of the symptoms listed below:

- **Difficulty concentrating:** This may affect many aspects of school activities, from following directions and completing assignments to paying attention in class. Concentration can be affected by persistent, repetitive thoughts that are not known to others. Finishing work in the appropriate time can be difficult, and just starting schoolwork can be difficult, too.

- **Social isolation:** Withdrawal from interactions with peers.

- **Low self-esteem:** In social and academic activities.

- **Problem behaviors:** Examples include fights or arguments, resulting from misunderstandings between the child and peers or staff. Unusual behaviors may be distressing to the child or peers and lead to clashes.

- **Medication side effects that can interfere with school performance:** Once a child is receiving medication treatment for OCD, the child should be monitored carefully for new mood changes or behaviors, which could potentially reflect medication side effects.

- **Other conditions, such as attention deficit/hyperactivity disorder (ADHD) which may also may be present, compounding any learning challenges:** Having one mental health condition does not "inoculate" the child from having other conditions as well.

- **Learning disorders and cognitive problems, which are often overlooked in this population:** A child's difficulties or frustrations in school should not be presumed to be due entirely to the OCD. If the child still has academic difficulty after OCD symptoms are treated, an educational evaluation for learning disabilities should be considered. A child's repeated reluctance to attend school may be an indicator of an undiagnosed learning disability.

At the Doctor's Office

A child's obsessive-compulsive symptoms often are not seen during an office visit. Clinicians may benefit from talking with parents, school staff, and other important caregivers to evaluate a child's functioning in each area to determine the underlying cause of the child's symptoms.

Clinicians may face some of the following challenges in diagnosing and treating a child or adolescent with OCD:

Obsessive-Compulsive Disorder

- **Varying symptoms:** Because of the variability of symptoms and their changing appearance as a child grows, a clinician may need to see a child over time to determine the appropriate diagnosis.

- **Other conditions may look like, or may accompany, obsessive-compulsive disorder:** These conditions include eating disorders (excessive focus on food habits and weight), phobias (excessive worry regarding a specific object or situation, such as spiders or flying), and psychotic disorders (preoccupation with unusual beliefs or fears).

- **Additional conditions often seen with obsessive-compulsive disorder should be considered:** These include Tourette disorder (a condition of repetitive, distressing motor and vocal tics), attention deficit/hyperactivity disorder (ADHD), depression, social phobia, and panic disorder.

- **Link to Strep Throat:** Researchers have identified a possible link between strep throat infections and the sudden onset of OCD symptoms in a very small number of children. The condition is known as PANDAS, an abbreviation for pediatric autoimmune neuropsychiatric disorders associated with streptococcal infections. The children usually have dramatic, "overnight" onset of symptoms, including motor or vocal tics, obsessions, and/or compulsions. Although this syndrome is a rare occurrence, it makes sense for families to discuss any recent illnesses with their child's clinician.

- **Young people are often ashamed and embarrassed about their OCD symptoms and may not volunteer information:** Phrasing questions with particular sensitivity and compassion may allow a more complete picture of symptoms to emerge, especially since obsessions or compulsions might involve distasteful thoughts or worries of a sexual nature. Children may be unaware, or unwilling to admit, that their behavior may indicate symptoms of a disorder.

- **Unreasonable expectations:** Families may need to be coached about what they can reasonably expect from their child. Children who suffer from OCD will benefit if their family understands that therapy and medicines may reduce, but do not cure, symptoms.

How Is Obsessive-Compulsive Disorder Treated?

Obsessive-compulsive disorder is treatable through ongoing interventions provided by a child's medical practitioners, therapists, school staff, and family. These treatments include psychological interventions (counseling), biological interventions (medicines), and accommodations at home and school that reduce sources of stress for the child. Open, collaborative communication between a child's family, school, and clinicians optimizes the care and quality of life for the child with obsessive-compulsive disorder.

Psychological Interventions (Counseling)

Counseling can help children with OCD, and everyone around them, to understand that OCD symptoms are caused by an illness with complex genetic and environmental origins—not by flawed attitude or personality. Counseling also can reduce the impact of symptoms on daily life. A variety of psychological interventions can be helpful, and parents should discuss their child's particular needs with their clinician to determine which psychological treatments could be most beneficial for their child.

Cognitive behavior therapy (CBT): This is usually recommended for children and adolescents with obsessive-compulsive disorder. In CBT, a young person is helped to become aware of problem behaviors or thoughts in particular situations and is then guided by the clinician to try alternative behaviors for those situations. With younger patients, personifying the obsessions (for example, "Germy" to describe the fear of germs) allows children to "fight back" against the thoughts or behaviors that could keep them away from peers or family activities. Cognitive behavior therapy focuses on changing behaviors and on developing more positive thinking patterns as alternatives to the negative thoughts that cause symptoms.

CBT and related treatments, such as exposure response prevention and behavior therapy, are based on well-researched methods that have successfully helped children and adolescents to increase healthy behaviors and thoughts. These therapy approaches can enable people with OCD to tolerate their worries without having to perform their rituals. Young people may benefit from behavior therapy or CBT on an ongoing basis.

Individual psychotherapy: This may be useful for young people with OCD, particularly when they have ongoing stressors in their lives that make symptoms worse. Children with obsessive-compulsive disorder often carry a sense of failure, as if the illness was their fault. In many cases, they know that their disturbing thoughts and rituals

Obsessive-Compulsive Disorder

are generated by their own mind, which can increase their sense of self-blame. Individual psychotherapy can help young people become aware of and address their feelings of failure and self-blame.

Parent guidance sessions: These can help parents to manage their child's illness, identify effective parenting skills, learn how to function as a family despite the illness, and address complex feelings that can arise when raising a child who has a psychiatric disorder. Family therapy may be beneficial when issues are affecting the family as a whole.

Group psychotherapy: This can be valuable to a child by providing a safe place to talk with other children who face adversity or allowing a child to practice social skills or symptom-combating skills in a carefully structured setting.

School-based counseling: This can be effective in helping a child with OCD navigate the social, behavioral, and academic demands of the school setting.

Biological Interventions (Medicines)

While psychotherapy may be sufficient to treat some children with OCD, other children's symptoms do not improve significantly with psychotherapy alone. These children may benefit from medications.

The U.S. Food and Drug Administration (FDA) has approved Anafranil®, Luvox®, Prozac® (fluoxetine), and Zoloft® for treating children and adolescents with OCD. Medications approved by the FDA for other uses and age groups are also prescribed for young people with OCD. The FDA allows doctors to use their best judgment to prescribe medication for conditions for which the medication has not specifically been approved.

The antidepressants Celexa®, Lexapro®, and Paxil® are also commonly prescribed to treat symptoms of OCD. These medications, along with Luvox, Prozac, and Zoloft, belong to a group of medications called selective serotonin reuptake inhibitors, or SSRIs. Anafranil, another type of antidepressant medication, has anti-obsessional properties.

Sometimes larger doses of antidepressants (up to four times the standard antidepressant dose) are prescribed to improve OCD symptoms. If OCD symptoms occur in children with autism spectrum disorders, sometimes very low doses (for example, 1 mg of Prozac) are prescribed.

In most cases these medicines begin to be effective in reducing symptoms after the child or adolescent has taken them for at least two to four weeks. Fully twelve weeks may be required in order to determine whether the medication is going to be effective for a particular individual. Medications should be started, stopped, or adjusted only under the direct supervision of a trained clinician.

There is no "best" medicine to treat OCD, and it is important to remember that medicines usually reduce rather than eliminate symptoms. Different medicines or dosages may be needed at different times in a child's life or to address the emergence of particular symptoms. Successful treatment requires taking medicine daily as prescribed, allowing time for the medicine to work, and monitoring for both effectiveness and side effects. The family, clinician, and school should maintain frequent communication to ensure that medications are working as intended and to monitor and manage side effects.

The following cautions should be observed when any child or adolescent is treated with antidepressants:

- **Benefits and risks should be evaluated:** Questions have arisen about whether antidepressants can cause some children or adolescents to have suicidal thoughts. The evidence to date shows that antidepressants, when carefully monitored, have safely helped many children and adolescents. The latest reports on this issue from the U.S. Food and Drug Administration can be found on its website at www.fda.gov. Consideration of any medicine deserves a discussion with the prescribing clinician about its risks and benefits.

- **Careful monitoring is recommended for any child receiving medication:** Though most side effects occur soon after starting a medicine, adverse reactions can occur months after medicines are introduced. Agitation, restlessness, increased irritability, or comments about self-harm should be addressed immediately with the clinician if any of these symptoms emerge after the child starts an antidepressant. Frequent follow-up (weekly for the first month) is now advocated by the FDA for children starting an antidepressant.

- **Some children who have OCD may also have bipolar disorder:** In some individuals with bipolar disorder, antidepressants may initially improve depressive symptoms but can sometimes worsen manic symptoms. While antidepressants do not "cause" bipolar disorder, they can unmask or worsen manic symptoms.

Obsessive-Compulsive Disorder

Interventions at Home

At home, as well as at school, providing a sympathetic and tolerant environment and making some adaptations may be helpful to aid a child or adolescent with OCD:

- **Understand the illness:** Understanding the nature of obsessive-compulsive disorder and its consequences will help parents sympathize with a child's struggles.

- **Listen to the child's feelings:** Isolation can foster depression in these children. The simple experience of being listened to empathically, without receiving advice, may have a powerful and helpful effect. Parents should not let their own worries prevent them from being a strong source of support for their child.

- **Plan for transitions:** Getting to school in the morning or preparing for bed in the evening may be complicated by the urge to complete rituals. Anticipating and planning for these transition times may be helpful for family members.

- **Adjust expectations until symptoms improve:** Helping a child make more attainable goals when symptoms are more severe is important, so that the child can have the positive experience of success.

- **Praise the child's efforts to resist symptoms:** Children often feel like they hear about only their mistakes. Even if improvements are small, every good effort deserves to be praised.

- **Talk as a family about what to say to people outside of the family:** Determine what feels comfortable for the child (for example, "I have this thing called OCD. I'm getting help for it, which is making things easier for me. I might do funny things sometimes, but we can still play together"). Even if the decision is made not to discuss this medical condition with others, having an agreed-on plan will make it easier to handle unexpected questions and minimize family conflicts.

- **Understand parental limits:** Fulfilling a child's extreme wishes related to symptoms (for example, showering for hours) may be neither possible nor advisable. Such well-intended efforts to support a child may actually delay the development of new coping strategies and reduce the benefits of behavior therapy. Finding the balance between supportive flexibility and appropriate limit setting is frequently challenging for parents and may be aided by the guidance of a trained professional.

- **"It's the OCD talking.":** Taking a supportive stance in which parents, child, and clinicians unite together to fight symptoms is an effective strategy to distinguish between symptoms, which are frustrating, and the child, who is doing the best he or she possibly can. Sometimes it is useful to help the child distinguish him- or herself from the illness ("It's the OCD talking").

Interventions at School

There are many ways that schools can help a child with obsessive-compulsive disorder succeed in the classroom. Meetings between parents and school staff, such as teachers, guidance counselors, or nurses, will allow for collaboration to develop helpful school structure for the child. The child may need particular changes (accommodations/modifications) within a classroom.

Examples of some accommodations, modifications, and school strategies include the following:

- Check in on arrival to see if the child can succeed in certain classes that day.
- Allow more time to complete certain types of assignments.
- Accommodate late arrival due to symptoms at home.
- Identify ways for teachers to assist the child in breaking out of an obsession or compulsion.
- Offer strategies for the child to resist uncomfortable thoughts.
- Allow the child to tape record homework if the child cannot touch writing materials.
- Give the child a choice of projects if the child has difficulty beginning a task.
- Suggest that the child change the sequence of homework problems or projects (for example, if the child has fears related to odd-numbers, start with even-numbered problems).
- Adjust the homework load to prevent the child from becoming overwhelmed. Academic stressors, along with other stresses, aggravate symptoms.

Obsessive-Compulsive Disorder

- Anticipate issues such as school avoidance if there are unresolved social and/or academic problems.

- If the child insists on certain OCD rituals at school, work with the child to identify less intrusive rituals (such as tapping one desk rather than tapping every desk).

- Assist with peer interactions in order to alleviate concerns for both the child and peers.

- Be aware that transitions may be particularly difficult for the child. Negotiate reasonable expectations for transitions within school hours. When a child with obsessive-compulsive disorder refuses to follow directions or to transition to the next task, for example, the reason may be anxiety rather than intentional oppositionality.

- Support and reinforce behavioral strategies developed by the clinician. This should be discussed with the child's parents and behavior therapist. Please refer to "Psychological Interventions" above, for details regarding behavior therapy.

- Encourage the child to help develop interventions. Enlisting the child in the task will lead to more successful strategies and will foster the child's ability to problem-solve.

Flexibility and a supportive environment are essential for a student with obsessive-compulsive disorder to achieve success in school. School faculty and parents together may be able to identify difficult situations and develop remedies to reduce a child's challenges at these times.

Sources

Information provided above on obsessive-compulsive disorder drew from sources including:

American Psychiatric Association, *Diagnostic and Statistical Manual of Mental Disorders,* 4th edition. Washington, DC: American Psychiatric Association, 1994.

Bostic, JQ, Bagnell, A. School Consultation. In Kaplan BJ, Sadock VA. *Comprehensive Textbook of Psychiatry*, 8th edition. Philadelphia: Lippincott Williams and Wilkins, 2005.

Dulcan, MK, Martini DR. *Concise Guide to Child and Adolescent Psychiatry,* 2nd edition. Washington, DC: American Psychiatric Association, 1999.

Lewis, Melvin (ed.) *Child and Adolescent Psychiatry: A Comprehensive Textbook*, 3rd edition. Philadelphia: Lippincott Williams and Wilkins, 2002.

Obsessive-Compulsive Foundation, OCD in Children. Internet location: www.ocfoundation.org/ocf1040a.htm September 17, 2004.

Chapter 46

Oppositional Defiant Disorder

Oppositional defiant disorder is a pattern of disobedient, hostile, and defiant behavior toward authority figures.

Causes

This disorder is more common in boys than in girls. Some studies have shown that it affects 20 percent of school-age children. However, most experts believe this figure is high due to changing definitions of normal childhood behavior, and possible racial, cultural, and gender biases.

This behavior typically starts by age eight. The cause of this disorder is unknown, and may be due to a combination of biology and parenting or environmental factors.

Symptoms

- Actively does not follow adults' requests
- Angry and resentful of others
- Argues with adults
- Blames others for own mistakes
- Has few or no friends or has lost friends
- Is in constant trouble in school

© 2008 A.D.A.M., Inc. Reprinted with permission. Updated February 6, 2008.

- Loses temper
- Spiteful or seeks revenge
- Touchy or easily annoyed

To fit this diagnosis, the pattern must last for at least six months and must be more than normal childhood misbehavior.

Exams and Tests

The pattern of behaviors must be different from those of other children around the same age and developmental level. The behavior must lead to significant problems in school or social activities.

It may help to get the child evaluated by a psychiatrist or psychologist. In children and adolescents, depression and attention deficit hyperactivity disorder (ADHD) can cause similar behavior problems, and should be considered as possibilities.

Treatment

The best treatment for the child is talking with a mental health professional (psychotherapy). The parents should also learn how to manage the child's behavior. Medication may be helpful if the behaviors occur as part of another condition (such as depression, childhood psychosis, or ADHD).

Outlook (Prognosis)

Some children respond well to treatment, while others do not.

Possible Complications

In many cases, children with oppositional defiant disorder grow up to have conduct disorder as adults.

When to Contact a Medical Professional

Call your health care provider if you have concerns about your child's development or behavior.

Prevention

Be consistent about rules and fair consequences at home. Don't make punishments too harsh or inconsistent.

Model the right behaviors for your child. Abuse and neglect increase the chances that this condition will occur.

References

Steiner H, Remsing L, Work Group on Quality Issues. Practice parameter for the assessment and treatment of children and adolescents with oppositional defiant disorder. *J Am Acad Child Adolesc Psychiatry*, 2007;46:126–41.

Part Five

Additional Help and Information

Chapter 47

Glossary of Terms Related to Childhood Diseases and Disorders

amblyopia: Poor vision caused by abnormal development of visual areas of the brain in response to abnormal visual stimulation during early development.[4]

anemia: Any condition in which the number of red blood cells per mm^3, the amount of hemoglobin in 100 ml of blood, or the volume of packed red blood cells per 100 ml of blood are less than normal.[4]

Apgar score: A numbered scoring system doctors use to assess a baby's physical state at the time of birth.[2]

applied behavior analysis: An intervention that relies on the theory that rewarded behavior is more likely to be repeated than ignored behavior. This theory provides the foundation of several different methods of behavioral management often used with persons who have autism and other developmental disorders.[1]

The terms in this glossary were excerpted from "Autism Overview: What We Know," National Institute of Child Health and Human Development, National Institutes of Health, NIH Publication No. 05-5592, updated January 2007 [marked 1]; "Cerebral Palsy: Hope through Research," National Institute of Neurological Disorders and Stroke, National Institutes of Health, NIH Publication No. 06-159, December 11, 2007 [marked 2]; "Muscular Dystrophy: Hope through Research," National Institute of Neurological Disorders and Stroke, National Institutes of Health, February 12, 2008 [marked 3]; and *Stedman's Electronic Medical Dictionary* v.5.0, © 2000 Lippincott Williams and Wilkins [marked 4].

asphyxia: A lack of oxygen due to trouble with breathing or poor oxygen supply in the air.[2]

ataxia: The loss of muscle control.[2]

athetoid: Making slow, sinuous, involuntary, writhing movements, especially with the hands.[2]

atrophy: A decrease in size or wasting away of a body part or tissue.[3]

autosomal dominant: A pattern of inheritance in which a child acquires a disease by receiving a normal gene from one parent and a defective gene from the other parent.[3]

autosomal recessive: A pattern of inheritance in which both parents carry and pass on a defective gene to their child.[3]

behavior management therapy: A method of therapy that focuses on managing behavior—that is, changing unwanted behaviors through rewards, reinforcements, and by confronting something that arouses anxiety, discomfort, or fear and overcoming the unwanted responses.[1]

bilirubin: A bile pigment produced by the liver of the human body as a byproduct of digestion.[2]

biopsy: A procedure in which tissue or other material is removed from the body and studied for signs of disease.[3]

cardiomyopathy: Heart muscle weakness that interferes with the heart's ability to pump blood.[3]

cerebral dysgenesis: Defective brain development.[2]

cerebral: Relating to the two hemispheres of the human brain.[2]

chromosome: One of the "packages" of genes and other DNA in the nucleus of a cell. Humans have twenty-three pairs of chromosomes, forty-six in all. Each parent contributes one chromosome to each pair, so children get half of their chromosomes from their mothers and half from their fathers.[1]

computed tomography (CT) scan: An imaging technique that uses x-rays and a computer to create a picture of the brain's tissues and structures.[2]

contracture: chronic shortening of a muscle or tendon that limits movement of a bony joint, such as the elbow.[3]

Glossary of Terms Related to Childhood Diseases

cytokines: Messenger cells that play a role in the inflammatory response to infection.[2]

developmental delay: Behind schedule in reaching the milestones of early childhood development.[2]

developmental screening: A check-up similar to the physical check-up a child gets from a health care provider, but that focuses on a child's social, emotional, and intellectual development. This screening monitors and charts development to make sure that the child is developing as expected for his or her age.[1]

dyskinetic: The impairment of the ability to perform voluntary movements, which results in awkward or incomplete movements.[2]

dyslexia: Impaired reading ability with a competence level below that expected on the basis of the individual's level of intelligence, and in the presence of normal vision and letter recognition and normal recognition of the meaning of pictures and objects.[4]

dystonia: A condition of abnormal muscle tone.[2]

electroencephalogram (EEG): A technique for recording the pattern of electrical currents inside the brain.[2]

electromyography: A recording and study of the electrical properties of skeletal muscle.[3]

epilepsy: A brain disorder in which clusters of nerve cells, or neurons, in the brain sometimes signal abnormally. In epilepsy, the normal pattern of neuronal activity becomes disturbed, causing strange sensations, emotions, and behavior or sometimes convulsions, muscle spasms, and loss of consciousness.[1]

failure to thrive: A condition characterized by a lag in physical growth and development.[2]

febrile: Denoting or relating to fever.[4]

focal (partial) seizure: A brief and temporary alteration in movement, sensation, or autonomic nerve function caused by abnormal electrical activity in a localized area of the brain.[2]

fragile X syndrome: The most common form of inherited mental retardation. A mutation in a single gene, the FMR1 gene located on the X chromosome, causes fragile X syndrome and can be passed from one generation to the next. Symptoms of fragile X syndrome occur because the mutated gene cannot produce enough of a protein that is needed by the body's cells, especially cells in the brain, to develop and function normally.[1]

gastroesophageal reflux disease (GERD): Also known as heartburn, which happens when stomach acids back up into the esophagus.[2]

gastrostomy: A surgical procedure that creates an artificial opening in the stomach for the insertion of a feeding tube.[2]

gene: Pieces of DNA. They contain the information for making a specific protein.[1]

hemophilia: an inherited disorder of blood coagulation characterized by a permanent tendency to hemorrhages, spontaneous or traumatic, because of a defect in the blood coagulating mechanism.[4]

hypertonia: Increased muscle tone.[2]

hypotonia: Decreased muscle tone.[2]

hypoxic-ischemic encephalopathy: Brain damage caused by poor blood flow or insufficient oxygen supply to the brain.[2]

infectious: A disease capable of being transmitted from person to person, with or without actual contact.[4]

intracranial hemorrhage: Bleeding in the brain.[2]

intrauterine infection: Infection of the uterus, ovaries, or fallopian tubes.[2]

jaundice: A blood disorder caused by the abnormal buildup of bilirubin in the bloodstream.[2]

linkage studies: Tests conducted among family members to determine how a genetic trait is passed on through generations.[3]

lordosis: An abnormal forward curving of the spine.[3]

magnetic resonance imaging (MRI): An imaging technique that uses radio waves, magnetic fields, and computer analysis to create a picture of body tissues and structures.[2]

mental retardation: A term used when a person has certain limitations in mental functioning and in skills such as communicating, taking care of him or herself, and social skills.[1]

myopathy: Any disorder of muscle tissue or muscles.[3]

Glossary of Terms Related to Childhood Diseases

myotonia: An inability to relax muscles following a sudden contraction.[3]

nerve entrapment: Repeated or prolonged pressure on a nerve root or peripheral nerve.[2]

off-label drugs: Drugs prescribed to treat conditions other than those that have been approved by the Food and Drug Administration.[2]

orthotic devices: Special devices, such as splints or braces, used to treat posture problems involving the muscles, ligaments, or bones.[2]

palsy: Paralysis, or the lack of control over voluntary movement.[2]

periventricular leukomalacia (PVL): "Peri" means near; "ventricular" refers to the ventricles or fluid spaces of the brain; and "leukomalacia" refers to softening of the white matter of the brain. PVL is a condition in which the cells that make up white matter die near the ventricles. Under a microscope, the tissue looks soft and sponge-like.[2]

ptosis: An abnormal drooping of the eyelids.[3]

quadriplegia: Paralysis of both the arms and legs.[2]

Rett syndrome: Mostly caused by mutations in the MECP2 gene on the X chromosome. Rett syndrome is a disorder of brain development that occurs almost exclusively in girls. After a few months of apparently normal development, affected girls develop problems with language, learning, coordination, and other brain functions.[1]

Rh incompatibility: A blood condition in which antibodies in a pregnant woman's blood attack fetal blood cells and impair an unborn baby's supply of oxygen and nutrients.[2]

rubella (also known as German measles): A viral infection that can damage the nervous system of an unborn baby if a mother contracts the disease during pregnancy.[2]

scoliosis: A disease of the spine in which the spinal column tilts or curves to one side of the body.[2]

seizure: A sudden attack, often one of convulsions, as in epilepsy. Seizures don't necessarily involve movement or thrashing; they can also make someone seem as though they are frozen, unmoving.[1]

selective dorsal rhizotomy: A surgical procedure in which selected nerves are severed to reduce spasticity in the legs.[2]

spastic: Describes stiff muscles and awkward movements.[2]

stereognosia: Difficulty perceiving and identifying objects using the sense of touch.[2]

strabismus: Misalignment of the eyes, also known as cross eyes.[2]

streptococcal: Relating to or caused by any organism of the genus *Streptococcus*.[4]

susceptibility: The state of being predisposed to, sensitive to, or of lacking the ability to resist manifestations of something (such as a pathogen, familial disease, or a drug); a person who is susceptible is more likely to show symptoms of a disorder.[1]

thrombocytopenia: A condition in which there is an abnormally small number of platelets in the circulating blood.[4]

thrombosis: Formation or presence of a thrombus; clotting within a blood vessel which may cause infarction of tissues supplied by the vessel.[4]

tonic-clonic seizure: A type of seizure that results in loss of consciousness, generalized convulsions, loss of bladder control, and tongue biting followed by confusion and lethargy when the convulsions end.[2]

tremor: An involuntary trembling or quivering.[2]

tuberous sclerosis: A rare, multi-system genetic disease that causes noncancerous tumors to grow in the brain and on other vital organs such as the kidneys, heart, eyes, lungs, and skin. It commonly affects the central nervous system and results in symptoms including seizures, developmental delay, behavioral problems, skin abnormalities, and kidney disease.[1]

ultrasound: A technique that bounces sound waves off tissue and bone and uses the pattern of echoes to form an image, called a sonogram.[2]

X-linked recessive: A pattern of disease inheritance in which the mother carries the affected gene on the chromosome that determines the child's sex and passes it to her son.[3]

Chapter 48

Resource List for Parents

General

American Academy of Pediatrics
National Headquarters
141 Northwest Point Boulevard
Elk Grove Village, IL 60007-1098
Phone: 847-434-4000
Fax: 847-434-8000
Website: www.aap.org

Centers for Disease Control and Prevention
1600 Clifton Road
Atlanta, GA 30333
Toll-Free: 800-311-3435
Phone: 404-498-1515
Website: http://www.cdc.gov
E-mail: cdcinfo@cdc.gov

National Digestive Diseases Information Clearinghouse
2 Information Way
Bethesda, MD 20892-3570
Toll-Free: 800-891-5389
Fax: 703-738-4929
TTY: 866-569-1162
Website: http://digestive.niddk.nih.gov
E-mail: nddic@info.niddk.nih.gov

National Heart, Lung, and Blood Institute (NHLBI)
NHLBI Health Information Ctr.
P.O. Box 30105
Bethesda, MD 20824-0105
Phone: 301-592-8573
Fax: 240-629-3246
TTY: 240-629-3255
Website: http://www.nhlbi.nih.gov
E-mail: nhlbiinfo@nhlbi.nih.gov

The information in this chapter was compiled from various sources deemed accurate. All contact information was verified and updated in July 2008. Inclusion does not imply endorsement. This list is intended to serve as a starting point for information gathering; it is not comprehensive.

National Institute of Arthritis and Musculoskeletal and Skin Diseases (NIAMS)
Information Clearinghouse
National Institutes of Health
1 AMS Circle
Bethesda, MD 20892-3675
Toll Free: 877-22-NIAMS (226-4267)
Phone: 301-495-4484
Fax: 301-718-6366
TTY: 301-565-2966
Website: http://www.niams.nih.gov
E-mail: NIAMSinfo@mail.nih.gov

National Institute of Child Health and Human Development (NICHD)
NICHD Information Resource Center
P.O. Box 3006
Rockville, MD 20847
Toll-Free: 800-370-2943
Fax: 301-984-1473
TTY: 888-320-6942
Website: http://www.nichd.nih.gov
E-mail: NICHDIRC@mail.nih.gov

National Institute of Neurological Disorders and Stroke
NIH Neurological Institute
P.O. Box 5801
Bethesda, MD 20824
Toll-Free: 800-352-9424
Phone: 301-496-5751
TTY: 301-468-5981
Website: http://www.ninds.nih.gov
E-mail: braininfo@ninds.nih.gov

Nemours Foundation
1600 Rockland Road
Wilmington, DE 19803
Phone: 302-651-4000
Website: http://www.kidshealth.org
E-mail: info@kidshealth.org

U.S. Food and Drug Administration
5600 Fishers Lane
Rockville, MD 20857-0001
Toll-Free: 888-INFO-FDA (888-463-6332)
Website: http://www.fda.gov

Acquired Immune Deficiency Syndrome (AIDS)

Elizabeth Glaser Pediatric AIDS Foundation
1140 Connecticut Avenue N.W., Suite 200
Washington, D.C. 20036
Toll-Free: 888-499-HOPE (4673)
Phone: 202-296-9165
Fax: 202-296-9185
Website: http://www.pedaids.org
E-mail: info@pedaids.org

National Pediatric AIDS Network
P.O. Box 1032
Boulder, CO 80306
Toll-Free: 800-646-1001
Website: http://www.npan.org

Resource List for Parents

Arthritis

American College of Rheumatology
1800 Century Place, Suite 250
Atlanta, GA 30345-4300
Phone: 404-633-3777
Fax: 404-633-1870
Website: http://www.rheumatology.org

Arthritis Foundation
P.O. Box 7669
Atlanta, GA 30357-0669
Toll-Free: 800-283-7800
Website: http://www.arthritis.org

Asthma and Allergies

Asthma and Allergy Foundation of America
1233 20th Street, N.W., Suite 402
Washington, DC 20036
Toll-Free: 800-7-ASTHMA (800-727-8462)
Website: http://www.aafa.org
E-mail: info@aafa.org

Blood Disorders

National Hemophilia Foundation
116 West 32nd Street, 11th Floor
New York, NY 10001
Phone: 212-328-3700
Fax: 212-328-3777
Website: http://www.hemophilia.org
E-mail: handi@hemophilia.org

National Human Genome Research Institute
National Institutes of Health
Building 31, Room 4B09
31 Center Drive, MSC 2152
Bethesda, MD 20892-2152
Phone: 301-402-0911
Fax: 301-402-0837
Website: http://www.genome.gov

Cancer

American Cancer Society
250 Williams Street N.W.
Atlanta, GA 30303
Toll-Free: 800-ACS-2345 (227-2345)
TTY: 866-228-4327
Website: http://www.cancer.org

Candlelighters Childhood Cancer Foundation
P.O. Box 498
Kensington, MD 20895-0498
Toll-Free: 800-366-CCCF (366-2223)
Phone: 301-962-3520
Fax: 301-962-3521
Website: http://www.candlelighters.org
E-mail: staff@candlelighters.org

Leukemia and Lymphoma Society
1311 Mamaroneck Avenue
Suite 310
White Plains, NY 10605-5221
Toll-Free: 800-955-4LSA
(955-4572)
Phone: 914-949-5213
Fax: 914-949-6691
Website: http://www.leukemia-lymphoma.org

National Brain Tumor Foundation
22 Battery Street, Suite 612
San Francisco, CA 94111
Toll-Free: 800-934-2873
Phone: 415-834-9970
Website: http://www.braintumor.org
E-mail: nbtf@braintumor.org

National Cancer Institute
NCI Public Inquiries Office
6116 Executive Boulevard
Room 3036A
Bethesda, MD 20892-8322
Toll-Free: 800-4-CANCER
(800-422-6237)
TTY: 800-332-8615
Website: http://www.cancer.gov
E-mail: cancergovstaff@mail.nih.gov

National Children's Cancer Society
1 South Memorial Drive, Suite 800
St. Louis, MO 63102
Toll-Free: 800-5-FAMILY
(800-532-6459)
Phone: 314-241-1600
Fax: 314-241-1996
Website: http://www.children-cancer.com

Pediatric Brain Tumor Foundation
302 Ridgefield Court
Asheville, NC 28806
Toll-Free: 800-253-6530
Phone: 828-665-6891
Fax: 828-665-6894
Website: http://www.pbtfus.org

Cardiovascular Disorders

American Heart Association
National Center
7272 Greenville Avenue
Dallas, TX 75231
Toll-Free: 800-AHA-USA-1
(800-242-8721)
Website: http://www.americanheart.org

Cystic Fibrosis

Cystic Fibrosis Foundation
6931 Arlington Road
Bethesda, MD 20814
Toll-Free: 800-FIGHT CF
(344-4823)
Phone: 301-951-4422
Fax: 301-951-6378
Website: http://www.cff.org
E-mail: info@cff.org

Resource List for Parents

Developmental Disorders

Association for Science in Autism Treatment
P.O. Box 188
Crosswicks, NJ 08515-0188
Phone: 781-397-8943
Fax: 781-397-8887
Website: http://www.asatonline.org
E-mail: info@asatonline.org

Autism National Committee (AUTCOM)
P.O. Box 429
Forest Knolls, CA 94933
Website: http://www.autcom.org

Autism Network International (ANI)
P.O. Box 35448
Syracuse, NY 13235-5448
Website: http://ani.autistics.org
E-mail: jisincla@mailbox.syr.edu

Autism Research Institute (ARI)
4182 Adams Avenue
San Diego, CA 92116
Phone: 619-281-7165
Fax: 619-563-6840
Website: http://www.autism.com
E-mail: director@autism.com

Autism Society of America
7910 Woodmont Avenue
Suite 300
Bethesda, MD 20814-3067
Toll-Free: 800-3AUTISM (328-8476)
Phone: 301-657-0881
Fax: 301-657-0869
Website: http://www.autism-society.org

Attention Deficit Disorder Association (ADDA)
15000 Commerce Parkway
Suite C
Mount Laurel, NJ 08054
Phone: 856-439-9099
Fax: 856-439-0525
Website: http://www.add.org
E-mail: adda@add.org

Autism Speaks, Inc.
2 Park Avenue, 11th Floor
New York, NY 10016
Phone: 212-252-8584
Fax: 212-252-8676
Website: http://www.autismspeaks.org
E-mail: contactus@autismspeaks.org

Brain Resources and Information Network (BRAIN)
P.O. Box 5801
Bethesda, MD 20824
Toll-Free: 800-352-9424
Website: http://www.ninds.nih.gov

Learning Disabilities Association of America
4156 Library Road
Pittsburgh, PA 15234-1349
Phone: 412-341-1515
Fax: 412-344-0224
Website: http://www.ldaamerica.org
E-mail: info@ldaamerica.org

MAAP Services for Autism, Asperger's, and PDD
P.O. Box 524
Crown Point, IN 46308
Phone: 219-662-1311
Fax: 219-662-0638
Website: http://www.maapservices.org
E-mail: info@maapservices.org

National Center for Learning Disabilities
381 Park Avenue South
Suite 1401
New York, NY 10016
Toll-Free: 888-575-7373
Phone: 212-545-7510
Fax: 212-545-9665
Website: http://www.ncld.org

National Institute of Mental Health (NIMH)
National Institutes of Health, DHHS
6001 Executive Boulevard
Bethesda, MD 20892-9663
Toll-Free: 866-615-NIMH (6464)
Phone: 301-443-4513
Fax: 301-443-4279
TTY: 301-443-8431
Website: http://www.nimh.nih.gov
E-mail: nimhinfo@nih.gov

National Institute on Deafness and Other Communication Disorders Information Clearinghouse
31 Center Drive, MSC 2320
Bethesda, MD 20892-2320
Toll-Free: 800-241-1044
TTD/TTY: 800-241-1055
Website: http://www.nidcd.nih.gov
E-mail: nidcdinfo@nidcd.nih.gov

Diabetes

American Diabetes Association
1701 North Beauregard Street
Alexandria, VA 22311
Toll-Free: 800-DIABETES (800-342-2383)
Website: http://www.diabetes.org
E-mail: AskADA@diabetes.org

Resource List for Parents

Juvenile Diabetes Research Foundation International
120 Wall Street, 19th Floor
New York, NY 10005
Toll-Free: 800-533-CURE (2873)
Fax: 212-785-9595
Website: http://www.jdrf.org
E-mail: info@jdrf.org

National Diabetes Education Program
1 Diabetes Way
Bethesda, MD 20892-3560
Toll-Free: 800-438-5383
Phone: 301-496-3583
Website: http://www.ndep.nih.gov
E-mail: ndep@mail.nih.gov

National Diabetes Information Clearinghouse
1 Information Way
Bethesda, MD 20892-3560
Toll-Free: 800-860-8747
Phone: 301-654-3327
Fax: 301-907-8906
Website: www.diabetes.niddk.nih.gov
E-mail: ndic@info.niddk.nih.gov

Gastrointestinal Disorders

American College of Gastroenterology
6400 Goldsboro, Suite 450
Bethesda, MD 20817
Phone: 301-263-9000
Website: www.acg.gi.org

International Foundation for Functional Gastrointestinal Disorders (IFFGD) Inc.
P.O. Box 170864
Milwaukee, WI 53217-8076
Toll-Free: 888-964-2001
Phone: 414-964-1799
Fax: 414-964-7176
Website: www.iffgd.org
E-mail: iffgd@iffgd.org

National Digestive Diseases Information Clearinghouse
2 Information Way
Bethesda, MD 20892-3570
Toll-Free: 800-891-5389
Phone: 301-654-3810
Fax: 301-907-8906
Website: www.digestive.niddk.nih.gov
E-mail: nddic@info.niddk.nih.gov

North American Society for Pediatric Gastroenterology, Hepatology, and Nutrition (NASPGHAN)
P.O. Box 6
Flourtown, PA 19031
Phone: 215-233-0808
Fax: 215-233-3918
Website: www.NASPGHAN.org
E-mail: naspghan@naspghan.org

Growth Disorders

Hormone Foundation
8401 Connecticut Avenue
Suite 900
Chevy Chase, MD 20815-5817
Toll-Free: 800-HORMONE
(467-6663)
Fax: 301-941-0259
Website: http://
www.hormone.org
E-mail:
hormone@endo-society.org

Human Growth Foundation
997 Glen Cove Avenue
Suite 5
Glen Head, NY 11545
Toll-Free: 800-451-6434
Fax: 516-671-4055
Website: http://www.hgfound.org

MAGIC Foundation
6645 W. North Avenue
Oak Park, IL 60302
Toll-Free: 800-3-MAGIC-3
(800-362-4423)
Phone: 708-383-0808
Website: http://
www.magicfoundation.org
E-mail:
ContactUs@magicfoundation.org

Hearing Disorders

National Institute on Deafness and Other Communication Disorders
NIDCD Information Clearinghouse
31 Center Drive, MSC 2320
Bethesda, MD 20892-2320
Toll-free: 800-241-1044
Fax: 301-770-8977
TTY: 800-241-1055
Website: http://
www.nidcd.nih.gov
E-mail: nidcdinfo@nidcd.nih.gov

Infectious Diseases

National Institute of Allergies and Infectious Diseases
NIAID Office of Communications and Government Relations
6610 Rockledge Drive, MSC 6612
Bethesda, MD 20892-6612
Toll-Free: 866-284-4107
Phone: 301-496-5717
Fax: 301-402-3573
TDD: 800-877-8339
Website: http://
www3.niaid.nih.gov

New York State Department of Health
Corning Tower
Empire State Plaza,
Albany, NY 12237
Website: http://
www.health.state.ny.us/diseases

Resource List for Parents

Wisconsin Department of Health and Family Services
Communicable Disease Epidemiology Section
1 West Wilson Street
Madison, WI 53703
Phone: 608-267-7321 or
608-267-9003
Fax: 608-266-2906
Website: http://dhs.wisconsin.gov/communicable

Injury Prevention

Safe Kids Worldwide
1301 Pennsylvania Avenue, N.W.
Suite 1000
Washington, DC 20004-1707
Phone: 202-662-0600
Fax 202-393-2072
Website: http://www.usa.safekids.org

Kidney and Urological Disorders

American Society of Pediatric Nephrology
3400 Research Forest Drive
The Woodlands, TX 77381
Phone: 281-419-0052
Website: www.aspneph.com
E-mail: info@aspneph.com

American Urological Association Foundation
1000 Corporate Boulevard
Linthicum, MD 21090
Toll-Free: 800-Ring-AUA (746-4282)
Phone: 410-689-3700
Fax: 410-689-3800
Website: www.auafoundation.org
E-mail: auafoundation@auanet.org

National Association for Continence
P.O. Box 1019
Charleston, SC 29402-1019
Toll-Free: 800-BLADDER (252-3337)
Phone: 843-377-0900
Website: www.nafc.org
E-mail: memberservices@nafc.org

National Kidney Foundation
30 East 33rd Street
New York, NY 10016
Toll-Free: 800-622-9010
Phone: 212-889-2210
Website: www.kidney.org
E-mail: info@kidney.org

Simon Foundation for Continence
P.O. Box 815
Wilmette, IL 60091
Toll-Free: 800-23-SIMON (237-4666)
Website: www.simonfoundation.org
E-mail: simoninfo@simonfoundation.org

Society of Urologic Nurses and Associates
P.O. Box 56
East Holly Avenue
Pitman, NJ 08071-0056
Toll-Free: 888-TAP-SUNA (827-7862)
Phone: 856-256-2335
Website: www.suna.org
E-mail: suna@ajj.com

Liver Disease

American Liver Foundation
75 Maiden Lane, Suite 603
New York, NY 10038
Phone: 212-668-1000
Fax: 212-483-8179
Website: http://www.liverfoundation.org

Mental Health

American Academy of Child & Adolescent Psychiatry
3615 Wisconsin Avenue, N.W.
Washington, DC 20016-3007
Phone: 202-966-7300
Fax: 202-966-2891
Website: http://www.aacap.org
E-mail: communications@aacap.org

American Psychological Association
750 First Street, N.E.
Washington, DC 20002-4242
Toll-Free: 800-374-2721
Phone: 202-336-5500
Website: http://www.apa.org

Children and Adults with Attention-Deficit/Hyperactivity Disorder
8181 Professional Place
Suite 150
Landover, MD 20785
Toll-Free: 800-233-4050
Phone: 301-306-7070
Fax: 301-306-7090
Website: www.chadd.org

Federation of Families for Children's Mental Health
9605 Medical Center Drive
Suite 280
Rockville, MD 20850
Phone: 240-403-1901
Fax: 240-403-1909
Website: http://www.ffcmh.org
E-mail: ffcmh@ffcmh.org

Mental Health America
2000 N. Beauregard Street
6th Floor
Alexandria, VA 22311
Toll-Free: 800-969-6642
Phone: 703-684-7722
TTY: 800-433-5959
Fax: 703-684-5968
Website: http://www.mentalhealthamerica.net

National Alliance on Mental Illness (NAMI)
Colonial Place Three
2107 Wilson Blvd., Suite 300
Arlington, VA 22201-3042
Toll-Free: 800-950-NAMI (6264)
Phone: 703-524-7600
Fax: 703-524-9094
Website: http://www.nami.org

Resource List for Parents

National Association for Children's Behavioral Health
1025 Connecticut Avenue, N.W.
Suite 1012
Washington, DC 20036
Phone: 202-857-9735
Fax: 202-362-5145
Website: http://www.nacbh.org
E-mail: naptcc@aol.com

National Association of School Psychologists
4340 East West Highway
Suite 402
Bethesda, MD 20814
Toll-Free: 866-331-NASP (6277)
Phone: 301-657-0270
Fax: 301-657-0275
TTY: 301-657-4155
Website: http://www.nasponline.org

Substance Abuse and Mental health Services Administrations (SAMHSA)'s National Mental Health Information Center
P.O. Box 42557
Washington, DC 20015
Toll-Free: 800-789-2647
Phone: 240-221-4022
Fax: 240-221-4295
TDD: 866-889-2647
Website: http://mentalhealth.samhsa.gov

Muscular Dystrophy

Facioscapulohumeral Muscular Dystrophy (FSHD) Society
64 Grove Street
Watertown, MA 02472
Phone: 617-658-7878 or 781-275-7781
Fax: 617-658-7879 or 781-275-7789
Website: http://www.fshsociety.org
E-mail: info@fshsociety.org

Muscular Dystrophy Association
3300 East Sunrise Drive
Tucson, AZ 85718-3208
Toll-Free: 800-572-1717
Phone: 520-529-2000
Fax: 520-529-5300
Website: http://www.mda.org
E-mail: mda@mdausa.org

Parent Project Muscular Dystrophy (PPMD)
158 Linwood Plaza, Suite 220
Fort Lee, NJ 07024
Toll-Free: 800-714-KIDS (5437)
Phone: 201-944-9985
Fax: 201-944-9987
Website: http://www.parentprojectmd.org
E-mail: info@parentprojectmd.org

Neurological Disorders

Charlie Foundation to Help Cure Pediatric Epilepsy
1223 Wilshire Blvd., Suite 815
Santa Monica, CA 90403
Fax: 310-393-1978
Website: http://www.charliefoundation.org

Children's Neurobiological Solutions (CNS) Foundation
1826 State Street
Santa Barbara, CA 93101
Toll-Free: 866-CNS-5580 (267-5580)
Phone: 805-898-4442
Fax: 805-898-4448
Website: http://www.cnsfoundation.org
E-mail: info@cnsfoundation.org

Citizens United for Research in Epilepsy (CURE)
730 N. Franklin, Suite 404
Chicago, IL 60654
Phone: 312-255-1801
Fax: 312-255-1809
Website: http://www.CUREepilepsy.org
E-mail: info@CUREepilepsy.org

Epilepsy Foundation
8301 Professional Place East
Landover, MD 20785-7223
Toll-Free: 800-EFA-1000 (332-1000)
Phone: 301-459-3700
Fax: 301-577-2684
Website: http://www.epilepsyfoundation.org
E-mail: postmaster@efa.org

Epilepsy Foundation of Metropolitan New York
257 Park Avenue South
Suite 302
New York, NY 10010
Phone: 212-677-8550
Fax: 212-677-5825
Website: http://www.epilepsyinstitute.org
E-mail: website@epilepsyinstitute.org

People Against Childhood Epilepsy (PACE)
7 East 85th Street, Suite A3
New York, NY 10028
Phone: 212-665-PACE (7223)
Fax: 212-327-3075
Website: http://www.paceusa.org
E-mail: pacenyemail@aol.com

Pathways Awareness Foundation
150 N. Michigan Avenue
Suite 2100
Chicago, IL 60601
Toll-Free: 800-955-CHILD
Phone: 312-893-6620
Fax: 312-893-6621
Website: http://www.pathwaysawareness.org
E-mail: friends@pathwaysawareness.org

Resource List for Parents

United Cerebral Palsy (UCP)
1660 L Street, N.W., Suite 700
Washington, DC 20036
Toll-Free: 800-USA-5UCP (872-5827)
Phone: 202-776-0406
Fax: 202-776-0414
Website: http://www.ucp.org
E-mail: info@ucp.org

Oral Health

American Academy of Pediatric Dentistry
211 East Chicago Avenue
Suite 1700
Chicago, IL 60611-2637
Phone: 312-337-2169
Fax: 312-337-6329
Website: http://www.aapd.org

Reye Syndrome

National Reye's Syndrome Foundation, Inc.
Toll-Free: 800-233-7393 (U.S. only)
Phone: 419-636-2679
Fax: 419-636-9897
Website: http://www.reyessyndrome.org
E-mail: nrsf@reyessyndrome.org

Scoliosis

American Physical Therapy Association
1111 North Fairfax Street
Alexandria, VA 22314-1488
Toll Free: 800-999-2782, ext. 3395
Phone: 703-684-2782
TDD: 703-683-6748
Fax: 703-684-7343
Website: http://www.apta.org

National Scoliosis Foundation
5 Cabot Place
Stoughton, MA 02072
Toll Free: 800-NSF-MYBACK (673-6922)
Website: http://www.scoliosis.org
E-mail: nsf@scoliosis.org

Scoliosis Association, Inc.
P.O. Box 811705
Boca Raton, FL 33481-1705
Toll Free: 800-800-0669
Phone: 561-994-4435
Fax: 561-994-2455
Website: http://www.scoliosis-assoc.org

Scoliosis Research Society
555 East Wells Street
Suite 1100
Milwaukee, WI 53202
Phone: 414-289-9107
Fax: 414-276-3349
Website: http://www.srs.org
E-mail: info@srs.org

Skin Disorders

American Academy of Dermatology
P.O. Box 4014
Schaumburg, IL 60618-4014
Toll-free: 866-503-SKIN (7546)
Phone: 847-240-1280
Fax: 847-240-1859
Website: http://www.aad.org
E-mail: MRC@aad.org

National Psoriasis Foundation
6600 S.W. 92nd Avenue
Suite 300
Portland, OR 97223-7195
Toll-Free: 800-723-9166
Phone: 503-244-7404
Fax: 503-245-0626
Website: http://www.psoriasis.org
E-mail: getinfo@psoriasis.org

Sleep Disorders

National Sleep Foundation
1522 K Street, N.W., Suite 500
Washington, DC 20005
Phone: 202-347-3471
Fax: 202-347-3472
Website: http://www.sleepfoundation.org
E-mail: nsf@sleepfoundation.org

Vision Disorders

National Eye Institute
Information Office
31 Center Drive MSC 2510
Bethesda, MD 20892-2510
Phone: 301-496-5248
Website: http://www.nei.nih.gov
E-mail: 2020@nei.nih.gov

Index

Index

Index

Page numbers followed by 'n' indicate a footnote. Page numbers in *italics* indicate a table or illustration.

A

A-200 (pyrethrin) 200
AAFA *see* Asthma and Allergy Foundation of America
AAFP *see* American Academy of Family Physicians
AATD *see* alpha-1 antitrypsin deficiency
"Abdominal Pain" (Boyse) 366n
abdominal pain, overview 366–70
"About Bone Cancer and Soft Tissue Sarcoma" (Seattle Cancer Care Alliance) 279n
"About Lymphoma" (Seattle Cancer Care Alliance) 269n
acanthosis nigricans 307
Aciphex (rabeprazole) 396
ACTH *see* adrenocorticotropin hormone
acute bronchitis 528
acute lymphocytic leukemia (ALL) 264–68
acute myelogenous leukemia (AML) 264–68

acute sinusitis
  described 336–37
  treatment 340
acute streptococcal pharyngitis 88
acyclovir 161
Adacel 21
A.D.A.M., Inc., publications
  appendicitis 370n
  encephalitis 159n
  epilepsy 492n
  flat feet 435n
  growth hormone deficiency 354n
  oppositional defiant disorder 641n
  perforated eardrum 333n
  rheumatic fever 83n
  swimmer's ear 344n
  tonsillitis 347n
adenoidectomy
  obstructive sleep apnea 326
  otitis media 331–32
adenoids, described 316–18
adenoviruses 125
ADHD *see* attention deficit hyperactivity disorder
adrenocorticotropin hormone (ACTH) 355, 358
adverse reactions, vaccinations 20
Afrin (oxymetazoline) 323

669

Childhood Diseases and Disorders Sourcebook, Second Edition

airway injury prevention,
  described 48–49
albendazole 180
ALL *see* acute lymphocytic leukemia
Allen ENT and Allergy, nosebleeds
  publication 322n
allergic asthma
  described 218
  food allergy 230
allergic conjunctivitis, described 220
allergic rhinitis, described 218
allergies
  overview 218–27
  sinusitis 337
  see also food allergy
allergy shots *see* immunotherapy
allogeneic stem cell transplantation,
  leukemia 268
alpha-1 antitrypsin deficiency
  (AATD), overview 424–27
"Alpha-1 Antitrypsin Deficiency
  (AATD)" (Cincinnati Children's
  Hospital Medical Center) 424n
Alphanate 260
amblyopia
  defined 647
  overview 548–49
"Amblyopia" (National
  Eye Institute) 548n
American Academy of Child and
  Adolescent Psychiatry, contact
  information 662
American Academy of Dermatology,
  contact information 666
American Academy of Dermatology,
  warts publication 155n
American Academy of Family
  Physicians (AAFP), publications
  bipolar disorder 615n
  tinea infections 209n
American Academy of Pediatric
  Dentistry, contact information 665
American Academy of Pediatrics,
  contact information 653
American Cancer Society, contact
  information 655
American College of
  Gastroenterology, contact
  information 659

American College of Rheumatology,
  contact information 655
American Diabetes Association,
  contact information 658
American Headache Society,
  pediatric headache publication
  503n
American Heart Association
  contact information 656
  publications
    arrhythmia 284n
    Kawasaki disease 302n
American Liver Foundation
  contact information 662
  Reye syndrome publication 173n
American Physical Therapy
  Association, contact information 665
American Psychological Association,
  contact information 662
American Society of Pediatric
  Nephrology, contact information 661
American Urological Association
  Foundation, contact information 661
AML *see* acute myelogenous leukemia
Anafranil 635
anaphylaxis
  described 219
  food allergy 229
anemia
  defined 647
  overview 234–38
  see also sickle cell disease
animal bites, first aid 61
antibiotic medications
  bronchitis 530
  encephalitis 162
  foodborne illness 69–70
  Lyme disease 104
  meningitis 164–65
  otitis media 331
  perforated eardrum 334
  pertussis 119
  pneumonia 170–71
  rheumatic fever 84–85
  scarlet fever 87
  staph infections 109
  strep throat 89
  tonsillitis 348
  urinary tract infections 419

Index

anxiety disorders, overview 611–14
APD *see* auditory processing disorder
Apgar score, defined 647
aplastic anemia
  described 235
  thrombocytopenia 249
"Appendicitis" (A.D.A.M., Inc.) 370n
appendicitis, overview 370–73
applied behavior analysis, defined 647
arrhythmia, overview 284–90
Arthritis Foundation, contact information 655
"Ascariasis" (NIAID) 178n
ascariasis, overview 178–80
Ascaris lumbricoides 178
asphyxia, defined 648
aspirin
  fever 55
  Reye syndrome 173–75
  thrombocytopenia 254
Association for Science in Autism Treatment, contact information 657
asthma
  overview 524–27
  statistics 4
  see also allergic asthma
Asthma and Allergy Foundation of America (AAFA)
  allergic reactions publication 218n
  contact information 655
astrocytomas, described 479–80
ataxia, defined 648
ataxic cerebral palsy 486
athetoid, defined 648
athetoid cerebral palsy 486
athlete's foot 209
atrophy, defined 648
atropine, amblyopia 549
Attention Deficit Disorder Association, contact information 657
attention deficit hyperactivity disorder (ADHD), overview 577–81
auditory processing disorder (APD), overview 583–86
"Auditory Processing Disorder in Children" (NIDCD) 583n

aura
  migraine headache 505–6
  seizures 494
autism
  fragile X syndrome 595
  overview 561–76
Autism National Committee, contact information 657
Autism Network International, contact information 657
"Autism Overview: What We Know" (NICHD) 561n, 647n
Autism Research Institute, contact information 657
Autism Society of America, contact information 657
Autism Speaks, Inc., contact information 657
"Autoimmune Hepatitis" (Cincinnati Children's Hospital Medical Center) 428n
autoimmune hepatitis, overview 428–30
automobile safety seats
  children 52
  infants 51
autosomal dominant, defined 648
autosomal recessive, defined 648
Axid (nizatidine) 395
Ayr nasal gel 324
azathioprine 430
azithromycin 119

B

Bacille Calmette-Guérin (BCG) 117
bacteremia, pneumococcal disease 80–81
Bactroban 109
Bartonella henselae 94
"Basic First Aid Procedures" (City of Miami) 61n
Baylisascaris procyonis 180–81
"*Baylisascaris procyonis* (Raccoon Round Worm)" (Wisconsin Department of Health and Family Services) 180n
Baylor, Norman 19

671

BCG *see* Bacille Calmette-Guérin
Becker muscular dystrophy 455–57
bedwetting, overview 404–8
behavioral therapy, autism 569
behavior management therapy, defined 648
Bell's palsy, Lyme disease 103
bethanechol 396
bicycle injury prevention, described 50–51
bilirubin, defined 648
biopsy
    brain tumors 473
    defined 648
    lymphoma 272
bipolar disorder
    depression 624
    obsessive compulsive disorder 636
    overview 615–17
"Bipolar Disorder" (AAFP) 615n
bismuth subsalicylate 69
bleomycin 157
blood pressure
    described 297
    diabetes mellitus 311
blood stream infections, pneumococcal disease 80
Boeckner, Linda 28n
bone marrow, thrombocytopenia 248
bone marrow transplantation
    neuroblastoma 278
    sickle cell disease 240
Boostrix 21
Borrelia burgdorferi 102, 104
"Bowlegs" (Dartmouth-Hitchcock Medical Center) 432n
bowlegs, described 432–33
Boyse, Kyla 366n, 387n, 587n
bradycardia 288
Brain Resources and Information Network, contact information 657
brain stem glioma, described 477–78
brain tumors, overview 470–84
bronchi, described 167
bronchioles, described 167
"Bronchitis" (Cedars-Sinai Medical Center) 528n
bronchitis, overview 528–31
bruises, first aid 62

burn prevention, described 40–41
burns, first aid 62

C

calcium, diet and nutrition 28
calcium deposits, described 449
calcivirus, described 66
Campylobacter
    described 66, 68
    diarrhea 381
cancer, brain tumors 471
Candlelighters Childhood Cancer Foundation, contact information 655
CAPD *see* central auditory processing disorder
carbohydrates, diet and nutrition 28
cardiomyopathy, defined 648
cardiovascular disorders *see* arrhythmia; hyperlipidemia; hypertension
CAT scan *see* computed axial tomography scan
"Cat Scratch Disease" (Nemours Foundation) 94n
cat scratch disease, overview 94–97
CBT *see* cognitive behavioral therapy
CDC *see* Centers for Disease Control and Prevention
Cedars-Sinai Medical Center, publications
    bronchitis 528n
    pneumonia 167n
Celexa 635
celiac disease, overview 374–76
Centany 109
Centers for Disease Control and Prevention (CDC)
    contact information 653
    publications
        asthma 524n
        Cryptosporidium infection 182n
        dwarf tapeworm 193n
        Epstein-Barr virus 140n
        fifth disease 133n
        foodborne illness 65n
        fragile X syndrome 595n

Index

Centers for Disease Control and Prevention (CDC), continued
publications, continued
giardiasis 188n
group A streptococcal disease 76n
hand, foot, mouth disease 136n
head lice 195n
Hymenolepis infection 193n
infectious mononucleosis 140n
influenza 142n
measles 145n
meningococcal disease 163n
mumps 147n
physical fitness 33n
pneumococcal disease 79n
scabies 204n
scarlet fever 86n
toxocariasis 212n
tuberculosis 115n
central auditory processing disorder (CAPD) 583
CeraLyte 69
cerebral, defined 648
cerebral dysgenesis, defined 648
"Cerebral Palsy" (March of Dimes Birth Defects Foundation) 485n
cerebral palsy, overview 485–91
"Cerebral Palsy: Hope through Research" (NINDS) 647n
Charlie Foundation to Help Cure Pediatric Epilepsy, contact information 664
chemotherapy
brain tumors 474–75
lymphoma 274–75
neuroblastoma 278
chicken pox *see* varicella
"Chickenpox (Varicella)" (Wisconsin Department of Health and Family Services) 122n
"Child Health USA 2005" (DHHS) 3n
"Childhood Nephrotic Syndrome" (NIDDK) 409n
"Children and Adolescents with Anxiety Disorders" (SAMHSA) 611n
"Children and Adolescents with Attention-Deficit/Hyperactivity Disorder" (DHHS) 577n

"Children and Adolescents with Conduct Disorder" (SAMHSA) 619n
Children and Adults with Attention-Deficit/Hyperactivity Disorder, contact information 662
"Children and Arrhythmia" (American Heart Association) 284n
Children's Healthcare of Atlanta, publications
heart murmur 290n
hypertension 297n
neuroblastoma 276n
Osgood-Schlatter disease 460n
Children's Neurobiological Solutions Foundation, contact information 664
"Children's Sleep Habits" (National Sleep Foundation) 35n
chloramphenicol 249
cholesterol, described 292–93
Christmas disease 244
chromosome, defined 648
chronic bronchitis 528
chronic lymphocytic leukemia (CLL) 264–68
chronic myelogenous leukemia (CML) 264–68
chronic sinusitis
described 337–38
treatment 340–41
cimetidine 395
Cincinnati Children's Hospital Medical Center, publications
alpha-1 antitrypsin deficiency 424n
antibiotic resistant staph 107n
autoimmune hepatitis 428n
croup 131n
fever 53n
hyperlipidemia 292n
juvenile dermatomyositis 446n
cisapride 396
Citizens United for Research in Epilepsy, contact information 664
City of Miami, first aid publication 61n
clarithromycin 119

673

classic hemophilia 244
Cleveland Clinic, gastroenteritis publication 390n
"Clinical Hypothyroidism: General Information" (Magic Foundation) 357n
clinical trials
  amblyopia 549
  cystic fibrosis 538
  Tourette syndrome 521
CLL *see* chronic lymphocytic leukemia
Clostridium botulinum 67, 71
Clostridium tetani 112
CML *see* chronic myelogenous leukemia
coagulation, thrombophilia 256
cognitive behavioral therapy (CBT)
  anxiety disorders 614
  depression 625
  obsessive compulsive disorder 634
  recurrent abdominal pain 368
"Common Cold" (NIAID) 124n
common cold, overview 124–30
complete heart block 288
computed axial tomography scan (CAT scan; CT scan)
  alpha-1 antitrypsin deficiency 426
  brain tumors 472
  defined 648
  encephalitis 161
  flat feet 436
  lymphoma 272
  sarcoma 281
  Tourette syndrome 517
  urinary tract infections 420
conduct disorder, overview 619–22
conductive hearing loss, described 320
cone-rod dystrophy 555
congenital neuropathy 411–12
congenital rubella syndrome (CRS) 153
"Conjunctivitis" (Illinois Department of Public Health) 550n
conjunctivitis, overview 550–52
constipation, overview 387–89
constitutional growth delay, overview 352–53

"Constitutional Growth Delay in Children" (Magic Foundation) 352n
contact dermatitis, described 219–20
continuous murmur 291
continuous positive airway pressure (CPAP), obstructive sleep apnea 327
contractures
  defined 648
  described 448
  muscular dystrophy 458
Cooke, David A. 193n, 327n, 377n, 397n, 462n, 577n, 583n, 601n, 607n, 611n, 619n, 623n
coprolalia, Tourette syndrome 516
coronaviruses 125
corticosteroids, allergies 224
Coumadin (warfarin) 257
coxsackie viruses
  described 125
  hand foot mouth disease 136–37
CPAP *see* continuous positive airway pressure
craniopharyngioma, described 478
cromolyn sodium 224
"Croup" (Cincinnati Children's Hospital Medical Center) 131n
croup, overview 131–33
CRS *see* congenital rubella syndrome
Cryptosporidia 67
cryptosporidiosis, overview 182–87
Cryptosporidium 182–87
"*Cryptosporidium* Infection" (CDC) 182n
CT scan *see* computed axial tomography scan
CVS *see* cyclic vomiting syndrome
cyclic vomiting syndrome (CVS), overview 377–80
"Cyclic Vomiting Syndrome" (NIDDK) 377n
Cyclospora, described 67
cyclosporine 451
cystic fibrosis, overview 531–38

Index

Cystic Fibrosis Foundation
  contact information 656
  cystic fibrosis publication 531n
cystitis, described 416
cytokines, defined 649

D

DAPTACEL 21
Dartmouth-Hitchcock Medical
  Center, publications
  bowlegs 432n
  intoeing 440n
  knock knee 432n
dasatinib 268
DDAVP *see* desmopressin
deep-vein thrombosis (DVT)
  256–57
deer ticks, Lyme disease 102
DEET, Lyme disease 105
dehydration
  diarrhea 383–84
  fever 56
dehydroepiandrosterone
  (DHEA) 355
Department of Health and
  Human Services (DHHS; HHS)
  see US Department of Health
  and Human Services
depression, overview 623–27
"Depression in Children and
  Adolescents" (Ryan) 623n
desmopressin (DDAVP)
  hemophilia 246
  von Willebrand disease 260
developmental delay
  defined 649
  overview 587–89
"Developmental Delay" (Boyse) 587n
developmental disability 595
developmental screening, defined 649
dextroamphetamine 519
DHEA *see* dehydroepiandrosterone
DHHS *see* US Department of Health
  and Human Services
diabetes mellitus, overview 305–13
diabetic ketoacidosis (DKA) 306
"Diagnosis" (AAFA) 218n

diarrhea
  cryptosporidiosis 183
  foodborne illness 69–70
  gastroenteritis 390–91
  overview 381–86
"Diarrhea" (NIDDK) 381n
diastolic blood pressure,
  described 297
diastolic murmur 291
DIC *see* disseminated
  intravascular clotting
diet and nutrition
  cholesterol levels 295–96
  daily food choices *30*
  diarrhea 385–86
  encopresis 389
  food fat levels *31*
  gastroenteritis 392
  gluten allergy 374–76
  lactose intolerance 399–401
  recurrent abdominal pain 367–68
  school-aged children 28–32
Dietary Guidelines for Americans 30
diphtheria
  overview 98–99
  vaccine 21
"Diphtheria" (Virginia Department
  of Health) 98n
diphtheria tetanus pertussis
  vaccine (DTaP), described 21, 120
Dispertab (erythromycin) 396
disseminated intravascular
  clotting (DIC) 250
diurnal enuresis 408
DKA *see* diabetic ketoacidosis
doctor visits, preparations 9–14
dolichostenomelia 452
drowning prevention, described 42–44
drug allergy, described 219
DTaP *see* diphtheria tetanus
  pertussis vaccine
DTP vaccine 99
Duchenne muscular dystrophy
  455–56
Duvoid (bethanechol) 396
dwarfism 354
dwarf tapeworm, overview 193–94
dysfunctional voiding, described 421
dyskinetic, defined 649

dyskinetic cerebral palsy 486
dyslexia
 defined 649
 overview 591–94
"Dyslexia" (National Center for Learning Disabilities) 591n
dysrhythmias 284
dystonia, defined 649

E

E. coli see Escherichia coli
EBV *see* Epstein-Barr virus
echinacea, common cold 129
echolalia, Tourette syndrome 516
echoviruses 125
ectopia lentis 452
"Eczema/Atopic Dermatitis" (New Zealand Dermatological Society) 540n
EEG *see* electroencephalogram
Elavil 626
electroencephalogram (EEG)
 defined 649
 encephalitis 161
 Tourette syndrome 517
electrolyte replacement, diarrhea 69
electromyography, defined 649
elevated temperature *see* fever
emergency departments, described 58–60
encephalitis
 hand foot mouth disease 137
 overview 159–62
 rubella 153
"Encephalitis" (A.D.A.M., Inc.) 159n
"Encopresis (Constipation and Soiling)" (Boyse) 387n
encopresis, overview 387–89
endocrinologists
 constitutional growth delay 353
 growth hormone deficiency 356
 idiopathic short stature 360
Engerix-B 22
"Enlarged Adenoids" (Nemours Foundation) 316n
enterobiasis 202
Enterobius vermicularis 202

enteroviruses
 described 125
 encephalitis 159
 hand foot mouth disease 136
enuresis, described 408
environmental bronchitis 528
ependymoma, described 478–79
epilepsy
 autism 573
 defined 649
 overview 492–99
"Epilepsy" (A.D.A.M., Inc.) 492n
Epilepsy Foundation, contact information 664
Epilepsy Foundation of Metropolitan New York, contact information 664
epinephrine, allergies 224
Epstein-Barr virus (EBV), overview 140–41
"Epstein-Barr Virus and Infectious Mononucleosis" (CDC) 140n
erythema migrans 103
erythromycin 119, 396
Escherichia coli infections
 described 65–66, 68
 diarrhea 381
esomeprazole 396
ethmoid sinuses, described 336
Ewing sarcomas, described 279–82
eye allergy, described 220

F

Facioscapulohumeral Muscular Dystrophy Society, contact information 663
"The Facts about Anemia" (Medical College of Wisconsin) 234n
failure to thrive, defined 649
FALCPA *see* Food Allergen Labeling and Consumer Protection Act
fall prevention, described 44–45
falls, first aid 61
famotidine 395
farsightedness 553–54
"Farsightedness (Hyperopia)" (St. Luke's Cataract and Laser Institute) 553n

Index

FDA *see* US Food and Drug Administration
febrile, defined 649
febrile seizures, overview 499–502
"Febrile Seizures Fact Sheet" (NINDS) 499n
fecal incontinence, described 387–89
Federation of Families for Children's Mental Health, contact information 662
fever
  common cold 126
  overview 53–56
  see also rheumatic fever; scarlet fever
"Fever" (Cincinnati Children's Hospital Medical Center) 53n
fifth disease, overview 133–36
first aid, common emergencies 61–62
first aid kit, described 62
flat feet, overview 435–37
flesh-eating bacteria
  see necrotizing fasciitis
Florida Department of Health, hearing loss publication 319n
"Florida Resource Guide for Families of Young Children with Hearing Loss" (Florida Department of Health) 319n
flu *see* influenza
"The Flu: A Guide for Parents" (CDC) 142n
FluMist 23
fluoxetine 626, 635
flu vaccine, described 23
focal segmental glomerulosclerosis (FSGS) 411
focal seizure, defined 649
follicle stimulating hormone (FSH) 358
Food Allergen Labeling and Consumer Protection Act (FALCPA) 231
food allergy
  described 218
  diarrhea 382
  overview 228–32
Food and Drug Administration (FDA) *see* US Food and Drug Administration

foodborne diseases, overview 65–73
"Foodborne Illness" (CDC) 65n
foot warts *see* plantar warts
foscarnet 161
Foscavir (foscarnet) 161
"Fragile X Syndrome" (CDC) 595n
fragile X syndrome (FXS)
  autism 573
  defined 649–50
  overview 595–600
"Frequently Asked Questions" (Cystic Fibrosis Foundation) 531n
frontal sinuses, described 336
FSGS *see* focal segmental glomerulosclerosis
FSH *see* follicle stimulating hormone
fundoplication, gastroesophageal reflux disease 397
FXS *see* fragile X syndrome

G

GABS *see* group A beta-hemolytic streptococci
gallium scan, lymphoma 272
Gardasil 22
GAS *see* group A streptococcal infections
"Gastroenteritis" (Cleveland Clinic) 390n
gastroenteritis, overview 390–93
gastroesophageal reflux disease (GERD)
  defined 650
  overview 393–97
"Gastroesophageal Reflux in Children and Adolescents" (NIDDK) 393n
gastrostomy, defined 650
Gatorade, diarrhea 69
generalized anxiety disorder, described 611–12
genes
  cystic fibrosis 531–32
  defined 650
  fragile X syndrome 596–97
  Marfan syndrome 452–53
  Tourette syndrome 520–21

gene therapy
  cystic fibrosis 536
  hemophilia 246
  sickle cell disease 240–41
GERD *see* gastroesophageal reflux disease
German measles
  defined 651
  overview 152–54
Giardia intestinalis 188
Giardia lamblia 67, 188
"Giardiasis" (CDC) 188n
giardiasis, overview 188–93
Elizabeth Glaser Pediatric AIDS Foundation, contact information 654
Gleevec (imatinib mesylate) 268
glomerulonephritis, impetigo 91
gluten allergy 374–76
gonadotropins, described 354
grand mal seizures, described 495
group A beta-hemolytic streptococci (GABS) 90–91
"Group A Streptococcal (GAS) Disease" (CDC) 76n
group A streptococcal infections (GAS), overview 76–79
  see also impetigo; necrotizing fasciitis; scarlet fever; strep throat; streptococcal infections; streptococcal toxic shock syndrome
"Growing Pains" (Nemours Foundation) 438n
growing pains, overview 438–40
growth hormone deficiency
  idiopathic short stature 360
  overview 354–56
"Growth Hormone Deficiency" (A.D.A.M., Inc.) 354n
Guillain-Barré syndrome, foodborne illness 68

H

"Haemophilus Influenzae Type B (HIB Disease)" (Wisconsin Department of Health and Family Services) 100n

Haemophilus influenzae type B (Hib disease)
  meningitis 163
  otitis media 329
  overview 100–101
haemophilus influenzae Type b vaccine (Hib), described 21–22
"Hand, Foot, and Mouth Disease" (CDC) 136n
hand foot mouth disease (HFMD), overview 136–39
Handler, Steven D. 324n
handwashing
  common cold 126
  cryptosporidiosis 186
  foodborne illness 73
  giardiasis 191
  influenza 143
  overview 37–38
  pneumonia 172
Havrix 22
HDL *see* high-density lipoprotein (HDL) cholesterol
headache, overview 503–7
"Headaches in Children" (American Headache Society) 503n
head lice, overview 195–201
"Head Lice Infestation" (CDC) 195n
hearing loss, overview 319–22
heart disorders *see* arrhythmia; hyperlipidemia; hypertension; Marfan syndrome
heart murmurs, overview 290–91
"Heart Murmurs in Pediatric Patients" (Children's Healthcare of Atlanta) 290n
hemolytic uremic syndrome (HUS)
  described 66, 68
  overview 413–15
"Hemolytic Uremic Syndrome" (NIDDK) 413n
hemophilia
  defined 650
  overview 244–47
heparin-induced thrombocytopenia (HIT) 250
hepatitis A, foodborne illness 67
hepatitis A vaccine, described 22

Index

heredity
  allergy 221
  anemia 235
  bedwetting 406
  cystic fibrosis 531–32
  fragile X syndrome 597–98
  hemophilia 244–47
  hyperlipidemia 294
  juvenile dermatomyositis 447
  Marfan syndrome 452, 454–55
  nephrotic syndrome 411–12
  retinitis pigmentosa 555–56
  sickle cell disease 239–40
  thalassemia 242–44
  thrombocytopenia 248
  Tourette syndrome 519–20
  von Willebrand disease 260
herpes zoster (shingles), varicella 123
HFMD see hand foot mouth disease
HHS see US Department of Health and Human Services
Hib see haemophilus influenzae Type b vaccine
Hib disease see *Haemophilus influenzae* type B
Hibiclens 109
high blood pressure *see* hypertension
high-density lipoprotein (HDL) cholesterol, described 293
HIT see heparin-induced thrombocytopenia
Hodgkin lymphoma, described 270–75
honey, common cold 129–30
Hormone Foundation, contact information 660
hormones
  bedwetting 405
  precocious puberty 361–62
"How to Give Medicine to Children" (FDA) 15n
Human Growth Foundation, contact information 660
human papillomavirus (HPV), vaccine 22–23
Humate-P 260
HUS see hemolytic uremic syndrome
hybrid diabetes 307–8

hydrocephalus
  brain tumors 474
  neurofibromatosis 509
hydroxychloroquine 450–51
"Hymenolepis Infection" (CDC) 193n
Hymenolepis nana 193–94
hypercoagulability 256
hyperglycemia, described 310
hyperlipidemia, overview 292–96
"Hyperlipidemia/Cholesterol Problems in Children" (Cincinnati Children's Hospital Medical Center) 292n
hyperopia 553–54
hypertension (high blood pressure)
  diabetes mellitus 311
  overview 297–301
"Hypertension in Pediatric Patients" (Children's Healthcare of Atlanta) 297n
hypertonia, defined 650
hypoglycemia, described 309–10
hypothalamus, hypothyroidism 358
hypothyroidism, overview 357–59
hypotonia, defined 650
hypoxic-ischemic encephalopathy, defined 650

I

IBS see irritable bowel syndrome
"Idiopathic Short Stature" (Magic Foundation) 359n
idiopathic short stature, overview 359–61
idiopathic thrombocytopenic purpura 254
Illinois Department of Public Health, conjunctivitis publication 550n
imatinib mesylate 268
Immunization Action Coalition, publications
  German measles 152n
  rubella 152n
  tetanus 112n

Childhood Diseases and Disorders Sourcebook, Second Edition

immunizations
 diphtheria 99
 Haemophilus influenzae
  type B 101
 see also vaccinations
immunotherapy
 described 224
 warts 157
impetigo
 described 76
 overview 90–91
"Impetigo" (Wisconsin Department
 of Health and Family Services)
 90n
inactivated polio vaccine (IPV),
 described 25
incontinence *see* bedwetting; fecal
 incontinence; urinary incontinence
incubation period, foodborne illness
 68
Indiana State Department of
 Health, handwashing
 publication 37n
industrial bronchitis 528
Infanrix 21
infectious, defined 650
infectious bronchitis 528
infectious mononucleosis,
 overview 140–41
influenza (flu), overview 142–44
influenza vaccine, described 23
injury prevention, overview 40–52
inoculation lesion, cat scratch
 disease 94–95
insect stings, described 219
insulin, described 305
insulin resistance, described 305,
 306, 307
interferon, warts 157
International Food Information
 Council Foundation, food allergy
 publication 228n
International Foundation for
 Functional Gastrointestinal
 Disorders, contact information 659
interpersonal therapy
 depression 625
 obsessive compulsive disorder 634–
  35

"Intoeing" (Dartmouth-Hitchcock
 Medical Center) 440n
intoeing, overview 440–41
intracranial hemorrhage,
 defined 650
intrauterine infection, defined 650
intravenous immunoglobulin (IVIG)
 451
invasive group A streptococcal
 infections 77–78
IPV *see* inactivated polio vaccine
iron
 anemia 237–38
 diet and nutrition 28–29
iron deficiency anemia, described
 234
irritable bowel syndrome (IBS),
 overview 397–98
"Irritable Bowel Syndrome in
 Children" (NIDDK) 397n
irritative bronchitis 528
"Is It a Medical Emergency?"
 (Nemours Foundation) 58n
IVIG *see* intravenous
 immunoglobulin
Ixodes ticks, Lyme disease 102

J

jaundice, defined 650
JDM *see* juvenile dermatomyositis
JIA *see* juvenile idiopathic arthritis
JPA *see* juvenile pilocytic
 astrocytoma
JRA *see* juvenile rheumatoid
 arthritis
juvenile dermatomyositis
 (JDM) 446–51
"Juvenile Dermatomyositis (JDM)"
 (Cincinnati Children's Hospital
 Medical Center) 446n
Juvenile Diabetes Research
 Foundation International, contact
 information 659
juvenile idiopathic arthritis
 (JIA) 442
juvenile pilocytic astrocytoma
 (JPA) 479–80

Index

juvenile rheumatoid arthritis (JRA), overview 442–45
"Juvenile Rheumatoid Arthritis" (Nemours Foundation) 442n

K

"Kawasaki Disease" (American Heart Association) 302n
Kawasaki disease, overview 302–3
"Knock Knee" (Dartmouth-Hitchcock Medical Center) 432n
knock-knee, described 433–34
Koate DVI 260
Kwell (lindane) 201

L

lactose intolerance
  described 230
  overview 399–401
lansoprazole 396
laryngospasm, tetanus 113
late bloomers, described 352
latent TB infection 116–17
latex allergy, described 219
LDL see low-density lipoprotein (LDL) cholesterol
"Learning about Hemophilia" (National Human Genome Research Institute) 244n
"Learning about Marfan Syndrome" (National Human Genome Research Institute) 452n
"Learning about Retinitis Pigmentosa" (National Human Genome Research Institute) 555n
"Learning About Sickle Cell Disease" (National Human Genome Research Institute) 239n
"Learning About Thalassemia" (National Human Genome Research Institute) 242n
"Learning Disabilities" (National Dissemination Center for Children with Disabilities) 601n
learning disabilities, overview 601–6
Learning Disabilities Association of America, contact information 658
"Leukemia" (Leukemia and Lymphoma Society) 264n
leukemia, overview 264–69
Leukemia and Lymphoma Society
  contact information 656
  leukemia publication 264n
Levothroid 359
Levoxyl 359
Lexapro 635
LH see luteinizing hormone
lindane 201
linkage studies, defined 650
lipids, described 311
Lippincott Williams and Wilkins, dictionary publication 647n
Listeria monocytogenes 71
liver transplantation, autoimmune hepatitis 430
lockjaw see tetanus
loperamide 392
lorazepam 380
lordosis, defined 650
low-density lipoprotein (LDL) cholesterol, described 293
lumbar puncture
  encephalitis 161
  lymphoma 272
lungs
  asthma 524–27
  bronchitis 528–30
  cystic fibrosis 531–38
  described 167
luteinizing hormone (LH) 358
Luvox 635
"Lyme Disease" (Nemours Foundation) 102n
Lyme disease, overview 102–6
lymph nodes
  cat scratch disease 94–95
  infectious mononucleosis 140
lymphoma, overview 269–75
"Lymphoma Treatment" (Seattle Cancer Care Alliance) 269n

M

MAAP Services for Autism, Asperger's, and PDD, contact information 658
Magic Foundation
  contact information 660
  publications
    constitutional growth delay 352n
    hypothyroidism 357n
    idiopathic short stature 359n
    precocious puberty 361n
magnetic resonance imaging (MRI)
  brain tumors 472
  defined 650
  encephalitis 161
  flat feet 436
  Marfan syndrome 453
  neurofibromatosis 512
  sarcoma 281
  Tourette syndrome 517
  urinary tract infections 420
malathion 201
manic depressive disorder 624
March of Dimes Birth Defects Foundation, cerebral palsy publication 485n
Marcus, Carole L. 324n
Marfan syndrome, overview 452–55
Massachusetts General Hospital Department of Psychiatry, obsessive-compulsive disorder publication 629n
maturity-onset diabetes of young (MODY) 308
maxillary sinuses, described 336
MCV4 165
measles
  overview 145–46
  vaccine 24
"Measles" (CDC) 145n
measles mumps rubella vaccine (MMR), described 24, 146, 148
mebendazole 180, 203
Medical College of Wisconsin, anemia publication 234n
medical emergencies, overview 58–61
medical examinations, preparations 9–14

"Medical Facts about Psoriasis in Children" (National Psoriasis Foundation) 543n
medications
  allergies 223–24
  arrhythmias 288–89
  autism 571–72
  autoimmune hepatitis 430
  bedwetting 407–8
  bipolar disorder 616
  bronchitis 530
  cat scratch disease 97
  cerebral palsy 489
  common cold 127–28
  conjunctivitis 551
  cyclic vomiting syndrome 379–80
  cystic fibrosis 534, 535
  diabetes mellitus 313
  diarrhea 382
  dispensing procedures 15–17
  encephalitis 161–62
  fever 54–55
  fifth disease 135
  gastroesophageal reflux disease 395–96
  giardiasis 190
  head lice 200–201
  influenza 143
  juvenile rheumatoid arthritis 445
  leukemia 268
  nosebleeds 323
  obsessive compulsive disorder 635–36
  Osgood-Schlatter disease 461–62
  perforated eardrum 334
  pertussis 119
  pinworms 203
  pneumonia 170–71
  rheumatic fever 84–85
  scabies 206
  sinusitis 340–41
  thrombocytopenia 250, 253–55
  tinea infections 210
  tonsillitis 348
  Tourette syndrome 518–19
  tuberculosis 117
  urinary tract infections 419
  warts 157
medulloblastoma, described 481

Index

megaloblastic anemia, described 234–35
membranoproliferative glomerulonephritis (MPGN) 411
Menactra 24
MenactraT 165
meningitis
  overview 163–66
  pneumococcal disease 80, 81
meningococcal conjugate vaccine 165
"Meningococcal Disease" (CDC) 163n
meningococcal disease vaccine, described 24
meningococcal meningitis 164
meningococcal polysaccharide vaccine 165
Menomune 165
Mental Health America, contact information 662
mental retardation
  autism 573
  defined 650
  fragile X syndrome 595
metastases, described 277
metatarsus adductus 441
methicillin resistant *Staphylococcus aureus* (MRSA), described 107–9
methotrexate 445, 450
methylphenidate 519
metoclopramide 396
microbes, foodborne illness 67–68
middle ear infections *see* otitis media
migraine headache, described 505–6
minimal change disease 410–11
mixed diabetes 307–8
mixed hearing loss, described 321–22
MMR *see* measles mumps rubella vaccine
MODY *see* maturity-onset diabetes of young
moisture alarms, bedwetting 408
mosaic warts 155
Moseley, C. 455n
motor vehicle accident prevention, described 51–52
MPGN *see* membranoproliferative glomerulonephritis
MPSV4 165
MRI *see* magnetic resonance imaging

MRSA *see* methicillin resistant *Staphylococcus aureus*
mumps
  overview 147–49
  vaccine 24
"Mumps: Q&A about the Disease" (CDC) 147n
mupirocin cream 109
"Muscular Dystrophy" (Moseley) 455n
muscular dystrophy, overview 455–59
Muscular Dystrophy Association, contact information 663
"Muscular Dystrophy: Hope through Research" (NINDS) 647n
mycoplasma infection 110–11
"*Mycoplasma pneumonia* (New Hampshire Department of Health and Human Services)" 110n
Mycoplasma pneumoniae 110–11
myopathy, defined 650
myopia 452, 554
myotonia, defined 651

N

nasal polyps, sinusitis 337–38
nasopharyngeal tonsils 316
National Alliance on Mental Illness, contact information 662
National Association for Children's Behavioral Health, contact information 663
National Association for Continence, contact information 661
National Association of School Psychologists, contact information 663
National Brain Tumor Foundation
  contact information 656
  pediatric brain tumors publication 470n
National Cancer Institute, contact information 656
National Center for Learning Disabilities
  contact information 658
  dyslexia publication 591n

Childhood Diseases and Disorders Sourcebook, Second Edition

National Children's Cancer Society, contact information 656
National Diabetes Education Program
  contact information 659
  pediatric diabetes publication 305n
National Diabetes Information Clearinghouse, contact information 659
National Dissemination Center for Children with Disabilities, learning disabilities publication 601n
National Eye Institute
  amblyopia publication 548n
  contact information 666
National Heart, Lung, and Blood Institute (NHLBI)
  contact information 653
  thrombocytopenia publication 247n
National Hemophilia Foundation
  contact information 655
  von Willebrand disease publication 259n
National Human Genome Research Institute
  contact information 655
  publications
    hemophilia 244n
    Marfan syndrome 452n
    retinitis pigmentosa 555n
    sickle cell disease 239n
    thalassemia 242n
National Institute of Allergy and Infectious Diseases (NIAID)
  contact information 660
  publications
    ascariasis 178n
    common cold 124n
    pinworm infection 202n
    sinusitis 335n
    strep throat 88n
National Institute of Arthritis and Musculoskeletal and Skin Diseases (NIAMS)
  contact information 654
  scoliosis publication 462n
National Institute of Child Health and Human Development (NICHD)
  autism publications 561n, 647n
  contact information 654

National Institute of Diabetes and Digestive and Kidney Diseases (NIDDK)
  contact information 653, 659
  publications
    bedwetting 404n
    celiac disease 374n
    childhood nephrotic syndrome 409n
    cyclic vomiting syndrome 377n
    diarrhea 381n
    gastroesophageal reflux 393n
    hemolytic uremic syndrome 413n
    irritable bowel syndrome 397n
    lactose intolerance 399n
    urinary incontinence 404n
    urinary tract infections 415n
National Institute of Mental Health, contact information 658
National Institute of Neurological Disorders and Stroke (NINDS)
  contact information 654
  publications
    cerebral palsy 647n
    febrile seizures 499n
    muscular dystrophy 647n
    neurofibromatosis 508n
    Tourette syndrome 515n
National Institute on Deafness and Other Communication Disorders (NIDCD)
  contact information 658, 660
  publications
    auditory processing disorder 583n
    otitis media 327n
    stuttering 607n
National Kidney Foundation, contact information 661
National Pediatric AIDS Network, contact information 654
National Psoriasis Foundation
  contact information 666
  pediatric psoriasis publication 543n
National Reye's Syndrome Foundation, Inc., contact information 665
National Scoliosis Foundation, contact information 665

Index

National Sleep Foundation
  contact information 666
  sleep habits publication 35n
nearsightedness 554
"Nearsightedness (Myopia)" (St. Luke's Cataract and Laser Institute) 553n
necrotizing fasciitis, described 77–79
Neisseria meningitidis 163–65
Nemours Foundation
  contact information 654
  publications
    cat scratch disease 94n
    doctor visits 9n
    enlarged adenoids 316n
    growing pains 438n
    juvenile rheumatoid arthritis 442n
    Lyme disease 102n
    medical emergency 58n
neonatal tetanus 114–15
Neoral (cyclosporine) 451
nephropathy, described 310–11
nephrotic syndrome, overview 409–12
nerve entrapment, defined 651
"Neuroblastoma" (Children's Healthcare of Atlanta) 276n
neuroblastoma, overview 276–78
neurofibromatosis, overview 508–15
"Neurofibromatosis Fact Sheet" (NINDS) 508n
neuropathy, described 311
New Hampshire Department of Health and Human Services, mycoplasma infection publications 110n
New York State Department of Health, contact information 660
New Zealand Dermatological Society, eczema publication 540n
Nexium (esomeprazole) 396
NF1 508–10
NF2 511–12
NHLBI *see* National Heart, Lung, and Blood Institute
NIAID *see* National Institute of Allergy and Infectious Diseases
NIAMS *see* National Institute of Arthritis and Musculoskeletal and Skin Diseases
NICHD *see* National Institute of Child Health and Human Development
NIDCD *see* National Institute on Deafness and Other Communication Disorders
NIDDK *see* National Institute of Diabetes and Digestive and Kidney Diseases
nitazoxanide 185
Nix (permethrin) 200
nizatidine 395
non-Hodgkin lymphoma, described 270–75
non-rapid eye movement (NREM), described 35
nonstructural scoliosis 463
North American Society for Pediatric Gastroenterology, Hepatology, and Nutrition, contact information 659
Norwalk viruses, described 66
nosebleeds
  first aid 61
  overview 322–24
"Nosebleeds" (Allen ENT and Allergy) 322n
NREM *see* non-rapid eye movement
nutrition *see* diet and nutrition
"Nutrition for the School-Aged Child" (Boeckner; Schledewitz) 28n

O

"Obsessive-Compulsive Disorder" (Massachusetts General Hospital Department of Psychiatry) 629n
obsessive compulsive disorder (OCD)
  described 612
  overview 629–40
"Obstructive Sleep Apnea" (Handler; Marcus) 324n

Childhood Diseases and Disorders Sourcebook, Second Edition

obstructive sleep apnea (OSA)
  bedwetting 406
  overview 324–27
occupational therapy, autism 569–70
OCD *see* obsessive compulsive disorder
ocular larva migrans (OLM) 212–13
off-label drugs, defined 651
oligoarticular juvenile rheumatoid arthritis 443
OLM *see* ocular larva migrans
omeprazole 379, 396
oppositional defiant disorder 619, 641–43
"Oppositional Defiant Disorder" (A.D.A.M., Inc.) 641n
optic nerve glioma, described 481–82
Oralyte 69
ORSA *see* oxacillin resistant *Staphylococcus aureus*
orthomyxoviruses 125
orthotic devices, defined 651
OSA *see* obstructive sleep apnea
"Osgood-Schlatter Disease" (Children's Healthcare of Atlanta) 460n
Osgood-Schlatter disease, overview 460–62
osteosarcoma, described 279–82
otitis media
  overview 327–32
  pneumococcal disease 80
"Otitis Media (Ear Infection)" (NIDCD) 327n
over-the-counter medications, dispensing procedures 15–16
"Overview of Diabetes in Children and Adolescents" (National Diabetes Education Program) 305n
Ovide (malathion) 201
"Oxacillin Resistant *Staph aureus* (ORSA) / Methicillin Resistant *Staph aureus* (MRSA)" (Cincinnati Children's Hospital Medical Center) 107n
oxacillin resistant *Staphylococcus aureus* (ORSA), described 107–9
oxymetazoline 323

P

PAC *see* premature atrial contraction
pacemakers, arrhythmias 289–90
palsy, defined 651
panhypopituitarism 354
panic disorder, described 612
pantoprazole 396
paramyxoviruses 125
parasites, foodborne illness 68–69
Parent Project Muscular Dystrophy, contact information 663
"A Parent's Guide to Kids' Vaccines" (FDA) 19n
Parinaud oculoglandular syndrome 95
paroxetine 626
paroxysmal atrial tachycardia (PAT) 286
paroxysmal supraventricular tachycardia (PSVT) 286
partial seizures
  defined 649
  described 495–96
partial thromboplastin time (PTT) 253
"Parvovirus B19 (Fifth Disease)" (CDC) 133n
parvovirus B19, overview 133–36
PAT *see* paroxysmal atrial tachycardia
patch test, allergies 222
Pathways Awareness Foundation, contact information 664
Paxil 635
PDD *see* pervasive developmental disorders
pectus carinatum 452
pectus excavatum 452
Pedialyte 69
Pediatric Brain Tumor Foundation, contact information 656
"Pediatric FAQ" (National Brain Tumor Foundation) 470n

Index

pediculosis, overview 195–201
People Against Childhood Epilepsy, contact information 664
Pepcid (famotidine) 395
Pepto-Bismol (bismuth subsalicylate) 69
perforated eardrum, overview 333–35
periventricular leukomalacia (PVL), defined 651
permethrin 200
persistent femoral anteversion 441
personal flotation devices (PFD), described 43–44
"Pertussis (Whooping Cough)" (Wisconsin Department of Health and Family Services) 118n
pertussis (whooping cough)
 overview 118–20
 vaccine 21
pervasive developmental disorders (PDD) 562
"Pes Planus" (A.D.A.M., Inc.) 435n
pes planus, overview 435–37
petit mal seizures, described 494–95
PET scan *see* positron emission tomography
PFD *see* personal flotation devices
phenobarbital 501
pHisoHex 109
phobias, described 612
physical activity
 overweight children 29–32
 recommendations 33–34
"Physical Activity for Everyone: Are There Special Recommendations for Young People?" (CDC) 33n
physical examinations, preparations 9–14
physical fitness
 health 33–34
 overweight children 29–32
physical therapy
 autism 570
 juvenile rheumatoid arthritis 445
pica 212
pineal tumor, described 482–83
pinkeye 550–52
"Pinworm Infection" (NIAID) 202n
pinworms, overview 202–4

piperonyl butoxide 200
pituitary dwarfism 354
pituitary gland
 hypothyroidism 358
 precocious puberty 361
plantar warts, described 155, 157
Plaquenil (hydroxychloroquine) 450–51
PNET *see* primitive neuroectodermal tumor
pneumococcal conjugate vaccine
 described 25, 81–82
 otitis media 329
pneumococcal disease, overview 79–82
"Pneumococcal Disease in Children: Q&A" (CDC) 79n
pneumococcal vaccine polyvalent, described 25
pneumonia
 overview 167–72
 pneumococcal disease 80
"Pneumonia" (Cedars-Sinai Medical Center) 167n
Pneumovax 82
Pneumovax 23 25
Pnu-Immune 82
poisoning prevention, described 46–47
polio vaccine, described 25
polyarticular arthritis 443
Polysporin 324
positron emission tomography (PET scan)
 lymphoma 272
 sarcoma 281
posttraumatic stress disorder (PTSD), described 612–13
"Precocious Puberty" (Magic Foundation) 361n
precocious puberty, overview 361–64
prednisone
 autoimmune hepatitis 430
 juvenile dermatomyositis 450
 thrombocytopenia 254
premature atrial contraction (PAC) 285
premature ventricular contraction (PVC) 285

"Preparing Your Child for Visits to the Doctor" (DHHS) 9n
preschoolers, sleep habits 35–36
prescription medications, dispensing procedures 16–17
Prevacid (lansoprazole) 396
"Preventing Childhood Airway Obstruction Injuries" (Safe Kids Worldwide) 48n
"Preventing Childhood Burns" (Safe Kids Worldwide) 40n
"Preventing Childhood Drowning" (Safe Kids Worldwide) 42n
"Preventing Childhood Falls" (Safe Kids Worldwide) 44n
"Preventing Childhood Poisoning" (Safe Kids Worldwide) 46n
"Preventing Injuries to Children in Motor Vehicle Crashes" (Safe Kids Worldwide) 51n
"Preventing Injuries to Children Riding Bicycles" (Safe Kids Worldwide) 50n
"Prevention" (AAFA) 218n
Prevnar 25, 81–82, 329
Prilosec (omeprazole) 379, 396
primary enuresis 408
primary headache, described 503
primitive neuroectodermal tumor (PNET) 483–84
proglottids 193
Pronto (pyrethrin) 200
Propulsid (cisapride) 396
protein, diet and nutrition 28
prothrombin time (PT) 253
Protonix (pantoprazole) 396
Prozac (fluoxetine) 626, 635
psoriasis, overview 543–45
PSVT see paroxysmal supraventricular tachycardia
PT see prothrombin time
ptosis, defined 651
PTT see partial thromboplastin time
puberty, described 362
PVC see premature ventricular contraction
PVL see periventricular leukomalacia
pyrantel pamoate 180, 203
pyrethrins 200

Q

quadriplegia, defined 651
Quanti-FERON TB Gold Test 116–17
"Questions and Answers about Scoliosis in Children and Adolescents" (NIAMS) 462n
"Quick Facts About ... Handwashing" (Indiana State Department of Health) 37n

R

rabeprazole 396
"Rabies" (Wisconsin Department of Health and Family Services) 149n
rabies, overview 149–51
raccoon roundworms 180–81
radiation therapy
  brain tumors 474
  lymphoma 274–75
  neuroblastoma 278
radiofrequency ablation, arrhythmias 289
ranitidine 379, 395
RAP see recurrent abdominal pain
rapid eye movement (REM), described 35
R&C (pyrethrin) 200
Recombivax HB 22
recurrent abdominal pain (RAP), overview 366–69
reflux see gastroesophageal reflux disease
Reglan (metoclopramide) 396
REM see rapid eye movement
respiratory syncytial viruses 125
retinitis pigmentosa, overview 555–57
retinopathy, described 310
Rett syndrome, defined 651
Reye syndrome
  aspirin 123
  overview 173–75
  salicylates 16
"Reye Syndrome" (American Liver Foundation) 173n
rhabdoid tumor, described 484

Index

"Rheumatic Fever"
  (A.D.A.M., Inc.) 83n
rheumatic fever, overview 83–85
rheumatoid arthritis, overview 442–45
Rh incompatibility, defined 651
rhinoviruses 125
Rid (pyrethrin) 200
ringworm 209–11
Robimycin (erythromycin) 396
RotaTeq 26
rotavirus vaccine, described 26
roundworms 178–81, 202–4
rubella
  defined 651
  overview 152–54
  vaccine 24
"Ruptured Eardrum"
  (A.D.A.M., Inc.) 333n
Ryan, Neal 623n

S

Safe Kids Worldwide
  contact information 661
  publications
    airway obstruction prevention 48n
    bicycle injury prevention 50n
    burn prevention 40n
    drowning prevention 42n
    fall prevention 44n
    motor vehicle injury
      prevention 51n
    poisoning prevention 46n
safety considerations
  airway injury prevention 48–49
  bicycle injury prevention 50–51
  burn prevention 40–41
  drowning prevention 42–44
  fall prevention 44–45
  motor vehicle accident
    prevention 51–52
  poisoning prevention 46–47
safety helmets
  bicycles 50
  children 45
Salmonella
  described 66, 68, 70
  diarrhea 381

SAMHSA *see* Substance Abuse
  and Mental Health Services
  Administration
Sandimmune (cyclosporine) 451
sarcoma, overview 279–82
"Sarcoma Treatment" (Seattle
  Cancer Care Alliance) 279n
Sarcoptes scabei 204
"Scabies" (CDC) 204n
scabies, overview 204–6
scarlet fever
  impetigo 91
  overview 86–87
"Scarlet Fever" (CDC) 86n
schistosomes, swimmers itch 207
Schledewitz, Karen 28n
schwannomatosis 512–13
scoliosis
  defined 651
  Marfan syndrome 452
  muscular dystrophy 459
  overview 462–68
Scoliosis Association, Inc.,
  contact information 665
Scoliosis Research Society,
  contact information 665
Seattle Cancer Care Alliance,
  publications
  lymphoma 269n
  sarcoma 279n
secondary diabetes 308
secondary headache, described 503
secretin, autism 572
seizure disorder 492
seizures
  defined 651
  described 492
selective dorsal rhizotomy,
  defined 651
sensorineural hearing loss,
  described 320
separation anxiety disorder,
  described 612
sertraline 626
Shigella
  described 67, 70
  diarrhea 381
shingles *see* herpes zoster
sickle cell disease, overview 239–41

Childhood Diseases and Disorders Sourcebook, Second Edition

sick sinus syndrome 288
Simon Foundation for Continence,
  contact information 661
sinuses, described 336
"Sinus Infection (Sinusitis)"
  (NIAID) 335n
sinusitis, overview 335–43
skin test, allergies 222
sleep habits, described 35–36
sleep studies, described 326
snacks, recommendations 29
Society of Urologic Nurses and
  Associates
  contact information 662
soft tissue sarcomas, described 279–82
soiling, described 387–89
spastic, defined 651
spastic cerebral palsy 485–86
speech-language therapy
  auditory processing disorder 585
  autism 569
  stuttering 608–9
sphenoid sinuses, described 336
spinal meningitis 163
spleen, thrombocytopenia 248, 251
splenectomy, idiopathic
  thrombocytopenic purpura 254
Sprycel (dasatinib) 268
SRS *see* stereotactic radiosurgery
St. Luke's Cataract and Laser
  Institute, publications
  farsightedness 553n
  nearsightedness 553n
  strabismus 557n
Staphylococcus aureus
  described 67, 71, 107
  impetigo 90
statistics
  AIDS 5
  amblyopia 548
  ascariasis 178
  asthma 4
  attention deficit hyperactivity
    disorder 578
  cerebral palsy 485
  child mortality 7
  common cold 124
  conduct disorder 620
  cystic fibrosis 534

statistics, continued
  encephalitis 160
  febrile seizures 499
  fragile X syndrome 595
  hemophilia 245
  hospitalizations 6
  influenza 5–6
  injuries 7
  juvenile dermatomyositis 446
  measles 145
  mental health 4–5
  neuroblastoma 276–77
  neurofibromatosis 508
  otitis media 327
  pneumococcal disease 80
  pneumonia 167
  tetanus 113, 114
  urinary tract infections 415
*Stedman's Electronic Medical
  Dictionary* (Lippincott Williams
  and Wilkins) 647n
stem cell transplantation
  leukemia 268
  lymphoma 275
stereoagnosia, defined 652
stereotactic radiosurgery (SRS),
  brain tumors 474
strabismus
  defined 652
  overview 557–58
"Strabismus (Crossed or Turned
  Eye)" (St. Luke's Cataract and
  Laser Institute) 557n
strep throat
  described 76, 78–79
  foodborne illness 67
  obsessive compulsive disorder 633
  overview 88–89
  rheumatic fever 83, 85
"Strep Throat" (NIAID) 88n
streptococcal infections
  defined 652
  overview 76–91
  see also group A streptococcal
    infections
streptococcal toxic shock syndrome
  (STSS), described 77–79
Streptococcus pneumoniae 79–80, 163
Streptococcus pyogenes 90

Index

stridor, croup 131
structural scoliosis 463
STSS *see* streptococcal toxic shock syndrome
"Stuttering" (NIDCD) 607n
stuttering, overview 607–10
Substance Abuse and Mental Health Services Administration (SAMHSA)
  contact information 663
  publications
    anxiety disorders 611n
    conduct disorder 619n
sulfite sensitivity, described 230
supraventricular tachycardia (SVT) 286–87
surgical procedures
  appendicitis 371–72
  arrhythmias 289
  cerebral palsy 489
  enlarged adenoids 317–18
  gastroesophageal reflux disease 396–97
  muscular dystrophy 458–59
  neuroblastoma 278
  obstructive sleep apnea 326
  scoliosis 465–67
  sinusitis 341
  see also biopsy
susceptibility, defined 652
SVT *see* supraventricular tachycardia
sweat test, cystic fibrosis 532–33
"Swimmer's Ear" (A.D.A.M., Inc.) 344n
swimmer's ear, overview 344–45
"Swimmer's Itch" (Wisconsin Department of Health and Family Services) 207n
swimmer's itch, overview 207–8
swimming pool safety measures 42–43
Synthroid 359
systemic juvenile rheumatoid arthritis 443
systolic blood pressure, described 297
systolic murmur 291

T

tachycardia 286
Tagamet (cimetidine) 395
tapeworms 193–94
tarsal coalition 435–36
TB *see* tuberculosis
Tdap *see* tetanus diphtheria pertussis vaccine
temperature *see* fever
tension-type headache, described 504–5
tests
  allergies 222–23
  alpha-1 antitrypsin deficiency 426
  anemia 236
  appendicitis 371
  celiac disease 375
  cerebral palsy 488–89
  cyclic vomiting syndrome 379
  cystic fibrosis 532–33
  diarrhea 384–85
  encephalitis 161
  epilepsy 496
  febrile seizures 501
  fifth disease 134–35
  food allergy 230–31
  fragile X syndrome 599–600
  gastroesophageal reflux disease 394–95
  giardiasis 190, 192–93
  growth hormone deficiency 355
  hemophilia 245
  hypertension 300–301
  infectious mononucleosis 141
  juvenile dermatomyositis 449
  juvenile rheumatoid arthritis 444
  leukemia 267
  Lyme disease 104
  lymphoma 272
  Marfan syndrome 453
  muscular dystrophy 457–58
  neurofibromatosis 513–14
  perforated eardrum 334
  pertussis 119–20
  pneumonia 170
  rheumatic fever 84
  sarcoma 280–81
  scarlet fever 87
  scoliosis 464
  sickle cell disease 241
  sinusitis 339–70

Childhood Diseases and Disorders Sourcebook, Second Edition

tests, continued
  strep throat 89
  swimmer's ear 344–45
  thalassemia 243–44
  thrombocytopenia 252–53
  Tourette syndrome 517–18
  tuberculosis 116–17
  urinary tract infections 420
tetanus
  overview 112–15
  vaccine 21, 114
tetanus diphtheria pertussis vaccine (Tdap)
  described 21, 114, 120
"Tetanus Disease: Questions and Answers" (Immunization Action Coalition) 112n
tetanus immune globulin (TIG) 114
thalassemia, overview 242–44
thoracolumbosacral orthosis (TLSO) 466
thrombocytopenia
  defined 652
  overview 247–55
"Thrombocytopenia" (NHLBI) 247n
"Thrombophilia" (University of Colorado Denver) 256n
thrombophilia, overview 256–58
thrombosis, defined 652
thrombotic thrombocytopenic purpura (TTP) 250
thyroid disorders *see* growth hormone deficiency; hypothyroidism
thyrotropins, described 354
tibial torsion 441
ticks, Lyme disease 102–6
tics, Tourette syndrome 515–16
TIG *see* tetanus immune globulin
tinea, overview 209–11
"Tinea Infections: Athlete's Foot, Jock Itch and Ringworm" (AAFP) 209n
TLSO *see* thoracolumbosacral orthosis
TMP/SMX *see* trimethoprim/ sulfamethoxazole
Tofranil 625

tonic clonic seizures
  defined 652
  described 495
tonsillectomy, obstructive sleep apnea 326
"Tonsillitis" (A.D.A.M., Inc.) 347n
tonsillitis, overview 347–49
Tourette syndrome, overview 515–21
"Tourette Syndrome Fact Sheet" (NINDS) 515n
"Toxocariasis" (CDC) 212n
toxocariasis, overview 212–13
trachea (windpipe)
  bronchitis 528
  described 167
travel concerns
  allergies 226–27
  diarrhea 386
  food safety 187
"Treating Arrhythmias in Children" (American Heart Association) 284n
"Treating Head Lice Infestation" (CDC) 195n
"Treatment" (AAFA) 218n
tremor, defined 652
triggers, asthma 526–27
trimethoprim/sulfamethoxazole (TMP/SMX), pertussis 119
Tripedia 21
Triple X (pyrethrin) 200
TTP *see* thrombotic thrombocytopenic purpura
tuberculin skin test 116–17
tuberculosis (TB), overview 115–17
"Tuberculosis: General Information" (CDC) 115n
tuberous sclerosis
  autism 573
  defined 652
tympanostomy tubes, pneumococcal disease 81
type 1 diabetes mellitus, described 305–6
type 2 diabetes mellitus, described 306–7
"Types of Arrhythmia in Children" (American Heart Association) 284n

Index

U

ulcers, described 448
ultrasound
  defined 652
  urinary tract infections 420
"Understanding Food Allergy"
  (International Food Information
  Council Foundation) 228n
unipolar depression 624
United Cerebral Palsy, contact
  information 665
University of Colorado Denver,
  thrombophilia publication 256n
Urecholine (bethanechol) 396
urgent care centers, described 58,
  60–61
urinary incontinence, overview
  404–8
urinary obstruction, described 421
urinary tract, depicted *416*, *417*
urinary tract infections (UTI),
  overview 415–22
"Urinary Tract Infections in
  Children" (NIDDK) 415n
urticaria, described 219
US Department of Health and
  Human Services (DHHS; HHS),
  publications
    attention deficit hyperactivity
      disorder 577n
    child health statistics 3n
US Food and Drug Administration
  (FDA)
    contact information 654
    publications
      medication dispensing 15n
      vaccinations 19n
UTI *see* urinary tract infections

V

vaccinations
  adverse reactions 20
  diphtheria 99
  influenza 142–43
  measles 146
  meningitis 165

vaccinations, continued
  mumps 147–49
  otitis media 329
  pneumococcal disease 81–82
  pneumonia 171–72
  recommendations overview
    19–26
  rubella 153
  tetanus 114
  varicella 123
vaccine information sheets,
  described 20
valproate 501
VAQTA 22
varicella (chicken pox)
  overview 122–24
  vaccine 26
varicella vaccine, described 26
varicella zoster immune globulin
  (VZIG) 123
Varivax 26
vasopressin, described 354
venlafaxine 626
ventricular tachycardia
  (VT) 287–88
ventriculoperitoneal shunt 474
very low density lipoprotein
  (VLDL) cholesterol, described
  293
vesicles, varicella 122
vesicoureteral reflux (VUR) 421
Vibrio parahaemolyticus,
  described 67, 70
viral meningitis, hand foot
  mouth disease 137
Virginia Department of Health,
  diphtheria publication 98n
viruses
  common cold 125
  diarrhea 382
visceral larva migrans
  (VLM) 212–13
vitamin C, common cold 129
vitamins, recommendations 28–29
VLDL *see* very low density
  lipoprotein (VLDL) cholesterol
VLM *see* visceral larva migrans
"von Willebrand Disease" (National
  Hemophilia Foundation) 259n

von Willebrand disease, overview 259–61
VT *see* ventricular tachycardia
VUR *see* vesicoureteral reflux

W

warfarin 257
"Warts" (American Academy of Dermatology) 155n
warts, overview 155–58
water sports, safety considerations 42–44
WBRT *see* whole brain radiation therapy
wellness promotion, overview 28–38
"What Are Allergies?" (AAFA) 218n
"What Causes Allergies?" (AAFA) 218n
"What I Need to Know about Celiac Disease" (NIDDK) 374n
whole brain radiation therapy (WBRT) 474
whooping cough *see* pertussis
"Why Does Milk Bother Me?" (NIDDK) 399n
Wisconsin Department of Health and Family Services
  contact information 661
  publications
    Baylisascaris procyonis 180n
    chickenpox 122n
Wisconsin Department of Health and Family Services, continued
  publications, continued
    haemophilus influenza type B 100n
    impetigo 90n
    rabies 149n
    raccoon round worm 180n
    swimmer's itch 207n
    varicella 122n
    whooping cough 118n
Wolff-Parkinson-White syndrome 287
wounds, first aid 61

X

X-linked recessive, defined 652

Y

Yersinia enterocolitica, described 71
"You Can Control Your Asthma" (CDC) 524n

Z

Zantac (ranitidine) 379, 395
zinc, common cold 130
Zoloft (sertraline) 626, 635
Zovirax (acyclovir) 161

Health Reference Series
COMPLETE CATALOG
List price $87 per volume. **School and library price $78 per volume.**

Adolescent Health Sourcebook, 2nd Edition
Basic Consumer Health Information about the Physical, Mental, and Emotional Growth and Development of Adolescents, Including Medical Care, Nutritional and Physical Activity Requirements, Puberty, Sexual Activity, Acne, Tanning, Body Piercing, Common Physical Illnesses and Disorders, Eating Disorders, Attention Deficit Hyperactivity Disorder, Depression, Bullying, Hazing, and Adolescent Injuries Related to Sports, Driving, and Work

Along with Substance Abuse Information about Nicotine, Alcohol, and Drug Use, a Glossary, and Directory of Additional Resources

Edited by Joyce Brennfleck Shannon. 683 pages. 2006. 978-0-7808-0943-7.

"It is written in clear, nontechnical language aimed at general readers. . . . Recommended for public libraries, community colleges, and other agencies serving health care consumers."
—*American Reference Books Annual, 2003*

"Recommended for school and public libraries. Parents and professionals dealing with teens will appreciate the easy-to-follow format and the clearly written text. This could become a 'must have' for every high school teacher." —*E-Streams, Jan '03*

"A good starting point for information related to common medical, mental, and emotional concerns of adolescents." —*School Library Journal, Nov '02*

"This book provides accurate information in an easy to access format. It addresses topics that parents and caregivers might not be aware of and provides practical, useable information."
—*Doody's Health Sciences Book Review Journal, Sep-Oct '02*

"Recommended reference source."
—*Booklist, American Library Association, Sep '02*

AIDS Sourcebook, 3rd Edition
Basic Consumer Health Information about Acquired Immune Deficiency Syndrome (AIDS) and Human Immunodeficiency Virus (HIV) Infection, Including Facts about Transmission, Prevention, Diagnosis, Treatment, Opportunistic Infections, and Other Complications, with a Section for Women and Children, Including Details about Associated Gynecological Concerns, Pregnancy, and Pediatric Care

Along with Updated Statistical Information, Reports on Current Research Initiatives, a Glossary, and Directories of Internet, Hotline, and Other Resources

Edited by Dawn D. Matthews. 664 pages. 2003. 978-0-7808-0631-3.

"The 3rd edition of the *AIDS Sourcebook*, part of Omnigraphics' *Health Reference Series*, is a welcome update. . . . This resource is highly recommended for academic and public libraries."
—*American Reference Books Annual, 2004*

"Excellent sourcebook. This continues to be a highly recommended book. There is no other book that provides as much information as this book provides."
—*AIDS Book Review Journal, Dec-Jan '00*

"Recommended reference source."
—*Booklist, American Library Association, Dec '99*

Alcoholism Sourcebook, 2nd Edition
Basic Consumer Health Information about Alcohol Use, Abuse, and Dependence, Featuring Facts about the Physical, Mental, and Social Health Effects of Alcohol Addiction, Including Alcoholic Liver Disease, Pancreatic Disease, Cardiovascular Disease, Neurological Disorders, and the Effects of Drinking during Pregnancy

Along with Information about Alcohol Treatment, Medications, and Recovery Programs, in Addition to Tips for Reducing the Prevalence of Underage Drinking, Statistics about Alcohol Use, a Glossary of Related Terms, and Directories of Resources for More Help and Information

Edited by Amy L. Sutton. 653 pages. 2006. 978-0-7808-0942-0.

"This title is one of the few reference works on alcoholism for general readers. For some readers this will be a welcome complement to the many self-help books on the market. Recommended for collections serving general readers and consumer health collections."
—*E-Streams, Mar '01*

"This book is an excellent choice for public and academic libraries."
—*American Reference Books Annual, 2001*

"Recommended reference source."
—*Booklist, American Library Association, Dec '00*

"Presents a wealth of information on alcohol use and abuse and its effects on the body and mind, treatment, and prevention." —*SciTech Book News, Dec '00*

"Important new health guide which packs in the latest consumer information about the problems of alcoholism." —*Reviewer's Bookwatch, Nov '00*

SEE ALSO *Drug Abuse Sourcebook*

695

Allergies Sourcebook, 3rd Edition

Basic Consumer Health Information about Allergic Disorders, Such as Anaphylaxis, Hives, Eczema, Rhinitis, Sinusitis, and Conjunctivitis, and Their Triggers, Including Pollen, Mold, Dust Mites, Animal Dander, Insects, Chemicals, Food, Food Additives, and Medications;

Along with Advice about the Diagnosis and Treatment of Allergy Symptoms, a Glossary of Related Terms, a Directory of Resources for Help and Information, and Suggestions for Additional Reading

Edited by Amy L. Sutton. 598 pages. 2007. 978-0-7808-0950-5.

"This book brings a great deal of useful material together.... This is an excellent addition to public and consumer health library collections."

—*American Reference Books Annual, 2003*

"This second edition would be useful to laypersons with little or advanced knowledge of the subject matter. This book would also serve as a resource for nursing and other health care professions students. It would be useful in public, academic, and hospital libraries with consumer health collections." —*E-Streams, Jul '02*

Alternative Medicine Sourcebook

SEE *Complementary & Alternative Medicine Sourcebook*

Alzheimer's Disease Sourcebook, 3rd Edition

Basic Consumer Health Information about Alzheimer's Disease, Other Dementias, and Related Disorders, Including Multi-Infarct Dementia, AIDS Dementia Complex, Dementia with Lewy Bodies, Huntington's Disease, Wernicke-Korsakoff Syndrome (Alcohol-Related Dementia), Delirium, and Confusional States

Along with Information for People Newly Diagnosed with Alzheimer's Disease and Caregivers, Reports Detailing Current Research Efforts in Prevention, Diagnosis, and Treatment, Facts about Long-Term Care Issues, and Listings of Sources for Additional Information

Edited by Karen Bellenir. 645 pages. 2003. 978-0-7808-0666-5.

"This very informative and valuable tool will be a great addition to any library serving consumers, students and health care workers."
—*American Reference Books Annual, 2004*

"This is a valuable resource for people affected by dementias such as Alzheimer's. It is easy to navigate and includes important information and resources."
—*Doody's Review Service, Feb '04*

"Recommended reference source."
—*Booklist, American Library Association, Oct '99*

SEE ALSO *Brain Disorders Sourcebook*

Arthritis Sourcebook, 2nd Edition

Basic Consumer Health Information about Osteoarthritis, Rheumatoid Arthritis, Other Rheumatic Disorders, Infectious Forms of Arthritis, and Diseases with Symptoms Linked to Arthritis, Featuring Facts about Diagnosis, Pain Management, and Surgical Therapies

Along with Coping Strategies, Research Updates, a Glossary, and Resources for Additional Help and Information

Edited by Amy L. Sutton. 593 pages. 2004. 978-0-7808-0667-2.

"This easy-to-read volume is recommended for consumer health collections within public or academic libraries." —*E-Streams, May '05*

"As expected, this updated edition continues the excellent reputation of this series in providing sound, usable health information.... Highly recommended."
—*American Reference Books Annual, 2005*

"Excellent reference." —*The Bookwatch, Jan '05*

Asthma Sourcebook, 2nd Edition

Basic Consumer Health Information about the Causes, Symptoms, Diagnosis, and Treatment of Asthma in Infants, Children, Teenagers, and Adults, Including Facts about Different Types of Asthma, Common Co-Occurring Conditions, Asthma Management Plans, Triggers, Medications, and Medication Delivery Devices

Along with Asthma Statistics, Research Updates, a Glossary, a Directory of Asthma-Related Resources, and More

Edited by Karen Bellenir. 609 pages. 2006. 978-0-7808-0866-9.

"A worthwhile reference acquisition for public libraries and academic medical libraries whose readers desire a quick introduction to the wide range of asthma information." —*Choice, Association of College & Research Libraries, Jun '01*

"Recommended reference source."
—*Booklist, American Library Association, Feb '01*

"Highly recommended." —*The Bookwatch, Jan '01*

"There is much good information for patients and their families who deal with asthma daily."
—*American Medical Writers Association Journal, Winter '01*

"This informative text is recommended for consumer health collections in public, secondary school, and community college libraries and the libraries of universities with a large undergraduate population."
—*American Reference Books Annual, 2001*

Attention Deficit Disorder Sourcebook

Basic Consumer Health Information about Attention Deficit/Hyperactivity Disorder in Children and Adults,

Including Facts about Causes, Symptoms, Diagnostic Criteria, and Treatment Options Such as Medications, Behavior Therapy, Coaching, and Homeopathy

Along with Reports on Current Research Initiatives, Legal Issues, and Government Regulations, and Featuring a Glossary of Related Terms, Internet Resources, and a List of Additional Reading Material

Edited by Dawn D. Matthews. 470 pages. 2002. 978-0-7808-0624-5.

"Recommended reference source."
—*Booklist, American Library Association, Jan '03*

"This book is recommended for all school libraries and the reference or consumer health sections of public libraries." —*American Reference Books Annual, 2003*

Back & Neck Sourcebook, 2nd Edition

Basic Consumer Health Information about Spinal Pain, Spinal Cord Injuries, and Related Disorders, Such as Degenerative Disk Disease, Osteoarthritis, Scoliosis, Sciatica, Spina Bifida, and Spinal Stenosis, and Featuring Facts about Maintaining Spinal Health, Self-Care, Pain Management, Rehabilitative Care, Chiropractic Care, Spinal Surgeries, and Complementary Therapies

Along with Suggestions for Preventing Back and Neck Pain, a Glossary of Related Terms, and a Directory of Resources

Edited by Amy L. Sutton. 633 pages. 2004. 978-0-7808-0738-9.

"Recommended . . . an easy to use, comprehensive medical reference book." —*E-Streams, Sep '05*

"The strength of this work is its basic, easy-to-read format. Recommended." —*Reference and User Services Quarterly, American Library Association, Winter '97*

Blood & Circulatory Disorders Sourcebook, 2nd Edition

Basic Consumer Health Information about the Blood and Circulatory System and Related Disorders, Such as Anemia and Other Hemoglobin Diseases, Cancer of the Blood and Associated Bone Marrow Disorders, Clotting and Bleeding Problems, and Conditions That Affect the Veins, Blood Vessels, and Arteries, Including Facts about the Donation and Transplantation of Bone Marrow, Stem Cells, and Blood and Tips for Keeping the Blood and Circulatory System Healthy

Along with a Glossary of Related Terms and Resources for Additional Help and Information

Edited by Amy L. Sutton. 659 pages. 2005. 978-0-7808-0746-4.

"Highly recommended pick for basic consumer health reference holdings at all levels."
—*The Bookwatch, Aug '05*

"Recommended reference source."
—*Booklist, American Library Association, Feb '99*

"An important reference sourcebook written in simple language for everyday, non-technical users."
—*Reviewer's Bookwatch, Jan '99*

Brain Disorders Sourcebook, 2nd Edition

Basic Consumer Health Information about Acquired and Traumatic Brain Injuries, Infections of the Brain, Epilepsy and Seizure Disorders, Cerebral Palsy, and Degenerative Neurological Disorders, Including Amyotrophic Lateral Sclerosis (ALS), Dementias, Multiple Sclerosis, and More

Along with Information on the Brain's Structure and Function, Treatment and Rehabilitation Options, Reports on Current Research Initiatives, a Glossary of Terms Related to Brain Disorders and Injuries, and a Directory of Sources for Further Help and Information

Edited by Sandra J. Judd. 625 pages. 2005. 978-0-7808-0744-0.

"Highly recommended pick for basic consumer health reference holdings at all levels."
—*The Bookwatch, Aug '05*

"Belongs on the shelves of any library with a consumer health collection." —*E-Streams, Mar '00*

"Recommended reference source."
—*Booklist, American Library Association, Oct '99*

SEE ALSO Alzheimer's Disease Sourcebook

Breast Cancer Sourcebook, 2nd Edition

Basic Consumer Health Information about Breast Cancer, Including Facts about Risk Factors, Prevention, Screening and Diagnostic Methods, Treatment Options, Complementary and Alternative Therapies, Post-Treatment Concerns, Clinical Trials, Special Risk Populations, and New Developments in Breast Cancer Research

Along with Breast Cancer Statistics, a Glossary of Related Terms, and a Directory of Resources for Additional Help and Information

Edited by Sandra J. Judd. 595 pages. 2004. 978-0-7808-0668-9.

"This book will be an excellent addition to public, community college, medical, and academic libraries."
—*American Reference Books Annual, 2006*

"It would be a useful reference book in a library or on loan to women in a support group."
—*Cancer Forum, Mar '03*

"Recommended reference source."
—*Booklist, American Library Association, Jan '02*

"This reference source is highly recommended. It is quite informative, comprehensive and detailed in nature, and yet it offers practical advice in easy-to-read language. It could be thought of as the 'bible' of breast cancer for the consumer." — *E-Streams, Jan '02*

"From the pros and cons of different screening methods and results to treatment options, *Breast Cancer Sourcebook* provides the latest information on the subject."
— *Library Bookwatch, Dec '01*

"This thoroughgoing, very readable reference covers all aspects of breast health and cancer.... Readers will find much to consider here. Recommended for all public and patient health collections."
— *Library Journal, Sep '01*

SEE ALSO Cancer Sourcebook for Women, Women's Health Concerns Sourcebook

Breastfeeding Sourcebook

Basic Consumer Health Information about the Benefits of Breastmilk, Preparing to Breastfeed, Breastfeeding as a Baby Grows, Nutrition, and More, Including Information on Special Situations and Concerns Such as Mastitis, Illness, Medications, Allergies, Multiple Births, Prematurity, Special Needs, and Adoption

Along with a Glossary and Resources for Additional Help and Information

Edited by Jenni Lynn Colson. 388 pages. 2002. 978-0-7808-0332-9.

"Particularly useful is the information about professional lactation services and chapters on breastfeeding when returning to work.... *Breastfeeding Sourcebook* will be useful for public libraries, consumer health libraries, and technical schools offering nurse assistant training, especially in areas where Internet access is problematic."
— *American Reference Books Annual, 2003*

SEE ALSO Pregnancy & Birth Sourcebook

Burns Sourcebook

Basic Consumer Health Information about Various Types of Burns and Scalds, Including Flame, Heat, Cold, Electrical, Chemical, and Sun Burns

Along with Information on Short-Term and Long-Term Treatments, Tissue Reconstruction, Plastic Surgery, Prevention Suggestions, and First Aid

Edited by Allan R. Cook. 604 pages. 1999. 978-0-7808-0204-9.

"This is an exceptional addition to the series and is highly recommended for all consumer health collections, hospital libraries, and academic medical centers."
— *E-Streams, Mar '00*

"This key reference guide is an invaluable addition to all health care and public libraries in confronting this ongoing health issue."
— *American Reference Books Annual, 2000*

"Recommended reference source."
— *Booklist, American Library Association, Dec '99*

SEE ALSO Dermatological Disorders Sourcebook

Cancer Sourcebook, 5th Edition

Basic Consumer Health Information about Major Forms and Stages of Cancer, Featuring Facts about Head and Neck Cancers, Lung Cancers, Gastrointestinal Cancers, Genitourinary Cancers, Lymphomas, Blood Cell Cancers, Endocrine Cancers, Skin Cancers, Bone Cancers, Metastatic Cancers, and More

Along with Facts about Cancer Treatments, Cancer Risks and Prevention, a Glossary of Related Terms, Statistical Data, and a Directory of Resources for Additional Information

Edited by Karen Bellenir. 1,133 pages. 2007. 978-0-7808-0947-5.

"With cancer being the second leading cause of death for Americans, a prodigious work such as this one, which locates centrally so much cancer-related information, is clearly an asset to this nation's citizens and others."
— *Journal of the National Medical Association, 2004*

"This title is recommended for health sciences and public libraries with consumer health collections."
— *E-Streams, Feb '01*

"... can be effectively used by cancer patients and their families who are looking for answers in a language they can understand. Public and hospital libraries should have it on their shelves."
— *American Reference Books Annual, 2001*

"Recommended reference source."
— *Booklist, American Library Association, Dec '00*

SEE ALSO Breast Cancer Sourcebook, Cancer Sourcebook for Women, Pediatric Cancer Sourcebook, Prostate Cancer Sourcebook

Cancer Sourcebook for Women, 3rd Edition

Basic Consumer Health Information about Leading Causes of Cancer in Women, Featuring Facts about Gynecologic Cancers and Related Concerns, Such as Breast Cancer, Cervical Cancer, Endometrial Cancer, Uterine Sarcoma, Vaginal Cancer, Vulvar Cancer, and Common Non-Cancerous Gynecologic Conditions, in Addition to Facts about Lung Cancer, Colorectal Cancer, and Thyroid Cancer in Women

Along with Information about Cancer Risk Factors, Screening and Prevention, Treatment Options, and Tips on Coping with Life after Cancer Treatment, a Glossary of Cancer Terms, and a Directory of Resources for Additional Help and Information

Edited by Amy L. Sutton. 715 pages. 2006. 978-0-7808-0867-6.

"An excellent addition to collections in public, consumer health, and women's health libraries."
— *American Reference Books Annual, 2003*

"Overall, the information is excellent, and complex topics are clearly explained. As a reference book for the consumer it is a valuable resource to assist them to make informed decisions about cancer and its treatments."
— *Cancer Forum, Nov '02*

"Highly recommended for academic and medical reference collections."
— *Library Bookwatch, Sep '02*

"This is a highly recommended book for any public or consumer library, being reader friendly and containing accurate and helpful information."
— *E-Streams, Aug '02*

"Recommended reference source."
— *Booklist, American Library Association, Jul '02*

SEE ALSO Breast Cancer Sourcebook, Women's Health Concerns Sourcebook

Cancer Survivorship Sourcebook

Basic Consumer Health Information about the Physical, Educational, Emotional, Social, and Financial Needs of Cancer Patients from Diagnosis, through Cancer Treatment, and Beyond, Including Facts about Researching Specific Types of Cancer and Learning about Clinical Trials and Treatment Options, and Featuring Tips for Coping with the Side Effects of Cancer Treatments and Adjusting to Life after Cancer Treatment Concludes

Along with Suggestions for Caregivers, Friends, and Family Members of Cancer Patients, a Glossary of Cancer Care Terms, and Directories of Related Resources

Edited by Karen Bellenir. 6561 pages. 2007. 978-0-7808-0985-7.

Cardiovascular Diseases & Disorders Sourcebook, 3rd Edition

Basic Consumer Health Information about Heart and Vascular Diseases and Disorders, Such as Angina, Heart Attacks, Arrhythmias, Cardiomyopathy, Valve Disease, Atherosclerosis, and Aneurysms, with Information about Managing Cardiovascular Risk Factors and Maintaining Heart Health, Medications and Procedures Used to Treat Cardiovascular Disorders, and Concerns of Special Significance to Women

Along with Reports on Current Research Initiatives, a Glossary of Related Medical Terms, and a Directory of Sources for Further Help and Information

Edited by Sandra J. Judd. 713 pages. 2005. 978-0-7808-0739-6.

"This updated sourcebook is still the best first stop for comprehensive introductory information on cardiovascular diseases."
— *American Reference Books Annual, 2006*

"Recommended for public libraries and libraries supporting health care professionals."
— *E-Streams, Sep '05*

"This should be a standard health library reference."
— *The Bookwatch, Jun '05*

"Recommended reference source."
— *Booklist, American Library Association, Dec '00*

". . . comprehensive format provides an extensive overview on this subject."
— *Choice, Association of College & Research Libraries*

Caregiving Sourcebook

Basic Consumer Health Information for Caregivers, Including a Profile of Caregivers, Caregiving Responsibilities and Concerns, Tips for Specific Conditions, Care Environments, and the Effects of Caregiving

Along with Facts about Legal Issues, Financial Information, and Future Planning, a Glossary, and a Listing of Additional Resources

Edited by Joyce Brennfleck Shannon. 600 pages. 2001. 978-0-7808-0331-2.

"Essential for most collections."
— *Library Journal, Apr 1, 2002*

"An ideal addition to the reference collection of any public library. Health sciences information professionals may also want to acquire the Caregiving Sourcebook for their hospital or academic library for use as a ready reference tool by health care workers interested in aging and caregiving." — *E-Streams, Jan '02*

"Recommended reference source."
— *Booklist, American Library Association, Oct '01*

Child Abuse Sourcebook

Basic Consumer Health Information about the Physical, Sexual, and Emotional Abuse of Children, with Additional Facts about Neglect, Munchausen Syndrome by Proxy (MSBP), Shaken Baby Syndrome, and Controversial Issues Related to Child Abuse, Such as Withholding Medical Care, Corporal Punishment, and Child Maltreatment in Youth Sports, and Featuring Facts about Child Protective Services, Foster Care, Adoption, Parenting Challenges, and Other Abuse Prevention Efforts

Along with a Glossary of Related Terms and Resources for Additional Help and Information

Edited by Dawn D. Matthews. 620 pages. 2004. 978-0-7808-0705-1.

"A valuable and highly recommended resource for school, academic and public libraries whether used on its own or as a starting point for more in-depth research."
— *E-Streams, Apr '05*

"Every week the news brings cases of child abuse or neglect, so it is useful to have a source that supplies so much helpful information. . . . Recommended. Public and academic libraries, and child welfare offices."
— *Choice, Association of College & Research Libraries, Mar '05*

"Packed with insights on all kinds of issues, from foster care and adoption to parenting and abuse prevention."
— *The Bookwatch, Nov '04*

SEE ALSO: Domestic Violence Sourcebook

Childhood Diseases & Disorders Sourcebook

Basic Consumer Health Information about Medical Problems Often Encountered in Pre-Adolescent Children, Including Respiratory Tract Ailments, Ear Infections, Sore Throats, Disorders of the Skin and Scalp, Digestive and Genitourinary Diseases, Infectious Diseases, Inflammatory Disorders, Chronic Physical and Developmental Disorders, Allergies, and More

Along with Information about Diagnostic Tests, Common Childhood Surgeries, and Frequently Used Medications, with a Glossary of Important Terms and Resource Directory

Edited by Chad T. Kimball. 662 pages. 2003. 978-0-7808-0458-6.

"This is an excellent book for new parents and should be included in all health care and public libraries."
—American Reference Books Annual, 2004

SEE ALSO: Healthy Children Sourcebook

Colds, Flu & Other Common Ailments Sourcebook

Basic Consumer Health Information about Common Ailments and Injuries, Including Colds, Coughs, the Flu, Sinus Problems, Headaches, Fever, Nausea and Vomiting, Menstrual Cramps, Diarrhea, Constipation, Hemorrhoids, Back Pain, Dandruff, Dry and Itchy Skin, Cuts, Scrapes, Sprains, Bruises, and More

Along with Information about Prevention, Self-Care, Choosing a Doctor, Over-the-Counter Medications, Folk Remedies, and Alternative Therapies, and Including a Glossary of Important Terms and a Directory of Resources for Further Help and Information

Edited by Chad T. Kimball. 638 pages. 2001. 978-0-7808-0435-7.

"A good starting point for research on common illnesses. It will be a useful addition to public and consumer health library collections."
—American Reference Books Annual, 2002

"Will prove valuable to any library seeking to maintain a current, comprehensive reference collection of health resources. . . . Excellent reference."
—The Bookwatch, Aug '01

"Recommended reference source."
—Booklist, American Library Association, Jul '01

Communication Disorders Sourcebook

Basic Information about Deafness and Hearing Loss, Speech and Language Disorders, Voice Disorders, Balance and Vestibular Disorders, and Disorders of Smell, Taste, and Touch

Edited by Linda M. Ross. 533 pages. 1996. 978-0-7808-0077-9.

"This is skillfully edited and is a welcome resource for the layperson. It should be found in every public and medical library." —Booklist Health Sciences Supplement, American Library Association, Oct '97

Complementary & Alternative Medicine Sourcebook, 3rd Edition

Basic Consumer Health Information about Complementary and Alternative Medical Therapies, Including Acupuncture, Ayurveda, Traditional Chinese Medicine, Herbal Medicine, Homeopathy, Naturopathy, Biofeedback, Hypnotherapy, Yoga, Art Therapy, Aromatherapy, Clinical Nutrition, Vitamin and Mineral Supplements, Chiropractic, Massage, Reflexology, Crystal Therapy, Therapeutic Touch, and More

Along with Facts about Alternative and Complementary Treatments for Specific Conditions Such as Cancer, Diabetes, Osteoarthritis, Chronic Pain, Menopause, Gastrointestinal Disorders, Headaches, and Mental Illness, a Glossary, and a Resource List for Additional Help and Information

Edited by Sandra J. Judd. 657 pages. 2006. 978-0-7808-0864-5.

"Recommended for public, high school, and academic libraries that have consumer health collections. Hospital libraries that also serve the public will find this to be a useful resource." —E-Streams, Feb '03

"Recommended reference source."
—Booklist, American Library Association, Jan '03

"An important alternate health reference."
—MBR Bookwatch, Oct '02

"A great addition to the reference collection of every type of library." —American Reference Books Annual, 2000

Congenital Disorders Sourcebook, 2nd Edition

Basic Consumer Health Information about Nonhereditary Birth Defects and Disorders Related to Prematurity, Gestational Injuries, Congenital Infections, and Birth Complications, Including Heart Defects, Hydrocephalus, Spina Bifida, Cleft Lip and Palate, Cerebral Palsy, and More

Along with Facts about the Prevention of Birth Defects, Fetal Surgery and Other Treatment Options, Research Initiatives, a Glossary of Related Terms, and Resources for Additional Information and Support

Edited by Sandra J. Judd. 647 pages. 2006. 978-0-7808-0945-1.

"Recommended reference source."
—Booklist, American Library Association, Oct '97

SEE ALSO Pregnancy & Birth Sourcebook

Contagious Diseases Sourcebook

Basic Consumer Health Information about Infectious Diseases Spread by Person-to-Person Contact through

Direct Touch, Airborne Transmission, Sexual Contact, or Contact with Blood or Other Body Fluids, Including Hepatitis, Herpes, Influenza, Lice, Measles, Mumps, Pinworm, Ringworm, Severe Acute Respiratory Syndrome (SARS), Streptococcal Infections, Tuberculosis, and Others

Along with Facts about Disease Transmission, Antimicrobial Resistance, and Vaccines, with a Glossary and Directories of Resources for More Information

Edited by Karen Bellenir. 643 pages. 2004. 978-0-7808-0736-5.

"This easy-to-read volume is recommended for consumer health collections within public or academic libraries." — E-Streams, May '05

"This informative book is highly recommended for public libraries, consumer health collections, and secondary schools and undergraduate libraries."
— American Reference Books Annual, 2005

"Excellent reference." — The Bookwatch, Jan '05

Death & Dying Sourcebook, 2nd Edition

Basic Consumer Health Information about End-of-Life Care and Related Perspectives and Ethical Issues, Including End-of-Life Symptoms and Treatments, Pain Management, Quality-of-Life Concerns, the Use of Life Support, Patients' Rights and Privacy Issues, Advance Directives, Physician-Assisted Suicide, Caregiving, Organ and Tissue Donation, Autopsies, Funeral Arrangements, and Grief

Along with Statistical Data, Information about the Leading Causes of Death, a Glossary, and Directories of Support Groups and Other Resources

Edited by Joyce Brennfleck Shannon. 653 pages. 2006. 978-0-7808-0871-3.

"Public libraries, medical libraries, and academic libraries will all find this sourcebook a useful addition to their collections."
— American Reference Books Annual, 2001

"An extremely useful resource for those concerned with death and dying in the United States."
— Respiratory Care, Nov '00

"Recommended reference source."
— Booklist, American Library Association, Aug '00

"This book is a definite must for all those involved in end-of-life care." — Doody's Review Service, 2000

Dental Care & Oral Health Sourcebook, 2nd Edition

Basic Consumer Health Information about Dental Care, Including Oral Hygiene, Dental Visits, Pain Management, Cavities, Crowns, Bridges, Dental Implants, and Fillings, and Other Oral Health Concerns, Such as Gum Disease, Bad Breath, Dry Mouth, Genetic and Developmental Abnormalities, Oral Cancers, Orthodontics, and Temporomandibular Disorders

Along with Updates on Current Research in Oral Health, a Glossary, a Directory of Dental and Oral Health Organizations, and Resources for People with Dental and Oral Health Disorders

Edited by Amy L. Sutton. 609 pages. 2003. 978-0-7808-0634-4.

"This book could serve as a turning point in the battle to educate consumers in issues concerning oral health."
— American Reference Books Annual, 2004

"Unique source which will fill a gap in dental sources for patients and the lay public. A valuable reference tool even in a library with thousands of books on dentistry. Comprehensive, clear, inexpensive, and easy to read and use. It fills an enormous gap in the health care literature." — Reference & User Services Quarterly, American Library Association, Summer '98

"Recommended reference source."
— Booklist, American Library Association, Dec '97

Depression Sourcebook

Basic Consumer Health Information about Unipolar Depression, Bipolar Disorder, Postpartum Depression, Seasonal Affective Disorder, and Other Types of Depression in Children, Adolescents, Women, Men, the Elderly, and Other Selected Populations

Along with Facts about Causes, Risk Factors, Diagnostic Criteria, Treatment Options, Coping Strategies, Suicide Prevention, a Glossary, and a Directory of Sources for Additional Help and Information

Edited by Karen Bellenir. 602 pages. 2002. 978-0-7808-0611-5.

"*Depression Sourcebook* is of a very high standard. Its purpose, which is to serve as a reference source to the lay reader, is very well served."
— Journal of the National Medical Association, 2004

"Invaluable reference for public and school library collections alike." — Library Bookwatch, Apr '03

"Recommended for purchase."
— American Reference Books Annual, 2003

Dermatological Disorders Sourcebook, 2nd Edition

Basic Consumer Health Information about Conditions and Disorders Affecting the Skin, Hair, and Nails, Such as Acne, Rosacea, Rashes, Dermatitis, Pigmentation Disorders, Birthmarks, Skin Cancer, Skin Injuries, Psoriasis, Scleroderma, and Hair Loss, Including Facts about Medications and Treatments for Dermatological Disorders and Tips for Maintaining Healthy Skin, Hair, and Nails

Along with Information about How Aging Affects the Skin, a Glossary of Related Terms, and a Directory of Resources for Additional Help and Information

Edited by Amy L. Sutton. 645 pages. 2005. 978-0-7808-0795-2.

"... comprehensive, easily read reference book."
—Doody's Health Sciences Book Reviews, Oct '97

SEE ALSO Burns Sourcebook

Diabetes Sourcebook, 3rd Edition

Basic Consumer Health Information about Type 1 Diabetes (Insulin-Dependent or Juvenile-Onset Diabetes), Type 2 Diabetes (Noninsulin-Dependent or Adult-Onset Diabetes), Gestational Diabetes, Impaired Glucose Tolerance (IGT), and Related Complications, Such as Amputation, Eye Disease, Gum Disease, Nerve Damage, and End-Stage Renal Disease, Including Facts about Insulin, Oral Diabetes Medications, Blood Sugar Testing, and the Role of Exercise and Nutrition in the Control of Diabetes

Along with a Glossary and Resources for Further Help and Information

Edited by Dawn D. Matthews. 622 pages. 2003. 978-0-7808-0629-0.

"This edition is even more helpful than earlier versions. . . . It is a truly valuable tool for anyone seeking readable and authoritative information on diabetes."
— American Reference Books Annual, 2004

"An invaluable reference." — Library Journal, May '00

Selected as one of the 250 "Best Health Sciences Books of 1999." — Doody's Rating Service, Mar-Apr '00

"Provides useful information for the general public."
— Healthlines, University of Michigan Health Management Research Center, Sep/Oct '99

". . . provides reliable mainstream medical information . . . belongs on the shelves of any library with a consumer health collection." — E-Streams, Sep '99

"Recommended reference source."
— Booklist, American Library Association, Feb '99

Diet & Nutrition Sourcebook, 3rd Edition

Basic Consumer Health Information about Dietary Guidelines and the Food Guidance System, Recommended Daily Nutrient Intakes, Serving Proportions, Weight Control, Vitamins and Supplements, Nutrition Issues for Different Life Stages and Lifestyles, and the Needs of People with Specific Medical Concerns, Including Cancer, Celiac Disease, Diabetes, Eating Disorders, Food Allergies, and Cardiovascular Disease

Along with Facts about Federal Nutrition Support Programs, a Glossary of Nutrition and Dietary Terms, and Directories of Additional Resources for More Information about Nutrition

Edited by Joyce Brennfleck Shannon. 633 pages. 2006. 978-0-7808-0800-3.

"This book is an excellent source of basic diet and nutrition information." — Booklist Health Sciences Supplement, American Library Association, Dec '00

"This reference document should be in any public library, but it would be a very good guide for beginning students in the health sciences. If the other books in this publisher's series are as good as this, they should all be in the health sciences collections."
—American Reference Books Annual, 2000

"This book is an excellent general nutrition reference for consumers who desire to take an active role in their health care for prevention. Consumers of all ages who select this book can feel confident they are receiving current and accurate information." —Journal of Nutrition for the Elderly, Vol. 19, No. 4, 2000

SEE ALSO Digestive Diseases & Disorders Sourcebook, Eating Disorders Sourcebook, Gastrointestinal Diseases & Disorders Sourcebook, Vegetarian Sourcebook

Digestive Diseases & Disorders Sourcebook

Basic Consumer Health Information about Diseases and Disorders that Impact the Upper and Lower Digestive System, Including Celiac Disease, Constipation, Crohn's Disease, Cyclic Vomiting Syndrome, Diarrhea, Diverticulosis and Diverticulitis, Gallstones, Heartburn, Hemorrhoids, Hernias, Indigestion (Dyspepsia), Irritable Bowel Syndrome, Lactose Intolerance, Ulcers, and More

Along with Information about Medications and Other Treatments, Tips for Maintaining a Healthy Digestive Tract, a Glossary, and Directory of Digestive Diseases Organizations

Edited by Karen Bellenir. 335 pages. 2000. 978-0-7808-0327-5.

"This title would be an excellent addition to all public or patient-research libraries."
— American Reference Books Annual, 2001

"This title is recommended for public, hospital, and health sciences libraries with consumer health collections." — E-Streams, Jul-Aug '00

"Recommended reference source."
— Booklist, American Library Association, May '00

SEE ALSO Eating Disorders Sourcebook, Gastrointestinal Diseases & Disorders Sourcebook

Disabilities Sourcebook

Basic Consumer Health Information about Physical and Psychiatric Disabilities, Including Descriptions of Major Causes of Disability, Assistive and Adaptive Aids, Workplace Issues, and Accessibility Concerns

Along with Information about the Americans with Disabilities Act, a Glossary, and Resources for Additional Help and Information

Edited by Dawn D. Matthews. 616 pages. 2000. 978-0-7808-0389-3.

"It is a must for libraries with a consumer health section." — American Reference Books Annual, 2002

"A much needed addition to the Omnigraphics *Health Reference Series*. A current reference work to provide people with disabilities, their families, caregivers or those who work with them, a broad range of information in one volume, has not been available until now. . . . It is recommended for all public and academic library reference collections." —*E-Streams, May '01*

"An excellent source book in easy-to-read format covering many current topics; highly recommended for all libraries." —*Choice, Association of College & Research Libraries, Jan '01*

"Recommended reference source."
—*Booklist, American Library Association, Jul '00*

Domestic Violence Sourcebook, 2nd Edition

Basic Consumer Health Information about the Causes and Consequences of Abusive Relationships, Including Physical Violence, Sexual Assault, Battery, Stalking, and Emotional Abuse, and Facts about the Effects of Violence on Women, Men, Young Adults, and the Elderly, with Reports about Domestic Violence in Selected Populations, and Featuring Facts about Medical Care, Victim Assistance and Protection, Prevention Strategies, Mental Health Services, and Legal Issues

Along with a Glossary of Related Terms and Resources for Additional Help and Information

Edited by Dawn D. Matthews. 628 pages. 2004. 978-0-7808-0669-6.

"Educators, clergy, medical professionals, police, and victims and their families will benefit from this realistic and easy-to-understand resource."
—*American Reference Books Annual, 2005*

"Recommended for all collections supporting consumer health information. It should also be considered for any collection needing general, readable information on domestic violence." —*E-Streams, Jan '05*

"This sourcebook complements other books in its field, providing a one-stop resource . . . Recommended."
—*Choice, Association of College & Research Libraries, Jan '05*

"Interested lay persons should find the book extremely beneficial. . . . A copy of *Domestic Violence and Child Abuse Sourcebook* should be in every public library in the United States."
—*Social Science & Medicine, No. 56, 2003*

"This is important information. The Web has many resources but this sourcebook fills an important societal need. I am not aware of any other resources of this type." —*Doody's Review Service, Sep '01*

"Recommended reference source."
—*Booklist, American Library Association, Apr '01*

"Important pick for college-level health reference libraries." —*The Bookwatch, Mar '01*

"Because this problem is so widespread and because this book includes a lot of issues within one volume, this work is recommended for all public libraries."
—*American Reference Books Annual, 2001*

SEE ALSO Child Abuse Sourcebook

Drug Abuse Sourcebook, 2nd Edition

Basic Consumer Health Information about Illicit Substances of Abuse and the Misuse of Prescription and Over-the-Counter Medications, Including Depressants, Hallucinogens, Inhalants, Marijuana, Stimulants, and Anabolic Steroids

Along with Facts about Related Health Risks, Treatment Programs, Prevention Programs, a Glossary of Abuse and Addiction Terms, a Glossary of Drug-Related Street Terms, and a Directory of Resources for More Information

Edited by Catherine Ginther. 607 pages. 2004. 978-0-7808-0740-2.

"Commendable for organizing useful, normally scattered government and association-produced data into a logical sequence."
—*American Reference Books Annual, 2006*

"This easy-to-read volume is recommended for consumer health collections within public or academic libraries." —*E-Streams, Sep '05*

"An excellent library reference."
—*The Bookwatch, May '05*

"Containing a wealth of information, this book will be useful to the college student just beginning to explore the topic of substance abuse. This resource belongs in libraries that serve a lower-division undergraduate or community college clientele as well as the general public." — *Choice, Association of College & Research Libraries, Jun '01*

"Recommended reference source."
—*Booklist, American Library Association, Feb '01*

SEE ALSO Alcoholism Sourcebook

Ear, Nose & Throat Disorders Sourcebook, 2nd Edition

Basic Consumer Health Information about Disorders of the Ears, Hearing Loss, Vestibular Disorders, Nasal and Sinus Problems, Throat and Vocal Cord Disorders, and Otolaryngologic Cancers, Including Facts about Ear Infections and Injuries, Genetic and Congenital Deafness, Sensorineural Hearing Disorders, Tinnitus, Vertigo, Ménière Disease, Rhinitis, Sinusitis, Snoring, Sore Throats, Hoarseness, and More

Along with Reports on Current Research Initiatives, a Glossary of Related Medical Terms, and a Directory of Sources for Further Help and Information

Edited by Sandra J. Judd. 659 pages. 2006. 978-0-7808-0872-0.

"Overall, this sourcebook is helpful for the consumer seeking information on ENT issues. It is recommended for public libraries."
—American Reference Books Annual, 1999

"Recommended reference source."
—Booklist, American Library Association, Dec '98

Eating Disorders Sourcebook, 2nd Edition

Basic Consumer Health Information about Anorexia Nervosa, Bulimia Nervosa, Binge Eating, Compulsive Exercise, Female Athlete Triad, and Other Eating Disorders, Including Facts about Body Image and Other Cultural and Age-Related Risk Factors, Prevention Efforts, Adverse Health Effects, Treatment Options, and the Recovery Process

Along with Guidelines for Healthy Weight Control, a Glossary, and Directories of Additional Resources

Edited by Joyce Brennfleck Shannon. 585 pages. 2007. 978-0-7808-0948-2.

"Recommended for health science libraries that are open to the public, as well as hospital libraries. This book is a good resource for the consumer who is concerned about eating disorders." —E-Streams, Mar '02

"This volume is another convenient collection of excerpted articles. Recommended for school and public library patrons; lower-division undergraduates; and two-year technical program students."
—Choice, Association of College & Research Libraries, Jan '02

"Recommended reference source."
—Booklist, American Library Association, Oct '01

SEE ALSO Diet & Nutrition Sourcebook, Digestive Diseases & Disorders Sourcebook, Gastrointestinal Diseases & Disorders Sourcebook

Emergency Medical Services Sourcebook

Basic Consumer Health Information about Preventing, Preparing for, and Managing Emergency Situations, When and Who to Call for Help, What to Expect in the Emergency Room, the Emergency Medical Team, Patient Issues, and Current Topics in Emergency Medicine

Along with Statistical Data, a Glossary, and Sources of Additional Help and Information

Edited by Jenni Lynn Colson. 494 pages. 2002. 978-0-7808-0420-3.

"Handy and convenient for home, public, school, and college libraries. Recommended."
—Choice, Association of College & Research Libraries, Apr '03

"This reference can provide the consumer with answers to most questions about emergency care in the United States, or it will direct them to a resource where the answer can be found."
—American Reference Books Annual, 2003

"Recommended reference source."
—Booklist, American Library Association, Feb '03

Endocrine & Metabolic Disorders Sourcebook

Basic Information for the Layperson about Pancreatic and Insulin-Related Disorders Such as Pancreatitis, Diabetes, and Hypoglycemia; Adrenal Gland Disorders Such as Cushing's Syndrome, Addison's Disease, and Congenital Adrenal Hyperplasia; Pituitary Gland Disorders Such as Growth Hormone Deficiency, Acromegaly, and Pituitary Tumors; Thyroid Disorders Such as Hypothyroidism, Graves' Disease, Hashimoto's Disease, and Goiter; Hyperparathyroidism; and Other Diseases and Syndromes of Hormone Imbalance or Metabolic Dysfunction

Along with Reports on Current Research Initiatives

Edited by Linda M. Shin. 574 pages. 1998. 978-0-7808-0207-0.

"Omnigraphics has produced another needed resource for health information consumers."
—American Reference Books Annual, 2000

"Recommended reference source."
—Booklist, American Library Association, Dec '98

Environmental Health Sourcebook, 2nd Edition

Basic Consumer Health Information about the Environment and Its Effect on Human Health, Including the Effects of Air Pollution, Water Pollution, Hazardous Chemicals, Food Hazards, Radiation Hazards, Biological Agents, Household Hazards, Such as Radon, Asbestos, Carbon Monoxide, and Mold, and Information about Associated Diseases and Disorders, Including Cancer, Allergies, Respiratory Problems, and Skin Disorders

Along with Information about Environmental Concerns for Specific Populations, a Glossary of Related Terms, and Resources for Further Help and Information

Edited by Dawn D. Matthews. 673 pages. 2003. 978-0-7808-0632-0.

"This recently updated edition continues the level of quality and the reputation of the numerous other volumes in Omnigraphics' **Health Reference Series**."
—American Reference Books Annual, 2004

"An excellent updated edition."
—The Bookwatch, Oct '03

"Recommended reference source."
—Booklist, American Library Association, Sep '98

"This book will be a useful addition to anyone's library." —Choice Health Sciences Supplement, Association of College & Research Libraries, May '98

". . . a good survey of numerous environmentally induced physical disorders . . . a useful addition to anyone's library."
—Doody's Health Sciences Book Reviews, Jan '98

Ethnic Diseases Sourcebook

Basic Consumer Health Information for Ethnic and Racial Minority Groups in the United States, Including General Health Indicators and Behaviors, Ethnic Diseases, Genetic Testing, the Impact of Chronic Diseases, Women's Health, Mental Health Issues, and Preventive Health Care Services

Along with a Glossary and a Listing of Additional Resources

Edited by Joyce Brennfleck Shannon. 664 pages. 2001. 978-0-7808-0336-7.

"Recommended for health sciences libraries where public health programs are a priority."
— *E-Streams, Jan '02*

"Not many books have been written on this topic to date, and the *Ethnic Diseases Sourcebook* is a strong addition to the list. It will be an important introductory resource for health consumers, students, health care personnel, and social scientists. It is recommended for public, academic, and large hospital libraries."
— *American Reference Books Annual, 2002*

"Recommended reference source."
— *Booklist, American Library Association, Oct '01*

"Will prove valuable to any library seeking to maintain a current, comprehensive reference collection of health resources. . . . An excellent source of health information about genetic disorders which affect particular ethnic and racial minorities in the U.S."
— *The Bookwatch, Aug '01*

Eye Care Sourcebook, 2nd Edition

Basic Consumer Health Information about Eye Care and Eye Disorders, Including Facts about the Diagnosis, Prevention, and Treatment of Common Refractive Problems Such as Myopia, Hyperopia, Astigmatism, and Presbyopia, and Eye Diseases, Including Glaucoma, Cataract, Age-Related Macular Degeneration, and Diabetic Retinopathy

Along with a Section on Vision Correction and Refractive Surgeries, Including LASIK and LASEK, a Glossary, and Directories of Resources for Additional Help and Information

Edited by Amy L. Sutton. 543 pages. 2003. 978-0-7808-0635-1.

". . . a solid reference tool for eye care and a valuable addition to a collection."
— *American Reference Books Annual, 2004*

Family Planning Sourcebook

Basic Consumer Health Information about Planning for Pregnancy and Contraception, Including Traditional Methods, Barrier Methods, Hormonal Methods, Permanent Methods, Future Methods, Emergency Contraception, and Birth Control Choices for Women at Each Stage of Life

Along with Statistics, a Glossary, and Sources of Additional Information

Edited by Amy Marcaccio Keyzer. 520 pages. 2001. 978-0-7808-0379-4.

"Recommended for public, health, and undergraduate libraries as part of the circulating collection."
— *E-Streams, Mar '02*

"Information is presented in an unbiased, readable manner, and the sourcebook will certainly be a necessary addition to those public and high school libraries where Internet access is restricted or otherwise problematic." — *American Reference Books Annual, 2002*

"Recommended reference source."
— *Booklist, American Library Association, Oct '01*

"Will prove valuable to any library seeking to maintain a current, comprehensive reference collection of health resources. . . . Excellent reference."
— *The Bookwatch, Aug '01*

SEE ALSO *Pregnancy & Birth Sourcebook*

Fitness & Exercise Sourcebook, 3rd Edition

Basic Consumer Health Information about the Physical and Mental Benefits of Fitness, Including Cardiorespiratory Endurance, Muscular Strength, Muscular Endurance, and Flexibility, with Facts about Sports Nutrition and Exercise-Related Injuries and Tips about Physical Activity and Exercises for People of All Ages and for People with Health Concerns

Along with Advice on Selecting and Using Exercise Equipment, Maintaining Exercise Motivation, a Glossary of Related Terms, and a Directory of Resources for More Help and Information

Edited by Amy L. Sutton. 663 pages. 2007. 978-0-7808-0946-8.

"This work is recommended for all general reference collections."
— *American Reference Books Annual, 2002*

"Highly recommended for public, consumer, and school grades fourth through college." — *E-Streams, Nov '01*

"Recommended reference source."
— *Booklist, American Library Association, Oct '01*

"The information appears quite comprehensive and is considered reliable. . . . This second edition is a welcomed addition to the series."
— *Doody's Review Service, Sep '01*

Food Safety Sourcebook

Basic Consumer Health Information about the Safe Handling of Meat, Poultry, Seafood, Eggs, Fruit Juices, and Other Food Items, and Facts about Pesticides, Drinking Water, Food Safety Overseas, and the Onset, Duration, and Symptoms of Foodborne Illnesses, Including Types of Pathogenic Bacteria, Parasitic Protozoa, Worms, Viruses, and Natural Toxins

Along with the Role of the Consumer, the Food Handler, and the Government in Food Safety; a Glossary, and Resources for Additional Help and Information

Edited by Dawn D. Matthews. 339 pages. 1999. 978-0-7808-0326-8.

"This book is recommended for public libraries and universities with home economic and food science programs."
— *E-Streams, Nov '00*

"Recommended reference source."
— *Booklist, American Library Association, May '00*

"This book takes the complex issues of food safety and foodborne pathogens and presents them in an easily understood manner. [It does] an excellent job of covering a large and often confusing topic."
— *American Reference Books Annual, 2000*

Forensic Medicine Sourcebook

Basic Consumer Information for the Layperson about Forensic Medicine, Including Crime Scene Investigation, Evidence Collection and Analysis, Expert Testimony, Computer-Aided Criminal Identification, Digital Imaging in the Courtroom, DNA Profiling, Accident Reconstruction, Autopsies, Ballistics, Drugs and Explosives Detection, Latent Fingerprints, Product Tampering, and Questioned Document Examination

Along with Statistical Data, a Glossary of Forensics Terminology, and Listings of Sources for Further Help and Information

Edited by Annemarie S. Muth. 574 pages. 1999. 978-0-7808-0232-2.

"Given the expected widespread interest in its content and its easy to read style, this book is recommended for most public and all college and university libraries."
— *E-Streams, Feb '01*

"Recommended for public libraries."
— *Reference & User Services Quarterly, American Library Association, Spring 2000*

"Recommended reference source."
— *Booklist, American Library Association, Feb '00*

"A wealth of information, useful statistics, references are up-to-date and extremely complete. This wonderful collection of data will help students who are interested in a career in any type of forensic field. It is a great resource for attorneys who need information about types of expert witnesses needed in a particular case. It also offers useful information for fiction and nonfiction writers whose work involves a crime. A fascinating compilation. All levels."
— *Choice, Association of College & Research Libraries, Jan '00*

"There are several items that make this book attractive to consumers who are seeking certain forensic data.... This is a useful current source for those seeking general forensic medical answers."
— *American Reference Books Annual, 2000*

Gastrointestinal Diseases & Disorders Sourcebook, 2nd Edition

Basic Consumer Health Information about the Upper and Lower Gastrointestinal (GI) Tract, Including the Esophagus, Stomach, Intestines, Rectum, Liver, and Pancreas, with Facts about Gastroesophageal Reflux Disease, Gastritis, Hernias, Ulcers, Celiac Disease, Diverticulitis, Irritable Bowel Syndrome, Hemorrhoids, Gastrointestinal Cancers, and Other Diseases and Disorders Related to the Digestive Process

Along with Information about Commonly Used Diagnostic and Surgical Procedures, Statistics, Reports on Current Research Initiatives and Clinical Trials, a Glossary, and Resources for Additional Help and Information

Edited by Sandra J. Judd. 681 pages. 2006. 978-0-7808-0798-3.

"... very readable form. The successful editorial work that brought this material together into a useful and understandable reference makes accessible to all readers information that can help them more effectively understand and obtain help for digestive tract problems."
— *Choice, Association of College & Research Libraries, Feb '97*

SEE ALSO *Diet & Nutrition Sourcebook, Digestive Diseases & Disorders Sourcebook, Eating Disorders Sourcebook*

Genetic Disorders Sourcebook, 3rd Edition

Basic Consumer Health Information about Hereditary Diseases and Disorders, Including Facts about the Human Genome, Genetic Inheritance Patterns, Disorders Associated with Specific Genes, Such as Sickle Cell Disease, Hemophilia, and Cystic Fibrosis, Chromosome Disorders, Such as Down Syndrome, Fragile X Syndrome, and Turner Syndrome, and Complex Diseases and Disorders Resulting from the Interaction of Environmental and Genetic Factors, Such as Allergies, Cancer, and Obesity

Along with Facts about Genetic Testing, Suggestions for Parents of Children with Special Needs, Reports on Current Research Initiatives, a Glossary of Genetic Terminology, and Resources for Additional Help and Information

Edited by Karen Bellenir. 777 pages. 2004. 978-0-7808-0742-6.

"This text is recommended for any library with an interest in providing consumer health resources."
— *E-Streams, Aug '05*

"This is a valuable resource for anyone wishing to have an understandable description of any of the topics or disorders included. The editor succeeds in making complex genetic issues understandable."
— *Doody's Book Review Service, May '05*

"A good acquisition for public libraries."
— *American Reference Books Annual, 2005*

"Excellent reference." —*The Bookwatch, Jan '05*

"Recommended reference source."
—*Booklist, American Library Association, Apr '01*

"Important pick for college-level health reference libraries." —*The Bookwatch, Mar '01*

Head Trauma Sourcebook

Basic Information for the Layperson about Open-Head and Closed-Head Injuries, Treatment Advances, Recovery, and Rehabilitation

Along with Reports on Current Research Initiatives

Edited by Karen Bellenir. 414 pages. 1997. 978-0-7808-0208-7.

Headache Sourcebook

Basic Consumer Health Information about Migraine, Tension, Cluster, Rebound and Other Types of Headaches, with Facts about the Cause and Prevention of Headaches, the Effects of Stress and the Environment, Headaches during Pregnancy and Menopause, and Childhood Headaches

Along with a Glossary and Other Resources for Additional Help and Information

Edited by Dawn D. Matthews. 362 pages. 2002. 978-0-7808-0337-4.

"Highly recommended for academic and medical reference collections." —*Library Bookwatch, Sep '02*

Healthy Aging Sourcebook

Basic Consumer Health Information about Maintaining Health through the Aging Process, Including Advice on Nutrition, Exercise, and Sleep, Help in Making Decisions about Midlife Issues and Retirement, and Guidance Concerning Practical and Informed Choices in Health Consumerism

Along with Data Concerning the Theories of Aging, Different Experiences in Aging by Minority Groups, and Facts about Aging Now and Aging in the Future; and Featuring a Glossary, a Guide to Consumer Help, Additional Suggested Reading, and Practical Resource Directory

Edited by Jenifer Swanson. 536 pages. 1999. 978-0-7808-0390-9.

"Recommended reference source."
—*Booklist, American Library Association, Feb '00*

SEE ALSO *Physical & Mental Issues in Aging Sourcebook*

Healthy Children Sourcebook

Basic Consumer Health Information about the Physical and Mental Development of Children between the Ages of 3 and 12, Including Routine Health Care, Preventative Health Services, Safety and First Aid,

Healthy Sleep, Dental Care, Nutrition, and Fitness, and Featuring Parenting Tips on Such Topics as Bedwetting, Choosing Day Care, Monitoring TV and Other Media, and Establishing a Foundation for Substance Abuse Prevention

Along with a Glossary of Commonly Used Pediatric Terms and Resources for Additional Help and Information

Edited by Chad T. Kimball. 647 pages. 2003. 978-0-7808-0247-6.

"It is hard to imagine that any other single resource exists that would provide such a comprehensive guide of timely information on health promotion and disease prevention for children aged 3 to 12."
—*American Reference Books Annual, 2004*

"The strengths of this book are many. It is clearly written, presented and structured."
—*Journal of the National Medical Association, 2004*

SEE ALSO *Childhood Diseases & Disorders Sourcebook*

Healthy Heart Sourcebook for Women

Basic Consumer Health Information about Cardiac Issues Specific to Women, Including Facts about Major Risk Factors and Prevention, Treatment and Control Strategies, and Important Dietary Issues

Along with a Special Section Regarding the Pros and Cons of Hormone Replacement Therapy and Its Impact on Heart Health, and Additional Help, Including Recipes, a Glossary, and a Directory of Resources

Edited by Dawn D. Matthews. 336 pages. 2000. 978-0-7808-0329-9.

"A good reference source and recommended for all public, academic, medical, and hospital libraries."
—*Medical Reference Services Quarterly, Summer '01*

"Because of the lack of information specific to women on this topic, this book is recommended for public libraries and consumer libraries."
—*American Reference Books Annual, 2001*

"Contains very important information about coronary artery disease that all women should know. The information is current and presented in an easy-to-read format. The book will make a good addition to any library." —*American Medical Writers Association Journal, Summer '00*

"Important, basic reference."
—*Reviewer's Bookwatch, Jul '00*

SEE ALSO *Cardiovascular Diseases & Disorders Sourcebook, Women's Health Concerns Sourcebook*

Hepatitis Sourcebook

Basic Consumer Health Information about Hepatitis A, Hepatitis B, Hepatitis C, and Other Forms of Hepatitis, Including Autoimmune Hepatitis, Alcoholic Hepatitis, Nonalcoholic Steatohepatitis, and Toxic Hepatitis, with

Facts about Risk Factors, Screening Methods, Diagnostic Tests, and Treatment Options

Along with Information on Liver Health, Tips for People Living with Chronic Hepatitis, Reports on Current Research Initiatives, a Glossary of Terms Related to Hepatitis, and a Directory of Sources for Further Help and Information

Edited by Sandra J. Judd. 597 pages. 2005. 978-0-7808-0749-5.

"Highly recommended."
—*American Reference Books Annual, 2006*

Household Safety Sourcebook

Basic Consumer Health Information about Household Safety, Including Information about Poisons, Chemicals, Fire, and Water Hazards in the Home

Along with Advice about the Safe Use of Home Maintenance Equipment, Choosing Toys and Nursery Furniture, Holiday and Recreation Safety, a Glossary, and Resources for Further Help and Information

Edited by Dawn D. Matthews. 606 pages. 2002. 978-0-7808-0338-1.

"This work will be useful in public libraries with large consumer health and wellness departments."
—*American Reference Books Annual, 2003*

"As a sourcebook on household safety this book meets its mark. It is encyclopedic in scope and covers a wide range of safety issues that are commonly seen in the home." —*E-Streams, Jul '02*

Hypertension Sourcebook

Basic Consumer Health Information about the Causes, Diagnosis, and Treatment of High Blood Pressure, with Facts about Consequences, Complications, and Co-Occurring Disorders, Such as Coronary Heart Disease, Diabetes, Stroke, Kidney Disease, and Hypertensive Retinopathy, and Issues in Blood Pressure Control, Including Dietary Choices, Stress Management, and Medications

Along with Reports on Current Research Initiatives and Clinical Trials, a Glossary, and Resources for Additional Help and Information

Edited by Dawn D. Matthews and Karen Bellenir. 613 pages. 2004. 978-0-7808-0674-0.

"Academic, public, and medical libraries will want to add the *Hypertension Sourcebook* to their collections."
—*E-Streams, Aug '05*

"The strength of this source is the wide range of information given about hypertension."
—*American Reference Books Annual, 2005*

Immune System Disorders Sourcebook, 2nd Edition

Basic Consumer Health Information about Disorders of the Immune System, Including Immune System Function and Response, Diagnosis of Immune Disorders, Information about Inherited Immune Disease, Acquired Immune Disease, and Autoimmune Diseases, Including Primary Immune Deficiency, Acquired Immunodeficiency Syndrome (AIDS), Lupus, Multiple Sclerosis, Type 1 Diabetes, Rheumatoid Arthritis, and Graves' Disease

Along with Treatments, Tips for Coping with Immune Disorders, a Glossary, and a Directory of Additional Resources.

Edited by Joyce Brennfleck Shannon. 671 pages. 2005. 978-0-7808-0748-8.

"Highly recommended for academic and public libraries." —*American Reference Books Annual, 2006*

"The updated second edition is a 'must' for any consumer health library seeking a solid resource covering the treatments, symptoms, and options for immune disorder sufferers.... An excellent guide."
—*MBR Bookwatch, Jan '06*

Infant & Toddler Health Sourcebook

Basic Consumer Health Information about the Physical and Mental Development of Newborns, Infants, and Toddlers, Including Neonatal Concerns, Nutrition Recommendations, Immunization Schedules, Common Pediatric Disorders, Assessments and Milestones, Safety Tips, and Advice for Parents and Other Caregivers

Along with a Glossary of Terms and Resource Listings for Additional Help

Edited by Jenifer Swanson. 585 pages. 2000. 978-0-7808-0246-9.

"As a reference for the general public, this would be useful in any library." —*E-Streams, May '01*

"Recommended reference source."
—*Booklist, American Library Association, Feb '01*

"This is a good source for general use."
—*American Reference Books Annual, 2001*

Infectious Diseases Sourcebook

Basic Consumer Health Information about Non-Contagious Bacterial, Viral, Prion, Fungal, and Parasitic Diseases Spread by Food and Water, Insects and Animals, or Environmental Contact, Including Botulism, E. Coli, Encephalitis, Legionnaires' Disease, Lyme Disease, Malaria, Plague, Rabies, Salmonella, Tetanus, and Others, and Facts about Newly Emerging Diseases, Such as Hantavirus, Mad Cow Disease, Monkeypox, and West Nile Virus

Along with Information about Preventing Disease Transmission, the Threat of Bioterrorism, and Current Research Initiatives, with a Glossary and Directory of Resources for More Information

Edited by Karen Bellenir. 634 pages. 2004. 978-0-7808-0675-7.

"This reference continues the excellent tradition of the *Health Reference Series* in consolidating a wealth of information on a selected topic into a format that is easy to use and accessible to the general public."
— *American Reference Books Annual, 2005*

"Recommended for public and academic libraries."
— *E-Streams, Jan '05*

Injury & Trauma Sourcebook

Basic Consumer Health Information about the Impact of Injury, the Diagnosis and Treatment of Common and Traumatic Injuries, Emergency Care, and Specific Injuries Related to Home, Community, Workplace, Transportation, and Recreation

Along with Guidelines for Injury Prevention, a Glossary, and a Directory of Additional Resources

Edited by Joyce Brennfleck Shannon. 696 pages. 2002. 978-0-7808-0421-0.

"This publication is the most comprehensive work of its kind about injury and trauma."
— *American Reference Books Annual, 2003*

"This sourcebook provides concise, easily readable, basic health information about injuries. . . . This book is well organized and an easy to use reference resource suitable for hospital, health sciences and public libraries with consumer health collections."
— *E-Streams, Nov '02*

"Practitioners should be aware of guides such as this in order to facilitate their use by patients and their families."
— *Doody's Health Sciences Book Review Journal, Sep-Oct '02*

"Recommended reference source."
— *Booklist, American Library Association, Sep '02*

"Highly recommended for academic and medical reference collections."
— *Library Bookwatch, Sep '02*

Kidney & Urinary Tract Diseases & Disorders Sourcebook

SEE Urinary Tract & Kidney Diseases & Disorders Sourcebook

Learning Disabilities Sourcebook, 2nd Edition

Basic Consumer Health Information about Learning Disabilities, Including Dyslexia, Developmental Speech and Language Disabilities, Non-Verbal Learning Disorders, Developmental Arithmetic Disorder, Developmental Writing Disorder, and Other Conditions That Impede Learning Such as Attention Deficit/Hyperactivity Disorder, Brain Injury, Hearing Impairment, Klinefelter Syndrome, Dyspraxia, and Tourette's Syndrome

Along with Facts about Educational Issues and Assistive Technology, Coping Strategies, a Glossary of Related Terms, and Resources for Further Help and Information

Edited by Dawn D. Matthews. 621 pages. 2003. 978-0-7808-0626-9.

"The second edition of Learning Disabilities Sourcebook far surpasses the earlier edition in that it is more focused on information that will be useful as a consumer health resource."
— *American Reference Books Annual, 2004*

"Teachers as well as consumers will find this an essential guide to understanding various syndromes and their latest treatments. [An] invaluable reference for public and school library collections alike."
— *Library Bookwatch, Apr '03*

Named "Outstanding Reference Book of 1999."
— *New York Public Library, Feb '00*

"An excellent candidate for inclusion in a public library reference section. It's a great source of information. Teachers will also find the book useful. Definitely worth reading."
— *Journal of Adolescent & Adult Literacy, Feb 2000*

"Readable . . . provides a solid base of information regarding successful techniques used with individuals who have learning disabilities, as well as practical suggestions for educators and family members. Clear language, concise descriptions, and pertinent information for contacting multiple resources add to the strength of this book as a useful tool."
— *Choice, Association of College & Research Libraries, Feb '99*

"Recommended reference source."
— *Booklist, American Library Association, Sep '98*

"A useful resource for libraries and for those who don't have the time to identify and locate the individual publications."
— *Disability Resources Monthly, Sep '98*

Leukemia Sourcebook

Basic Consumer Health Information about Adult and Childhood Leukemias, Including Acute Lymphocytic Leukemia (ALL), Chronic Lymphocytic Leukemia (CLL), Acute Myelogenous Leukemia (AML), Chronic Myelogenous Leukemia (CML), and Hairy Cell Leukemia, and Treatments Such as Chemotherapy, Radiation Therapy, Peripheral Blood Stem Cell and Marrow Transplantation, and Immunotherapy

Along with Tips for Life During and After Treatment, a Glossary, and Directories of Additional Resources

Edited by Joyce Brennfleck Shannon. 587 pages. 2003. 978-0-7808-0627-6.

"Unlike other medical books for the layperson, . . . the language does not talk down to the reader. . . . This volume is highly recommended for all libraries."
— *American Reference Books Annual, 2004*

". . . a fine title which ranges from diagnosis to alternative treatments, staging, and tips for life during and after diagnosis."
— *The Bookwatch, Dec '03*

Liver Disorders Sourcebook

Basic Consumer Health Information about the Liver and How It Works; Liver Diseases, Including Cancer, Cirrhosis, Hepatitis, and Toxic and Drug Related Diseases; Tips for Maintaining a Healthy Liver; Laboratory Tests, Radiology Tests, and Facts about Liver Transplantation

Along with a Section on Support Groups, a Glossary, and Resource Listings

Edited by Joyce Brennfleck Shannon. 591 pages. 2000. 978-0-7808-0383-1.

"A valuable resource."
—*American Reference Books Annual, 2001*

"This title is recommended for health sciences and public libraries with consumer health collections."
—*E-Streams, Oct '00*

"Recommended reference source."
—*Booklist, American Library Association, Jun '00*

■

Lung Disorders Sourcebook

Basic Consumer Health Information about Emphysema, Pneumonia, Tuberculosis, Asthma, Cystic Fibrosis, and Other Lung Disorders, Including Facts about Diagnostic Procedures, Treatment Strategies, Disease Prevention Efforts, and Such Risk Factors as Smoking, Air Pollution, and Exposure to Asbestos, Radon, and Other Agents

Along with a Glossary and Resources for Additional Help and Information

Edited by Dawn D. Matthews. 678 pages. 2002. 978-0-7808-0339-8.

"This title is a great addition for public and school libraries because it provides concise health information on the lungs."
—*American Reference Books Annual, 2003*

"Highly recommended for academic and medical reference collections." —*Library Bookwatch, Sep '02*

SEE ALSO Respiratory Diseases & Disorders Sourcebook

■

Medical Tests Sourcebook, 2nd Edition

Basic Consumer Health Information about Medical Tests, Including Age-Specific Health Tests, Important Health Screenings and Exams, Home-Use Tests, Blood and Specimen Tests, Electrical Tests, Scope Tests, Genetic Testing, and Imaging Tests, Such as X-Rays, Ultrasound, Computed Tomography, Magnetic Resonance Imaging, Angiography, and Nuclear Medicine

Along with a Glossary and Directory of Additional Resources

Edited by Joyce Brennfleck Shannon. 654 pages. 2004. 978-0-7808-0670-2.

"Recommended for hospital and health sciences libraries with consumer health collections."
—*E-Streams, Mar '00*

"This is an overall excellent reference with a wealth of general knowledge that may aid those who are reluctant to get vital tests performed."
—*Today's Librarian, Jan '00*

"A valuable reference guide."
—*American Reference Books Annual, 2000*

■

Men's Health Concerns Sourcebook, 2nd Edition

Basic Consumer Health Information about the Medical and Mental Concerns of Men, Including Theories about the Shorter Male Lifespan, the Leading Causes of Death and Disability, Physical Concerns of Special Significance to Men, Reproductive and Sexual Concerns, Sexually Transmitted Diseases, Men's Mental and Emotional Health, and Lifestyle Choices That Affect Wellness, Such as Nutrition, Fitness, and Substance Use

Along with a Glossary of Related Terms and a Directory of Organizational Resources in Men's Health

Edited by Robert Aquinas McNally. 644 pages. 2004. 978-0-7808-0671-9.

"A very accessible reference for non-specialist general readers and consumers."   — *The Bookwatch, Jun '04*

"This comprehensive resource and the series are highly recommended."
—*American Reference Books Annual, 2000*

"Recommended reference source."
— *Booklist, American Library Association, Dec '98*

■

Mental Health Disorders Sourcebook, 3rd Edition

Basic Consumer Health Information about Mental and Emotional Health and Mental Illness, Including Facts about Depression, Bipolar Disorder, and Other Mood Disorders, Phobias, Post-Traumatic Stress Disorder (PTSD), Obsessive-Compulsive Disorder, and Other Anxiety Disorders, Impulse Control Disorders, Eating Disorders, Personality Disorders, and Psychotic Disorders, Including Schizophrenia and Dissociative Disorders

Along with Statistical Information, a Special Section Concerning Mental Health Issues in Children and Adolescents, a Glossary, and Directories of Resources for Additional Help and Information

Edited by Karen Bellenir. 661 pages. 2005. 978-0-7808-0747-1.

"Recommended for public libraries and academic libraries with an undergraduate program in psychology."
—*American Reference Books Annual, 2006*

"Recommended reference source."
—*Booklist, American Library Association, Jun '00*

Mental Retardation Sourcebook

Basic Consumer Health Information about Mental Retardation and Its Causes, Including Down Syndrome, Fetal Alcohol Syndrome, Fragile X Syndrome, Genetic Conditions, Injury, and Environmental Sources Along with Preventive Strategies, Parenting Issues, Educational Implications, Health Care Needs, Employment and Economic Matters, Legal Issues, a Glossary, and a Resource Listing for Additional Help and Information

Edited by Joyce Brennfleck Shannon. 642 pages. 2000. 978-0-7808-0377-0.

"Public libraries will find the book useful for reference and as a beginning research point for students, parents, and caregivers."
— *American Reference Books Annual, 2001*

"The strength of this work is that it compiles many basic fact sheets and addresses for further information in one volume. It is intended and suitable for the general public. This sourcebook is relevant to any collection providing health information to the general public."
— *E-Streams, Nov '00*

"From preventing retardation to parenting and family challenges, this covers health, social and legal issues and will prove an invaluable overview."
— *Reviewer's Bookwatch, Jul '00*

Movement Disorders Sourcebook

Basic Consumer Health Information about Neurological Movement Disorders, Including Essential Tremor, Parkinson's Disease, Dystonia, Cerebral Palsy, Huntington's Disease, Myasthenia Gravis, Multiple Sclerosis, and Other Early-Onset and Adult-Onset Movement Disorders, Their Symptoms and Causes, Diagnostic Tests, and Treatments Along with Mobility and Assistive Technology Information, a Glossary, and a Directory of Additional Resources

Edited by Joyce Brennfleck Shannon. 655 pages. 2003. 978-0-7808-0628-3.

"... a good resource for consumers and recommended for public, community college and undergraduate libraries." — *American Reference Books Annual, 2004*

Muscular Dystrophy Sourcebook

Basic Consumer Health Information about Congenital, Childhood-Onset, and Adult-Onset Forms of Muscular Dystrophy, Such as Duchenne, Becker, Emery-Dreifuss, Distal, Limb-Girdle, Facioscapulohumeral (FSHD), Myotonic, and Ophthalmoplegic Muscular Dystrophies, Including Facts about Diagnostic Tests, Medical and Physical Therapies, Management of Co-Occurring Conditions, and Parenting Guidelines Along with Practical Tips for Home Care, a Glossary, and Directories of Additional Resources

Edited by Joyce Brennfleck Shannon. 577 pages. 2004. 978-0-7808-0676-4.

"This book is highly recommended for public and academic libraries as well as health care offices that support the information needs of patients and their families."
— *E-Streams, Apr '05*

"Excellent reference." — *The Bookwatch, Jan '05*

Obesity Sourcebook

Basic Consumer Health Information about Diseases and Other Problems Associated with Obesity, and Including Facts about Risk Factors, Prevention Issues, and Management Approaches Along with Statistical and Demographic Data, Information about Special Populations, Research Updates, a Glossary, and Source Listings for Further Help and Information

Edited by Wilma Caldwell and Chad T. Kimball. 376 pages. 2001. 978-0-7808-0333-6.

"The book synthesizes the reliable medical literature on obesity into one easy-to-read and useful resource for the general public."
— *American Reference Books Annual, 2002*

"This is a very useful resource book for the lay public."
— *Doody's Review Service, Nov '01*

"Well suited for the health reference collection of a public library or an academic health science library that serves the general population." — *E-Streams, Sep '01*

"Recommended reference source."
— *Booklist, American Library Association, Apr '01*

"Recommended pick both for specialty health library collections and any general consumer health reference collection." — *The Bookwatch, Apr '01*

Oral Health Sourcebook

SEE Dental Care & Oral Health Sourcebook

Osteoporosis Sourcebook

Basic Consumer Health Information about Primary and Secondary Osteoporosis and Juvenile Osteoporosis and Related Conditions, Including Fibrous Dysplasia, Gaucher Disease, Hyperthyroidism, Hypophosphatasia, Myeloma, Osteopetrosis, Osteogenesis Imperfecta, and Paget's Disease

Along with Information about Risk Factors, Treatments, Traditional and Non-Traditional Pain Management, a Glossary of Related Terms, and a Directory of Resources

Edited by Allan R. Cook. 584 pages. 2001. 978-0-7808-0239-1.

"This would be a book to be kept in a staff or patient library. The targeted audience is the layperson, but the therapist who needs a quick bit of information on a particular topic will also find the book useful."
— *Physical Therapy, Jan '02*

"This resource is recommended as a great reference source for public, health, and academic libraries, and is another triumph for the editors of Omnigraphics."
— *American Reference Books Annual, 2002*

"Recommended for all public libraries and general health collections, especially those supporting patient education or consumer health programs."
— *E-Streams, Nov '01*

"Will prove valuable to any library seeking to maintain a current, comprehensive reference collection of health resources.... From prevention to treatment and associated conditions, this provides an excellent survey."
— *The Bookwatch, Aug '01*

"Recommended reference source."
— *Booklist, American Library Association, Jul '01*

SEE ALSO *Healthy Aging Sourcebook, Physical & Mental Issues in Aging Sourcebook, Women's Health Concerns Sourcebook*

Pain Sourcebook, 2nd Edition

Basic Consumer Health Information about Specific Forms of Acute and Chronic Pain, Including Muscle and Skeletal Pain, Nerve Pain, Cancer Pain, and Disorders Characterized by Pain, Such as Fibromyalgia, Shingles, Angina, Arthritis, and Headaches

Along with Information about Pain Medications and Management Techniques, Complementary and Alternative Pain Relief Options, Tips for People Living with Chronic Pain, a Glossary, and a Directory of Sources for Further Information

Edited by Karen Bellenir. 670 pages. 2002. 978-0-7808-0612-2.

"A source of valuable information.... This book offers help to nonmedical people who need information about pain and pain management. It is also an excellent reference for those who participate in patient education."
— *Doody's Review Service, Sep '02*

"Highly recommended for academic and medical reference collections."   — *Library Bookwatch, Sep '02*

"The text is readable, easily understood, and well indexed. This excellent volume belongs in all patient education libraries, consumer health sections of public libraries, and many personal collections."
— *American Reference Books Annual, 1999*

"The information is basic in terms of scholarship and is appropriate for general readers. Written in journalistic style... intended for non-professionals. Quite thorough in its coverage of different pain conditions and summarizes the latest clinical information regarding pain treatment."   — *Choice, Association of College and Research Libraries, Jun '98*

"Recommended reference source."
— *Booklist, American Library Association, Mar '98*

Pediatric Cancer Sourcebook

Basic Consumer Health Information about Leukemias, Brain Tumors, Sarcomas, Lymphomas, and Other Cancers in Infants, Children, and Adolescents, Including Descriptions of Cancers, Treatments, and Coping Strategies

Along with Suggestions for Parents, Caregivers, and Concerned Relatives, a Glossary of Cancer Terms, and Resource Listings

Edited by Edward J. Prucha. 587 pages. 1999. 978-0-7808-0245-2.

"An excellent source of information. Recommended for public, hospital, and health science libraries with consumer health collections."   — *E-Streams, Jun '00*

"Recommended reference source."
— *Booklist, American Library Association, Feb '00*

"A valuable addition to all libraries specializing in health services and many public libraries."
— *American Reference Books Annual, 2000*

SEE ALSO *Childhood Diseases & Disorders Sourcebook, Healthy Children Sourcebook*

Physical & Mental Issues in Aging Sourcebook

Basic Consumer Health Information on Physical and Mental Disorders Associated with the Aging Process, Including Concerns about Cardiovascular Disease, Pulmonary Disease, Oral Health, Digestive Disorders, Musculoskeletal and Skin Disorders, Metabolic Changes, Sexual and Reproductive Issues, and Changes in Vision, Hearing, and Other Senses

Along with Data about Longevity and Causes of Death, Information on Acute and Chronic Pain, Descriptions of Mental Concerns, a Glossary of Terms, and Resource Listings for Additional Help

Edited by Jenifer Swanson. 660 pages. 1999. 978-0-7808-0233-9.

"This is a treasure of health information for the layperson."   — *Choice Health Sciences Supplement, Association of College & Research Libraries, May '00*

"Recommended for public libraries."
— *American Reference Books Annual, 2000*

"Recommended reference source."
— *Booklist, American Library Association, Oct '99*

SEE ALSO *Healthy Aging Sourcebook*

Podiatry Sourcebook, 2nd Edition

Basic Consumer Health Information about Disorders, Diseases, Deformities, and Injuries that Affect the Foot and Ankle, Including Sprains, Corns, Calluses, Bunions, Plantar Warts, Plantar Fasciitis, Neuromas, Clubfoot, Flat Feet, Achilles Tendonitis, and Much More

Along with Information about Selecting a Foot Care Specialist, Foot Fitness, Shoes and Socks, Diagnostic Tests and Corrective Procedures, Financial Assistance for Corrective Devices, a Glossary of Related Terms, and a Directory of Resources for Additional Help and Information

Edited by Ivy L. Alexander. 543 pages. 2007. 978-0-7808-0944-4.

"Recommended reference source."
— *Booklist, American Library Association, Feb '02*

"There is a lot of information presented here on a topic that is usually only covered sparingly in most larger comprehensive medical encyclopedias."
— *American Reference Books Annual, 2002*

Pregnancy & Birth Sourcebook, 2nd Edition

Basic Consumer Health Information about Conception and Pregnancy, Including Facts about Fertility, Infertility, Pregnancy Symptoms and Complications, Fetal Growth and Development, Labor, Delivery, and the Postpartum Period, as Well as Information about Maintaining Health and Wellness during Pregnancy and Caring for a Newborn

Along with Information about Public Health Assistance for Low-Income Pregnant Women, a Glossary, and Directories of Agencies and Organizations Providing Help and Support

Edited by Amy L. Sutton. 626 pages. 2004. 978-0-7808-0672-6.

"Will appeal to public and school reference collections strong in medicine and women's health.... Deserves a spot on any medical reference shelf."
— *The Bookwatch, Jul '04*

"A well-organized handbook. Recommended."
— *Choice, Association of College & Research Libraries, Apr '98*

"Recommended reference source."
— *Booklist, American Library Association, Mar '98*

"Recommended for public libraries."
— *American Reference Books Annual, 1998*

SEE ALSO *Breastfeeding Sourcebook, Congenital Disorders Sourcebook, Family Planning Sourcebook*

Prostate & Urological Disorders Sourcebook

Basic Consumer Health Information about Urogenital and Sexual Disorders in Men, Including Prostate and Other Andrological Cancers, Prostatitis, Benign Prostatic Hyperplasia, Testicular and Penile Trauma, Cryptorchidism, Peyronie Disease, Erectile Dysfunction, and Male Factor Infertility, and Facts about Commonly Used Tests and Procedures, Such as Prostatectomy, Vasectomy, Vasectomy Reversal, Penile Implants, and Semen Analysis

Along with a Glossary of Andrological Terms and a Directory of Resources for Additional Information

Edited by Karen Bellenir. 631 pages. 2005. 978-0-7808-0797-6.

Prostate Cancer Sourcebook

Basic Consumer Health Information about Prostate Cancer, Including Information about the Associated Risk Factors, Detection, Diagnosis, and Treatment of Prostate Cancer

Along with Information on Non-Malignant Prostate Conditions, and Featuring a Section Listing Support and Treatment Centers and a Glossary of Related Terms

Edited by Dawn D. Matthews. 358 pages. 2001. 978-0-7808-0324-4.

"Recommended reference source."
— *Booklist, American Library Association, Jan '02*

"A valuable resource for health care consumers seeking information on the subject.... All text is written in a clear, easy-to-understand language that avoids technical jargon. Any library that collects consumer health resources would strengthen their collection with the addition of the *Prostate Cancer Sourcebook*."
— *American Reference Books Annual, 2002*

SEE ALSO *Men's Health Concerns Sourcebook*

Reconstructive & Cosmetic Surgery Sourcebook

Basic Consumer Health Information on Cosmetic and Reconstructive Plastic Surgery, Including Statistical Information about Different Surgical Procedures, Things to Consider Prior to Surgery, Plastic Surgery Techniques and Tools, Emotional and Psychological Considerations, and Procedure-Specific Information

Along with a Glossary of Terms and a Listing of Resources for Additional Help and Information

Edited by M. Lisa Weatherford. 374 pages. 2001. 978-0-7808-0214-8.

"An excellent reference that addresses cosmetic and medically necessary reconstructive surgeries.... The style of the prose is calm and reassuring, discussing the many positive outcomes now available due to advances in surgical techniques."
— *American Reference Books Annual, 2002*

"Recommended for health science libraries that are open to the public, as well as hospital libraries that are open to the patients. This book is a good resource for the consumer interested in plastic surgery."
— *E-Streams, Dec '01*

"Recommended reference source."
— *Booklist, American Library Association, Jul '01*

Rehabilitation Sourcebook

Basic Consumer Health Information about Rehabilitation for People Recovering from Heart Surgery, Spinal Cord Injury, Stroke, Orthopedic Impairments, Amputation, Pulmonary Impairments, Traumatic Injury, and More, Including Physical Therapy, Occupational Therapy, Speech/Language Therapy, Massage Therapy, Dance Therapy, Art Therapy, and Recreational Therapy

Along with Information on Assistive and Adaptive Devices, a Glossary, and Resources for Additional Help and Information

Edited by Dawn D. Matthews. 531 pages. 1999. 978-0-7808-0236-0.

"This is an excellent resource for public library reference and health collections."
— *American Reference Books Annual, 2001*

"Recommended reference source."
— *Booklist, American Library Association, May '00*

Respiratory Diseases & Disorders Sourcebook

Basic Information about Respiratory Diseases and Disorders, Including Asthma, Cystic Fibrosis, Pneumonia, the Common Cold, Influenza, and Others, Featuring Facts about the Respiratory System, Statistical and Demographic Data, Treatments, Self-Help Management Suggestions, and Current Research Initiatives

Edited by Allan R. Cook and Peter D. Dresser. 771 pages. 1995. 978-0-7808-0037-3.

"Designed for the layperson and for patients and their families coping with respiratory illness. . . . an extensive array of information on diagnosis, treatment, management, and prevention of respiratory illnesses for the general reader." — *Choice, Association of College & Research Libraries, Jun '96*

"A highly recommended text for all collections. It is a comforting reminder of the power of knowledge that good books carry between their covers."
— *Academic Library Book Review, Spring '96*

"A comprehensive collection of authoritative information presented in a nontechnical, humanitarian style for patients, families, and caregivers."
— *Association of Operating Room Nurses, Sep/Oct '95*

SEE ALSO Lung Disorders Sourcebook

Sexually Transmitted Diseases Sourcebook, 3rd Edition

Basic Consumer Health Information about Chlamydial Infections, Gonorrhea, Hepatitis, Herpes, HIV/AIDS, Human Papillomavirus, Pubic Lice, Scabies, Syphilis, Trichomoniasis, Vaginal Infections, and Other Sexually Transmitted Diseases, Including Facts about Risk Factors, Symptoms, Diagnosis, Treatment, and the Prevention of Sexually Transmitted Infections

Along with Updates on Current Research Initiatives, a Glossary of Related Terms, and Resources for Additional Help and Information

Edited by Amy L. Sutton. 629 pages. 2006. 978-0-7808-0824-9.

"Recommended for consumer health collections in public libraries, and secondary school and community college libraries."
— *American Reference Books Annual, 2002*

"Every school and public library should have a copy of this comprehensive and user-friendly reference book."
— *Choice, Association of College & Research Libraries, Sep '01*

"This is a highly recommended book. This is an especially important book for all school and public libraries."
— *AIDS Book Review Journal, Jul-Aug '01*

"Recommended reference source."
— *Booklist, American Library Association, Apr '01*

Sleep Disorders Sourcebook, 2nd Edition

Basic Consumer Health Information about Sleep and Sleep Disorders, Including Insomnia, Sleep Apnea, Restless Legs Syndrome, Narcolepsy, Parasomnias, and Other Health Problems That Affect Sleep, Plus Facts about Diagnostic Procedures, Treatment Strategies, Sleep Medications, and Tips for Improving Sleep Quality

Along with a Glossary of Related Terms and Resources for Additional Help and Information

Edited by Amy L. Sutton. 567 pages. 2005. 978-0-7808-0743-3.

"This book will be useful for just about everybody, especially the 40 million Americans with sleep disorders."
— *American Reference Books Annual, 2006*

"Recommended for public libraries and libraries supporting health care professionals." — *E-Streams, Sep '05*

". . . key medical library acquisition."
— *The Bookwatch, Jun '05*

Smoking Concerns Sourcebook

Basic Consumer Health Information about Nicotine Addiction and Smoking Cessation, Featuring Facts about the Health Effects of Tobacco Use, Including Lung and Other Cancers, Heart Disease, Stroke, and Respiratory Disorders, Such as Emphysema and Chronic Bronchitis

Along with Information about Smoking Prevention Programs, Suggestions for Achieving and Maintaining a Smoke-Free Lifestyle, Statistics about Tobacco Use, Reports on Current Research Initiatives, a Glossary of Related Terms, and Directories of Resources for Additional Help and Information

Edited by Karen Bellenir. 621 pages. 2004. 978-0-7808-0323-7.

"Provides everything needed for the student or general reader seeking practical details on the effects of tobacco use." — *The Bookwatch, Mar '05*

"Public libraries and consumer health care libraries will find this work useful."
— *American Reference Books Annual, 2005*

Sports Injuries Sourcebook, 3rd Edition

Basic Consumer Health Information about Sprains and Strains, Fractures, Growth Plate Injuries, Overtraining Injuries, and Injuries to the Head, Face, Shoulders, Elbows, Hands, Spinal Column, Knees, Ankles, and Feet, and with Facts about Heat-Related Illness, Steroids and Sport Supplements, Protective Equipment, Diagnostic Procedures, Treatment Options, and Rehabilitation

Along with a Glossary of Related Terms and a Directory of Resources for Additional Help and Information

Edited by Sandra J. Judd. 651 pages. 2007. 978-0-7808-0949-9.

"This is an excellent reference for consumers and it is recommended for public, community college, and undergraduate libraries."
— *American Reference Books Annual, 2003*

"Recommended reference source."
— *Booklist, American Library Association, Feb '03*

■

Stress-Related Disorders Sourcebook

Basic Consumer Health Information about Stress and Stress-Related Disorders, Including Stress Origins and Signals, Environmental Stress at Work and Home, Mental and Emotional Stress Associated with Depression, Post-Traumatic Stress Disorder, Panic Disorder, Suicide, and the Physical Effects of Stress on the Cardiovascular, Immune, and Nervous Systems

Along with Stress Management Techniques, a Glossary, and a Listing of Additional Resources

Edited by Joyce Brennfleck Shannon. 610 pages. 2002. 978-0-7808-0560-6.

"Well written for a general readership, the *Stress-Related Disorders Sourcebook* is a useful addition to the health reference literature."
— *American Reference Books Annual, 2003*

"I am impressed by the amount of information. It offers a thorough overview of the causes and consequences of stress for the layperson. . . . A well-done and thorough reference guide for professionals and nonprofessionals alike." — *Doody's Review Service, Dec '02*

■

Stroke Sourcebook

Basic Consumer Health Information about Stroke, Including Ischemic, Hemorrhagic, Transient Ischemic Attack (TIA), and Pediatric Stroke, Stroke Triggers and Risks, Diagnostic Tests, Treatments, and Rehabilitation Information

Along with Stroke Prevention Guidelines, Legal and Financial Information, a Glossary, and a Directory of Additional Resources

Edited by Joyce Brennfleck Shannon. 606 pages. 2003. 978-0-7808-0630-6.

"This volume is highly recommended and should be in every medical, hospital, and public library."
— *American Reference Books Annual, 2004*

"Highly recommended for the amount and variety of topics and information covered." — *Choice, Nov '03*

■

Surgery Sourcebook

Basic Consumer Health Information about Inpatient and Outpatient Surgeries, Including Cardiac, Vascular, Orthopedic, Ocular, Reconstructive, Cosmetic, Gynecologic, and Ear, Nose, and Throat Procedures and More

Along with Information about Operating Room Policies and Instruments, Laser Surgery Techniques, Hospital Errors, Statistical Data, a Glossary, and Listings of Sources for Further Help and Information

Edited by Annemarie S. Muth and Karen Bellenir. 596 pages. 2002. 978-0-7808-0380-0.

"Large public libraries and medical libraries would benefit from this material in their reference collections."
— *American Reference Books Annual, 2004*

"Invaluable reference for public and school library collections alike." — *Library Bookwatch, Apr '03*

■

Thyroid Disorders Sourcebook

Basic Consumer Health Information about Disorders of the Thyroid and Parathyroid Glands, Including Hypothyroidism, Hyperthyroidism, Graves Disease, Hashimoto Thyroiditis, Thyroid Cancer, and Parathyroid Disorders, Featuring Facts about Symptoms, Risk Factors, Tests, and Treatments

Along with Information about the Effects of Thyroid Imbalance on Other Body Systems, Environmental Factors That Affect the Thyroid Gland, a Glossary, and a Directory of Additional Resources

Edited by Joyce Brennfleck Shannon. 599 pages. 2005. 978-0-7808-0745-7.

"Recommended for consumer health collections."
— *American Reference Books Annual, 2006*

"Highly recommended pick for basic consumer health reference holdings at all levels."
— *The Bookwatch, Aug '05*

■

Transplantation Sourcebook

Basic Consumer Health Information about Organ and Tissue Transplantation, Including Physical and Financial Preparations, Procedures and Issues Relating to Specific Solid Organ and Tissue Transplants, Rehabilitation, Pediatric Transplant Information, the Future of Transplantation, and Organ and Tissue Donation

Along with a Glossary and Listings of Additional Resources

Edited by Joyce Brennfleck Shannon. 628 pages. 2002. 978-0-7808-0322-0.

"Along with these advances [in transplantation technology] have come a number of daunting questions for potential transplant patients, their families, and their health care providers. This reference text is the best single tool to address many of these questions. . . . It will be a much-needed addition to the reference collections in health care, academic, and large public libraries."
—American Reference Books Annual, 2003

"Recommended for libraries with an interest in offering consumer health information." —E-Streams, Jul '02

"This is a unique and valuable resource for patients facing transplantation and their families."
—Doody's Review Service, Jun '02

Traveler's Health Sourcebook

Basic Consumer Health Information for Travelers, Including Physical and Medical Preparations, Transportation Health and Safety, Essential Information about Food and Water, Sun Exposure, Insect and Snake Bites, Camping and Wilderness Medicine, and Travel with Physical or Medical Disabilities

Along with International Travel Tips, Vaccination Recommendations, Geographical Health Issues, Disease Risks, a Glossary, and a Listing of Additional Resources

Edited by Joyce Brennfleck Shannon. 613 pages. 2000. 978-0-7808-0384-8.

"Recommended reference source."
—Booklist, American Library Association, Feb '01

"This book is recommended for any public library, any travel collection, and especially any collection for the physically disabled."
—American Reference Books Annual, 2001

SEE ALSO Worldwide Health Sourcebook

Urinary Tract & Kidney Diseases & Disorders Sourcebook, 2nd Edition

Basic Consumer Health Information about the Urinary System, Including the Bladder, Urethra, Ureters, and Kidneys, with Facts about Urinary Tract Infections, Incontinence, Congenital Disorders, Kidney Stones, Cancers of the Urinary Tract and Kidneys, Kidney Failure, Dialysis, and Kidney Transplantation

Along with Statistical and Demographic Information, Reports on Current Research in Kidney and Urologic Health, a Summary of Commonly Used Diagnostic Tests, a Glossary of Related Terms, and a Directory of Resources for Additional Help and Information

Edited by Ivy L. Alexander. 649 pages. 2005. 978-0-7808-0750-1.

"A good choice for a consumer health information library or for a medical library needing information to refer to their patients."
—American Reference Books Annual, 2006

Vegetarian Sourcebook

Basic Consumer Health Information about Vegetarian Diets, Lifestyle, and Philosophy, Including Definitions of Vegetarianism and Veganism, Tips about Adopting Vegetarianism, Creating a Vegetarian Pantry, and Meeting Nutritional Needs of Vegetarians, with Facts Regarding Vegetarianism's Effect on Pregnant and Lactating Women, Children, Athletes, and Senior Citizens

Along with a Glossary of Commonly Used Vegetarian Terms and Resources for Additional Help and Information

Edited by Chad T. Kimball. 360 pages. 2002. 978-0-7808-0439-5.

"Organizes into one concise volume the answers to the most common questions concerning vegetarian diets and lifestyles. This title is recommended for public and secondary school libraries." —E-Streams, Apr '03

"Invaluable reference for public and school library collections alike." —Library Bookwatch, Apr '03

"The articles in this volume are easy to read and come from authoritative sources. The book does not necessarily support the vegetarian diet but instead provides the pros and cons of this important decision. The Vegetarian Sourcebook is recommended for public libraries and consumer health libraries."
—American Reference Books Annual, 2003

SEE ALSO Diet & Nutrition Sourcebook

Women's Health Concerns Sourcebook, 2nd Edition

Basic Consumer Health Information about the Medical and Mental Concerns of Women, Including Maintaining Health and Wellness, Gynecological Concerns, Breast Health, Sexuality and Reproductive Issues, Menopause, Cancer in Women, Leading Causes of Death and Disability among Women, Physical Concerns of Special Significance to Women, and Women's Mental and Emotional Health

Along with a Glossary of Related Terms and Directories of Resources for Additional Help and Information

Edited by Amy L. Sutton. 746 pages. 2004. 978-0-7808-0673-3.

"This is a useful reference book, which makes the reader knowledgeable about several issues that concern women's health. It is recommended for public libraries and home library collections." —E-Streams, May '05

"A useful addition to public and consumer health library collections."
—American Reference Books Annual, 2005

"A highly recommended title."
—The Bookwatch, May '04

"Handy compilation. There is an impressive range of diseases, devices, disorders, procedures, and other physical and emotional issues covered . . . well organized, illustrated, and indexed." —Choice, Association of College & Research Libraries, Jan '98

SEE ALSO Breast Cancer Sourcebook, Cancer Sourcebook for Women, Healthy Heart Sourcebook for Women, Osteoporosis Sourcebook

Workplace Health & Safety Sourcebook

Basic Consumer Health Information about Workplace Health and Safety, Including the Effect of Workplace Hazards on the Lungs, Skin, Heart, Ears, Eyes, Brain, Reproductive Organs, Musculoskeletal System, and Other Organs and Body Parts

Along with Information about Occupational Cancer, Personal Protective Equipment, Toxic and Hazardous Chemicals, Child Labor, Stress, and Workplace Violence

Edited by Chad T. Kimball. 626 pages. 2000. 978-0-7808-0231-5.

"As a reference for the general public, this would be useful in any library." —*E-Streams, Jun '01*

"Provides helpful information for primary care physicians and other caregivers interested in occupational medicine.... General readers; professionals."
—*Choice, Association of College & Research Libraries, May '01*

"Recommended reference source."
—*Booklist, American Library Association, Feb '01*

"Highly recommended." —*The Bookwatch, Jan '01*

Worldwide Health Sourcebook

Basic Information about Global Health Issues, Including Malnutrition, Reproductive Health, Disease Dispersion and Prevention, Emerging Diseases, Risky Health Behaviors, and the Leading Causes of Death

Along with Global Health Concerns for Children, Women, and the Elderly, Mental Health Issues, Research and Technology Advancements, and Economic, Environmental, and Political Health Implications, a Glossary, and a Resource Listing for Additional Help and Information

Edited by Joyce Brennfleck Shannon. 614 pages. 2001. 978-0-7808-0330-5.

"Named an Outstanding Academic Title."
—*Choice, Association of College & Research Libraries, Jan '02*

"Yet another handy but also unique compilation in the extensive **Health Reference Series,** this is a useful work because many of the international publications reprinted or excerpted are not readily available. Highly recommended." —*Choice, Association of College & Research Libraries, Nov '01*

"Recommended reference source."
—*Booklist, American Library Association, Oct '01*

SEE ALSO Traveler's Health Sourcebook

Teen Health Series
Helping Young Adults Understand, Manage, and Avoid Serious Illness

List price $65 per volume. **School and library price $58 per volume.**

Alcohol Information for Teens
Health Tips about Alcohol and Alcoholism
Including Facts about Underage Drinking, Preventing Teen Alcohol Use, Alcohol's Effects on the Brain and the Body, Alcohol Abuse Treatment, Help for Children of Alcoholics, and More

Edited by Joyce Brennfleck Shannon. 370 pages. 2005. 978-0-7808-0741-9.

"Boxed facts and tips add visual interest to the well-researched and clearly written text."
— *Curriculum Connection*, Apr '06

Allergy Information for Teens
Health Tips about Allergic Reactions Such as Anaphylaxis, Respiratory Problems, and Rashes
Including Facts about Identifying and Managing Allergies to Food, Pollen, Mold, Animals, Chemicals, Drugs, and Other Substances

Edited by Karen Bellenir. 410 pages. 2006. 978-0-7808-0799-0.

Asthma Information for Teens
Health Tips about Managing Asthma and Related Concerns
Including Facts about Asthma Causes, Triggers, Symptoms, Diagnosis, and Treatment

Edited by Karen Bellenir. 386 pages. 2005. 978-0-7808-0770-9.

"Highly recommended for medical libraries, public school libraries, and public libraries."
— *American Reference Books Annual*, 2006

"It is so clearly written and well organized that even hesitant readers will be able to find the facts they need, whether for reports or personal information.... A succinct but complete resource."
— *School Library Journal*, Sep '05

Body Information for Teens
Health Tips about Maintaining Well-Being for a Lifetime
Including Facts about the Development and Functioning of the Body's Systems, Organs, and Structures and the Health Impact of Lifestyle Choices

Edited by Sandra Augustyn Lawton. 458 pages. 2007. 978-0-7808-0443-2.

Cancer Information for Teens
Health Tips about Cancer Awareness, Prevention, Diagnosis, and Treatment
Including Facts about Frequently Occurring Cancers, Cancer Risk Factors, and Coping Strategies for Teens Fighting Cancer or Dealing with Cancer in Friends or Family Members

Edited by Wilma R. Caldwell. 428 pages. 2004. 978-0-7808-0678-8.

"Recommended for school libraries, or consumer libraries that see a lot of use by teens."
— *E-Streams*, May '05

"A valuable educational tool."
— *American Reference Books Annual*, 2005

"Young adults and their parents alike will find this new addition to the *Teen Health Series* an important reference to cancer in teens."
— *Children's Bookwatch*, Feb '05

Complementary and Alternative Medicine Information for Teens
Health Tips about Non-Traditional and Non-Western Medical Practices
Including Information about Acupuncture, Chiropractic Medicine, Dietary and Herbal Supplements, Hypnosis, Massage Therapy, Prayer and Spirituality, Reflexology, Yoga, and More

Edited by Sandra Augustyn Lawton. 405 pages. 2006. 978-0-7808-0966-6.

Diabetes Information for Teens
Health Tips about Managing Diabetes and Preventing Related Complications
Including Information about Insulin, Glucose Control, Healthy Eating, Physical Activity, and Learning to Live with Diabetes

Edited by Sandra Augustyn Lawton. 410 pages. 2006. 978-0-7808-0811-9.

Diet Information for Teens, 2nd Edition

Health Tips about Diet and Nutrition

Including Facts about Dietary Guidelines, Food Groups, Nutrients, Healthy Meals, Snacks, Weight Control, Medical Concerns Related to Diet, and More

Edited by Karen Bellenir. 432 pages. 2006. 978-0-7808-0820-1.

"Full of helpful insights and facts throughout the book. ... An excellent resource to be placed in public libraries or even in personal collections."
—*American Reference Books Annual, 2002*

"Recommended for middle and high school libraries and media centers as well as academic libraries that educate future teachers of teenagers. It is also a suitable addition to health science libraries that serve patrons who are interested in teen health promotion and education." —*E-Streams, Oct '01*

"This comprehensive book would be beneficial to collections that need information about nutrition, dietary guidelines, meal planning, and weight control. ... This reference is so easy to use that its purchase is recommended." —*The Book Report, Sep-Oct '01*

"This book is written in an easy to understand format describing issues that many teens face every day, and then provides thoughtful explanations so that teens can make informed decisions. This is an interesting book that provides important facts and information for today's teens." —*Doody's Health Sciences Book Review Journal, Jul-Aug '01*

"A comprehensive compendium of diet and nutrition. The information is presented in a straightforward, plain-spoken manner. This title will be useful to those working on reports on a variety of topics, as well as to general readers concerned about their dietary health."
—*School Library Journal, Jun '01*

Drug Information for Teens, 2nd Edition

Health Tips about the Physical and Mental Effects of Substance Abuse

Including Information about Marijuana, Inhalants, Club Drugs, Stimulants, Hallucinogens, Opiates, Prescription and Over-the-Counter Drugs, Herbal Products, Tobacco, Alcohol, and More

Edited by Sandra Augustyn Lawton. 468 pages. 2006. 978-0-7808-0862-1.

"A clearly written resource for general readers and researchers alike." —*School Library Journal*

"This book is well-balanced. ... a must for public and school libraries."
—*VOYA: Voice of Youth Advocates, Dec '03*

"The chapters are quick to make a connection to their teenage reading audience. The prose is straightforward and the book lends itself to spot reading. It should be useful both for practical information and for research, and it is suitable for public and school libraries."
—*American Reference Books Annual, 2003*

"Recommended reference source."
—*Booklist, American Library Association, Feb '03*

"This is an excellent resource for teens and their parents. Education about drugs and substances is key to discouraging teen drug abuse and this book provides this much needed information in a way that is interesting and factual." —*Doody's Review Service, Dec '02*

Eating Disorders Information for Teens

Health Tips about Anorexia, Bulimia, Binge Eating, and Other Eating Disorders

Including Information on the Causes, Prevention, and Treatment of Eating Disorders, and Such Other Issues as Maintaining Healthy Eating and Exercise Habits

Edited by Sandra Augustyn Lawton. 337 pages. 2005. 978-0-7808-0783-9.

"An excellent resource for teens and those who work with them."
—*VOYA: Voice of Youth Advocates, Apr '06*

"A welcome addition to high school and undergraduate libraries." —*American Reference Books Annual, 2006*

"This book covers the topic in a lucid manner but delves deeper into every aspect of an eating disorder. A solid addition for any nonfiction or reference collection." —*School Library Journal, Dec '05*

Fitness Information for Teens

Health Tips about Exercise, Physical Well-Being, and Health Maintenance

Including Facts about Aerobic and Anaerobic Conditioning, Stretching, Body Shape and Body Image, Sports Training, Nutrition, and Activities for Non-Athletes

Edited by Karen Bellenir. 425 pages. 2004. 978-0-7808-0679-5.

"Another excellent offering from Omnigraphics in their Teen Health Series. ... This book will be a great addition to any public, junior high, senior high, or secondary school library."
—*American Reference Books Annual, 2005*

Learning Disabilities Information for Teens

Health Tips about Academic Skills Disorders and Other Disabilities That Affect Learning

Including Information about Common Signs of Learning Disabilities, School Issues, Learning to Live with a Learning Disability, and Other Related Issues

Edited by Sandra Augustyn Lawton. 337 pages. 2005. 978-0-7808-0796-9.

"This book provides a wealth of information for any reader interested in the signs, causes, and consequences

of learning disabilities, as well as related legal rights and educational interventions.... Public and academic libraries should want this title for both students and general readers."
— *American Reference Books Annual, 2006*

Mental Health Information for Teens, 2nd Edition
Health Tips about Mental Wellness and Mental Illness
Including Facts about Mental and Emotional Health, Depression and Other Mood Disorders, Anxiety Disorders, Behavior Disorders, Self-Injury, Psychosis, Schizophrenia, and More

Edited by Karen Bellenir. 400 pages. 2006. 978-0-7808-0863-8.

"In both language and approach, this user-friendly entry in the *Teen Health Series* is on target for teens needing information on mental health concerns."
— *Booklist, American Library Association, Jan '02*

"Readers will find the material accessible and informative, with the shaded notes, facts, and embedded glossary insets adding appropriately to the already interesting and succinct presentation."
— *School Library Journal, Jan '02*

"This title is highly recommended for any library that serves adolescents and parents/caregivers of adolescents." — *E-Streams, Jan '02*

"Recommended for high school libraries and young adult collections in public libraries. Both health professionals and teenagers will find this book useful."
— *American Reference Books Annual, 2002*

"This is a nice book written to enlighten the society, primarily teenagers, about common teen mental health issues. It is highly recommended to teachers and parents as well as adolescents."
— *Doody's Review Service, Dec '01*

Sexual Health Information for Teens
Health Tips about Sexual Development, Human Reproduction, and Sexually Transmitted Diseases
Including Facts about Puberty, Reproductive Health, Chlamydia, Human Papillomavirus, Pelvic Inflammatory Disease, Herpes, AIDS, Contraception, Pregnancy, and More

Edited by Deborah A. Stanley. 391 pages. 2003. 978-0-7808-0445-6.

"This work should be included in all high school libraries and many larger public libraries.... highly recommended."
— *American Reference Books Annual, 2004*

"*Sexual Health* approaches its subject with appropriate seriousness and offers easily accessible advice and information." — *School Library Journal, Feb '04*

Skin Health Information for Teens
Health Tips about Dermatological Concerns and Skin Cancer Risks
Including Facts about Acne, Warts, Hives, and Other Conditions and Lifestyle Choices, Such as Tanning, Tattooing, and Piercing, That Affect the Skin, Nails, Scalp, and Hair

Edited by Robert Aquinas McNally. 429 pages. 2003. 978-0-7808-0446-3.

"This volume, as with others in the series, will be a useful addition to school and public library collections." — *American Reference Books Annual, 2004*

"There is no doubt that this reference tool is valuable."
— *VOYA: Voice of Youth Advocates, Feb '04*

"This volume serves as a one-stop source and should be a necessity for any health collection."
— *Library Media Connection*

Sports Injuries Information for Teens
Health Tips about Sports Injuries and Injury Protection
Including Facts about Specific Injuries, Emergency Treatment, Rehabilitation, Sports Safety, Competition Stress, Fitness, Sports Nutrition, Steroid Risks, and More

Edited by Joyce Brennfleck Shannon. 405 pages. 2003. 978-0-7808-0447-0.

"This work will be useful in the young adult collections of public libraries as well as high school libraries."
— *American Reference Books Annual, 2004*

Suicide Information for Teens
Health Tips about Suicide Causes and Prevention
Including Facts about Depression, Risk Factors, Getting Help, Survivor Support, and More

Edited by Joyce Brennfleck Shannon. 368 pages. 2005. 978-0-7808-0737-2.

Tobacco Information for Teens
Health Tips about the Hazards of Using Cigarettes, Smokeless Tobacco, and Other Nicotine Products
Including Facts about Nicotine Addiction, Immediate and Long-Term Health Effects of Tobacco Use, Related Cancers, Smoking Cessation, Tobacco Use Prevention, and Tobacco Use Statistics

Edited by Karen Bellenir. 440 pages. 2007. 978-0-7808-0976-5.

Health Reference Series

Adolescent Health Sourcebook, 2nd Edition
Adult Health Concerns Sourcebook
AIDS Sourcebook, 4th Edition
Alcoholism Sourcebook, 2nd Edition
Allergies Sourcebook, 3rd Edition
Alzheimer Disease Sourcebook, 4th Edition
Arthritis Sourcebook, 2nd Edition
Asthma Sourcebook, 2nd Edition
Attention Deficit Disorder Sourcebook
Autism & Pervasive Developmental Disorders Sourcebook
Back & Neck Sourcebook, 2nd Edition
Blood & Circulatory Disorders Sourcebook, 2nd Edition
Brain Disorders Sourcebook, 2nd Edition
Breast Cancer Sourcebook, 2nd Edition
Breastfeeding Sourcebook
Burns Sourcebook
Cancer Sourcebook, 5th Edition
Cancer Sourcebook for Women, 3rd Edition
Cancer Survivorship Sourcebook
Cardiovascular Diseases & Disorders Sourcebook, 3rd Edition
Caregiving Sourcebook
Child Abuse Sourcebook
Childhood Diseases & Disorders Sourcebook
Colds, Flu & Other Common Ailments Sourcebook
Communication Disorders Sourcebook
Complementary & Alternative Medicine Sourcebook, 3rd Edition
Congenital Disorders Sourcebook, 2nd Edition
Contagious Diseases Sourcebook
Cosmetic & Reconstructive Surgery Sourcebook, 2nd Edition
Death & Dying Sourcebook, 2nd Edition
Dental Care and Oral Health Sourcebook, 3rd Edition

Depression Sourcebook, 2nd Edition
Dermatological Disorders Sourcebook, 2nd Edition
Diabetes Sourcebook, 4th Edition
Diet & Nutrition Sourcebook, 3rd Edition
Digestive Diseases & Disorder Sourcebook
Disabilities Sourcebook
Disease Management Sourcebook
Domestic Violence Sourcebook, 2nd Edition
Drug Abuse Sourcebook, 2nd Edition
Ear, Nose & Throat Disorders Sourcebook, 2nd Edition
Eating Disorders Sourcebook, 2nd Edition
Emergency Medical Services Sourcebook
Endocrine & Metabolic Disorders Sourcebook, 2nd Edition
EnvironmentalHealth Sourcebook, 2nd Edition
Ethnic Diseases Sourcebook
Eye Care Sourcebook, 3rd Edition
Family Planning Sourcebook
Fitness & Exercise Sourcebook, 3rd Edition
Food Safety Sourcebook
Forensic Medicine Sourcebook
Gastrointestinal Diseases & Disorders Sourcebook, 2nd Edition
Genetic Disorders Sourcebook, 3rd Edition
Head Trauma Sourcebook
Headache Sourcebook
Health Insurance Sourcebook
Healthy Aging Sourcebook
Healthy Children Sourcebook
Healthy Heart Sourcebook for Women
Hepatitis Sourcebook
Household Safety Sourcebook
Hypertension Sourcebook
Immune System Disorders Sourcebook, 2nd Edition
Infant & Toddler Health Sourcebook
Infectious Diseases Sourcebook